The Complete Procedure Coding Solution

Third Edition

Shelley C. Safian, PhD, RHIA
MAOM/HSM, CCS-P, CPC-H, CPC-I,
AHIMA-Approved ICD-10-CM/PCS Trainer

Mary A. Johnson, CPC
Central Carolina Technical College

THE COMPLETE PROCEDURE CODING SOLUTION, THIRD EDITION

Published by McGraw-Hill Education, 2 Penn Plaza, New York, NY 10121. Copyright © 2016 by McGraw-Hill Education. All rights reserved. Printed in the United States of America. Previous editions © 2012 and 2009. No part of this publication may be reproduced or distributed in any form or by any means, or stored in a database or retrieval system, without the prior written consent of McGraw-Hill Education, including, but not limited to, in any network or other electronic storage or transmission, or broadcast for distance learning.

Some ancillaries, including electronic and print components, may not be available to customers outside the United States.

This book is printed on acid-free paper.

1 2 3 4 5 6 7 8 9 0 RMN/RMN 1 0 9 8 7 6 5

ISBN   978-0-07-802071-1
MHID   0-07-802071-9

Senior Vice President, Products & Markets: *Kurt L. Strand*
Vice President, General Manager, Products & Markets: *Marty Lange*
Vice President, Content Design & Delivery: *Kimberly Meriwether David*
Managing Director: *Chad Grall*
Brand Manager: *William Mulford*
Director, Product Development: *Rose Koos*
Senior Product Developer: *Michelle Flomenhoft*
Executive Marketing Manager: *Roxan Kinsey*

Market Development Manager: *Kimberly Bauer*
Digital Product Analyst: *Katherine Ward*
Director, Content Design & Delivery: *Linda Avenarius*
Program Manager: *Faye M. Herrig*
Content Project Managers: *Jane Mohr, Brent Dela Cruz, and Judi David*
Buyer: *Susan K. Culbertson*
Design: *Studio Montage, St. Louis, MO*
Content Licensing Specialist: *Lorraine Buczek*
Compositor: *SPi Global*
Printer: *R. R. Donnelley*

Library of Congress Cataloging-in-Publication Data

Safian, Shelley C.
    [Complete procedure coding book]
    The complete procedure coding solution / Shelley C. Safian, PhD, RHIA, MAOM/HSM, CCS-P,
CPC-H, CPC-I, AHIMA-approved ICD-10-CM/PCS trainer, Mary A. Johnson, CPC,
Central Carolina Technical College.—Third edition.
        pages cm
    ISBN 978-0-07-802071-1 (alk. paper)
    1. Medicine—Terminology—Code numbers. I. Johnson, Mary A. (Medical record
coding program manager) II. Title.
    R123.S184 2016
    610.1'4—dc23

                                                          2014046120

mheducation.com/highered

ABOUT THE AUTHORS

Shelley C. Safian

Shelley Safian has been teaching medical coding and health information management for more than a decade, at both on ground and on-line campuses. In addition to her regular teaching responsibilities at Herzing University and Berkeley College Online, she often presents seminars sponsored by AHIMA and AAPC, writes regularly about coding for the *Just Coding* newsletter, and has written articles published in *AAPC Healthcare Business Monthly, SurgiStrategies,* and *HFM (Healthcare Financial Management)* magazine. Safian is the course author for multiple distance education courses on various coding topics, including ICD-10-CM, ICD-10-PCS, CPT, and HCPCS Level II coding.

Safian is a Registered Health Information Administrator (RHIA) and Certified Coding Specialist–Physician-based (CCS-P) from the American Health Information Management Association and a Certified Professional Coder–Hospital (CPC-H), and a Certified Professional Coding Instructor (CPC-I) from the American Academy of Professional Coders. She has earned the designation of AHIMA-Approved ICD-10-CM/PCS Trainer.

Safian completed her Graduate Certificate in healthcare management at Keller Graduate School of Management. The University of Phoenix awarded her Master of Arts/Organizational Management degree. She earned her PhD in healthcare administration with a focus in health information management.

Mary A. Johnson

Mary Johnson is currently the Medical Record Coding Program Director at Central Carolina Technical College, Sumter, South Carolina. Her background includes corporate training as well as on-campus and on-line platforms. Johnson also designs and implements customized coding curricula. Johnson received her Bachelor of Arts dual degree in Business Administration and Marketing from Columbia College, Columbia, South Carolina. Johnson is a Certified Professional Coder (CPC) credentialed through the American Academy of Professional Coders and is ICD-10-CM proficient.

Acknowledgements

—This book is dedicated to *Joshua* and *Roxie*, without whose love and support I could not accomplish all that I do - *Shelley*.

—This book is dedicated in loving memory of my parents, *Dr. and Mrs. Clarence J. Johnson, Sr.* and to my Aunt Wanda for their love and support. Also, to those students that I have had the privilege to work with and to those students who are beginning their journey into the world of medical coding - *Mary*

BRIEF CONTENTS

CONTENTS

Welcome to *The Complete Procedure Coding Solution*. This product is part of a three-part series that instructs students on how to become proficient in medical coding—a healthcare field that continues to be in high demand. The Bureau of Labor Statistics notes the demand for health information management professionals (which includes coders) will continue to increase incredibly through 2018 and beyond.

This series was written to speak directly to the medical coding student using step-by-step instructions and conversational language to maximize understanding. Built into the structure of these solutions are many opportunities for students to practice coding and apply what they have learned. Students will also have the chance to practice abstracting with real-world health professionals' documentation and accurately translating these facts into the best, most accurate codes.

To the Student

Your medical coding classes introduce you to the skills you will need to work in the health information management field. A fundamental role of an insurance coding and medical billing specialist's job is to work with the insurance companies that will reimburse the healthcare facility for the services and treatments provided to patients. You may be employed by a hospital, clinic, doctor's office, health maintenance organization, mental health care facility, insurance company, government agency, or long-term care facility. Your career will be challenging, interesting, and one of the top 10 fastest-growing Allied Health professions.

Before you begin your adventure, here are some tips to help you succeed:

- First, take a deep breath. Coding is complex and is not like anything else you have tackled before. Remember that you are learning a new skill! Give yourself some time to become proficient.

- Second, *never* code directly from the Alphabetic Index. *Always* look the code up in the Tabular list before deciding on a code. If you remember this rule, you will always head in the right direction.

- Third, when you encounter a word or an abbreviation that you don't understand, stop and look it up in your medical dictionary.

- Fourth, after you finish coding the case studies, scenarios, or whatever you are coding, put it all aside. Then, later or the next day, go back and do "back coding." In the Tabular list, look up each code you came up with and match the code description carefully with the case study or scenario words. Remember the importance of documentation by the healthcare provider—this is more important than ever with the implementation of ICD-10-CM and ICD-10-PCS! This process is a very effective way to double-check your answers. Your fresh eyes will enable you to see words and notations you may have missed before.

- Finally, reevaluate your work by checking every question to make certain you understand how you found your answer. When you find you have gotten an exercise, a test question, or another activity wrong, try to figure out what happened. Make sure you ask your instructor for help when you need it!

Good luck on your medical coding journey!

To the Instructor

The Safian/Johnson Medical Coding series includes three products:

The Complete Diagnosis Coding Solution, 3e
The Complete Procedure Coding Solution, 3e
You Code It! Abstracting Case Studies Practicum, 2e (Third edition coming soon!)

These solutions are designed to give your students the medical coding experience they need in order to pass their first medical coding certification exams, such as CCS/CCS-P or CPC/CPC-H. The products offer students a variety of practice opportunities by reinforcing the learning outcomes set forth in every chapter. The chapter materials are organized in short bursts of text followed by practice—keeping students active and coding throughout!

In addition to providing innovative approaches to learning medical coding, McGraw-Hill Education knows how much effort it takes to prepare for a new course. Through focus groups, symposia, reviews, and conversations with instructors like you, we have gathered information about the materials you need in order to facilitate successful courses. We are committed to providing you with high-quality, accurate instructor support.

Digital Resources

Knowing the importance of flexibility and digital learning, McGraw-Hill Education has created multiple assets to enhance the learning experience no matter the class format: traditional, on-line, or hybrid. This product is designed with digital solutions to help instructors and students be successful.

Learn Without Limits: McGraw-Hill *Connect*

Today's learning extends beyond the classroom, beyond one format, beyond a singular style. That's why we deliver everything instructors and students need directly to your fingertips, integrating education seamlessly into your lives. We don't just improve results, we make the everyday a little smoother by providing intuitive technology that enables learning and simplifies life.

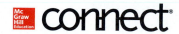

Students at the Center

To design a powerful learning experience that makes a palpable difference, we went straight to the source. Collecting and mining millions of data points, we partnered closely with students and educators globally, compiling feedback that revealed deep insights to inform the construction of each facet within this revolutionary learning environment. The result? An innovative synthesis of adaptive technology and learning resources perfectly calibrated to guide each student on a personalized path toward better grades.

Activate Learning

Learning doesn't just happen. To encourage achievement and evoke curiosity, it's essential to shift learning from a passive experience to one that is energetic and engaged—in and outside the classroom. By immersing students in their course content and prompting them to interact with key concepts, while continually adapting to their individual needs, *Connect* activates learning and empowers students to take control, raising grades and increasing retention and raising grades. *Connect* makes digital teaching and learning personal, easy, and effective. Learn more at **www.mcgrawhillconnect.com!**

Learning at the speed of you: The LearnSmart Advantage Suite

Connect's Superior Adaptive Technology 'Fills the Knowledge Gap' and Empowers Students Outside of Class for a More Engaging and Interactive Experience in Class. Connect builds student confidence outside of class with adaptive technology that pinpoints exactly what a student knows and what they don't, and then seamlessly offers up learning resources within the platform that are designed to have the greatest impact on that specific learning moment. With SmartBook, reading is an interactive and dynamic experience in which content is tailor-made for each student. Built with the unique LearnSmart adaptive technology, it focuses not only on addressing learning in the moment, but empowers students by helping them retain information over time, so that they are more prepared and engaged in class.

- **LearnSmart Advantage:** More than 2 million students have answered more than 1.3 billion questions in LearnSmart since 2009, making it the most widely used and intelligent adaptive study tool available on the market today. LearnSmart is proven to strengthen memory recall, keep students in class, and boost grades—students using LearnSmart are 13% more likely to pass their classes, and 35% less likely to dropout.

- **SmartBook [New Capabilities]:** SmartBook makes study time as productive and efficient as possible. It identifies and closes knowledge gaps through a continually adapting reading experience that provides introduces personalized learning resources at the precise moment of need. This ensures that every minute spent with SmartBook is returned to the student as the most value-added minute possible. The result? More confidence, better grades, and greater success.

Go to **www.LearnSmartAdvantage.com** for more information!

Record and distribute your lectures for multiple viewing: My Lectures—Tegrity

McGraw-Hill Tegrity records and distributes your class lecture with just a click of a button. Students can view it anytime and anywhere via computer, tablet, or other mobile device. It indexes as it records your PowerPoint presentations and anything shown on your computer, so students can use key words to find exactly what they want to study. Tegrity is available as an integrated feature of **McGraw-Hill *Connect* Medical Coding** and as a stand-alone product.

A single sign-on with Connect *and your Blackboard course:* McGraw-Hill Education and Blackboard—for a premium user experience

Blackboard, the web-based course management system, has partnered with McGraw-Hill Education to better allow students and faculty to use online materials and activities to complement face-to-face teaching. Blackboard features exciting social learning and teaching tools that foster active learning opportunities for students. You'll transform your closed-door classroom into communities where students remain connected to their educational experience 24 hours a day. This partnership allows you and your students access to McGraw-Hill's *Connect* and *Create* right from within your Blackboard course—all with a single sign-on. Not only do you get single sign-on with *Connect* and *Create,* but you also get deep integration of McGraw-Hill Education content and content engines right in Blackboard. Whether you're choosing a book for your course or building Connect assignments, all the tools you need are right where you want them—inside Blackboard. Gradebooks are now seamless. When a student completes an integrated Connect assignment, the grade for that assignment automatically (and instantly) feeds into your Blackboard grade center. McGraw-Hill Education and

Blackboard can now offer you easy access to industry-leading technology and content, whether your campus hosts it or we do. Be sure to ask your local McGraw-Hill Education representative for details.

Still want a single sign-on solution and using another learning management system?

See how **McGraw-Hill Campus** makes the grade by offering universal sign-on, automatic registration, gradebook synchronization and open access to a multitude of learning resources—all in one place. MH Campus supports Active Directory, Angel, Blackboard, Canvas, Desire2Learn, eCollege, IMS, LDAP, Moodle, Moodlerooms, Sakai, Shibboleth, WebCT, BrainHoney, Campus Cruiser, and Jenzibar eRacer. Additionally, MH Campus can be easily connected with other authentication authorities and LMSs. Visit **http://mhcampus.mhhe.com/** to learn more.

Create a textbook organized the way you teach: McGraw-Hill Education *Create*

With *Create,* you can easily rearrange chapters, combine material from other content sources, and quickly upload content you have written, such as your course syllabus or teaching notes. Find the content you need in *Create* by searching through thousands of leading McGraw-Hill Education textbooks. Arrange your book to fit your teaching style. *Create* even allows you to personalize your book's appearance by selecting the cover and adding your name, school, and course information. Order a *Create* book and you'll receive a complimentary print review copy in 3 to 5 business days or a complimentary electronic review copy (eComp) via e-mail in minutes. Go to **www.mcgrawhillcreate .com** today and register to experience how Create empowers you to teach *your* students *your* way.

Best-in-Class Digital Support

Based on feedback from our users, McGraw-Hill Education has developed Digital Success Programs that will provide you and your students the help you need, when you need it.

- *Training for instructors:* Get ready to drive classroom results with our **Digital Success Team**—ready to provide in-person, remote, or on-demand training as needed.
- *Peer support and training:* No one understands your needs like your peers. Get easy access to knowledgeable digital users by joining our Connect Community, or speak directly with one of our **Digital Faculty Consultants,** who are instructors using McGraw-Hill Education digital products.
- *Online training tools:* Get immediate anytime, anywhere access to modular tutorials on key features through our **Connect Success Academy.**

Get started today. Learn more about McGraw-Hill Education's Digital Success Programs by contacting your local sales representative or visit **http://connect.customer .mheducation.com/start.**

Need help? Contact the McGraw-Hill Education Customer Experience Group (CXG)

Visit the CXG website at **www.mhhe.com/support.** Browse our FAQs (frequently asked questions) and product documentation and/or contact a CXG representative. CXG is available Sunday through Friday.

Additional Instructor Resources

The following resources are available in the Instructor Resources located under the Library tab in Connect:

- **Instructor's manual and Tools to Plan Course** pages with course overview, lesson plans, and answers for end-of-chapter exercises, as well as competency correlations, sample syllabi, conversion guide (from 2nd edition to 3rd edition), asset map, and more. Answer keys are updated annually.
- **PowerPoint presentations** for each chapter correlated to learning outcomes. Each presentation seeks to reinforce key concepts and provide an additional visual aid for students.
- **Test bank** and answer key for use in class assessment. The comprehensive test bank includes a variety of question types, with each question linked directly to a learning outcome from the text. Questions are also tagged with relevant topic, Bloom's Taxonomy level, difficulty level, and competencies, where applicable. The test bank is available in Connect; Word and EZ Test versions are available.

What's New in Our Third Edition

The Complete Procedure Coding Solution, third edition, has been revised to include a greater number of realistic scenarios and case studies for students to gain hands-on learning with the popular **Let's Code It!** scenarios and **You Code It!** case studies. **Guidance Connection** boxes—a new feature for this edition—make it easier for students to connect learning concepts and specific official guidelines to critical thinking. **Keys to Coding** boxes also include additional helpful information to support students' learning. And, of course, we have added four new chapters covering **ICD-10-PCS** (using the 2015 code set version). Throughout the book, more anatomy and physiology descriptions, as well as more information on inclusive signs and symptoms, enhance your comprehension of the procedure coding process.

The entire text has been updated using CPT, ICD-10-PCS, and 2015 HCPCS Level II. The instructor's manual features a 2015-compliant answer key to all end-of-chapter tests: **Chapter Reviews** (matching, short answer, and multiple-choice questions), **You Code It! Practice** (short scenarios), and end-of-chapter **You Code It! Application** (full physician's notes/operative reports). Additional exercises, including several types of interactive exercises, are also available in Connect. Answer keys are also updated annually for the newest diagnosis codes and are made available in the password-protected Instructor Resources center on-line.

Chapter-by-Chapter Updates

Chapter 1: Legal and Ethical Issues
- Key terms include several additional terms
- The new Guidance Connection feature connects students to official guidelines
- Updated AHIMA Standards of Ethical Coding
- Updated AAPC Code of Ethical Standards

Chapter 2: Introduction to Coding and CPT
- Key terms include several additional terms
- The new Guidance Connection feature connects students to official guidelines

Chapter 3: Introduction to CPT Modifiers
- The new Guidance Connection feature connects students to official guidelines
- Additional Let's Code It! scenario and examples

Chapter 4: Evaluation and Management Codes, Part 1
- Key terms include additional terms
- The new Guidance Connection feature connects students to official guidelines

Chapter 5: Evaluation and Management Codes, Part 2
- Key terms include additional terms
- The new Guidance Connection feature connects students to official guidelines
- New section on complex chronic care coordination services and transitional care management services

Chapter 6: Anesthesia Coding
- The new Guidance Connection feature connects students to official guidelines

Chapter 7: Surgery Coding, Part 1
- The new Guidance Connection feature connects students to official guidelines
- New section on types of surgical procedures, including prophylactic procedures
- New subsections on surgical approaches
- Expanded section on repairs (closures)

Chapter 8: Surgery Coding, Part 2
- The new Guidance Connection feature connects students to official guidelines

Chapter 9: Radiology Coding
- The new Guidance Connection feature connects students to official guidelines

Chapter 10: Pathology and Laboratory Coding
- The new Guidance Connection feature connects students to official guidelines
- New example of an actual pathology report
- New section on bone marrow testing

Chapter 11: Medicine Coding
- The new Guidance Connection feature connects students to official guidelines

Chapter 12: Category II and Category III Coding
- The new Guidance Connection feature connects students to official guidelines

Chapter 13: HCPCS Level II Coding: Introduction and Guidelines
- The new Guidance Connection feature connects students to official guidelines

New! Chapter 14: HCPCS Level II Modifiers
- New chapter

Chapter 15: Coding Medical Supplies, Durable Medical Equipment (DME), Pharmaceutical, and Ambulance and Other Transportation Services
- General updates

Chapter 16: Introduction to ICD-10-PCS
- New section on ICD-10-PCS general conventions
- New section on selection of principal procedure

New! Chapter 17: ICD-10-PCS—Medical and Surgical Section (0)
- New chapter
- Includes character definitions, including root operation terms
- The new Guidance Connection feature connects students to official guidelines
- Includes Examples and Let's Code It! Scenarios
- Includes new You Interpret It! section

New! Chapter 18: ICD-10-PCS—Obstetrics (1), Placement (2), Administration (3), Measurement and Monitoring (4), Extracorporeal Assistance and Performance (5), Extracorporeal Therapies (6), Osteopathic (7), Other Procedures (8), and Chiropractic (9) Sections
- New chapter
- Includes character definitions, including root operation terms
- The new Guidance Connection feature connects students to official guidelines

- Includes Examples and Let's Code It! Scenarios
- Includes new You Interpret It! section

New! Chapter 19: ICD-10-PCS—Imaging (B), Nuclear Medicine (C), Radiation Oncology (D), Physical Rehabilitation and Diagnostic Audiology (F), Mental Health (G), and Substance Abuse Treatment (H) Sections
- New chapter
- Includes character definitions, including root operation terms
- The new Guidance Connection feature connects students to official guidelines
- Includes Examples and Let's Code It! Scenarios

Chapter 20: Procedure Coding Application
- New and additional exercises included to increase practice opportunities
- Fifty procedural case studies, including ICD-10-PCS
- All exercises also available in Connect

CodeitRightOnline™: Your Online Coding Tool

So that your students can gain experience with the use of an online coding tool, they will have access for a 29-day period to CodeitRightOnline, produced by Contexo Media, a division of Access Intelligence. CodeitRightOnline offers a comprehensive search function for CPT, HCPCS Level II, and ICD-10-CM/PCS code sets. It includes helpful tools like search indexing for easy reference and offers newsletter articles and other coding resources. For more information about the features of CodeitRightOnline and how to sign up for a trial, visit the Instructor Resource center, or talk to your local McGraw-Hill Education representative.

ACKNOWLEDGMENTS

Reviews

Many instructors reviewed the manuscript while it was in development and provided valuable feedback that directly affected the product's development. Their contributions are greatly appreciated.

Leslie Bishop, CMRS, MOL, MBA
Bryant & Stratton College

Dr. Lisa Campbell, CCS-P, CCS, CPC, CPC-H, CPC-I
South Suburban College

Rhonda Lively, B.S., RHIT, CPPM, CPC
Chattahoochee Technical College

Jane Mansell, CPC
Living Arts College

Emily Noel, CCA, MSM
Des Moines Area Community College

Irma Rodriguez, MEd, RHIA, CCS
South Texas College

Noreen Semanski, LPN, RHIT
McCann School of Business & Technology

Deborah Williams, RHIT
McLennan Community College

Technical Editing/Accuracy Panel

A panel of instructors completed a technical edit and review of all content in the page proofs to verify its accuracy.

Leathecia Arnold-Jackson, MHA, RHIA, CCS, CHTS-TR, Approved AHIMA ICD-10-CM/PCS Trainer
Peak Health Solutions

Kristi Couch, RHIA, CPC, CCA, CHP, CHA
Jefferson Community and Technical College

Angelia Hamilton, MHA, RHIA, CCS, CPC
South Suburban College

Susan Hawkins, M.S., M.B.A., M.H.A, CPC, CHTS-TR
Nashville State Community College

Christine Malone, MBA, MHA, CMPE, CPHRM, FACHE
Everett Community College

Digital Tool Development

Special thanks to the instructors who helped with the development of *Connect* and SmartBook. An expanded acknowledgments list is available in the Instructor Resources section of Connect.

GUIDED TOUR

The Complete Procedure Coding Solution was developed with student success in mind!

Chapter Openers

Each chapter begins by clearly identifying the **Learning Outcomes** students need to master along with the **Key Terms** they need to remember.

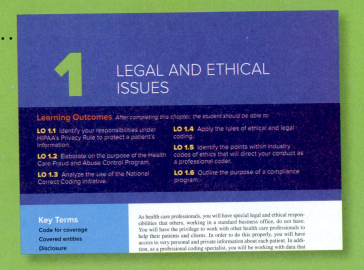

1

LEGAL AND ETHICAL ISSUES

Learning Outcomes *After completing this chapter, the student should be able to:*

LO 1.1 Identify your responsibilities under HIPAA's Privacy Rule to protect a patient's information.

LO 1.2 Elaborate on the purpose of the Health Care Fraud and Abuse Control Program.

LO 1.3 Analyze the use of the National Correct Coding Initiative.

LO 1.4 Apply the rules of ethical and legal coding.

LO 1.5 Identify the points within industry codes of ethics that will direct your conduct as a professional coder.

LO 1.6 Outline the purpose of a compliance program.

Key Terms
Code for coverage
Covered entities
Disclosure

As health care professionals, you will have special legal and ethical responsibilities that others, working in a standard business office, do not have. You will have the privilege to work with other health care professionals to help their patients and clients. In order to do this properly, you will have access to very personal and private information about each patient. In addition, as a professional coding specialist, you will be working with data that

Keys to Coding

These helpful tips appear periodically throughout the text to provide students with useful insights for ensuring their success and to illuminate strategies for avoiding the most common mistakes. These features also walk students through the critical thinking process required to make the necessary evaluations and determine the necessary specificities to code accurately.

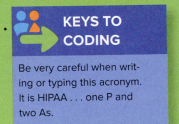

KEYS TO CODING

Be very careful when writing or typing this acronym. It is HIPAA . . . one P and two As.

Examples and Let's Code It! Scenarios

These features establish the connection between medical coding concepts and real-world application! Students experience guided practice and step-by-step examples that mirror situations they will most likely encounter in their professions.

Guidance Connection

connects the concepts students are learning about in the chapter to ICD-10-PCS official guidelines to further their knowledge and understanding of coding resources.

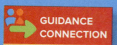

End-of-Chapter Review

Every chapter ends with Using Terminology (matching), Checking Your Understanding (multiple choice), and Applying your Knowledge (short answer) questions that reinforce the chapter learning outcomes.

Real Abstracting Practice with You Code It!

Exercises can be found at the end of each chapter. Plus, Chapter 20 consists solely of these activities.

You Code It! Practice

Practice diagnosis or procedure coding with these short coding scenarios.

YOU CODE IT! Practice
Chapter 6: Anesthesia Coding

Using the techniques described in this chapter, carefully read through the case studies and determine the most accurate anesthesia code(s) and modifier(s), if appropriate, for each case study.

1. Tammy Mirandosa, a healthy 31-year-old female, received anesthesia before delivering her daughter at the hospital. It was a vaginal delivery. The patient is otherwise healthy.

2. Dr. Adams administered general anesthesia to Manny Perez, an otherwise healthy 29-year-old firefighter. Dr. Zelmono performed a third-degree burn excision, followed by a skin grafting on Manny's chest where 9% of his body surface was burned while he was rescuing a little boy from a house fire.

3. Karen Walkins, a 41-year-old female, was previously diagnosed with benign hypertension due to morbid obesity. Dr. Masters administers general anesthesia so that Dr. Morgenstern can perform a direct venous thrombectomy on her lower left leg.

You Code It! Application

Using physicians' notes documenting realistic patient encounters, students gain experience with abstracting.

YOU CODE IT! Application
Chapter 4: Evaluation and Management Codes, Part 1

The following exercises provide practice in the application of abstracting the physicians' notes and learning to work with SOAP notes from our health care facility, Cipher, Victors & Associates. These case studies (SOAP notes) are modeled on real patient encounters. Using the techniques described in this chapter, carefully read through the case studies and determine the most accurate E/M code(s) for each case study.

CIPHER, VICTORS & ASSOCIATES
A Complete Health Care Facility
234 MAIN STREET • ANYTOWN, FL 32711 • 407-555-1234

PATIENT: OATES, MARLENE
ACCOUNT/EHR #: OATEMA001
DATE: 09/16/18

Attending Physician: James I. Cipher, MD

S: This new Pt is a 29-year-old female who was involved in a two-car motor vehicle accident (MVA) while driving on the job. She is complaining about some neck pain. She has tingling in her left hand and both feet. She states that her left arm hurts when she tries to pull it overhead. She apparently was told by a friend that she should likely need to see a spine doctor, but somehow she came to see me first. PMH is remarkable for kidney trouble. Past bronchoscopy, laparoscopy, and kidney stone surgery, otherwise noncontributory as per the medical history form completed by the patient and reviewed at this visit.

O: Ht 5'5" Wt 179 lb. R 16. Pt presented in a sling. She was told to use it by the same friend. She states if she does not use it, her arm does not feel any different, so I had her remove it. She states that she has not had any prior injury to this area and has no previous problems with her musculoskeletal system. On exam, HEENT is unremarkable. Neck muscles are taut, particularly on the left side. The left shoulder demonstrates full passive motion, with normal strength testing. No deformity is observable. Pt states there is some tenderness over the left trapezius area. The reflexes are brisk and symmetric. X-rays of her chest two views and C spine AP/LAT are relatively benign, as are complete x-rays of the shoulder.

A: Contusion of upper left arm and left shoulder

P: 1. MRI to rule out torn ligament
2. Rx Naprosyn
3. Referral to PT
4. Referral to orthopedist

James I. Cipher, MD

JIC/mg D: 09/16/18 09:50:16 T: 09/18/18 12:55:01

Determine the most accurate E/M code(s).

PART 1

CPT

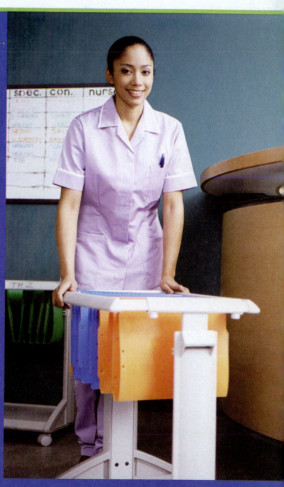

© image100/PunchStock

1 LEGAL AND ETHICAL ISSUES

Learning Outcomes
After completing this chapter, the student should be able to:

LO 1.1 Identify your responsibilities under HIPAA's Privacy Rule to protect a patient's information.

LO 1.2 Elaborate on the purpose of the Health Care Fraud and Abuse Control Program.

LO 1.3 Analyze the use of the National Correct Coding Initiative.

LO 1.4 Apply the rules of ethical and legal coding.

LO 1.5 Identify the points within industry codes of ethics that will direct your conduct as a professional coder.

LO 1.6 Outline the purpose of a compliance program.

Key Terms

Code for coverage

Covered entities

Disclosure

Ethical behaviors

Fraud

HIPAA's Privacy Rule

Mutually exclusive codes

Protected health information (PHI)

Supporting documentation

Unbundling

Upcoding

Use

Willful ignorance

As health care professionals, you will have special legal and ethical responsibilities that others, working in a standard business office, do not have. You will have the privilege to work with other health care professionals to help their patients and clients. In order to do this properly, you will have access to very personal and private information about each patient. In addition, as a professional coding specialist, you will be working with data that also directly relates to how much will be paid for the services provided—this is called reimbursement. As you can imagine, working with these two categories of information—personal information about an individual's health and how much professionals are being paid for their services—requires strict confidentiality, honesty, and accuracy.

What Is It?

Legal and ethical issues can be very complicated. This chapter helps you establish a solid foundation for your future career.

Let's begin with a shared understanding of what this all really means. Many professionals in all sections of the health care industry believe they do things legally and ethically each day, but in reality they do not. This may be because they are greedy or selfish. However, most often it is because they are not properly educated. What this means to you is that not only do you need to learn about ethics and legal concerns, but you also may need to share your knowledge with more experienced professionals when you get out into the industry.

Remember that just because someone has been in the business for 10 years does not mean he or she knows the newest laws and regulations or the proper way to comply. It may be important for you to not accept the explanation "This is the way we have always done this" because laws change, the industry changes, and a responsible professional must keep up.

Legal compliance keeps you on the right side of the law, whether it is civil or criminal, whether it is state or federal. An interesting inclusion in most laws is the specific mention of **willful ignorance.** What this means is that the excuse "I didn't know that was illegal" will not get anyone out of trouble. Many laws, such as the federal False Claims Act, include the phrase "know or should know," meaning that, if you are doing the job or the act, and as a part of that job or act you should know about what is legal or not, then you are as guilty if you do something illegal as someone who knows the law and does not comply on purpose.

Fraud is something you always want to avoid. This is claiming something is true when it is not. As coding specialists, it is our job to explain the entire story of what occurred during an encounter between a health care professional and a patient—what happened and why. We interpret the information provided by the professional into a new language—codes—to tell this story. Each code represents something different, with specifics that help you tell this story completely and honestly. If one number is different from the code you should be reporting, you are reporting something different.

EXAMPLE

21450 Closed treatment of mandibular fracture; *without* manipulation

21451 Closed treatment of mandibular fracture; *with* manipulation

These two CPT procedure codes report the same basic procedure on the same anatomical site, but they report a different level of work by the physician. If the physician *did* manipulate the fractured bone, and you report 21450, it is a lie, it is fraud, and it will deny the physician the proper level of reimbursement for the work provided. You want to get paid what you earn, and your physician and your facility do, too. If the physician *did not* manipulate the fractured bone and you report 21451, it is a lie, it is fraud, and it will provide the physician with more money wrongly.

In addition, professional coding specialists have an obligation, as do all other health care professionals, to always participate in **ethical behaviors.** This can sometimes be difficult to understand because most individuals gain their ethical compass from their personal culture, family, and religion. Later in this chapter, you will learn about the Standards of Ethical Coding and the Codes of Ethics that are used as guidance in our profession.

ethical behaviors
Actions that are in agreement with society's concept of right and wrong.

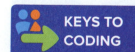

KEYS TO CODING

Be very careful when writing or typing this acronym. It is HIPAA . . . one P and two As.

LO 1.1 Health Insurance Portability and Accountability Act

The Health Insurance Portability and Accountability Act of 1996, known as HIPAA (pronounced *hip-aah*), was enacted by the federal government and directly applies to you as a coding professional. Like most federal laws, HIPAA covers many different issues and concerns. The Privacy Rule is one part of this law that you are obligated to know and understand.

HIPAA's Privacy Rule was written to protect an individual's privacy with regard to personal health information, without getting in the way of the flow of data that is necessary to provide appropriate care for that patient. Essentially, the lawmakers tried to make certain that *a patient's information is easily accessible to those who should have access to it* (such as the physician, insurance coder and biller, and therapist) *and, at the same time, keep it secured against unauthorized people* (such as potential employers, coworkers, or neighborhood gossips) so that they do not see things they have no business seeing.

HIPAA's Privacy Rule
A portion of HIPAA that ensures the availability of patient information for those who should see it while protecting that information from those who should not.

Who Is Responsible for Obeying This Law

HIPAA's Privacy Rule went into effect on April 14, 2003, and concerns every physician's office, clinic, hospital, and health insurance carrier—every type of business that is directly involved in the delivery of and/or payment for health care services, no matter how big or small. The largest of corporations owning hundreds of hospitals around the country and an office with one physician working alone are all included. HIPAA calls these businesses **covered entities,** and they all must comply with the terms of the law.

Covered entities are divided into three categories:

- Health care providers
- Health plans
- Health care clearinghouses

You probably already know the definition of a health care provider: any person or organization that gives health care services as the primary business purpose.

EXAMPLE

Health care providers as defined by HIPAA: physicians, dentists, hospitals, clinics, pharmacies, laboratories, etc.

Health plans are described as organizations that provide and/or pay for health care services as their main reason for being in business. They include health insurance carriers, HMOs, employee welfare benefit plans, government health plans (such as TriCare, Medicare, and Medicaid), and group health plans provided through employers and associations. It doesn't matter whether the plan is offered to an individual or a group—all companies offering this coverage are included.

EXAMPLE

Health care plans as defined by HIPAA: Medicare, Medicaid, TriCare, BlueCross BlueShield, Prudential, etc.

In addition, technology has created another type of organization involved in this process, called a health care clearinghouse. These companies help process electronic health insurance claims. Medical billing services, medical review services, and health information management system companies are included in this definition.

EXAMPLE

Health care clearinghouses as defined by HIPAA: National Clearinghouse, NDC Electronic Claims, WebMD Network Services, etc.

The workforces of covered entities are also included under HIPAA. A covered entity's workforce consists of every person who is involved with the company—full-time, part-time, volunteer, intern, extern, physician, nurse, assistant—and this has nothing to do with whether they are paid. Everyone must comply with the terms of this law.

---

covered entities
Health care providers, health plans, and health care clearinghouses—businesses that have access to the personal health information of patients.

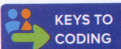

KEYS TO CODING

Respecting a patient's privacy is also a sign of respect for the person. When you are the patient, you want to be treated with respect. So following HIPAA's Privacy Rule is not just the law of the United States; it is the law of treating people fairly.

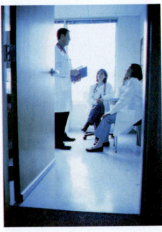

© Ryan McVay/Getty Images

What This Law Covers

You are certainly familiar with the topic of doctor-patient confidentiality. It means that anything a patient tells his or her doctor must be kept private. The doctor is not allowed, under most circumstances, to reveal to anyone what was said. This includes family members, parents (in many cases), and friends. This is important so that an individual will feel comfortable being open and honest and tell the physician things that are very, very personal, possibly even embarrassing or private facts that this person has never told anyone else. However, in order for the physician to properly treat this individual, the physician must know everything.

In order for you to do your job properly, you have access to all this confidential information. You need to know very personal and private facts about every one of your patients in order to accurately report the data.

You know what is wrong with them (their diagnoses) now and in the past; you know why they came to see this health care provider and why they saw others before they came to your facility, and you know what the health care provider thinks (observations and impressions) about these patients, as well as what has been done, is being done, and will be done to treat them. You know all these things because you have access to patients' health care records, including all the physician's notes. HIPAA calls this personal health care information (past, present, and future conditions) individually identifiable health information. In other words, it is information that anyone could look at and know exactly which individual is being discussed—one specific person. Specific pieces of data, called **protected health information (PHI),** are pieces of information related to an individual that must be kept confidential, the grouping of facts that might have someone say, "Oh, I know him! Oh, and he has that!"

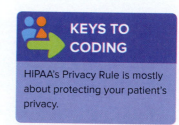

KEYS TO CODING

HIPAA's Privacy Rule is mostly about protecting your patient's privacy.

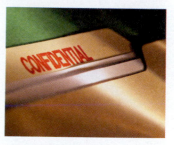

© Scott Speakes/Corbis

protected health information (PHI)
Any patient-identifiable health information regardless of the form in which it is stored (paper, computer file, etc.).

Evan's private health record is no longer private. His diagnosis of a sexually transmitted disease is health information. After discovering his gender, address, and birth date, someone can connect this diagnosis directly to one particular person. All these details, and any other pieces of information like these, are protected to be private under the law. This means that all this information is confidential, and it is against the law for you to reveal any of it, with only a few exceptions:

1. You can tell other health care professionals who are directly involved in the course of doing your job.
2. You can tell someone when given written permission from the patient to do so.
3. You can tell in situations, as outlined in the law, based on "best professional judgment."

The Use and Disclosure of PHI HIPAA's Privacy Rule is very specific as to how you can handle the PHI that you work with every day. The guidelines offer two terms to describe how you might deal with this data.

The term **use** (with regard to HIPAA) means that the information is being shared between people who work together in the same office and need to exchange PHI in order to better serve the patient.

use
The sharing of information between people working in the same health care facility for purposes of caring for the patient.

EXAMPLE

You are getting ready to code the diagnosis for Jayne Hite's recent visit and need additional information. You speak with the attending physician, Dr. Samson, to discuss Jayne's PHI so that you can make certain you find the best, most appropriate diagnosis code. You are using that patient's PHI because the information is being shared between you and the physician in the same office for the benefit of the patient.

disclosure
The sharing of information between health care professionals working in separate entities, or facilities, in the course of caring for the patient.

The second term is **disclosure.** HIPAA defines the term *disclosure* to mean that PHI is being revealed to someone outside the health care office or facility. For example, you prepare a health insurance claim form to send to the patient's insurance company so it will pay your office for the procedures provided. On that claim form, you must put the patient's full name and address, birth date, diagnosis codes, and procedure codes. As you learned earlier in this chapter, each piece of data is not necessarily confidential. When you put all this information together in one place, it becomes PHI because this health information (diagnosis and procedure codes) is now connected to a specific person (identified by the name, address, birth date, etc.) on one piece of paper. However, you must disclose this information to the insurance carrier in order to get paid. You are disclosing the information because the insurance company personnel who will read this claim form do not work for your health care facility—they are an outside company.

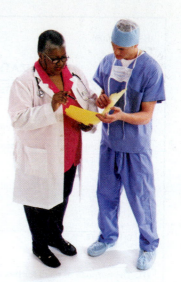

© PhotoDisc/Getty Images

EXAMPLE

Dr. Morton indicates that his patient, John Smith, needs some lab work. Dr. Morton will use Mr. Smith's PHI in his orders for which tests should be performed. Then you need to call the laboratory and disclose Mr. Smith's PHI (his name and diagnosis) along with what specific tests should be performed by the lab.

Remember that everyone in your office and everyone at the insurance carrier and the lab is a member of a covered entity's workforce. You are all bound by the same terms of the HIPAA law and cannot reveal any patient's PHI, except under particular circumstances (such as use and disclosure), unless you have the patient's written permission.

Getting Written Approval

In most situations, other than those already mentioned, the health care provider must get a patient's written permission to disclose the PHI. Although there are many preprinted forms that your office or facility may purchase, the Privacy Rule of HIPAA insists that all these documents have the following characteristics:

1. Are written in plain language (not legalese) so that the average person can understand what he or she is signing.
2. Are very specific as to exactly what information will be disclosed or used.
3. Specifically identify the person or organization that will be disclosing the information.
4. Specifically identify the person(s) who will be receiving the information.
5. Have a definite expiration date.
6. Clearly explain that the person signing this release may retract this authorization in writing at any time.

Figure 1-1 is an example of a form that your facility might use for this purpose.

Permitted Uses and Disclosures

The Privacy Rule outlines six circumstances in which health care professionals are permitted, with or without written patient permission, to use their best professional judgment as to whether or not they should use and/or disclose a patient's PHI.

1. *To the individual.* Health care professionals can *use their best professional judgment to decide whether or not a patient should be told* certain things contained in his or her health care record. Questions come up especially when mental health issues and terminal conditions (when a patient is almost certain to die in the near future) are concerned and there is doubt if the patient can deal with the medical facts. In almost all cases, providing patients with their own PHI is allowed.

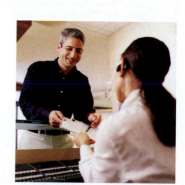

© Duncan Smith/Getty Images

2. *Treatment, payment, and/or operations (TPO).* This means that health care professionals are free to use and/or disclose PHI when it comes to making decisions, coordinating, and managing the *treatment* of a patient's condition.

   In addition, PHI can be disclosed for *payment* activities, such as billing and claims processing, as mentioned earlier in this chapter. In this description, the term *operations* refers to the health care facility's own management of case coordination and quality evaluations.

EXAMPLE

A physician needs to be able to discuss PHI details with a therapist so that together they can establish a proper course of treatment for the patient.

DEPARTMENT OF HEALTH AND HUMAN SERVICES
Indian Health Service

AUTHORIZATION FOR USE OR DISCLOSURE OF PROTECTED HEALTH INFORMATION

COMPLETE ALL SECTIONS, DATE, AND SIGN

I. I, _____ , hereby voluntarily authorize the disclosure of information from my
    health record.   *(Name of Patient)*

II. **The information is to be disclosed by:**   **And is to be provided to:**

NAME OF FACILITY	NAME OF PERSON/ORGANIZATION/FACILITY
ADDRESS	ADDRESS
CITY/STATE	CITY/STATE

III. **The purpose or need for this disclosure is:**

☐ Further Medical Care   ☐ Attorney   ☐ School   ☐ Research

☐ Personal Use   ☐ Insurance   ☐ Disability   ☐ Other *(Specify)* _____

IV. **The information to be disclosed from my health record:** *(check appropriate box(es))*

☐ Only information related to *(specify)* _____

☐ Only the period of events from _____ to _____

☐ Other *(specify) (CHS, Billing, etc.)* _____

☐ Entire Record

If you would like any of the following sensitive information disclosed, check the applicable box(es) below:

☐ Alcohol/Drug Abuse Treatment/Referral   ☐ HIV/AIDS-related Treatment

☐ Sexually Transmitted Diseases   ☐ Mental Health *(Other than Psychotherapy Notes)*

☐ Psychotherapy Notes ONLY (by checking this box, I am waiving any psychotherapist-patient privilege)

V. I understand that I may revoke this authorization in writing submitted at any time to the Health Information Management Department, except to the extent that action has been taken in reliance on this authorization. If this authorization was obtained as a condition of obtaining insurance coverage or a policy of insurance, other law may provide the insurer with the right to contest a claim under the policy. If this authorization has not been revoked, it will terminate one year from the date of my signature unless a different expiration date or *expiration event* is stated.

_____
(Specify new date)

I understand that IHS will not condition treatment or eligibility for care on my providing this authorization except if such care is:
(1) research related or (2) provided solely for the purpose of creating Protected Health Information for disclosure to a third party.

I understand that information disclosed by this authorization, except for Alcohol and Drug Abuse as defined in 42 CFR Part 2, may be subject to redisclosure by the recipient and may no longer be protected by the Health Insurance Portability and Accountability Act Privacy Rule [45 CFR Part 164] , and the Privacy Act of 1974 [5 USC 552a].

SIGNATURE OF PATIENT OR PERSONAL REPRESENTATIVE *(State relationship to patient)*	DATE
SIGNATURE OF WITNESS *(If signature of patient is a thumbprint or mark)*	DATE

This information is to be released for the purpose stated above and may not be used by the recipient for any other purpose. Any person who knowingly and willfully requests or obtains any record concerning an individual from a Federal agency under false pretenses shall be guilty of a misdemeanor (5 USC 552a(i)(3)).

PATIENT IDENTIFICATION	NAME *(Last, First, MI)*	RECORD NUMBER
	ADDRESS	
	CITY/STATE	DATE OF BIRTH

PSC Graphics (301) 443-1090   EF

FIGURE 1-1 Example of Authorization Form to Release Health Information

Source: Department of Health and Human Services, Form IHS-810 (4/09)

3. *Opportunity to agree or object.* This relates to a more informal situation where the patient is present and alert and has the ability to give verbal permission or not with regard to a specific disclosure.

One important point to remember: Although it is much easier to simply ask someone for his or her oral approval than to go get a form and make the patient sign first, it is in your best interest to get written approval whenever possible. People's memories may fail, or they may change their mind later about what they really did tell you. If there is nothing on paper, you cannot prove what was said. For your own protection, get it in writing whenever possible!

EXAMPLE

Harvey Jacobs is about to hear Dr. Arthur explain his test results. Harvey's wife is in the waiting room. Dr. Arthur may ask Harvey if it is okay to invite his wife in and permit her to hear this information. Harvey can then say, "Yes, that is fine" or "No, I don't want her to know about this." Dr. Arthur then must abide by what the patient requests.

4. *Incidental use and disclosure.* As long as reasonable safeguards are in place, this portion of the rule addresses the fact that information might accidentally be used or disclosed during the regular course of business.

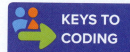

KEYS TO CODING

Incidental is close to the word *accidental*—if someone accidentally overhears what you say.

EXAMPLE

Dr. Peterson comes out of an examining room and approaches Nurse Matthews standing at the desk. This is a back area, and patients are not generally in this hallway, so Dr. Peterson speaks to the nurse in a normal tone of voice to instruct her on preparing Mrs. Riley for a procedure. All of a sudden, another patient comes around the corner, lost on her way back to the waiting room, and overhears the conversation.

This is called incidental use and is understandable in a working environment; therefore, it is not considered a violation of the law.

However, it is important for conversations like this to include only the minimum necessary PHI to accomplish the goal. *Minimum necessary* refers to the caution that should be used to release only the smallest amount of information required to accomplish the task and no more.

Not only is it unnecessary to release more, it is unprofessional.

EXAMPLE

In the hallway outside the exam room, the physician would only need to say, "Marilyn, please prepare Mrs. Riley for her examination." She would not need to include other details about Mrs. Riley, such as "Marilyn, please prepare Mrs. Riley for her examination. You know she has a terrible rash on her thighs. I suspect that it's poison ivy. However, it could be a sexually transmitted disease. We'll have to find out how many sexual partners she has had in the last 6 months."

5. *Public interest.* There are times when the public's best interest may prompt disclosing what you know about a patient. Very often, this is mandated by state laws, which would then take priority over the federal HIPAA law. In other words, if the federal law says you are allowed to tell, and your state's law says you must

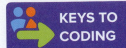
tell—then, you must! These situations include the reporting of suspected abuse (child abuse, elder abuse, neglect, domestic violence) and the reporting of sexually transmitted and other contagious diseases. You are included in the health care team and must think about the community, which must be warned if someone is walking around with a contagious (communicable) disease. Most states require notification to the police in cases where the patient has been shot or stabbed. It is your responsibility to find out what the laws are in your state and how to correctly file a report.

If the physician does not report suspected child abuse of one of your patients, it is your obligation to pick up the phone and call.

6. *Limited data set.* For research, public health statistics, or other health care operations, PHI can be revealed but only after it has been depersonalized. In other words, if the data that connects this information to a specific individual are removed or blacked out, the information is no longer individually identifiable health information, so it does not need to be protected any longer.

EXAMPLE

You can release a health record that has no name, address, telephone number, e-mail address, Social Security number, or photographs attached to it. Even certain physician's notes can be released after they have been stripped of personal data. Following is a sample portion of a record that can be shown without fear of violating anyone's privacy:

"_____ is 25 years old. Back in December, _____ was in a motor vehicle accident on the job. _____ is complaining about some neck pain. _____ has tingling into the right hand."

The example above is a direct quote from the medical record of an actual patient after the specified direct identifiers have been removed. You cannot connect this health information to any one particular person. Therefore, the information is no longer protected and can be used for research and in other ways that may help the community.

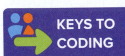
Privacy Notices HIPAA instructs all its covered entities to create policies and procedures with regard to the use and disclosure of PHI. In addition, the law actually states that, once policies and procedures are developed, the facilities must follow these policies. Copies of the written policy must be given to every patient and posted in a general area where it can be seen by all patients.

Notices of Privacy written in compliance with HIPAA's Privacy Rule must contain the following points:

1. A full description of how the covered entity may use and/or disclose a patient's PHI.
2. A statement about the covered entity's responsibility to protect a patient's privacy.
3. Complete information about the patient's rights, including contact information for the Department of Health and Human Services (HHS), should the patient wish to lodge a complaint that his or her privacy was violated.
4. The name of a specific employee of the covered entity must be named as *privacy officer*. This person's name, as well as contact information, must be included in the written notice to handle patients' questions and complaints.

The covered entity must receive written acknowledgment from each patient stating that he or she received the written privacy practices notice. This is usually one of the papers that a patient has to sign when going to a health care facility for the first time.

One of the most important aspects of this portion of the Privacy Rule is that the law specifically says that the covered entity not only has to create these policies and procedures but also has to abide by them. If it doesn't, it is considered to be in violation of federal law and punishable by fines and/or imprisonment.

Although some health care staff members feel that HIPAA and its Privacy Rule are a pain in the neck, think about what this law actually means: respecting your patients' privacy and dignity. Isn't that what you expect from your health care professionals when you go for help? It is not enough that only the doctor be bound to protect the patient's information as confidential because the doctor is no longer the only person who has access. Your health care facility is no place for gossip. You might find this person's hemorrhoids funny or that person's rash gross. As a professional, you should not be concerned with entertaining your friends with your patients' private circumstances. How would you feel if it were *your* personal problem that your health care team members were giggling about with their friends? Or you might consider telling your brother that his girlfriend came in with a sexually transmitted disease. You cannot! Everyone is entitled to privacy. As difficult as it may be, you must remain a professional.

Violating HIPAA's Privacy Rule

Any individual who discovers that his or her privacy has been misused or disclosed without permission can file a complaint with the Department of Health and Human Services (HHS) that the health care provider, health plan, or clearinghouse has not followed HIPAA's regulations. When writing this law, Congress included specifications for both civil and criminal penalties to be applied against any covered entity that fails to protect its patients' PHI. These penalties include fines—up to $250,000—and up to 10 years in prison (Figure 1-2).

A covered entity is responsible for any violation of HIPAA requirements by any of its employees, business associates, or other members of its workforce, such as interns and volunteers. Generally, the senior officials of the covered entity may be punished for the lack of compliance; however, middle managers and staff members are not exempt.

Civil Penalties

1. $100 with no prison for each single violation of a HIPAA regulation with a maximum of $25,000 for multiple violations of the same portion of the regulation during the same calendar year.

EXAMPLE

You tell your best friend that Alan Olin, whom you both went to school with, came into your physician's office and tested positive for a sexually transmitted disease. You, of course, swear her to secrecy. Later that day, she bumps into Alan's fiancée and feels obligated to tell her about Alan's condition. Alan puts two and two together, after his fiancée breaks up with him, and he files a complaint that you disclosed his PHI without permission. You and/or your physician is fined $100.

Criminal Penalties

2. Up to $50,000 *and* up to 1 year in jail for the unauthorized or inappropriate disclosure of individually identifiable health information.

EXAMPLE

After you are fined the $100 civil penalty for the inappropriate disclosure of Alan Olin's PHI, you and/or your physician is charged with criminal penalties for the same disclosure, including a fine of $50,000 and a year in jail.

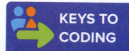

KEYS TO CODING

Just because you *can* take a look at any patient's chart doesn't mean you should. In your facility, you will probably be granted permission to access patients' charts so you can do your work. Under certain circumstances you may be tempted to look, not for your job but because the patient is your friend or neighbor or a celebrity. You may think no harm is being done, just caring or curiosity. But there is harm, and you shouldn't do it.

Back in October 2007, 27 employees of a New Jersey hospital were fired or put on suspension for looking at George Clooney's file after he was brought into the emergency department (ED) following a motorcycle accident.

You could be the president of the hospital and have your best friend come into the ED of your hospital. Without specific permission from that patient, you would be forbidden from looking at the record. Every individual has the right to make his or her own decision about who should know what about his or her own health information.

**HHS requires California medical center
to protect patients' right to privacy**

FOR IMMEDIATE RELEASE
Thursday, June 13, 2013

HHS Press Office
(202) 690-6343

News Release

Shasta Regional Medical Center (SRMC) has agreed to a comprehensive corrective action plan to settle a U.S. Department of Health and Human Services (HHS) investigation concerning potential violations of the Health Insurance Portability and Accountability Act (HIPAA) Privacy Rule.

The HHS Office for Civil Rights (OCR) opened a compliance review of SRMC following a Los Angeles Times article which indicated two SRMC senior leaders had met with media to discuss medical services provided to a patient. OCR's investigation indicated that SRMC failed to safeguard the patient's protected health information (PHI) from impermissible disclosure by intentionally disclosing PHI to multiple media outlets on at least three separate occasions, without a valid written authorization. OCR's review indicated that senior management at SRMC impermissibly shared details about the patient's medical condition, diagnosis and treatment in an email to the entire workforce. In addition, SRMC failed to sanction its workforce members for impermissibly disclosing the patient's records pursuant to its internal sanctions policy.

"When senior level executives intentionally and repeatedly violate HIPAA by disclosing identifiable patient information, OCR will respond quickly and decisively to stop such behavior," said OCR Director Leon Rodriguez. "Senior leadership helps define the culture of an organization and is responsible for knowing and complying with the HIPAA privacy and security requirements to ensure patients' rights are fully protected."

In addition to a $275,000 monetary settlement, a corrective action plan (CAP) requires SRMC to update its policies and procedures on safeguarding PHI from impermissible uses and disclosures and to train its workforce members. The CAP also requires fifteen other hospitals or medical centers under the same ownership or operational control as SRMC to attest to their understanding of permissible uses and disclosures of PHI, including disclosures to the media.

The Resolution Agreement can be found on the OCR website at:
http://www.hhs.gov/ocr/privacy/hipaa/enforcement/examples/shasta-agreement.pdf

FIGURE 1-2 Violators of HIPAA Face Consequences

3. Up to $100,000 *and* up to 5 years in prison for the unauthorized or inappropriate disclosure of individually identifiable health information through deception.

> ## EXAMPLE
>
> Your best friend since high school, Roxanne Rogers, just got a great job as a pharmaceutical representative. To help her, you give her a list of all the patients from your facility who have been diagnosed with diabetes so she can advertise her company's new drug to them. You and she both know this is illegal, so you tell Roxanne that you got permission from each of the patients to release the information (and that is a lie). After a patient complains to HHS, the investigation discovers your relationship with Roxanne. You and your physician are fined $100,000 per occurrence (that's for each person on the list), as well as sentenced to 5 years in prison.

4. Up to $250,000 *and* up to 10 years in prison for the unauthorized or inappropriate disclosure of individually identifiable health information through deception with intent to sell or use for business-related benefit, personal gain, or hateful detriment.

LO 1.2 Health Care Fraud and Abuse Control Program

HIPAA also created the Health Care Fraud and Abuse Control Program. This program, under the direction of the attorney general and the secretary of HHS, acts in association with the Office of the Inspector General (OIG) and coordinates with federal, state, and local law enforcement agencies to discover those who attempt to defraud or abuse the health care system, including Medicare and Medicaid patients and programs.

In 2003, approximately $723 million was returned to the Medicare Trust Fund and another $151.6 million was reimbursed to the Centers for Medicare and Medicaid Services (CMS). The federal government deposited approximately $2.51 billion in the Medicare Trust Fund in fiscal year 2009, plus more than $441 million of federal Medicaid funds were brought into the United States Treasury. Since it was created in 1997, the Health Care Fraud and Abuse Control Program has collected more than $15.6 billion for the Medicare Trust Fund—money improperly received by health care professionals filing fraudulent claims. The statistics show that, for every $1.00 (one dollar) spent to pay for these investigations and prosecutions, the government actually brings in about $4.00 (four dollars) in money returned.

Also, in 2003, 362 criminal indictments were filed in health care fraud cases, and 437 defendants were convicted for health care fraud–related crimes. Another 231 civil cases were filed, and 1,277 more civil matters were pending during this year. This program also prohibited 3,275 individuals and organizations from working with any federally sponsored programs (such as Medicare and Medicaid). Most of these were as a result of convictions for Medicare- or Medicaid-related crimes, including patient abuse and patient neglect, or as a result of providers' licenses having been revoked.

In 2009, 1,014 new investigations were started by the Fraud Section of the criminal division in conjunction with the U.S. Attorneys' offices. These investigations involve 1,786 defendants, while the federal prosecutors filed criminal charges involving 803 defendants in 481 cases and had another 1,621 health care fraud investigations involving 2,706 potential defendants. At the same time, the Department of Justice had 1,155 civil health care fraud cases pending and 886 new civil investigations opened.

When you compare the 2003 statistics with the 2009 statistics you can see that an increasing number of people are being caught trying to get money to which they are not entitled. This is an important reminder that, if individuals try to get you to participate in illegal or unethical behaviors, the question is not "will you be caught?" but "*when* will you be caught?".

LO 1.3 National Correct Coding Initiative

Reporting the procedures, services, and treatments provided to patients is a complex activity. Accuracy, or lack of accuracy, directly impacts reimbursement to providers and can incorrectly alter health care policies and guidelines as well as misdirect research endeavors. With this in mind, the Centers for Medicare and Medicaid Services (CMS) created the National Correct Coding Initiative (NCCI).

Annually, CMS updates its *National Correct Coding Initiative Coding Policy Manual for Medicare Services,* more commonly known as the *Coding Policy Manual,* on the basis of the coding conventions and guidelines determined by the American Medical Association's CPT manual, reviews of current coding practices, and accepted industry policies and guidelines. This manual is easily accessible on the CMS website.

Federal False Claims Act

The federal False Claims Act specifically forbids the submission of health care claims with the intention of gaining financial consideration by stating details that are not true and accurate. This regulation governs punishment of anyone who knows, or should know, that there is inaccurate information on any claim presented to a federal agency, such as CMS. Moreover, virtually every state has passed its own legislation to hold individuals liable for the same actions against state agencies and private organizations.

LO 1.4 Rules for Ethical and Legal Coding

As a coder, you have a very important responsibility—to yourself, your patients, and your facility. The work you do results in the creation of health claim forms, which are legal documents. Your responsibilities can help your facility stay healthy (business-wise) or contribute to the business's being fined and shut down by the OIG and your state's attorney general. It is important that you clearly understand the ethical and legal aspects of your new position. Following are some issues, with regard to the ethics and legalities of coding, with which you should become very familiar.

1. It is very important that the codes indicated on the health claim form represent the services actually performed and are supported by notes and other documentation in the patient's health record. Don't use a code on a claim form without having **supporting documentation** in the file.
2. Some health care providers instruct their coders to **code for coverage.** This means that codes (both diagnostic and procedural) are not chosen for the best, most accurate code available but, rather, with regard to the procedures the insurance company will pay for, or "cover." This is dishonest and is considered fraud. Some providers will rationalize this process by saying they are doing it so the patient can get the treatment he or she really needs to be paid for by the insurance company. Altruism aside, it is still illegal.
3. If you find yourself in an office or a facility that insists that you include codes for procedures that you know, or believe, were never performed, this might be a case of fraud. It might be that they just didn't know. However, sometimes this is done out in the open, even though it is illegal. Your participation in the process of getting money on false pretenses is serious. If you are found guilty of fraud, you might have to pay a fine and/or go to jail. This is not something to take lightly.
4. **Upcoding,** another illegal process, is using a code that reports a higher level of service than that which was actually provided. Upcoding is considered falsifying records. Even if all you do is fill out the claim form, it is still an unethical and illegal act.

supporting documentation
The paperwork in the patient's file that corroborates the codes presented on the claim form for a particular encounter.

code for coverage
To choose a code by the insurance company's rules of what it will pay for, rather than a code that accurately reflects the truth about the encounter.

upcoding
Using a code on a claim form that indicates a higher level of service than that which was actually performed.

EXAMPLE

Using a code for a colonoscopy when a sigmoidoscopy was actually done is an example of upcoding. A colonoscopy is a more complex procedure that requires patient preparation as well as a sedative. It also takes more time to perform. Therefore, the physician would be paid more to perform a colonoscopy than a sigmoidoscopy. You can see that it would be wrong to get paid for providing a more involved procedure when a simpler procedure was actually done.

5. If you resubmit a claim that has been lost, identify it as a "tracer" or "second submission." If you don't, you might be found guilty of double billing, billing the insurance company twice for a service provided only once. This also constitutes fraud.

6. It is not permissible to code and bill for individual (also known as component) services when a comprehensive or combination (bundle) code is available. This is referred to as **unbundling,** and it is illegal. For Medicare billing, refer to the Medicare National Correct Coding Initiative (CCI), which lists standardized bundled codes. The CCI is used to find coding conflicts, such as unbundling, the use of **mutually exclusive codes,** and other unacceptable reporting of CPT codes. When these errors are discovered, those claims are pulled for review and may be subject to possible suspension or rejection.

unbundling
Coding individual parts of a specific procedure rather than one combination, or bundle, that includes all the components.

mutually exclusive codes
Codes that are identified as those that are not permitted to be used on the same claim form with other codes.

EXAMPLE

Dr. Federman's notes indicate that Ellen Thompson, a 5-year-old female, received an MMR vaccine. Reporting 90704 Mumps virus vaccine, 90705 Measles virus vaccine, and 90706 Rubella virus vaccine separately—instead of the combination code of 90707 Measles, mumps, and rubella virus vaccine—is considered unbundling and is unethical.

EXAMPLE

In the CPT codebook, you'll find the instruction that tells you not to report one code with another. For example, "Do not report 43752 in conjunction with critical care codes 99291–99292." The "do not report" notation identifies mutually exclusive codes. This is the CPT book telling you it is unethical to place both 43752 and 99291 on the same claim form.

7. Separating the codes relating to one encounter and placing them on several claim forms over the course of several days is neither legal nor ethical. This not only indicates a lack of organization in the office but also can cause suspicion of duplicating service claims. Even if you are reporting procedures that were done for diagnoses that actually exist, remember that the claim form is a legal document. All data on that claim form, including dates of service, must be accurate. Do not submit the claim form until you are certain it is complete, with all diagnoses and procedures listed.

If, after you submit a claim, an additional service provided comes to light (such as a lab report with an extra charge), then you must file an amended claim. Although not illegal because you are identifying that this claim contains an adjustment, most third-party payers dislike amended claims. You can expect an amended claim to be scrutinized.

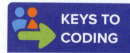

KEYS TO CODING

Always remember to read the complete descriptions in the provider's notes in addition to referencing the encounter form, and then, carefully, find the best available code, according to the documentation.

LO 1.5 Codes of Ethics

There are two premier trade organizations for professional coding specialists. Each has published a code of ethics to guide members of our industry on the best professional way to conduct themselves.

American Health Information Management Association Code of Ethics

The American Health Information Management Association (AHIMA) is the preeminent professional organization for health information workers, including insurance coding specialists. The AHIMA House of Delegates designated the elements in Box 1-1 as being critical to the highest level of honorable behavior for its members.

In this era of reimbursements based on diagnostic and procedural coding, the professional ethics of health information coding professionals continue to be challenged. Standards of ethical coding practices for coding professionals—developed by AHIMA's Coding Policy and Strategy Committee and approved by AHIMA's board of directors—are shown in Box 1-2.

AAPC Code of Ethical Standards

American Academy of Professional Coders (AAPC) is an influential organization in the health information management industry. Its members, and their certifications, are well respected throughout the United States and the world. Its Code of Ethical Standards, shown in Box 1-3, also illuminates the importance of an insurance coding and billing specialist's exhibiting the most ethical and moral conduct.

BOX 1-1 AHIMA Code of Ethics

This Code of Ethics sets forth ethical principles for the health information management profession. Members of this profession are responsible for maintaining and promoting ethical practices. This Code of Ethics, adopted by the American Health Information Management Association, shall be binding on health information management professionals who are members of the Association and all individuals who hold an AHIMA certification.

The following ethical principles are based on the core values of the American Health Information Management Association and apply to all health information management professionals. Health information management professionals must

1. Advocate, uphold, and defend the individual's right to privacy and the doctrine of confidentiality in the use and disclosure of information.

2. Put service and the health and welfare of persons before self-interest and conduct themselves in the practice of the profession so as to bring honor to themselves, their peers, and the health information management profession.

3. Preserve, protect, and secure personal health information in any form or medium and hold in the highest regard the contents of the records and other information of a confidential nature, taking into account the applicable statutes and regulations.

4. Refuse to participate in or conceal unethical practices or procedures.

5. Advance health information management knowledge and practice through continuing education, research, publications, and presentations.

6. Recruit and mentor students, peers, and colleagues to develop and strengthen a professional workforce.

7. Represent the profession accurately to the public.

8. Perform honorably health information management association responsibilities, either appointed or elected, and preserve the confidentiality of any privileged information made known in any official capacity.

9. State truthfully and accurately their credentials, professional education, and experiences.

10. Facilitate interdisciplinary collaboration in situations supporting health information practice.

11. Respect the inherent dignity and worth of every person.

Source: Reprinted with permission from the American Health Information Management Association. Copyright © 2015 by the American Health Information Management Association. All rights reserved. No part of this may be reproduced, reprinted, stored in a retrieval system, or transmitted, in any form or by any means, electronic photocopying, recording, or otherwise, without the prior written permission of the association. Adapted with permission from the Code of Ethics of the National Association of Social Workers.

BOX 1-2   AHIMA Standards of Ethical Coding

Coding professionals should:

1. Apply accurate, complete, and consistent coding practices for the production of high-quality health care data.

2. Report all health care data elements (e.g. diagnosis and procedure codes, present on admission indicator, discharge status) required for external reporting purposes (e.g. reimbursement and other administrative uses, population health, quality and patient safety measurement, and research) completely and accurately, in accordance with regulatory and documentation standards and requirements and applicable official coding conventions, rules, and guidelines.

3. Assign and report only the codes and data that are clearly and consistently supported by health record documentation in accordance with applicable code set and abstraction conventions, rules, and guidelines.

4. Query provider (physician or other qualified health care practitioner) for clarification and additional documentation prior to code assignment when there is conflicting, incomplete, or ambiguous information in the health record regarding a significant reportable condition or procedure or other reportable data element dependent on health record documentation (e.g. present on admission indicator).

5. Refuse to change reported codes or the narratives of codes so that meanings are misrepresented.

6. Refuse to participate in or support coding or documentation practices intended to inappropriately increase payment, qualify for insurance policy coverage, or skew data by means that do not comply with federal and state statutes, regulations and official rules and guidelines.

7. Facilitate interdisciplinary collaboration in situations supporting proper coding practices.

8. Advance coding knowledge and practice through continuing education.

9. Refuse to participate in or conceal unethical coding or abstraction practices or procedures.

10. Protect the confidentiality of the health record at all times and refuse to access protected health information not required for coding-related activities (examples of coding-related activities include completion of code assignment, other health record data abstraction, coding audits, and educational purposes).

11. Demonstrate behavior that reflects integrity, shows a commitment to ethical and legal coding practices, and fosters trust in professional activities.

BOX 1-3   AAPC Code of Ethical Standards

Members of the American Academy of Professional Coders shall be dedicated to providing the highest standard of professional coding and billing services to employers, clients and patients. Professional and personal behavior of AAPC members must be exemplary.

AAPC members shall maintain the highest standard of personal and professional conduct. Members shall respect the rights of patients, clients, employers and all other colleagues.

Members shall use only legal and ethical means in all professional dealings and shall refuse to cooperate with, or condone by silence, the actions of those who engage in fraudulent, deceptive or illegal acts.

Members shall respect and adhere to the laws and regulations of the land and uphold the mission statement of the AAPC.

Members shall pursue excellence through continuing education in all areas applicable to their profession.

Members shall strive to maintain and enhance the dignity, status, competence and standards of coding for professional services.

Members shall not exploit professional relationships with patients, employees, clients or employers for personal gain.

Above all else we will commit to recognizing the intrinsic worth of each member.

This code of ethical standards for members of the AAPC strives to promote and maintain the highest standard of professional service and conduct among its members. Adherence to these standards assures public confidence in the integrity and service of professional coders who are members of the AAPC.

Failure to adhere to these standards, as determined by AAPC, will result in the loss of credentials and membership with the American Academy of Professional Coders.

BOX 1-4 Federal Sentencing Guidelines Manual: The Seven Steps to Due Diligence

1. Establish compliance standards and procedures
2. Assign overall responsibility to specific high-level individual(s)
3. Use due care to avoid delegation of authority to individuals with an inclination to get involved in illegal actions
4. Effectively communicate standards and procedures to all staff
5. Utilize monitoring and auditing system to detect non-compliant conduct
6. Enforce adequate disciplinary sanctions when appropriate
7. Respond to episodes of non-compliance by modifying program, if necessary

Source: United States Sentencing Commission. (2014, November 1). 2014 USSC Guidelines Manual. Retrieved from http://www.ussc.gov/guidelines-manual/2014/2014-ussc-guidelines-manual

LO 1.6 Compliance Programs

A formal compliance program has been strongly recommended by the OIG of the HHS to help all health care facilities establish their organizations' respect for the laws and their agreement to follow the direction from those laws. However, there are certain health care providers for whom this is not only suggested but mandated by law.

The Deficit Reduction Act of 2005, which went into effect January 1, 2007, mandates a compliance program for all health care organizations that receive $5 million or more a year from Medicaid. This law is very specific that the facility's compliance program include written guidance and policies about employees' responsibilities under the False Claims Act.

On March 23, 2010, President Obama signed the Patient Protection and Affordable Care Act into law. Among the many other elements of health care covered by this law, there is a provision in Section 6401 that providers participating in Medicare and Medicaid create compliance programs. This includes physicians' offices and suppliers.

A compliance program will officially create policies and procedures; establish the structure to adhere to those policies; set up a monitoring system to ensure that it works; and correct conduct that does not comply. The foundation of the compliance program is the creation of an organizational culture of honesty and compliance with the laws, the discouragement of fraud, waste, and abuse, the discovery of any fraudulent activities as soon as possible using internal policies and audits, and immediate corrective action when fraud and abuse do occur.

The federal sentencing guidelines manual provides a seven-step list of the components of an effective compliance program. These are shown in Box 1-4 for you to review and understand.

Chapter Summary

Knowing your legal and ethical responsibilities as a health care professional will give you a strong foundation for a healthy career. HIPAA's Privacy Rule, along with the codes of ethics from both AHIMA and AAPC, should help guide you through any challenges. *Confidentiality, honesty,* and *accuracy* are three watchwords that all health information management professionals should live by.

CHAPTER 1 REVIEW
Legal and Ethical Issues

Mc Graw Hill Education **connect**®
Enhance your learning by completing these
exercises and more at mcgrawhillconnect.com!

Using Terminology

Match each key term to the appropriate definition.

_____ 1. LO 1.4 The paperwork in the patient's file that corroborates the codes presented on the claim form for a particular encounter.

_____ 2. LO 1.1 Any patient-identifiable health information regardless of the form in which it is stored (paper, computer file, etc.).

_____ 3. LO 1.1 Health care providers, health plans, and health care clearinghouses—businesses that have access to the personal health information of patients.

_____ 4. LO 1.1 The sharing of information between health care professionals working in separate entities, or facilities, in the course of caring for the patient.

_____ 5. LO 1.1 A portion of HIPAA that ensures the availability of patient information for those who should see it while protecting that information from those who should not.

_____ 6. LO 1.1 Purposely avoiding learning about a law to excuse not following that law.

_____ 7. LO 1.1 The sharing of information between people working in the same health care facility for purposes of caring for the patient.

_____ 8. LO 1.4 Coding individual parts of a specific procedure rather than one combination, or bundle, that includes all the components.

_____ 9. LO 1.4 Using a code on a claim form that indicates a higher level of service than that which was actually performed.

_____ 10. LO 1.1 Actions that are in agreement with society's concept of right and wrong.

_____ 11. LO 1.4 To choose a code by the insurance company's rules of what it will pay for, rather than a code that accurately reflects the truth about the encounter.

_____ 12. LO 1.1 Using inaccurate information or other dishonesty to wrongly gain money or other benefit.

_____ 13. LO 1.4 Codes that are identified as those that are not permitted to be used on the same claim form with other codes.

A. Code for coverage
B. Covered entities
C. Disclosure
D. Ethical behaviors
E. Fraud
F. HIPAA's Privacy Rule
G. Mutually exclusive codes
H. Protected health information (PHI)
I. Supporting documentation
J. Unbundling
K. Upcoding
L. Use
M. Willful ignorance

Checking Your Understanding

Choose the most appropriate answer for each of the following questions.

1. LO 1.1 According to HIPAA, covered entities include all *except*

   a. health care providers.
   b. health plans.
   c. health care computer software manufacturers.
   d. health care clearinghouses.

2. LO 1.1 HIPAA's Privacy Rule is all about the

    a. training of medical assistants.
    b. use and disclosure of protected health information.
    c. security of health records.
    d. insurance billing and coding issues.

3. LO 1.1 An example of protected health information is

    a. patient's Social Security number.
    b. patient's next of kin.
    c. all codes in the CPT book.
    d. patient's state of residence.

4. LO 1.1 HIPAA states that all covered entities must comply with the Privacy Rule as of

    a. October 16, 2003.
    b. April 14, 2003.
    c. September 15, 2003.
    d. March 1, 2004.

5. LO 1.1 A patient calls your office and asks for the results of her recent blood tests. You

    a. get her file and answer her questions honestly.
    b. tell her to hold on so that she can speak with the doctor.
    c. offer to make an appointment for her to come in to get the results.
    d. tell her she is breaking the law and hang up.

6. LO 1.1 Most state laws mandate that when a health care professional suspects abuse of any kind he or she *must*

    a. call the appropriate authorities.
    b. talk to the patient about the suspicions.
    c. wait until he or she is absolutely certain.
    d. talk to the patient's family.

7. LO 1.1 The intent of HIPAA's Privacy Rule is to

    a. protect an individual's privacy.
    b. not interfere with the flow of information necessary for care.
    c. restrict health care professionals from doing their jobs.
    d. protect an individual's privacy and not interfere with the flow of information necessary for care.

8. LO 1.1 All covered entities must create and implement written

    a. PHI information flow charts.
    b. customer service rules.
    c. privacy practices notices.
    d. coding guidelines.

9. LO 1.1 Protected health information (PHI) is

    a. any health information that can be connected to a specific individual.
    b. a listing of diagnosis codes.
    c. current procedural terminology.
    d. covered entity employee files.

10. LO 1.1 Taking authorization for the release of protected health information over the phone from an individual is
   a. acceptable, as long as you recognize the person's voice.
   b. never acceptable.
   c. acceptable, as long as someone else gets on the phone to vouch for the caller.
   d. acceptable under emergency situations.

11. LO 1.1 The term *use* per HIPAA's Privacy Rule refers to the exchange of information between health care personnel
   a. and health care personnel in other health care facilities.
   b. and family members.
   c. in the same office.
   d. and the pharmacist.

12. LO 1.1 The term *disclosure* per HIPAA's Privacy Rule refers to the exchange of information between health care personnel
   a. and health care personnel in other covered entities.
   b. and family members.
   c. in the same office.
   d. and the patient.

13. LO 1.1 Ensuring that patients' privacy is protected is the responsibility of
   a. the clinical staff.
   b. the attending physician.
   c. the registered nurse.
   d. all staff members.

14. LO 1.1 HIPAA is a _____ law.
   a. local.
   b. county.
   c. state.
   d. federal.

15. LO 1.1 Which of the following is *not* a covered entity under HIPAA?
   a. county hospital.
   b. BlueCross BlueShield.
   c. Physician Associates medical practice.
   d. computer technical support.

16. LO 1.1 A woman comes into the hospital emergency room. The attending physician suspects that her husband has been physically abusing her. The Privacy Rule says the physician is permitted, but not mandated, to disclose this information to the police. The state says the physician must report this to the police or lose his or her license. The physician should
   a. call his or her attorney.
   b. get the patient to sign a release form before telling anyone.
   c. call the police immediately.
   d. say nothing.

17. LO 1.1 A new Walgreen's store opens two blocks away from the office where you work. The manager of the store calls your medical practice and offers to pay for a copy of the names and addresses of your patients who have been taking prescribed medication on a regular basis. Do you

   a. meet with the doctor to determine how much to charge?
   b. explain that this would be against the law under HIPAA's Privacy Rule?
   c. provide the list for free to be a good neighbor?
   d. get the money for the list upfront?

18. LO 1.1 According to HIPAA's rules and regulations, a covered entity's workforce includes

   a. only paid, full-time employees.
   b. only licensed personnel working in the office.
   c. volunteers, trainees, and employees, part-time and full-time.
   d. business associates' employees.

19. LO 1.1 HIPAA's Privacy Rule has been carefully crafted to

   a. protect a patient's health care history.
   b. protect a patient's current medical issues.
   c. protect a patient's future health considerations.
   d. all of these.

20. LO 1.1 A written form to release PHI should include all *except*

   a. specific identification of the person who will be receiving the information.
   b. the specific information to be released.
   c. legal terminology so it will stand up in court.
   d. an expiration date.

21. LO 1.1 There can be _____ penalties for any violation of HIPAA's rules.

   a. civil.
   b. criminal.
   c. both civil and criminal.
   d. no.

22. LO 1.1 Those who are permitted to file an official complaint with HHS are

   a. health care providers.
   b. any individual.
   c. health plans.
   d. clearinghouses.

23. LO 1.1 Penalties for violating any portion of HIPAA apply to

   a. patients.
   b. patients' families.
   c. all covered entities.
   d. health care office managers.

24. LO 1.1 If you disclose unauthorized PHI through deception, you can

    a. be fined $100 for each occurrence.
    b. be fined $50,000 and get up to 1 year in jail.
    c. be fined $10,000 and get up to 5 years in prison.
    d. be fined $100,000 and get up to 5 years in prison.

25. LO 1.1 HHS stands for

    a. Department of Home and Health Services.
    b. Division of Health and Health Care Sciences.
    c. Department of Health and Human Services.
    d. District of Health and HIPAA Systems.

26. LO 1.4 Changing a code from one that is most accurate to one you know the insurance company will pay for is called

    a. coding for coverage.
    b. coding for packaging.
    c. unbundling.
    d. double billing.

27. LO 1.4 Unbundling is an illegal practice in which coders

    a. bill for services never provided.
    b. bill for services with no documentation.
    c. bill using several individual codes instead of one combination code.
    d. bill using a code for a higher level of service than what was actually provided.

28. LO 1.4 Upcoding is an illegal practice in which coders

    a. bill for services never provided.
    b. bill for services with no documentation.
    c. bill using several individual codes instead of one combination code.
    d. bill using a code for a higher level of service than what was actually provided.

29. LO 1.4 Medicare's CCI investigates claims that include

    a. unbundling.
    b. the improper use of mutually exclusive codes.
    c. unacceptable reporting of CPT codes.
    d. all of these.

30. LO 1.2 Coding improperly on a claim form can cause that claim to be

    a. rejected.
    b. reviewed.
    c. suspended.
    d. all of these.

Applying Your Knowledge

1. LO 1.1 What does HIPAA stand for? _____

_____

2. LO 1.1 Explain the HIPAA Privacy Rule. _____

_____

3. LO 1.1 Why was the HIPAA Privacy Rule written? _____

_____

4. LO 1.1 What is the definition of a health care provider? _____

_____

5. LO 1.2 Discuss health care fraud and explain why it is important to a professional coding specialist. _____

_____

6. LO 1.1 Define and explain PHI. _____

_____

7. LO 1.1 Discuss the difference between *use* and *disclosure* of PHI. _____

_____

8. LO 1.3 What is the National Correct Coding Initiative? Who created it and why was it created? How often is it updated? _____

_____

9. LO 1.4 What is the difference between upcoding and unbundling? Are they permissible practices for a professional coding specialist? _____

_____

10. LO 1.6 Explain the purpose of a compliance program. _____

_____

Following are some health care scenarios. Determine the best course of action that you, as the health information management professional for the facility, should take. Identify any legal and/or ethical issues that may need to be considered, and explain how you would deal with the situation.

CIPHER, VICTORS & ASSOCIATES
A Complete Health Care Facility
234 MAIN STREET • ANYTOWN, FL 32711 • 407-555-1234

PATIENT: SUSQUEHANNA, MARION
ACCOUNT/EHR #:   SUSQMA001
DATE: 09/17/18

Attending Physician: Valerie R. Victors, MD

This 25-year-old female is 21 weeks pregnant. She presents today in tears. She is suffering from hemorrhoids and cannot stand it anymore. The pain and itching are making life difficult for her, as it hurts to sit for any length of time, and she cannot sleep. As it is difficult for her to lie on her stomach, due to the pregnancy, she can only find some comfort by either walking around or lying on her side. She is asking (more like begging) for a hemorrhoidectomy—a simple surgical procedure that can be done in the office and will almost immediately provide her with complete relief.

The correct CPT code for the treatment of Marion's condition is

46260 Hemorrhoidectomy, internal and external, 2 or more columns/groups

However, Marion's insurance carrier will not pay for a hemorrhoidectomy with a diagnosis that indicates there are no complications. According to the insurance customer service representative, it will only pay in full for the procedure

46250 Hemorrhoidectomy, external, 2 or more columns/groups

Marion's husband, David, is a civilian who works for a defense contractor and is currently in Iraq supporting the troops. Money is tight for the family because David's paycheck has been delayed due to a mix-up in paperwork when he was transferred to the Middle East. There is no way they can afford to pay cash for the hemorrhoidectomy.

All you need to do is change the one number of the code and Marion can have the relief she so desperately needs. As the professional coding specialist in this office, what should you do?

_____

_____

_____

CIPHER, VICTORS & ASSOCIATES
A Complete Health Care Facility
234 MAIN STREET • ANYTOWN, FL 32711 • 407-555-1234

PATIENT: MARINOSCI, CHRISTOPHER
ACCOUNT/EHR #:   MARICH001
DATE: 10/05/18

Attending Physician: James I. Cipher, MD

As the coding specialist for this facility, you are given the chart for this patient after his recent encounter with Dr. Cipher. On the face sheet you notice that Dr. Cipher has indicated the procedure provided to this patient to be

Excision dermoid cyst, nose; simple, skin, subcutaneous

However, there is nothing at all in the rest of the documentation, including the encounter notes and lab reports, to support medical necessity for this procedure.

As the professional coding specialist in this office, what should you do?

_____

_____

_____

CIPHER, VICTORS & ASSOCIATES
A Complete Health Care Facility
234 MAIN STREET • ANYTOWN, FL 32711 • 407-555-1234

PATIENT: KELLOGG, JOAN
ACCOUNT/EHR #:   KELLJO001
DATE: 10/15/18

Attending Physician: James I. Cipher, MD

Today, Felicia Masterson comes into your office. She states that she is Joan Kellogg's sister and that she has been asked by her sister to collect a copy of her complete medical record. Ms. Masterson tells you that her sister has moved to another town and needs the records for an upcoming medical appointment with her new doctor. She hands you a printout of an e-mail, supposedly from Ms. Kellogg, to serve as documentation that she should have the records.

As the professional coding specialist in this office, what should you do?

_____

_____

_____

CIPHER, VICTORS & ASSOCIATES
A Complete Health Care Facility
234 MAIN STREET • ANYTOWN, FL 32711 • 407-555-1234

PATIENT: BORNER, EMILY
ACCOUNT/EHR #:   BORNEM001
DATE: 09/25/18

Attending Physician: James I. Cipher, MD

The patient is a 16-year-old female who came in for counseling on birth control.

Today, Glenda Borner came into the office. She stated that she is Emily's mother and found an appointment card for this facility in her daughter's jeans. She demands to know why her daughter came to see the physician. She is angry and frustrated and states that she will not leave until she is told why her daughter saw the doctor.

As the professional coding specialist in this office, what should you do?

_____

_____

_____

CIPHER, VICTORS & ASSOCIATES
A Complete Health Care Facility
234 MAIN STREET • ANYTOWN, FL 32711 • 407-555-1234

PATIENT: GRANGER, ALLEN
ACCOUNT/EHR #:   GRANAL001
DATE: 12/01/18

Attending Physician: Ronald Jones, MD

The patient came to see the physician because he hates his nose. His self-esteem is very low and, as a teenage boy, he has developed severe social anxiety. His family does not have the money to pay for a rhinoplasty (nose job) and the only way that the insurance company will pay for this cosmetic surgery is for medical necessity, such as a deviated septum.

You have been told to code the diagnosis of deviated septum to support medical necessity for the rhinoplasty. The doctor and office manager both tell you that this is the "right" thing to do.

As the professional coding specialist in this office, what should you do?

_____

_____

_____

2 INTRODUCTION TO CODING AND CPT

Learning Outcomes *After completing this chapter, the student should be able to:*

LO 2.1 Explain the purpose of diagnosis coding.

LO 2.2 Explain the purpose of procedure coding.

LO 2.3 Apply correctly the steps to accurate coding.

LO 2.4 Abstract documentation thoroughly.

LO 2.5 Use official guidelines provided to apply the best, most accurate code.

LO 2.6 Interpret notations and symbols to code accurately.

Key Terms

Abstracting

Diagnosis

Durable medical equipment (DME)

Inpatient

Medical necessity

Outpatient

Procedure

Query

Superbill

Supporting documentation

The purpose of coding is to make every effort to ensure clear and concise communication about health care issues among all parties involved. These parties include health care providers, the insurance companies (third-party payers), and government agencies.

The processing of health care information is an important part of our country's health care system. As you are probably aware, insurance carriers use this data to determine how much they should pay health care professionals for the attention and services provided to a patient. This is called the *reimbursement process.* The codes make it easier for the organizations involved to evaluate and manage all the data. In addition, these codes are used in the study of diseases and conditions that affect our population. Foundations and government agencies use statistical information to develop programs and policies that will best address the health of our residents. For example, they can only know that a disease such as Alzheimer's needs diagnostic tests, treatment, and possibly a vaccine or a cure by studying statistics to see what individuals are being diagnosed with around the country and the world.

Coding is simply interpreting health care terms and definitions into numbers or number-letter combinations (alphanumeric codes) that specifically relate to diagnoses and procedures.

LO 2.1 Medical Necessity

The International Classification of Diseases, 10th revision, Clinical Modification (ICD-10-CM) is a directory of every **diagnosis,** or reason a health care provider would spend time with and/or provide a service to a patient. Diagnosis codes are very important because they give the information about why the physician provided a particular service or treatment. These codes establish **medical necessity,** and every **procedure** code reported must be accompanied by a diagnosis code that justifies that specific procedure. Some examples of diagnoses are a broken ankle, diabetes, and the flu.

ICD-10-CM diagnosis codes are alphanumeric codes up to seven characters in length.

EXAMPLE

ICD-10-CM Diagnosis Codes

D15.0 Benign neoplasm of thymus

G93.0 Cerebral cysts

M79.601 Pain in right arm

S33.6xxA Sprain of sacroiliac joint, initial encounter

EXAMPLE

Diagnosis Codes Supporting Procedures Performed

Jerri Cavanaugh, a 13-year-old female, is brought to the emergency department by her mother after Jerri fell off her skateboard and hurt her ankle. Dr. Roberts orders x-rays that confirm Jerri's ankle is broken, and he applies a short leg (knee-to-toe) cast.

The diagnosis of a broken ankle makes the taking of the x-ray and the application of the lower leg cast good medical decisions. Dr. Roberts has a documented medical reason to provide these services.

EXAMPLE

Morris Cruz, a 65-year-old male, goes to see his physician, Dr. Bridges. Morris is complaining of pain upon urination. Dr. Bridges orders a urinalysis. The results of the test show that Morris has a urinary tract infection (UTI). Dr. Bridges is in a hurry and scribbles in his notes what looks like "URI."

The problem here is that URI stands for upper respiratory infection (chest congestion). You can see that the diagnosis of an upper respiratory infection does not justify the lab test that was ordered. This will be looked at as either an error or very poor medical judgment. In either case, the claim will be denied for lack of medical necessity.

LO 2.2 Procedures (Services and Treatments)

This and the following chapters in this text take you through three directories of code sets that you will use in the process of translating health care procedures (services and treatments) into codes. These three directories are *Current Procedural Terminology* (CPT), Health care Common Procedure Coding System (HCPCS) Level II, and ICD-10-PCS.

CPT, fourth edition, is similar to the ICD-10-CM, except that, instead of listing codes for diagnoses, the CPT catalogs codes for procedures, treatments, and services provided to patients, such as an x-ray, a vaccination, or the removal of a cyst. Technically, CPT codes are HCPCS Level I codes. However, professionals in the health care industry refer to these procedure codes simply as CPT codes.

CPT codes are chiefly five numbers, all in a row. Some CPT codes (known as category II codes and category III codes) can have four numbers followed by a letter. You will learn more about these codes later in this textbook.

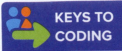

durable medical equipment (DME)
Items that are used in the care and treatment of a patient that either can last a long time or can be used again and again.

EXAMPLE

CPT Codes

31750 Tracheoplasty; cervical
0058T Cryopreservation; reproductive tissue, ovarian

The Health care Common Procedure Coding System (*HCPCS*) *Level II* lists codes used to identify **durable medical equipment (DME),** dental procedures, medications, and certain other services not listed in the CPT book. Items coded from HCPCS (pronounced *hick-picks*) might include a wheelchair, crutches, or a unit of blood for a transfusion. HCPCS Level II codes have one letter followed by four numbers.

EXAMPLE

HCPCS Codes

E0607 Home blood glucose monitor
D0120 Periodic oral examination
J0129 Injection, abatacept, 10 mg

inpatient
A patient admitted into a hospital for an overnight stay or longer.

When a hospital provides services and treatments to an individual who has been admitted into the hospital as an **inpatient,** codes will be used from ICD-10-PCS.

ICD-10-PCS procedure codes use a combination of letters and numbers. All codes are seven characters long. More about this code set appears in Part III of this resource.

EXAMPLE

ICD-10-PCS Codes

02QN0ZZ Repair of the pericardium, open approach
0BYF0Z0 Allogeneic transplantation of the lower right lung lobe

Specific Code Definitions

Each set of numbers or numbers/letters means something so specific that a code just one digit off could mean something totally unrelated. Transposing two numbers is a typical error. For example, when jotting down a phone number, you think one-seven-one but write down 711. However, instead of having a wrong phone number, an incorrect code could cause a claim to be rejected, denied, or pulled for investigation, resulting in your office's having to deal with delayed payment or no payment at all.

This is why it is critical to be careful and accurate when coding and *always* double-check your codes.

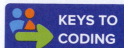

KEYS TO CODING

Documentation is your watchword. You must have the information *in writing*. If it is not written down (or in a computer document), then, as far as you are concerned, it never happened and therefore you cannot code it.

EXAMPLE

Specific Definitions: The Difference between 305 and 503

30520 Septoplasty or submucous resection, with or without cartilage scoring, contouring or replacement with graft . . . *nose surgery.*

50320 Donor nephrectomy (including cold preservation); open, from living donor . . . *the removal of a kidney from a live person to be transplanted into another.*

LO 2.3 Seven Steps to Accurate Coding

There is a seven-step process for coding a health care encounter in the approved manner. As you gain experience, coding a patient encounter will take less time. However, remember that time is not the number one consideration—no matter what anyone says; accuracy is the most important factor.

The steps are as follows:

1. *Read* the **superbill** and the physician's notes for this encounter completely, from beginning to end.

2. *Reread* the physician's notes, and *identify key words* regarding diagnoses and procedures directly relating to this encounter. Pulling out the key words is also called **abstracting** the physician's notes. You will need to evaluate the key words and distinguish between diagnostic statements and procedural statements.

3. *Make a list* of any questions you have regarding unclear or missing information necessary to code this encounter. **Query** the health care provider who treated the patient, and, if necessary, ask the provider to update the chart. Never assume. Code only what you know from actual documentation. As you read in Chap. 1, Box 1-2, "AHIMA Standards of Ethical Coding," the fourth standard directs you to have the **supporting documentation** to back up every code you submit on a claim form.

superbill
A form preprinted with the diagnosis codes and procedure codes most frequently used in a particular facility.

abstracting
The process of identifying the relevant words or phrases in health care documentation in order to determine the best, most appropriate code(s).

query
To ask.

supporting documentation
The written reports that provide evidence of what was provided to the patient and why.

EXAMPLE

The Importance of Querying the Physician

The documentation indicates that the physician performed a posterior vestibuloplasty on Marion Jones. You pull out the key words: vestibuloplasty; posterior. However, when you look up this procedure in the CPT book, you see that there are two codes to choose from:

40842 Vestibuloplasty; posterior, unilateral

40843 Vestibuloplasty; posterior, bilateral

You must query the physician to find out whether the procedure was done unilaterally (one side) or bilaterally (both sides). Make certain the physician answers your question *by entering* the information in the chart—and initials and dates it. Now you know which code is the best, most appropriate code.

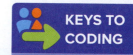

KEYS TO CODING

Use a medical dictionary to learn the true meaning of a medical term. If you don't know what the term means, you will have a problem interpreting it into an accurate code.

4. *Code the diagnosis or diagnoses* as stated by the physician. In the absence of a definitive diagnosis, code the identified signs and symptoms describing why the health care provider cared for this patient during this encounter. Use the best, most accurate code available based on the documentation.

5. *Code the procedure or procedures* as stated in the notes describing what the provider did for the patient during this encounter. Use the best, most appropriate codes available based on the documentation. When using the ICD-10-PCS for inpatient procedures or CPT for physician services and outpatient services, you will

   a. Dissect the procedural statement that you abstracted from the documentation. Identify the term that describes WHAT action was taken.

   Examples:

   i. Cranial nerve neuroplasty . . . the procedure is a "neuroplasty" and the anatomical site is the "cranial nerve".

   ii. Pelvic ultrasound (nonobstetrical) . . . the procedure is an "ultrasound" and the anatomical site is "pelvis"

   iii. Coronary thrombolysis . . . the procedure is a "thrombolysis" and the anatomical site is the "heart" (coronary refers to the heart).

   b. Look the main term up in the CPT alphabetic index. You may find the CPT index easier to deal with than ICD-10-CM's index. There are more items cross-listed. However, the same rule applies: if you can't decide which term to look up, look them all up until you find the right one.

   c. Look up the suggested code or codes in the numerical listing of CPT. Again, this is not a suggestion; this is a mandatory step. The main section of CPT, listing all the codes in numerical order (sort of), provides additional detail for the code description, as well as additional notations such as "Use this code with . . ." and directives for the requirement of additional codes. Often, the CPT alphabetic index will suggest several codes (12345, 12349, 25443) or a range of codes (12345–12357). You must look up ALL suggested codes in the numerical listing, not just the first, and then choose the most accurate from all the options. Do NOT use a range; the correct code is NEVER a range.

6. *Link every procedure code to at least one diagnosis code* shown on the same claim form to document medical necessity. Not only is this required, but also it is an excellent way to confirm that all your procedure codes are justified by a diagnosis code.

7. *Double-check your work by back coding* to ensure that you did not accidentally transpose any numbers, copy the wrong code, or misread a description.

Following these steps will help you code precisely, resulting in a greater number of your claims getting paid quickly, at the highest earned reimbursement rate.

LET'S CODE IT! SCENARIO

Luanne Cannellis, a 55-year-old female, has a family history of colon cancer, so she came in today for a screening colonoscopy. Dr. Cousins removed a polyp by snare during the examination.

Let's Code It!

Let's go through the steps to determine the codes that should be reported for this encounter between Dr. Cousins and Luanne Cannellis.

First, read the case completely. These notes are nice and short (whereas some notes can go on for many pages). Second, let's abstract the notes together. What key words identify the procedures performed? *Screening colonoscopy, removed a polyp by snare.*

Do you need to query the provider? For right now, all the information seems to be in the documentation. Sometimes, you may not know if information is missing until you get to the code descriptions.

Because the lessons here are all about coding the procedures, understand that the diagnosis is clearly stated in the notes: *family history of colon cancer.*

Now, you need to code the procedure or procedures. Turn to the alphabetic index in the CPT book, and find *Colonoscopy.* Below the subheading, read down the list of words, and find a word that was used in the description of the procedure. Do you see *Removal?* Indented underneath *Removal,* you will see the same term that Dr. Cousins wrote in his notes regarding what he removed: *Polyp.* The index suggests codes 45384–45385.

Turn to the page within the numerical listing of the CPT book, and look at the complete code descriptions.

45384 Colonoscopy, flexible, proximal to splenic flexure; with removal of tumor(s), polyp(s), or other lesion(s) by hot biopsy forceps or bipolar cautery

45385 Colonoscopy, flexible, proximal to splenic flexure; with removal of tumor(s), polyp(s), or other lesion(s) by snare technique

The difference between these two codes is the technique by which the physician removed the polyp. Which technique is documented? The notes state *by snare.* This means that the code description for 45385 matches the notes perfectly!

Next, you must link the procedure code to at least one diagnosis code. This step is pretty easy. There is only one diagnosis code, and it goes with the procedure code very well. The diagnosis of a family history of colon cancer establishes medical necessity for a colonoscopy.

The last step is to *always* double-check your answers. Just as you looked in the alphabetic index first, by the terms, and then found the numerical code, double-check your work by doing this process backward. My term for this is *back coding.* Look at the number and see if the code description matches your physician's notes. It does! Excellent.

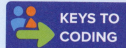

KEYS TO CODING

Never, never, never code directly from the alphabetic index. Always verify the suggested code in the numerical listing before using a code.

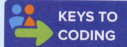

KEYS TO CODING

Patient = *who* came to see the provider for health care
Diagnosis = *why* the individual came to see the provider for this visit
Procedure = *what* the provider did for the individual

LO 2.4 Coding From Physician's Notes

As mentioned earlier in this chapter, you, as the professional coding specialist, will need all of the details and specifics about what occurred between a health care professional and a patient during an encounter, and why. The best way to gather this information is to review the physician's notes, lab reports, superbill/encounter form (Fig. 2-1), and *all* documentation for that encounter. When you read *exactly* what the physician thought, heard, observed, and did in his or her own words, you will have more specific information to use to help you determine the most accurate code. The more accurate the communication between the providing professional and the professional coding specialist, the more accurate the codes will be—ensuring optimal reimbursement.

Whether you are using CPT, HCPCS Level II, or ICD-10-PCS, your codes will be more accurate for the procedures, services, and treatments provided and they will all be supported for medical necessity when you access all the documentation. After all, how can you report the *whole story* if you don't know the *whole story?*

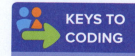

KEYS TO CODING

One absolute rule for professional coding specialists is . . . If it is not documented, it didn't happen! If it didn't happen, you can't code it.

Family Doctors Associates
123 Main Street • Anytown, FL 32711
(407) 555-1200

Date: September 16, 2016   Attending Physician: J. Healer, MD

Patient Name: Sasha White

CPT DESCRIPTION	CPT DESCRIPTION	CPT DESCRIPTION
OFFICE/HOSPITAL	**PATHOLOGY/LAB/RADIOLOGY**	**PROCEDURES/TESTS**
☐ 99201 OFFICE-NEW; FOCUSED	☒ 71020 X-RAY CHEST TWO VIEWS	☐ 12011 SIMPLE SUTURE, FACE
☒ 99202 OFFICE-NEW; EXPANDED	☒ 72040 X-RAY SPINE-C, TWO VIEWS	☐ 29125 SPLINT-SHORT ARM
☐ 99203 OFFICE-NEW; DETAILED	☒ 73030 X-RAY SHOULDER COMP	☐ 29355 WALKER CAST-LONG LEG
☐ 99204 OFFICE-NEW; COMPREHEN	☐ 76085 MAMMOGRAM-COMP DET	☐ 29540 STRAPPING-ANKLE
☐ 99205 OFFICE-NEW; COMPREHEN	☐ 76092 MAMMOGRAM SCREENING	☐ 45378 COLONOSCOPY-DIAGNOSTIC
☐ 99211 OFFICE-ESTB; MINIMAL	☐ 80050 BLOOD TEST-GEN HEALTH	☐ 45385 COLONOSCOPY-POLYP REM.
☐ 99212 OFFICE-ESTB; FOCUSED	☐ 80061 BLOOD TEST-LIPID PANEL	☐ 50390 ASPIRATION, RENAL CYST
☐ 99213 OFFICE-ESTB; EXPANDED	☐ 82947 BLOOD TEST-GLUCOSE	☐ 90703 TETANUS INJECTION
☐ 99214 OFFICE-ESTB; DETAILED	☐ 83718 BLOOD TEST-HDL	☐ 92081 VISUAL FIELD EXAM
☐ 99215 OFFICE-ESTB; COMPREHEN	☐ 85025 BLOOD TEST-CBC	☐ 93000 ECG, 12 LEADS, W/RPT
☐ 99281 EMER DEPT; FOCUSED	☐ 86403 STREP TEST, QUICK	☐ 93015 TREADMILL STRESS TEST
☐ 90844 COUNSELING – 50 MIN.	☐ 87430 ENZY IMMUNOASSAY-STREP	☐ 99173 VISUAL ACUITY SCREEN

FOLLOW-UP

PRN _____

WEEKS _____

NXT APPT. _____

TIME _____

FIGURE 2-1 An Example of a Superbill

LET'S CODE IT! SCENARIO

Jake Mathers, a 23-year-old male, came to see his regular physician, Dr. Patterson. Jake has 22 common warts and is very self-conscious of them. Dr. Patterson removes the warts. Dr. Patterson checked off the only code available on the screen, "17110 Destruct wart."

Let's Code It!

If you work only from the superbill, then all you know is what is checked off. Let's look up this code in the CPT book. The full description is

17110 Destruction (e.g., laser surgery, electrosurgery, cryosurgery, chemosurgery, surgical curettement), of benign lesions other than skin tags or cutaneous vascular proliferative lesions; up to 14 lesions

It is the only procedure code related to warts offered on the office's preprinted form. Let's read this code description, along with others near it in the CPT book. You will note a few facts:

- 17110 is used if the physician destroyed 14 lesions or fewer ["*up to* 14 lesions"].

- 17111 Destruction (e.g., laser surgery, electrosurgery, cryosurgery, chemosurgery, surgical curettement), of benign lesions other than skin tags or cutaneous vascular proliferative lesions; 15 or more lesions

If 15 or more lesions (warts) were destroyed, the physician did more work, entitling him or her to be paid more. The only way to report this would be to use code 17111.

If all you have is the check mark on the superbill, next to 17110 Destruct wart, you won't know which code is the most specific and the most accurate. You need to refer to the complete physician's notes of the encounter to answer these questions.

If this facility had a policy of creating claim forms only from superbills, the office would have received less payment than it actually deserved.

CPT Coding Book

The CPT book lists services, procedures, and treatments provided by all types of health care professionals. These codes may be used to report services provided in either inpatient facilities or **outpatient** facilities. Services such as counseling, treatments such as the application of a cast, and procedures such as the surgical removal of a mole are each assigned a special code to simplify reporting for purposes of reimbursement and statistical analysis. In addition, ancillary services, such as imaging (x-rays, CT scans, magnetic resonance imaging), pathology, and laboratory (biopsy analysis, blood tests, cultures), are also reported using CPT codes.

outpatient
A patient treated without being kept overnight.

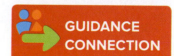

GUIDANCE CONNECTION

Review the CPT **Introduction**, subsection **Instructions for Use of the CPT Codebook**, for more input on how to properly read the information in this book.

EXAMPLE

Facilities

Inpatient facilities: acute care facility, a hospital.

Outpatient facilities: a physician's office, clinic, ambulatory care center, or emergency department.

The Organization of the CPT Book

The CPT book has two parts, which have many sections.

1. The main body of the CPT book has six sections, presented in numerical order (generally speaking) by code number:
   - Evaluation and Management: 99201–99499
   - Anesthesia: 00100–01999 and 99100–99140
   - Surgery: 10021–69990
   - Radiology: 70010–79999
   - Pathology and Laboratory: 80047–89398
   - Medicine: 90281–99199, 99500–99607

You may notice that, while each section within itself is in numerical order (for the most part), the sections are also in numerical order, for the most part. Bottom line . . . *read carefully.*

CPT Resequencing Initiative

The American Medical Association (AMA) implemented a new initiative with the 2010 CPT code set. Faced with the challenge of fitting new codes for evolving health care innovation and technology into a preexisting set of numbers, the AMA determined that resequencing codes would be easier for everyone to use rather than starting from scratch and renumbering the entire code set. (That certainly would have caused havoc!)

Therefore, when new codes were needed to be added to CPT and there were no more available numbers in the correct sequence, the next available code number was assigned. Different publishers of CPT books present this new information in various ways.

In the AMA-published CPT book, the new code is listed in two places:

1. In its correct numerical sequence. The code is shown in the correct numerical sequence with a notation that informs you where to find the code in its topic-related location.

> ### EXAMPLE
>
> Directly after code 46288 is code
> 46320 ► Code is out of numerical sequence. See 46200–46288 ◄

2. In its correct topic-related location. The code is placed with the other codes that report this procedure or service based on the specific code description. This is highlighted by a symbol to the left of the code number—# (the pound or number sign)—to bring your attention to the fact that this code is not in numerical order.

> ### EXAMPLE
>
> The codes in the subsection for Anus, Excision are listed:
>
> 46221   Hemorrhoidectomy, internal, by rubber band ligation(s)
> # 46945   Hemorrhoidectomy internal, by ligation other than rubber band; single hemorrhoid column/group
> # 46946   2 or more hemorrhoid columns/groups

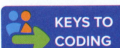

GUIDANCE CONNECTION

Review the CPT **Introduction,** subsection **Instructions for Use of the CPT Codebook— Code Symbols,** last paragraph, for more information on resequenced codes.

As you can see, it makes much more sense for all of the hemorrhoidectomy codes to be in the same place so that you can read through all of the code descriptions and choose the one that most accurately matches the physician's notes. If the new codes were just placed in numerical order, you would need to keep flipping back and forth.

3. The second part of the CPT book contains several sections, including
   - Category II codes: for supplemental tracking of performance measurement.
   - Category III codes: temporary codes for emerging technological procedures.
   - Appendixes A–M: modifiers and other relevant additional information.
   - Alphabetic index: all the CPT codes in alphabetical order by code description, presented in four classes of entries:
     a. Procedures or services, such as removal, implantation, or debridement.
     b. Anatomical site or organ, such as heart, mouth, or pharynx.
     c. Condition, such as miscarriage, cystitis, or abscess.
     d. Eponyms, synonyms, or abbreviations, such as Baker's cyst or EKG.

KEYS TO CODING

Not all publishers of CPT books present the information in this order. This is an excellent time to become familiar with the layout of your CPT book and know where you can find all of this key information.

LO 2.5 Guidelines, Formats, and Notations

Official Guidelines The official guidelines you will use to ensure that you are coding procedures correctly are presented right in your CPT. Notice the pages in front of each of the six sections of the main part of the book.

THE LAYOUT OF THE CPT BOOK

- Evaluation and Management Guidelines
- Evaluation and Management Numerical Listings
- Anesthesia Guidelines
- Anesthesia Numerical Listings
- Surgery Guidelines
- Surgery Numerical Listings
- Radiology Guidelines
- Radiology Numerical Listings
- Pathology and Laboratory Guidelines
- Pathology and Laboratory Numerical Listings
- Medicine Guidelines
- Medicine Numerical Listings

The guidelines identify important rules and directives that coders must follow when assigning codes from each section—for example,

- Evaluation and management services guidelines include the definitions of commonly used terms.
- Surgery guidelines include a listing of services that are bundled into the surgical package definition.
- Medicine guidelines include instructions on how to code multiple procedures and the proper use of add-on codes.

Also, there are additional guidelines and instructions throughout each section, shown in paragraphs under various subheadings. These instructional notations, ranging from a short sentence to several paragraphs, provide specific information regarding the proper coding appropriate to that anatomical site or type of procedure.

EXAMPLE

Instructional Notations in a Subsection
Biopsy
Directly above code 11100 is a paragraph containing important information for coders preparing to report a code from this subsection.
Cardiography
Above code 93000, critical coding guidelines in addition to important definitions and descriptions are provided at the beginning of this subsection.

Formats

The Formats of the Codes   As reviewed earlier in this chapter, the codes listed in the CPT book are structured as follows:

CPT codes (category I codes) are five-digit codes: all numbers with no punctuation: for example, 51100 Aspiration of bladder; by needle.

Category II codes are five-character codes: four numbers followed by the letter F: for example, 2001F Weight recorded.

Category III codes are five-character codes: four numbers followed by the letter T: for example, 0208T Pure tone audiometry.

Modifiers are two characters: two numbers, two letters, or one letter and one number. Modifiers are appended to a CPT code under special circumstances. When this is required, the modifier will be added, after a hyphen, after the main CPT code: for example, 47600-54 Cholecystectomy, surgical care only. [More about modifiers in Chap. 3.]

The Format of the Book   As you look through the CPT book, both the numerical listings and the alphabetic index show their data in columns. Notice that some information is indented under other descriptions or terms. An indented description or term attaches to the description or term that appears at the margin of the column above, or before, the indented words.

Turn to the numerical listing, in the surgery section, to code number
35501 Bypass graft, with vein; common carotid-ipsilateral internal carotid

Notice that this description is set at the inner margin of the column. The positioning indicates that it is the complete description of this code. Now, let's look right below this code, at the next code listed.

| 35501 | Bypass graft, with vein; common carotid-ipsilateral internal carotid |
| 35506 | carotid-subclavian or subclavian-carotid |

You can see that the description next to code 35506 is indented, not at the inner margin of the column. This means you must not only read 35506's description but also attach it to the description above. But before you do that, look at the punctuation of the first code:

| 35501 | Bypass graft, with vein; common carotid-ipsilateral internal carotid |

Notice the semicolon (the dot over the comma) after the word *vein*. The semicolon is very important. When you read the description for a code that has an indented term or phrase, attach it to the description of the code above, but only the part of the description *up to the semicolon*. Read it as shown by the underlines:

| 35501 | <u>Bypass graft, with vein;</u> common carotid-ipsilateral internal carotid |
| 35506 | <u>carotid-subclavian or subclavian-carotid</u> |

Putting both lines together means that the actual complete description of code 35506 is

| 35506 | Bypass graft, with vein; carotid-subclavian or subclavian-carotid |

The alphabetic index uses a similar type of space-saving formatting.

Find "excision" in the alphabetic index:

Excision
Abscess
    Brain 61514, 61522

Look at the words at the margin and those indented.

The term *Excision,* a type of procedure, is the heading of this part of the index. This heading is at the margin of the column, in bold. Beneath this, also at the margin of the column, is the word *Abscess.* Underneath this, indented, is the word *Brain,* followed by two suggested codes. Read backward, and you have *Brain, Abscess, Excision.* The physician's notes are more likely to read

<u>Excision</u> of an <u>abscess</u> in the <u>brain</u>

Just as with the descriptions in the numerical listing, you must be careful as you read and connect the indented words and phrases. Using a ruler or other straight edge may make it easier to see which words are indented and which are at the margins.

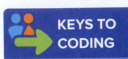

KEYS TO CODING

Remember, the rule is to read the part of the code *up to the semicolon* and then attach the indented description to it. The CPT book does this to save space.

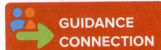

GUIDANCE CONNECTION

Review the CPT **Introduction,** subsection **Instructions for Use of the CPT Codebook—Format of the Terminology,** for more input on how to read the complete code descriptions when a portion is indented.

LO 2.6 Notations and Symbols

Throughout the CPT book, you will see notations and symbols. Let's review them together.

See A "see" reference is found under a heading in the alphabetic index. Let's review again an earlier example to better understand this reference.

In this example, under the heading "Excision," the notation "*See* Debridement; Destruction" provides two alternate terms that the physician may have used in his or her notes. The CPT book is suggesting that, if you cannot find a match to the documentation under "Excision," you might find it under the heading "Debridement" or the heading "Destruction."

+ The plus symbol (+) identifies an *add-on code*. An add-on procedure is most often performed with a main procedure. These services or treatments are additional to, and associated with, the main procedure and are never performed or reported alone (without the main procedure). Due to this relationship with the main procedure, add-on codes never use the modifier *51 Multiple Procedures*. (You will learn all about modifiers later in this book.) All the add-on codes are grouped and listed in Appendix D for additional reference.

> + 22328   each additional fractured vertebra or dislocated segment (List separately in addition to code for primary procedure)

EXAMPLE

Add-On Code Listing—the Plus Symbol
   +**22328**   each additional fractured vertebra or dislocated segment
   (List separately in addition to code for primary procedure)

(List Separately in Addition to Code for Primary Procedure) Seen at the end of the description of an add-on code, this notation reminds you that the code represents a procedure that is done as a part of another procedure, reported separately. Again, this should also remind you that this code cannot be used by itself.

EXAMPLE

Add-On Code Listing—the Parenthetical Notations
   22630 Arthrodesis, posterior interbody technique, including laminectomy and/or diskectomy to prepare interspace (other than for decompression), single interspace; lumbar
   +22632 each additional interspace (List separately in addition to code for primary procedure)
   (Use 22632 in conjunction with 22612, 22630, or 22633 when performed at a different level.)

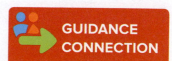

GUIDANCE CONNECTION

Review the CPT **Introduction**, subsection **Instructions for Use of the CPT Codebook— Add-On Codes,** for more input on how to properly report these codes.

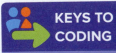
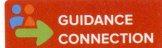
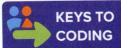
(Use . . . in Conjunction with . . .)   The notation "Use . . . in conjunction with . . ." is found below the description of an add-on code. Here, the CPT book is going one step further. In addition to the + symbol and the notation "List separately," the book states the primary procedure code or codes with which the add-on code may be reported.

•   The bullet symbol (•) identifies a new code, one that is in the CPT book for the first time. During the annual update of the CPT book, various codes and guidelines are added, deleted, or revised. The new, updated, printed version of CPT is effective every January 1.

▲   The triangle symbol (▲) distinguishes a code whose description has been changed since the last edition of CPT.

►◄   The double sideways triangles (►◄) mark the beginning and end of text that has been revised or is being shown for the first time in this year's CPT book. This symbol may highlight code descriptions, guidelines, and/or instructional paragraphs throughout the CPT book.

⊙   The bull's-eye symbol (⊙), a circle with a dot in the center, indicates that the code includes the administration of conscious sedation along with the procedure shown. The bull's-eye symbol tells you that you should not include a separate code when conscious sedation is provided during this treatment. All codes that include conscious sedation are grouped together and listed in Appendix G.

⊘   The symbol of a circle with a slash through it (⊘) identifies codes that are not permitted to be appended with modifier *51 Multiple Procedures.* These codes are procedures that are sometimes done at the same time as another procedure (like an add-on code) but can also be performed alone (unlike an add-on code). Consequently, when such a procedure is performed along with other procedures, you are not allowed to attach the multiple procedure modifier. All codes that are modifier 51 exempt are grouped and listed in Appendix E. There will be a lot more about modifiers as you go through this text.

⤶   Some versions of the CPT book may also include a circle with an arrow symbol (⤶). This symbol (⤶) points you toward an AMA-published reference that may be of additional guidance. The notation may direct you toward a particular edition of either the *CPT Assistant* newsletter or the book *CPT Changes: An Insider's View.*

YOU CODE IT! CASE STUDY

Melanie Terlington, a 23-year-old female, and her husband, Matthew, have been trying to have a baby. Melanie comes in so Dr. Petard can perform a pregnancy test (urine, by visual comparison).

You Code It!

Go through the steps to determine the procedure code(s) that should be reported for this encounter between Dr. Petard and Melanie Terlington.

  Step 1:   Read the case completely.
  Step 2:   Abstract the notes. Which key words can you identify relating to the procedure performed?

Step 3: Query the provider, if necessary.

Step 4: Diagnosis: Procreative consultation.

Step 5: Code the procedure(s).

Step 6: Link the procedure code(s) to at least one diagnosis code.

Step 7: Back code to double-check your choices.

Answer:

Did you determine the correct code?

81025 Urine pregnancy test, by visual color comparison methods

Excellent work!

Chapter Summary

In this chapter you learned about the important role that coding plays in our health care system. As a coding specialist, you must strive to accurately report the services and procedures provided to every patient. Health care professionals are responsible for ensuring that the supporting documentation is complete so that the coding specialist has the information necessary to find the best, most accurate code.

The seven steps to accurate coding may help you establish an effective sequence for reviewing the documentation and interpreting the information.

The *CPT,* fourth edition, contains thousands of codes for reporting services, treatments, and procedures. The book includes guidelines for each section, as well as additional notations, symbols, and references to assist you in your quest for the correct code or codes.

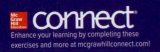

Using Terminology

Match each key term to the appropriate definition.

_____ **1.** LO 2.1 The assessment that the provider was acting according to standard practices in providing a procedure or service for an individual with a specific diagnosis.

_____ **2.** LO 2.3 A form preprinted with the diagnosis codes and procedure codes most frequently used in a particular facility.

_____ **3.** LO 2.4 A patient treated without being hospitalized.

_____ **4.** LO 2.3 To ask.

_____ **5.** LO 2.3 The process of identifying the relevant words or phrases in health care documentation in order to determine the best, most appropriate code(s).

_____ **6.** LO 2.1 A physician's determination of a patient's condition, illness, or injury.

_____ **7.** LO 2.2 Items that are used in the care and treatment of a patient that can either last a long time or can be used again and again.

_____ **8.** LO 2.1 A treatment or service provided by a health care professional.

_____ **9.** LO 2.2 A patient admitted into a hospital for an overnight stay or longer.

_____ **10.** LO 2.3 The written reports that provide evidence of what was provided to the patient and why.

A. Abstracting
B. Diagnosis
C. Durable medical equipment (DME)
D. Inpatient
E. Medical necessity
F. Outpatient
G. Procedure
H. Query
I. Superbill
J. Supporting documentation

Checking Your Understanding

Choose the most appropriate answer for each of the following questions.

1. LO 2.3 The seven steps to accurate coding are

a. _____

b. _____

c. _____

d. _____

e. _____

f. _____

g. _____

2. LO 2.3 The most important factor in coding is the

a. speed of coding process.
b. accuracy of codes.
c. quantity of codes.
d. level of codes.

3. LO 2.3 When you find unclear or missing information in the physician's notes, you should

    a. ask a coworker.
    b. figure out the information yourself; you should know what the doctor is thinking.
    c. query the physician.
    d. place the file at the bottom of the pile.

4. LO 2.1 Diagnosis codes identify

    a. what the provider did for the patient.
    b. who the policyholder is.
    c. at which facility the patient was seen by the provider.
    d. why the patient saw the provider.

5. LO 2.2 Procedure codes identify

    a. what the provider did for the patient.
    b. who the policyholder is.
    c. at which facility the patient was seen by the provider.
    d. why the patient saw the provider.

6. LO 2.4 Coding from superbills instead of physician's notes can cause the facility to

    a. lose time.
    b. lose money by undercoding.
    c. lose money by delaying payments received.
    d. all of these.

7. LO 2.5 CPT guidelines

    a. must be memorized by professional coders.
    b. can be found in the front of every CPT section.
    c. can be found in a separate guidelines book.
    d. change every 2 months.

8. LO 2.5 An example of a CPT guideline is a description of

    a. the proper way to read a superbill.
    b. the way to determine the principal diagnosis.
    c. the alphabetic listing of procedures and services.
    d. the proper use of add-on codes.

9. LO 2.5 A CPT category I code has

    a. five numbers.
    b. five letters.
    c. three numbers followed by three letters.
    d. the letter *P* followed by four numbers.

10. LO 2.2 HCPCS Level II codes may be used to report

    a. evaluation services.
    b. blood tests.
    c. durable medical equipment.
    d. diagnoses.

11. LO 2.1 ICD stands for

   a. International Classification of Diseases.
   b. International Classification of Diagnoses.
   c. International Categories of Drugs.
   d. Internal Classification of Diseases.

12. LO 2.2 CPT stands for

   a. Current Procedural Trailers.
   b. Classification of Procedural Techniques.
   c. Current Procedural Terminology.
   d. Classification of Procedural Terms.

13. LO 2.2 ICD-10-PCS procedure codes are used to report

   a. procedures done for inpatients.
   b. procedures done in a physician's office.
   c. diagnoses for inpatients.
   d. diagnoses of patients seen in an ambulatory care center.

14. LO 2.3 A superbill is

   a. a claim form for a major surgical procedure.
   b. a form preprinted with the most often used codes in a facility.
   c. a claim form for more than $5,000.
   d. a claim form issued from a hospital with more than 200 beds.

15. LO 2.6 The plus symbol (+) identifies

   a. a new code.
   b. an add-on code.
   c. a revised code.
   d. a code that includes conscious sedation.

16. LO 2.6 The circle with a dot in the center symbol identifies

   a. a new code.
   b. an add-on code.
   c. a revised code.
   d. a code that includes conscious sedation.

17. LO 2.4 A patient is considered an outpatient at any of these facilities *except*

   a. doctor's office.
   b. emergency room.
   c. after admission into a hospital.
   d. same-day surgery center.

18. LO 2.2 CPT codes are used for

   a. reimbursement from third-party payers.
   b. government agencies for funding allotment.
   c. foundations for research directions.
   d. all of these.

19. LO 2.4 The term *procedure* can also mean

    a. treatment.

    b. counseling.

    c. surgery.

    d. all of these.

20. LO 2.6 The CPT book is revised and in effect beginning each year on

    a. October 1.

    b. November 1.

    c. December 1.

    d. January 1.

Applying Your Knowledge

1. LO 2.1 Why are diagnosis codes important? _____

_____

2. LO 2.2 What does CPT stand for? _____

_____

3. LO 2.3 Why is it so critical to be careful and accurate when coding? _____

_____

4. LO 2.3 What does *abstracting the physician's notes* mean? _____

_____

5. LO 2.3 What is a superbill? _____

_____

6. LO 2.3/2.4 What is the one absolute rule for a professional coding specialist concerning documentation? _____

_____

7. LO 2.2/2.4 Explain the difference between *inpatient* and *outpatient*. _____

_____

8. LO 2.4 List the six sections of the main part of the CPT book. _____

_____

9. LO 2.6 What does a + (plus symbol) mean? _____

_____

10. LO 2.6 What does a ⊙ (bull's-eye symbol) mean? _____

_____

11. LO 2.6 What does a • (bullet symbol) mean? _____

_____

Using the techniques described in this chapter, carefully read through the case studies and determine the most accurate CPT code(s) and HCPCS code(s), if appropriate, for each case study.

1. Anna Samuels was taken to the operating room (OR) for an anterior cervical diskectomy with decompression of a single interspace of the spinal cord and nerve roots and including osteophytectomy. She is a healthy, 37-year-old female.

   _____

2. Robert Mourning, a 25-year-old male, was taken to the OR for a corneal transplant, lamellar, to the left eye.

   _____

3. Stuart Pencil, an 87-year-old male, was taken to the OR for a single lung transplant with a cardiopulmonary bypass. Dr. Labelle was concerned because Stuart was not expected to survive without the transplant.

   _____

4. Marlene Stapleton, an otherwise healthy 16-year-old female, was taken to the OR for a total thyroidectomy to remove a left thyroid mass.

   _____

5. Dr. Shoun inserted a nontunneled centrally inserted central venous catheter into Ted Thomas, a 4-year-old male. Ted was given conscious sedation so he could more easily withstand the procedure.

   _____

6. Barbara Dunedun, a 17-year-old female who is an amateur gymnast, was brought to the OR for the insertion of a plate with screws to assist the healing of the malunion of a humeral shaft fracture. An open procedure began.

   _____

7. Elaine Avalino, a 31-year-old female, was brought to the OR for a C-section. Anesthesia was administered. She has type 1 diabetes that is currently under control. Dr. Benito came to perform the cesarean delivery only.

   _____

8. John Johnson, a 39-year-old male, was rushed to the hospital by ambulance and taken directly to the OR for an appendectomy for a ruptured appendix and generalized peritonitis. The patient is otherwise healthy.

   _____

9. Dr. Cordoba performed a spigelian hernia repair in the lower abdomen on Michael Dollern, an 8-month-old male.

_____

10. Viviana Markum, a 13-year-old female, came to see her physician, Dr. Lovern. She had something in her eye, and it was irritating her. Nothing she did could get it out. Dr. Lovern took a problem-focused history and examined the area. He then applied a topical anesthetic and removed the foreign body from the conjunctiva of her eye.

_____

11. Drew Hansen, a 73-year-old male, was seen by his physician at an ambulatory surgical center for the insertion of a temporary transvenous single-chamber cardiac electrode. Conscious sedation was administered. The patient tolerated the procedure well. Code the procedure only.

_____

12. Nancy Carrington, a 5-month-old female, was taken to the OR for an excision of a 1.3-cm malignant neoplasm on her left cheek right below her eye. It is expected that the carcinoma was caught before any spread. The patient is in otherwise healthy condition.

_____

13. Sunshine Cannin, an otherwise healthy 41-year-old female, was admitted to the same-day surgery center after having an abnormal shoulder x-ray in the clinic the week before. Dr. Provan decided to do a diagnostic arthroscopy.

_____

14. Jason Munsey, a 15-year-old male, had severe pain in his right thumb. His mother believes it was from too much Playstation. Dr. Wienert took an x-ray, two views, of Jason's finger.

_____

15. Lorraine Osage, a 5-year-old female, saw Dr. Blander for a screening audiologic function test, pure tone, air only, to check her hearing.

_____

The following exercises provide practice in the application of abstracting the physicians' notes and learning to work with SOAP notes from our health care facility, Cipher, Victors & Associates. These case studies (SOAP notes) are modeled on real patient encounters. Using the techniques described in this chapter, carefully read through the case studies and determine the most accurate CPT code(s) and HCPCS code(s), if appropriate, for each case study.

SOAP notes are a standardized documentation method used by health care providers to build a patient's chart. The SOAP note has four parts, and each part will vary in length depending on the patient's encounter for that day.

So what does the acronym SOAP stand for?

S = subjective
O = objective
A = assessment
P = plan

What does the **subjective** portion of the SOAP note include?
The chief complaint, a short statement in the patient's own words as to the reason for the encounter.

What does the **objective** portion of the SOAP note include?
The results of the physical examination, any measurable result; a few examples are vital signs, height, weight, lab and diagnostic results.

What does the **assessment** portion of the SOAP note include?
A brief summary of the physician's diagnosis.

What does the **plan** portion of the SOAP note include?
The physician's plan of care (treatment) for the patient's encounter.

CIPHER, VICTORS & ASSOCIATES
A Complete Health Care Facility
234 MAIN STREET • ANYTOWN, FL 32711 • 407-555-1234

PATIENT: STARKER, SHARON
ACCOUNT/EHR #:   STARSH001
DATE: 08/11/18

Attending Physician: Willard B. Reader, MD

S: This new* patient is a 41-year-old female, who comes in with a complaint of severe neck pain and difficulty turning her head. She states she was in a car accident 2 days ago; her car was struck from behind when she was driving home from work.

O: Physician completes an evaluation and management documenting a problem focused history and exam and straightforward medical decision making as follows: PE reveals tightness upon palpitation of ligaments in neck and shoulders, most pronounced C3 to C5. X-rays are taken of the cervical vertebrae, three views (AP, Lat, and PA). Radiologic review denies any fracture.

A: Anterior longitudinal cervical sprain

P: 1. Prescribed cervical collar to be worn during all waking hours.
   2. Rx Vicodin (hydrocodone) 500 mg po prn
   3. 1,000 mg aspirin qid
   4. Pt to return in 2 weeks for follow-up

Willard B. Reader, MD

DRC/pw   D: 08/11/18 09:50:16   T: 08/13/18 12:55:01

*A new patient is a person who has not received any professional services within the past 3 years from either the provider or another provider of the same specialty who belongs to the same group practice.

Determine the most accurate CPT code(s).

_____

_____

_____

CIPHER, VICTORS & ASSOCIATES
A Complete Health Care Facility
234 MAIN STREET • ANYTOWN, FL 32711 • 407-555-1234

PATIENT: WESTERBY, ELMO
ACCOUNT/EHR #:   WESTEL001
DATE: 09/16/18

Attending Physician: Suzanne R. Taylor, MD

Preoperative Dx: Orbital mass, OD

Postoperative Dx: Herniated orbital fat pad, OD

Procedure: Excision of lesion and repair, right superior conjunctiva

Surgeon: Raul Sanchez, MD

Anesthesia: Local

PROCEDURE: After proparacaine was instilled in the eye, it was prepped and draped in the usual sterile manner and 2 percent lidocaine with 1:200,000 epinephrine was injected into the superior aspect of the right orbit. A corneal protective shield was placed in the eye. The eye was placed in down-gaze.

    The upper lid was everted and the fornix examined. The herniating mass was viewed and measured at 0.75 cm in diameter. Westcott scissors were used to incise the fornix conjunctivae. The herniating mass was then clamped, excised, and cauterized. It appeared to contain mostly fat tissue, which was sent to pathology.

    The superior fornix was repaired using running suture of 6-0 plain gut. Bacitracin ointment was applied to the eye followed by an eye pad. The patient tolerated the procedure well and left the OR in good condition.

_____

Suzanne R. Taylor, MD

SRT/pw   D: 09/16/18 09:50:16   T: 09/18/18 12:55:01

Determine the most accurate CPT code(s).

_____

_____

_____

CIPHER, VICTORS & ASSOCIATES
A Complete Health Care Facility
234 MAIN STREET • ANYTOWN, FL 32711 • 407-555-1234

PATIENT: GAYLORD, NITA
ACCOUNT/EHR #:   GAYLNI001
DATE: 09/16/18

Attending Physician: Suzanne R. Taylor, MD

The patient is a 61-year-old female with a very long history of schizoaffective disorder with numerous hospitalizations who was brought in by ambulance from the YMCA where she resides for increasing paranoia; increasing arguments with other people; and, in general, an exacerbation of her psychotic symptoms, which had been worsening over the previous 2 weeks.

I am here to provide psychoanalysis.

Initially, the patient was very agitated and uncooperative. She refused medications. She wanted to leave the hospital. A 2PC* was done and the patient had a court hearing that results in retention. Eventually, the patient agreed to a trial of a Risperdal; she fairly rapidly improved once she was started on Risperdal 2 mg twice daily. At the time of discharge compared with admission, the patient is much improved. She is usually pleasant and cooperative, with occasional difficult moments and some continuing mild paranoia. She has no hallucinations. She has no thoughts of harming herself or anyone else. She has been compliant with her medication until she recently refused hydrochlorothiazide. She is irritable at times, but overall she is redirectable and is considered to be at or close to her best baseline. She is considered no imminent danger to herself nor to others at this time.

FINAL DX: Schizoaffective disorder; hypothyroidism; hypercholesterolemia; borderline hypertension.

Prescriptions for 30-day supplies were given:

Ativan 2 mg po tid; Celexa 40 mg po daily; Risperdal 2 mg po bid; Synthroid 0.088 mg po qam; Zocor 40 mg po qhs

_____

Suzanne R. Taylor, MD

SRT/pw D: 09/16/18 09:50:16 T: 09/18/18 12:55:01

---

*2PC stands for "two physicians certify"—a medical certification testifying that an individual requires involuntary treatment at a psychiatric facility.

Determine the most accurate CPT code(s).

_____

_____

_____

CIPHER, VICTORS & ASSOCIATES
A Complete Health Care Facility
234 MAIN STREET • ANYTOWN, FL 32711 • 407-555-1234

PATIENT: KELLO, JOAN
ACCOUNT/EHR #:   KELLOJO001
DATE: 09/16/18

Attending Physician: Suzanne R. Taylor, MD

S: This patient is a 25-year-old female whom I have not seen in 10 months.* She has been well until 5 days ago. She presents with fever, severe frontal headache, facial pain, and runny nose. Patient states she has been having difficulty concentrating. She has a history of recurrent sinus infections.

O: Physician completes an evaluation and management documenting a problem focused history and exam and straightforward medical decision making as follows: T 101.5° HEENT: Tenderness over frontal and left maxillary sinuses. Nasal congestion visible. CT scan of the maxillofacial area, without contrast, reveals opacification of both frontal, left maxillary, and sphenoid sinuses and a possible large nonenhanced lesion in the brain.

A: Epidural abscess with frontal lobe lesions caused by significant compression on frontal lobe.

P: Recommendation for surgery to evacuate the abscess. Patient will think about it and call in a day or two. Rx antibiotics and pseudoephedrine

_____

Suzanne R. Taylor, MD

SRT/pw   D: 09/16/18 09:50:16   T: 09/18/18 12:55:01

*An established patient is a person who has received professional services within the last 3 years from either this provider or another provider of the same specialty belonging to the same group practice.

Determine the most accurate CPT code(s).

_____

_____

_____

CIPHER, VICTORS & ASSOCIATES
A Complete Health Care Facility
234 MAIN STREET • ANYTOWN, FL 32711 • 407-555-1234

PATIENT: KLACKSON, KEVIN
ACCOUNT/EHR #:   KLACKE01
DATE: 09/15/18

Diagnosis: Primary cardiomyopathy with chest pain

Procedure: Arterial catheterization

Physician: Frank Vincent, MD

Anesthesia: Local

Procedure: The patient was placed on the table in supine position. Local anesthesia was administered. Once we were assured that the patient had achieved no nervous stimuli, the incision was made and the catheter was introduced percutaneously. The incision was sutured with a simple repair. The patient tolerated the procedure well and was transferred to the recovery room.

Frank Vincent, MD

FV/mg   D: 9/15/18 09:50:16   T: 09/15/18 12:55:010

Determine the most accurate CPT code(s).

_____

_____

_____

INTRODUCTION TO CPT MODIFIERS

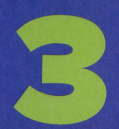

Learning Outcomes *After completing this chapter, the student should be able to:*

LO 3.1 Determine when a modifier is required.

LO 3.2 Apply personnel modifiers per the guidelines.

LO 3.3 Correctly use anesthesia physical status modifiers.

LO 3.4 Implement HCPCS modifiers correctly.

LO 3.5 Append multiple modifiers in the proper sequence.

LO 3.6 Identify circumstances that require a supplemental report.

In addition to the code for the specific procedure or service provided to the patient, there might be times when you will have to apply a **modifier.** Modifiers are two-character codes that add clarification and additional details to the procedure code's original description, as listed in the main portion of the *Current Procedural Terminology* (CPT) book. At times, the modifier provides necessary explanation to the third-party payer that directly relates to the reimbursement that the facility or physician will receive.

LO 3.1 Procedure Code Modifiers

Modifiers clarify a report, or claim form, in regard to the following:

- A service or procedure had both a professional component and a technical component.
- A service or procedure was performed by more than one physician.
- A service or procedure was performed in more than one location.
- A service or procedure was not performed in total (only part of it was done).
- An optional extra service was performed.
- A bilateral procedure was performed.
- A service or procedure was performed more than once.
- Unusual events arose.

One of the most important reasons to properly report a procedure code with a modifier is to provide more information about that procedure—additional details to the code description to make certain you are completely and accurately reporting the procedure, service, or treatment that was

Key Terms

Alphanumeric

Ambulatory surgery center (ASC)

CPT code modifier

HCPCS Level II modifier

Laterality

Modifier

Personnel modifier

Physical status modifier

Service-related modifier

Supplemental report

modifier
A two-character code that affects the meaning of another code; a code addendum that provides more meaning to the original code.

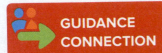
GUIDANCE CONNECTION

Review the CPT **Introduction,** subsection **Instructions for Use of the CPT Codebook— Modifiers,** for more input on how to properly use modifiers.

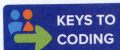
KEYS TO CODING

Bookmark **Appendix A** in your CPT code book. This is the section containing the CPT modifiers and their full descriptions. It is important that you reference these prior to using any modifier. Your HCPCS Level II book has its own section that lists those modifiers with their complete descriptions.

CPT code modifier
A two-character code that may be appended to a code from the main portion of the CPT book to provide additional information.

physical status modifier
A two-character alphanumeric code used to describe the condition of the patient at the time anesthesia services are administered.

alphanumeric
Containing both letters and numbers.

ambulatory surgery center (ASC)
A facility specially designed to provide surgical treatments without an overnight stay; also known as a *same-day surgery center.*

actually provided to the patient during the encounter. Some modifiers will result in the physician's or facility's getting paid more money because the circumstances resulted in their having to do more work than usual. For example, modifier 50 reports that the procedure was performed bilaterally.

Some modifiers will result in the physician's or facility's getting paid less money for the typical procedure but truthfully and accurately report that less work than usual was provided. For example, modifier 52 reports Reduced Services.

Some modifiers will prevent a claim for reimbursement from being denied because it brings attention to the fact that unusual circumstances required unusual work. For example, modifier 23 reports Unusual Anesthesia. (In these cases, you should also provide a letter or documentation to explain what those circumstances were so that you are telling the whole story.)

Some modifiers may have no effect at all on reimbursement but provide important details about the procedure that will be important for continuity of care, as well as for research and statistics. An example is modifier RC Right Coronary Artery.

All modifiers are listed in Appendix A, their own section of the CPT book. Listed in numerical order, each modifier is shown by category, accompanied by an explanation of when and how you should use that modifier.

There are four categories of modifiers:

- **CPT code modifiers** are two-character codes that can be attached to regular codes from the main portion of the CPT book and to HCPCS Level II codes.

EXAMPLE

CPT Modifiers

    23 Unusual Anesthesia
    66 Surgical Team

- Anesthesia **physical status modifiers** are two-character **alphanumeric** codes, used only with CPT codes reporting anesthesia services.

EXAMPLE

Physical Status Modifiers

    P1 A normal healthy patient
    P3 A patient with severe systemic disease

- **Ambulatory surgery center (ASC)** hospital outpatient *modifiers* are two-digit codes used only when reporting services provided at this type of outpatient facility.

EXAMPLE

ASC Modifiers

    27 Multiple outpatient hospital E/M encounters
    73 Discontinued outpatient procedure

- **HCPCS Level II modifiers** are two-character alphabetic or alphanumeric codes that are used to provide additional information about services when appended to CPT and HCPCS Level II codes. (There will be more about this later in this chapter and in Appendix B.)

HCPCS level II modifier
A two-character alphabetic or alphanumeric code that may be appended to a code from the main portion of the CPT book or a code from the HCPCS Level II book.

EXAMPLE

HCPCS Level II Modifiers

E1 Upper left eyelid
RT Right side (of body)

CPT Code Modifiers

Using modifiers is often a judgment that you, the coding specialist, will have to make as you review the details of each case. As you analyze the descriptions of the procedures performed as documented by the physician and compare them with the descriptions of the codes in the CPT book, you may find that there is more to the story. This is important because it is a coding professional's job to relate the whole story of the encounter. On occasion, the CPT book will remind you of a special circumstance that requires a modifier.

EXAMPLE

CPT Modifier Notation

68801 Dilation of lacrimal punctum, with or without irrigation
(To report a bilateral procedure, use 68801 with modifier 50.)

Modifier 50 is used to identify that a service or procedure was performed bilaterally (both sides).

EXAMPLE

CPT Instructional Paragraph

Paragraph above code 92550:

Audiologic Function Tests with Medical Diagnostic Evaluation

". . . All services include testing of both ears. Use modifier 52 if a test is applied to one ear instead of to two ears . . ."

Modifier 52 indicates that the service or procedure, as described, was not completed in full. If both ears are included in the code description but only one ear was tested, then a reduced service was provided.

YOU CODE IT! CASE STUDY

Arlene MacAvoy, a 37-year-old female, came into the emergency clinic with two lacerations: one on her right hand and the second on her right arm. Dr. Cherney debrided a complicated laceration, 3.1 cm long, on her upper right arm and a layered closure of a 2.5 cm laceration on her right hand, proximal to the second digit.

Go through the steps of coding, and determine the code or codes that should be reported for this encounter between Dr. Cherney and Arlene MacAvoy.

Step 1: Read the case completely.

Step 2: Abstract the notes: Which key words can you identify relating to why Dr. Cherney cared for Arlene?

_____

Step 3: Query the provider, if necessary.

Step 4: Code the diagnosis or diagnoses.

Step 5: Code the procedure(s): Repair of the lacerations to the hand and arm.

_____

Step 6: Link the procedure codes to at least one diagnosis code to confirm medical necessity.

Step 7: Back code to double-check your choices.

Answer:

Did you determine the correct code to be

13121 Repair, complex, scalp, arms, and/or legs; 2.6 cm to 7.5 cm

12041-59 Repair, intermediate, wounds of neck, hands, feet and/or external genitalia; 2.5 cm or less, distinct procedural service

GUIDANCE CONNECTION

Notice that the in-section official guidelines, in the subsection **Repair (Closure)**, paragraph 2, **When multiple wounds are repaired . . .**, state that the more complicated repair is reported as the primary procedure and the code for the second repair should be appended with modifier 59.

LO 3.2 Personnel Modifiers

As you read through the descriptions of the modifiers, most of them will seem very straightforward. **Personnel modifiers** explain special circumstances relating to the health care professionals involved in the treatment of the patient.

personnel modifier
A modifier adding information about the professional(s) attending to the provision of this procedure or treatment to the patient during this encounter.

EXAMPLE

Personnel Modifier

62 Two Surgeons

Modifier 62 clearly is used when the operative notes indicate that two surgeons worked side by side, both as primary surgeons, during a procedure. If the modifier is not there to explain that there *were* two primary surgeons involved, how else could the insurance carrier know that receiving two separate claim forms for the same patient on the same day is legitimate? The insurance carrier would certainly think that one of the physicians is fraudulently billing it for work done by another. The second claim filed, and possibly even the first one, might be denied or set aside for further investigation, and the carrier may even initiate a fraud investigation. This little two-digit code tells the insurance carrier that no one is cheating and both surgeons actually did provide for the patient.

The same scenario works for other personnel modifiers:

- 66 Surgical Team
- 80 Assistant Surgeon

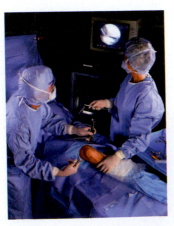
© Corbis

- 81 Minimum Assistant Surgeon
- 82 Assistant Surgeon (when qualified resident surgeon not available)

Using any of these modifiers provides an explanation, very directly and simply, why more than one health care professional is claiming reimbursement for providing service to the same patient on the same date.

YOU CODE IT! CASE STUDY

Reina Gold, a 39-year-old female, has been diagnosed with endometriosis and is admitted to Barton Hospital to have Dr. Thomas perform a vaginal, radical hysterectomy. While Reina is in the operating room (OR) and under anesthesia, Dr. Peters is going to perform an open sling operation for stress incontinence on her bladder. She tolerates both procedures well and is taken back to her room.

You Code It!

Go through the steps and determine the procedure code(s) that should be reported for this encounter between Reina Gold, Dr. Thomas, and Dr. Peters.

Step 1: Read the case completely.

Step 2: Abstract the notes: Which key words can you identify relating to the procedures performed?

_____

Step 3: Query the provider, if necessary.

Step 4: Diagnosis: Endometriosis, stress incontinence.

Step 5: Code the procedure(s).

_____

Step 6: Link the procedure codes to at least one diagnosis code.

Step 7: Back code to double-check your choices.

Answer:

Did you determine the correct codes?

58285-62 Vaginal hysterectomy, radical (Schauta type operation); two surgeons

57288-62 Sling operation for stress incontinence; two surgeons

Good job!

LO 3.3 Anesthesia Physical Status Modifiers

Anesthesia physical status modifiers are two-character alphanumeric codes: the letter *P* followed by a number. These modifiers identify the condition of the patient at the time anesthesia services are provided and highlight health circumstances that might dramatically affect the anesthesiologist's ability to successfully care for the patient. An explanation of the level of the patient's health at the time the anesthesiologist administers the service helps the third-party payer to better understand how hard this physician (anesthesiologist) had to work. For example, if a patient has uncontrolled hypertension at the time anesthesia is administered, the anesthesiologist must monitor

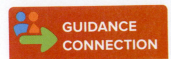
the patient more carefully, perhaps use a different type of anesthetic, and watch for possible complications that would not be an issue with an otherwise healthy patient. This status modifier, for the most part, does not relate to the reason the patient is having the anesthesia administered but is in relation to the patient's entire health. You can see that, without understanding the difference between treatment issue and overall health, it might be hard for you to identify a patient as "P1 A normal healthy patient" when the person is in your facility to have a diseased gallbladder removed. However, if the patient is *otherwise healthy,* P1 is the correct status modifier.

The physical status modifiers, P1–P6, may be appended only to codes from the Anesthesia section of the CPT book, codes 00100–01999.

EXAMPLE

Use of a Physical Status Modifier

Anesthesia for a diagnostic arthroscopy of the knee on a professional basketball player who is otherwise healthy.

01382-P1

There may be a case when a CPT modifier must also be used with an anesthesia code. When this is done, the physical status modifier is to be placed closest to the procedure code.

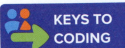
EXAMPLE

Using a Physical Status Modifier with a CPT Modifier

Anesthesia for a third-degree burn excision, 5% of total body surface area, for patient with uncontrolled diabetes and essential hypertension. The procedure was discontinued due to sudden onset of arrhythmia.

01952-P3-53

You will read more about the anesthesia physical status modifiers in Chap. 6, "Anesthesia Coding."

Ambulatory Surgery Center Hospital Outpatient Use Modifiers

Like the CPT modifiers, ambulatory surgery center (ASC)/hospital outpatient facilities use modifiers that are two-digit codes.

Many of the modifiers in this subheading are the same as the CPT modifiers. However, there are three additional modifiers specifically for ASC coders:

27 Multiple Outpatient Hospital E/M Encounters on the Same Date: *For hospital outpatient reporting purposes, utilization of hospital resources related to separate and distinct E/M encounters performed in multiple outpatient hospital settings on the same date may be reported by adding modifier 27 to each appropriate level outpatient and/ or emergency department E/M code(s). This modifier provides a means of reporting circumstances involving evaluation and management services provided by physician(s) in more than one (multiple) outpatient hospital setting(s) (e.g., hospital emergency department, clinic).*

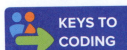

As the coding specialist for the hospital, you would be responsible for coding the services provided in all your facilities, including the clinic as well as the ED. Patricia Anatoly was seen in two different facilities on the same day for the same injury. First, you would code the services that Dr. Aden did—the E/M of Patricia's injury and his decision to send her to the ED for a higher level of care. Second, you would report the services that Patricia received in the ED, which certainly included additional evaluation and then the repair of her wound.

Without the use of modifier 27, you would have difficulty in getting the claim paid because the third-party payer may think that this is a case of duplicate billing or an error.

Occasionally, a planned surgical event is not performed due to circumstances that might put the patient in jeopardy. In such cases, all the preparation was done, the team was ready, and your facility needs to be reimbursed, even though you have not performed the service or treatment. Modifiers 73 and 74 will identify these unusual circumstances.

73 **Discontinued Outpatient Hospital/Ambulatory Surgery Center (ASC) Procedure Prior to the Administration of Anesthesia:** *Due to extenuating circumstances or those that threaten the well-being of the patient, the physician may cancel a surgical or diagnostic procedure subsequent to the patient's surgical preparation (including sedation when provided, and being taken to the room where the procedure is to be performed), but prior to the administration of anesthesia (local, regional block(s) or general). Under these circumstances, the intended service that is prepared for but canceled can be reported by its usual procedure number and the addition of modifier 73.*

74 **Discontinued Outpatient Hospital/Ambulatory Surgery Center (ASC) Procedure After Administration of Anesthesia:** *Due to extenuating circumstances or those that threaten the well-being of the patient, the physician may terminate a surgical or diagnostic procedure after the administration of anesthesia (local, regional block(s) or general), or after the procedure was started (incision made, intubation started, scope inserted, etc.). Under these circumstances, the procedure started, but terminated can be reported by its usual procedure number and the addition of modifier 74.*

LET'S CODE IT! SCENARIO

Kenneth Bonner, a 61-year-old male, was brought into Room 9 to be prepared for a bunionectomy. He changed into a gown, he got into bed, and the nurse took his vital signs. Kenneth's temperature was 38.9°C (102°F). Dr. Richter ordered a complete CBC, the results of which proved that Kenneth had an active infection in his system. The bunionectomy was canceled, and Kenneth was sent home.

Dr. Richter and her team were prepared and ready to perform a bunionectomy. However, it is not wise to operate on a patient with an active infection, so the procedure had to be canceled in the best interest of the patient. The facility still deserves to be reimbursed for its time, materials and supplies, and efforts. Therefore, the facility will submit a claim form to Kenneth's insurance carrier with the code for the bunionectomy and the modifier 73 to indicate that the procedure was canceled *prior to the administration of anesthesia:* 28290-73.

LO 3.4 HCPCS/National Level II Modifiers

The Health care Common Procedure Coding System (HCPCS) has two parts. The first (Level I) is the CPT. Even though all the codes come from HCPCS, only Level II codes are referred to as HCPCS, and they have their own modifiers. Part 2 of this text (Chaps. 13–14) goes into complete detail on HCPCS Level II codes, and Appendix B in this textbook reviews the HCPCS Level II modifiers.

A short list of HCPCS Level II modifiers is included in Appendix A of the CPT book. These modifiers are two-character codes, either one letter and one number or two letters. You'll notice that most of the HCPCS modifiers included in the CPT Appendix A specify **laterality.**

laterality
Relating to the side or sides of the body, *unilateral* meaning one side and *bilateral* meaning both sides.

- E1–E4 identify right/left/upper/lower eyelids.
- F1–FA identify each of the 10 fingers.
- T1–TA identify each of the 10 toes.
- LC–LD identify portions of the left coronary artery.
- RC identifies the right coronary artery.
- LT = left.
- RT = right.

Two of the modifiers shown have nothing to do with anatomical sites; QM and QN are related to the use of ambulance services.

It is very important that you know when you may or may not use HCPCS modifiers. Essentially, the insurance carrier to whom you are submitting the claim will either accept these codes and modifiers or not accept them. Medicare uses HCPCS codes and modifiers, along with CPT. This is true nationwide. However, it is your responsibility to find out whether other third-party payers with which you work want you to use them.

YOU CODE IT! CASE STUDY

Yamile Tourhy, a 67-year-old female, came to the Barton Ambulatory Surgery Center so that Dr. Bhmiami could excise a benign tumor from her right foot's big toe. She tolerated the procedure well and was discharged.

You Code It!

Go through the steps to determine the procedure code(s) that should be reported for this encounter between Dr. Bhmiami and Yamile Tourhy.

Step 1: Read the case completely.

Step 2: Abstract the notes: Which key words can you identify relating to the
procedures performed?

_____

Step 3: Query the provider, if necessary.

Step 4: Diagnosis: Benign neoplasm, great toe.

Step 5: Code the procedure(s).

_____

Step 6: Link the procedure codes to at least one diagnosis code.

Step 7: Back code to double-check your choices.

Answer:

Did you determine the correct codes?

**28108-T5 Excision or curettage of bone cyst or benign tumor,
phalanges of foot, right foot, great toe**

Terrific!

LO 3.5 Sequencing Multiple Modifiers

There may be circumstances where one case is so complex, unusual, or special that
you need more than one modifier to explain the whole scenario.

Two or Three Modifiers Needed

There are occasions when a particular procedure code will require the amendment
of more than one modifier. In these cases, you must place the modifiers in a particular order depending upon what each modifier represents. Let's review a few different
situations.

Generally, the CPT modifier that most directly changes, or modifies, the specific code description will be placed closest to the procedure code. These are called
service-related modifiers because they change, or alter, the description of the service
(such as -50 bilateral procedure), rather than those modifiers that explain personnel in
attendance (such as -62 Two Surgeons) or event (such as -57 Decision for Surgery).

service-related modifier
A modifier relating to a
change or adjustment of
a procedure or service
provided.

EXAMPLE

Dr. Hillman, and his surgical team, began the pancreatic transplantation procedure
on Lisa. Once the incision had been made, the patient's heartbeat became erratic
and could not be brought back under control, so the procedure was discontinued.
The procedure code reported requires two modifiers: 48554-53-66.

Modifier 53 explains that the procedure was discontinued. This modifier relates
the fact that everyone involved, including the facility, prepared for the surgery
and began the procedure but had to stop. This will explain why, sometime down
the road, this same patient may again go through a pancreatic transplantation.
In addition, this modifier will enable the health care professionals and the facility
to get some reimbursement to cover the cost of the services they did provide.
Modifier 66, on the other hand, explains that a surgical team was participating

in the surgery. This does not affect the specific code description of the procedure. It explains why the third-party payer will need to reimburse more than one surgeon. This modifier may also help to prevent the claim for each of those additional team members from being denied, or placed into determination, slowing the reimbursement process and avoiding an audit.

When a HCPCS Level II modifier is used in addition to a CPT modifier, the CPT modifier is placed closest to the procedure code, and the HCPCS Level II modifier follows.

EXAMPLE

24201-76-LT Removal of foreign body, upper arm or elbow area; deep, repeat procedure by same physician, left side

There is an exception to this rule when reporting anesthesia services. The physical status modifier always is reported closest to the anesthesia procedure code.

EXAMPLE

Dr. Morrissey administered the general anesthesia when Dr. Upton had to take the patient back into the surgery unexpectedly to attend to a problem with the replantation procedure for the patient's index finger of his right hand. For Dr. Morrissey, the code is 01810-P1-76.

© Chase Jarvis/Getty Images

LET'S CODE IT! SCENARIO

Dr. Lazenby performed a bilateral osteotomy on the shaft of Jack Banyon's femur. Another surgeon performed the same procedure on Jack two weeks ago but was unsuccessful, so Dr. Lazenby repeated the procedure. As an expert in this procedure, he was brought in to perform the surgery only and will not be involved in any preoperative or postoperative care of the patient.

Let's Code It!

To accurately report Dr. Lazenby's surgical services to Jack Banyon, you would need the following:

27448 Osteotomy, femur, shaft, or supracondylar; without fixation

-50 Modifier to report that it was a bilateral procedure

-54 Modifier to report Dr. Lazenby was providing surgical care only

-77 Modifier to report that this is a repeat procedure by another physician

Therefore, box 24D on the claim form CMS-1500 (find a sample of this form in Appendix A of this text) would look like this: 27448-50-54-77.

More Than Three Modifiers Needed

The CMS-1500 claim form, upon which you will record your chosen codes and other information to request reimbursement from the third-party payer, has a limited amount of space in which to place the necessary information, particularly when it comes to the inclusion of modifiers. Some third-party payers do not permit multiple modifiers to be listed on the same line as the CPT code. Therefore, should your case require three or more modifiers to completely explain all of the circumstances involved, you can use modifier 99.

> **99   Multiple Modifiers:** *Under certain circumstances two or more modifiers may be necessary to completely delineate a service. In such situations modifier 99 should be added to the basic procedure, and other applicable modifiers may be listed as part of the description of the service.*

LO 3.6 Supplemental Reports

Remember, *documentation* is your watchword. It is the backbone of the health information management industry. In many situations when a modifier is used, a **supplemental report** is needed for additional clarification.

Generally, the modifier itself provides a certain amount of explanation; however, the insurance carrier wants more details. You can be efficient and send the specific information along with the claim, or you can wait until the carrier requests additional information. Either way, you will have to supply all the facts. However, if you wait to be asked, you will be delaying payment to your facility.

supplemental report
A letter or report written by the attending physician or other health care professional to provide additional clarification or explanation.

LET'S CODE IT! SCENARIO

Leland Alexander, an 11-year-old boy, had a superficial cut, about 3.3 cm, on his left cheek, after being in a car accident and hit by broken glass. Dr. Chandra is ready to perform a simple repair of the wound, but she is very concerned. Leland has Tourette's syndrome, which causes him to jerk or move abruptly, especially when nervous. Although anesthesia is not typically used for a simple repair of a superficial wound, Dr. Chandra administers general anesthesia. Jacob Haverty, a CRNA, assists Dr. Chandra with monitoring Leland during the procedure.

Let's Code It!

Dr. Chandra performed a *simple repair* of Leland's *superficial wound* on his *face*. Go to the alphabetic index and look up *Repair*. As you look down the list of anatomical sites, you do not see face or cheek listed. You know that the repair was simple, and when you look at that listing, you note the direction "*See* Integumentary System, Repair, Simple." Once you go to that listing, you find the suggested codes 12001–12021. Let's take a look at the complete description in the numerical listing.

> **12011   Simple repair of superficial wounds of face, ears, eyelids, nose, lips and/or mucous membranes; 2.5 cm or less**

The basic description matches the notes exactly. However, several choices are determined by the size of the wound. The notes state that Leland's wound was 3.3 cm. This brings you to the correct code:

> **12013   Simple repair of superficial wounds of face, ears, eyelids, nose, lips and/or mucous membranes; 2.6 cm to 5.0 cm**

Great! Now, you have to address the fact that Dr. Chandra gave Leland *general anesthesia*. This was done for a very valid medical reason, and Dr. Chandra (and her facility) should be properly reimbursed for the service. Anesthesia is not included with code 12013 because it is not normally required. Leland's case is unusual. Unusual circumstances often require modifiers, so let's look at CPT's Appendix A to see if there is an applicable modifier. Modifier 23 seems to fit.

> **23   Unusual Anesthesia:** *Occasionally, a procedure, which usually requires either no anesthesia or local anesthesia, because of unusual circumstances must be done under general anesthesia. This circumstance may be reported by adding modifier 23 to the procedure code of the basic service.*

So modifier 23 should be appended, or attached, to the procedure code.

12013-23

You know that you have to code the anesthesia service as well.

00300   Anesthesia for all procedures on the integumentary system, muscles and nerves of head, neck, and posterior trunk, not otherwise specified

Let's look to see if there is an applicable CPT modifier to explain that an anesthesiologist was not involved. Modifier 47 seems to fit.

> **47   Anesthesia by surgeon:** *Regional or general anesthesia provided by the surgeon may be reported by adding modifier 47 to the basic service. (This does not include local anesthesia.) Note: Modifier 47 would not be used as a modifier for the anesthesia procedures.*

Well, the note within the description of modifier 47 tells you that this modifier is necessary but that it cannot be used with code 00300. You have to attach the modifier to the procedure code. Therefore, you submit the claim with one CPT code and two modifiers: 12013-23-47. In addition, it is smart to include a supplemental report with the claim to explain the use of general anesthesia. You are aware that the insurance company wants to know the details before paying the claim.

Chapter Summary

Modifiers provide additional explanation to the third-party payer so that it can fully appreciate any special circumstances that affected the procedures and services provided to the patient. In health care, as well as in so many other instances of our lives, most things do not fit neatly into predetermined descriptions. By using modifiers correctly, you provide an additional explanation and promote the efficient and more accurate reimbursement of your facility.

The following chapters in this text review, in detail, the proper use of all the modifiers listed in Appendix A of the CPT book, with reference to the specific type of procedure code each affects.

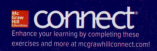

Using Terminology

Match each key term to the appropriate definition.

_____ **1.** LO 3.1 Containing both letters and numbers.

_____ **2.** LO 3.1 A two-character alphabetic or alphanumeric code that may be appended to a code from the main portion of the CPT book or a code from the HCPCS Level II book.

_____ **3.** LO 3.6 A letter or report written by the attending physician or other health care professional to provide additional clarification or explanation.

_____ **4.** LO 3.5 A modifier relating to a change or adjustment of a procedure or service provided.

_____ **5.** LO 3.4 Relating to the side or sides of the body, unilateral meaning one side and bilateral meaning both sides.

_____ **6.** LO 3.1 A two-character code that affects the meaning of another code; a code addendum that provides more meaning to the original code.

_____ **7.** LO 3.1 A facility specially designed to provide surgical treatments without an overnight stay; also known as a same-day surgery center.

_____ **8.** LO 3.2 A modifier adding information about the professional(s) attending to the provision of this procedure or treatment to the patient during this encounter.

_____ **9.** LO 3.1 A two-character code that may be appended to a code from the main portion of the CPT book to provide additional information.

_____ **10.** LO 3.1 A two-character alphanumeric code used to describe the condition of the patient at the time anesthesia services are administered.

A. Alphanumeric

B. Ambulatory surgery center (ASC)

C. CPT code modifier

D. HCPCS Level II modifier

E. Laterality

F. Modifier

G. Personnel modifier

H. Physical status modifier

I. Service-related modifier

J. Supplemental report

Checking Your Understanding

Choose the most appropriate answer for each of the following questions.

1. LO 3.1 A modifier explains

   a. the reason a procedure was performed.

   b. an unusual circumstance.

   c. the date of service.

   d. the level of education of the physician.

2. LO 3.1 Modifiers are attached to

   a. policy numbers.

   b. diagnosis codes.

   c. procedure codes.

   d. pharmaceutical codes.

3. LO 3.1 A modifier is a code made up of

   a. two numbers.
   b. two letters.
   c. one number and one letter.
   d. all of these.

4. LO 3.1/3.4 A physical status modifier may only be attached to

   a. anesthesia codes.
   b. surgical codes.
   c. radiology codes.
   d. evaluation and management codes.

5. LO 3.4 An example of a HCPCS Level II modifier is

   a. 23.
   b. P4.
   c. E2.
   d. 99.

6. LO 3.2 An example of a personnel modifier is

   a. 81.
   b. 47.
   c. LC.
   d. 57.

7. LO 3.5 If a third-party payer limits your use of multiple modifiers, you should use

   a. no modifiers.
   b. 91.
   c. 51.
   d. 99.

8. LO 3.3 P5 is an example of a

   a. HCPCS Level II modifier.
   b. CPT modifier.
   c. physical status modifier.
   d. personnel modifier.

9. LO 3.5 When appending both a CPT modifier and a HCPCS modifier to a procedure code,

   a. the HCPCS modifier comes first.
   b. the CPT modifier comes first.
   c. it doesn't matter which comes first.
   d. use neither—they cancel each other out.

10. LO 3.6 A(n) _____ is a letter or report written by the attending physician or other health care professional to provide additional clarification or explanation.

    a. supplemental report.
    b. service-related report.
    c. ambulatory surgery report.
    d. personnel report.

Applying Your Knowledge

1. **LO 3.1** Why are modifiers used? _____

   _____

2. **LO 3.3** What is a physical status modifier? _____

   _____

3. **LO 3.2** What is a personnel modifier? _____

   _____

4. **LO 3.3** Explain what an anesthesia physical status modifier is and why it is used. _____

   _____

5. **LO 3.4** Explain HCPCS/National Level II modifiers and why it is important to use them. Include an example. _____

   _____

6. **LO 3.5** What is a service-related modifier? _____

   _____

7. **LO 3.6** What is a supplemental report? Why would a supplemental report be needed, and when do you submit it? _____

   _____

8. **LO 3.1/3.5** What additional information does modifier -50 provide? _____

   _____

9. **LO 3.1/3.5** What additional information does modifier -54 provide? _____

   _____

10. **LO 3.3** What additional information does anesthesia physical status modifier P1 provide? _____

    _____

Using the techniques described in this chapter, carefully read through the case studies and determine the most accurate modifier for each case study.

1. Dr. White removed Vanetta Johns's gallbladder 10 days ago. Today, she comes to see Dr. White because of a problem in her knee. Which modifier should be appended to the encounter's E/M code?

   _____

2. Dr. Regis performed an appendectomy on Wilfred Maxell. However, the operation took twice as long as usual because Wilfred weighs 432 pounds. Which modifier should be appended to the code for the surgical procedure?

   _____

3. Dr. Calhoun performed a biopsy on the left external ear of Janise Smith, a 71-year-old female. Which HCPCS modifier will Medicare require you to append to the procedure code?

   _____

4. Adrian Matthews, a 15-year-old male, was brought into the OR in the Barton ASC to have a programmable pump inserted into his spine for pain control. After the anesthesia was administered and Adrian was fully unconscious, Dr. Clayton made the first incision. Adrian began to hemorrhage. The bleeding was stopped, the incision was closed, and the procedure was discontinued. Which modifier should be appended to the code for the insertion of the pump?

   _____

5. Elizabeth Julienne, a 53-year-old female, goes to see Dr. Rodriguez at the referral of her family physician, Dr. Roth, for his opinion as to whether or not she should have surgery. After the evaluation and Elizabeth's agreement, Dr. Rodriguez schedules surgery for Thursday. Which modifier should be appended to Dr. Rodriguez's consultation code for today's evaluation?

   _____

6. Sophia Alvera, a 71-year-old female, is having Dr. Young remove a cyst from her left ring finger. Which modifier does Medicare require you to append to the procedure code for the removal of the cyst?

   _____

7. John Jung, a 2-week-old male, was rushed into surgery for repair of a septal defect. If the repair is not completed successfully, he may not survive. What is the correct anesthesia physical status modifier?

   _____

8. Dr. Kidman is preparing to perform open-heart surgery on Frank Wenami. Dr. Fortner is asked to assist because a surgical resident is not available. Which modifier should be appended to the procedure code on Dr. Fortner's claim for services?

_____

9. Nancy Nemeir, a 41-year-old female, comes to see Dr. Parker for a complete physical examination, required by her insurance carrier. Which modifier should be appended to the code for the physical examination?

_____

10. Earl Hillier, a 5-week-old male, was born prematurely and weighs 3.8 kg. Dr. Volkesberg performs a cardiac catheterization on Earl. Which modifier should be appended to the procedure code?

_____

11. Dr. Koenig excised an abscess on Harold Crenshaw's great toe, right foot. Which modifier does Medicare require you to append to the procedure code?

_____

12. Debra Dumont, a 9-year-old female, has been complaining of hearing a constant ringing in her right ear. Dr. Lowell performs an assessment for tinnitus in the one ear only. Which modifier should be appended to the procedure code?

_____

13. Dr. Nevradi performed a percutaneous transluminal coronary atherectomy, by mechanical method, on Maxine Burwell's left circumflex artery. Which modifier does Medicare require you to append to the procedure code?

_____

14. Ronald Aswan, a 15-year-old male, came to Dr. Pollard to have corrective surgery on both of his eyes. Which modifier is appended to the procedure code?

_____

15. Carlo Yawya, a 19-year-old male, hurt his shoulder while camping. The clinic in the area took an x-ray but did not have a radiologist, so Carlo brought the films to Dr. Ellerton for interpretation and evaluation. Which modifier should Dr. Ellerton's coder append to the code for the x-rays?

_____

The following exercises provide practice in the application of abstracting the physician's notes and learning to work with SOAP notes from our health care facility, Cipher, Victors & Associates. These case studies (SOAP notes) are modeled on real patient encounters. Using the techniques described in this chapter, carefully read through the case studies and determine the most accurate CPT code(s), HCPCS code(s), and modifiers, if appropriate, for each case study.

CIPHER, VICTORS & ASSOCIATES
A Complete Health Care Facility
234 MAIN STREET • ANYTOWN, FL 32711 • 407-555-1234

PATIENT:	MORRISON, GARRET
ACCOUNT/EHR #:	MORRGA001
DATE:	11/13/18
Diagnosis:	Morbid obesity
Procedure:	Gastric bypass, secondary to skin infection—CANCELED
Physician:	Marion M. March, MD Anesthesiologist: George Harland, MD
Anesthesia:	General endotracheal anesthesia
Location:	AMBULATORY SURGICAL CENTER—EAST

PROCEDURE: Pt is a 30-year-old male with a long history of morbid obesity who recently underwent silastic gastric banding, and, due to reflux disease, subsequently required a procedure to loosen the band. Most recently, he has experienced significant reflux disease and presents for removal of his band and to have a short limb Roux-en-Y gastric bypass.

The patient was brought into the OR and placed in the supine position. General endotracheal anesthesia was administered. The patient's gown was removed for prepping, at which point clinicians noticed there were small, acne-like lesions over the anterior surface of his abdomen, his inguinal areas, and on his legs. Several of the lesions fell on the incision line.

Additionally, there was a large midline abdominal wall defect, which was assumed to represent an abdominal wall hernia, and most likely will require a mesh repair. For these two reasons the case was canceled after general anesthesia was administered. The patient was awakened from anesthesia and taken to the recovery room. There were no immediate complications evident.

Marion M. March, MD

MMM/mg   D: 11/13/18 09:50:16   T: 11/13/18 12:55:01

Determine the most accurate CPT code(s) and modifiers, as appropriate.

_____

_____

_____

CIPHER, VICTORS & ASSOCIATES
A Complete Health Care Facility
234 MAIN STREET • ANYTOWN, FL 32711 • 407-555-1234

PATIENT: ATWELL, SARAH

ACCOUNT/EHR #:   ATWESA001

DATE: 10/03/18

Diagnosis: Fecal incontinence, diarrhea, constipation

Procedure: Total colonoscopy with hot biopsy destruction of sessile 3-mm mid-sigmoid colon polyp and multiple cold biopsies taken randomly throughout the colon

Physician: Marion M. March, MD

Anesthesia: Demerol 50 mg and Versed 3 mg both given IV

PROCEDURE: Pt is a 43-year-old female. Patient was placed into position. Digital examination revealed no masses. The pediatric variable flexion Olympus colonoscope was introduced into the rectum and advanced to the cecum. A picture was taken of the appendiceal orifice and the ileocecal valve.

The scope was then carefully extubated. The mucosa looked normal. Random biopsies were taken from the ascending colon, the transverse colon, the descending colon, the sigmoid colon, and the rectum. There was a 3-mm sessile polyp in the mid-sigmoid colon that a hot biopsy destroyed.

IMPRESSION: Sigmoid colon polyp destroyed by hot biopsy
RECOMMENDATIONS: The physician asked the patient to call the office in a week to get the results of the pathology. At a later time, take cold biopsies because of history of diarrhea.

_____

Marion M. March, MD

MMM/mg   D: 10/03/18 09:50:16   T: 10/05/18 12:55:01

Determine the most accurate CPT code(s) and modifiers as appropriate.

_____

_____

_____

CIPHER, VICTORS & ASSOCIATES
A Complete Health Care Facility
234 MAIN STREET • ANYTOWN, FL 32711 • 407-555-1234

PATIENT: TACOMA, THOMAS

ACCOUNT/EHR #:   TACOTH001

DATE: 09/13/18

Diagnosis: Family history of colon cancer

Procedure: Colonoscopy

Physician: Marion M. March, MD

Anesthesia: Versed 4 mg, Demerol 75 mg

PROCEDURE: Pt is a 75-year-old male presenting for a colonoscopy. He understands the nature of the procedure, the risks and consequences, and alternative procedures and consents to the procedure. The patient receives educational materials, information on the risks of the procedure, and answers to frequently asked questions.

   The patient is placed in the left lateral decubitus position. The rectal exam reveals normal sphincter tone and no masses. A colonoscope is introduced into the rectum and advanced to the distal sigmoid colon. Further advancement is impossible due to the marked fixation and severe angulation of the rectosigmoid colon.

   On withdrawal, no masses or polyps are noted, and the mucosa is normal throughout. Rectal vault is unremarkable. The patient tolerates the procedure without difficulty.

IMPRESSION: Normal colonoscopy, only to the distal sigmoid colon
PLAN: Strong recommendation for a barium enema

_____

Marion M. March, MD

MMM/mg   D: 09/13/18 09:50:16   T: 09/13/18 12:55:01

Determine the most accurate CPT code(s) and modifiers as appropriate.

_____

_____

_____

CIPHER, VICTORS & ASSOCIATES
A Complete Health Care Facility
234 MAIN STREET • ANYTOWN, FL 32711 • 407-555-1234

PATIENT: STERLING, KRISTA

ACCOUNT/EHR #:   STERKR001

DATE: 12/01/18

Diagnosis: Obstructive sleep apnea

Procedure: Aborted uvulopalatopharyngoplasty

Physician: Marion M. March, MD

Anesthesia: Bilateral superior laryngeal nerve blocks

Location: AMBULATORY SURGICAL CENTER–EAST

PROCEDURE: After obtaining informed consent, the patient was taken to the operating room and placed in a supine position. The patient was properly identified, and Versed 4 mg was injected.
   Prior to the anesthesia service being performed, the patient exhibited significant coughing and gagging. After multiple attempts to calm the response, the procedure was aborted. The patient was taken to the recovery room.

IMPRESSION: Aborted uvulopalatopharyngoplasty

_____

Marion M. March, MD

MMM/mg   D: 12/01/18 09:50:16   T: 12/07/18 12:55:01

Determine the most accurate CPT code(s) and modifiers as appropriate.

_____

_____

_____

CIPHER, VICTORS & ASSOCIATES
A Complete Health Care Facility
234 MAIN STREET • ANYTOWN, FL 32711 • 407-555-1234

PATIENT: ULVERTON, NATALIE

ACCOUNT/EHR #:   ULVENA001

DATE: 11/09/18

Diagnosis: Chronic obstructive lung disease

Procedure: Lung transplant, single, with cardiopulmonary bypass

Surgical Team: Marion M. March, MD, primary; Fredrick Avatar, MD; Gene Lavelle, MD

Anesthesia: General

PROCEDURE: Pt is a 37-year-old female brought into the OR, placed on the table, and draped in sterile fashion. Anesthesia was administered. At thoracotomy, the left lung was removed by dividing the left main stem bronchus at the level of the left upper lobe. The two pulmonary veins and single pulmonary artery were divided distally. An allograft left lung was inserted. The recipient left main stem bronchus and pulmonary artery were re-resected to accommodate the transplant. The recipient pulmonary veins were opened into the left atrium. An end-to-end anastomosis of the recipient's respective structures (pulmonary artery, main stem bronchus, and left atrial cuffs) was made to the similar donor structures. Two chest tubes were inserted. Bronchoscopy was performed in the OR. Cardiopulmonary bypass was successfully completed.

    Patient tolerated the procedure well and was taken to the recovery room.

_____

Marion M. March, MD

MMM/mg   D: 11/09/18 09:50:16   T: 11/13/18 12:55:01

Determine the most accurate CPT code(s) and modifiers as appropriate.

_____

_____

_____

EVALUATION AND MANAGEMENT CODES, PART 1

4

Learning Outcomes *After completing this chapter, the student should be able to:*

LO 4.1 Abstract documentation to identify the location of the encounter.

LO 4.2 Distinguish between new and established patients.

LO 4.3 Calculate the appropriate level of service.

LO 4.4 Determine when to report prolonged services.

LO 4.5 Ascertain the appropriate way to report a consultation.

LO 4.6 Determine the appropriate level of medical decision making provided by the physician.

Evaluation and Management (E/M) is the first section in the CPT book and lists codes numbered 99201–99499. These codes are used to report and reimburse physicians for their expertise and thought processes involved in diagnosing and treating patients, such as

- Talking with the patient and his or her family.
- Reviewing data such as complaints, signs, symptoms, and examination results.
- Doing research in medical books and journals.
- Consulting with other health care professionals.

All these elements, including the training and education that this health care professional has had, go into the decision of what to do next for the patient—what advice, what prescription, what test, what treatment, what procedure. E/M codes provide a way to reimburse the health care professional for his or her assessment and supervision of the patient and the determination of the best course for his or her care.

E/M Codes

As you just read, E/M codes are used to describe specifically the physician's expertise and assessment that was provided during an encounter between him or her and a patient. There are many different types of E/M codes, as you will learn throughout this and the next chapter. Let's begin by reviewing the pieces of information you will need to abstract from the physician's documentation to code the E/M portion of the encounter properly.

LO 4.1 Location

The first element you must identify is the location of the encounter. Exactly where did the provider see the patient: in an outpatient location

Key Terms

Consultation

Established patient

Evaluation and Management (E/M)

Level of patient history

Level of physical examination

Medical decision making (MDM)

New patient

PFSH

Relationship

Transfer of care

evaluation and management (E/M)
Specific characteristics of a face-to-face meeting between a health care professional and a patient.

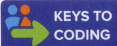

KEYS TO CODING

Should a patient be seen by the physician in the office and then be admitted into the hospital on the same day by that physician, the entire encounter for the day, including the office visit, would be reported with a hospital code, under either *Hospital Observation Services* or *Hospital Inpatient Services—Initial Hospital Care.*

relationship
The level of familiarity between provider and patient.

new patient
A person who has not received any professional services within the past 3 years from either the provider or another provider of the same specialty who belongs to the same group practice.

established patient
A person who has received professional services within the last 3 years from either this provider or another provider of the same specialty belonging to the same group practice.

consultation
An encounter for purposes of a second physician's opinion or advice, requested by another physician, regarding the management of a patient's specific health concern. A consultation is planned to be a short-term relationship between a health care professional and a patient.

(such as a physician's office), in the hospital, in a skilled nursing facility? Did they just speak on the phone, or did the provider see the patient somewhere else?

Unlike when you are coding other procedures, it can be more efficient to go directly to the E/M section of CPT rather than beginning with the alphabetic index. Knowing where this encounter took place between the provider and the patient will enable you to narrow down the range of possible codes and get to the accurate one more effectively. In addition, going to the location subsection of the E/M section will let you know what additional information you need to determine the right code. For example, when the encounter occurs at the physician's office, you will need to know the level of history taken, the level of examination performed, and the complexity of medical decision making (MDM). However, when the encounter occurs on the telephone, you will need to know how long the physician was on the phone and the date of the most recent face-to-face E/M service. You will learn more about these later in this chapter and in the next chapter.

Take out your copy of the *Current Procedural Terminology* (CPT) codebook so we can go through this together. Go to the **Evaluation and Management (E/M)** section of the CPT book. Look at the first subheading on the first page:

Office or Other Outpatient Services

This header, like many others throughout the section, identifies the location of the encounter—where the physician met with the patient. Other location-specific headings in the E/M section are shown in Box 4-1.

Once you are in the subsection that identifies where the encounter happened, you can see what additional information you will need to gather from the physician's notes to determine the correct code. For example, in the Office or Other Outpatient Services subsection, you can see that the next piece of data you need to know is the relationship between this provider and this patient—whether this patient is a new patient or an established patient. However, under the Hospital Inpatient Services subsection, the next piece of information you will need to cull from the documentation is whether this is the initial hospital care visit or a subsequent hospital care visit.

EXAMPLES

Maxwell Edison, a 61-year-old male, was brought into the emergency department (ED) with sharp pain in his chest radiating downward into his left arm. The best, most appropriate E/M code will be found in the 99281–99288 range of codes, under *Emergency Department Services.*

Dr. Farber goes to the Suniland Nursing Home to see his patient, Gail Robbins, a 93-year-old female. The best, most appropriate E/M code will be found in the 99304–99318 range of codes, under *Nursing Facility Services.*

Amanda Carter, a 21-year-old female, comes to see Dr. Atwater at his office. The best, most appropriate E/M code will be found in the 99201–99215 range of codes, under *Office or Other Outpatient Services.*

LO 4.2 Relationship

As you can see in Figure 4-1, throughout the E/M section of the CPT book, subheadings identify the **relationship** between the provider and the individual. E/M codes use three types of relationship for determining the best, most appropriate code. The three relationships are **new patient, established patient,** and **consultation.**

In the hospital, nursing facility, intensive neonatal and pediatric critical care, and intensive care locations, you will need to identify whether the encounter is the initial or subsequent visit rather than if the relationship is new or established.

You must know the relationship between the patient and the provider so that you can communicate an understanding of how familiar the physician is with the patient;

BOX 4-1   Location-Specific Headings in the E/M Section

Office or Other Outpatient Services
Hospital Observation Services
Hospital Inpatient Services
Office or Other Outpatient Consultations
Inpatient Consultations
Emergency Department Services

Nursing Facility Services
Domiciliary, Rest Home (e.g., Boarding Home), or Custodial Care Services
Domiciliary, Rest Home (e.g., Assisted Living Facility), or Home Care Plan Oversight Services
Home Services

New Patient

99201   **Office or other outpatient visit** for the evaluation and management of a new patient, which requires these three key components:

- **a problem focused history;**
- **a problem focused examination; and**
- **straightforward medical decision making.**

Counseling and/or coordination of care with other providers or agencies are provided consistent with the nature of the problem(s) and the patient's and/or family's needs.

Usually, the presenting problems are self limited or minor. Physicians typically spend 10 minutes face-to-face with the patient and/or family.

FIGURE 4-1 E/M Section Subheadings Show the Relationship between Physician and Patient

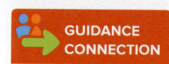

GUIDANCE CONNECTION

Additional explanations can be found in the **Evaluation and Management (E/M) Services Guidelines,** subhead **Definitions of Commonly Used Terms—New and Established Patient,** in your CPT book directly in front of the E/M section that lists all the codes.

the patient's personal history, social history, and family history; and other elements that may affect the physician's decisions regarding the patient's health. Certainly you can understand that, the first time they meet, the physician knows absolutely nothing about the patient. He or she must spend time asking questions to help collect the information that will be critical to determining the correct diagnosis and course of treatment. When the physician sees the patient again, however, all the doctor will need to do is quickly read through the patient's file to refresh his or her memory of past conditions and issues.

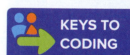

KEYS TO CODING

Some location subsections have different codes for a new patient and an established patient, and others do not. You must read the descriptions at the beginning of each subsection to be certain whether this is a criterion for a particular E/M code. For example, the subheading *Emergency Department Services* offers the same codes whether the individual is a new or an established patient.

EXAMPLE

Amanda Carter, a 21-year-old female, comes to see Dr. Atwater at his office and complains of severe pain in her right wrist and forearm. She just moved to the area, and this is the first time Dr. Atwater has seen her. The E/M codes applicable for this encounter are now in the smaller range of 99201–99205, Office or Other Outpatient Services, New Patient.

LET'S CODE IT! SCENARIO

Margaret Tanner, an 83-year-old female, broke her hip one month ago. She has been a patient of Dr. Rodriquez for several years. Since her release from the hospital, Margaret has been homebound until her hip completely heals. Therefore, Dr. Rodriquez went to her home to check on her progress.

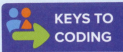

Initial care visits are reported for the first time your physician, the one for whom you are coding, sees the patient at this location for this course of treatment or care. Subsequent care visits are reported for the second time and all visits thereafter that your physician sees the patient at this location during this course of treatment or care.

For example, Aaron is admitted to the hospital on Saturday after having a myocardial infarction (MI) while playing tennis. His regular cardiologist is Dr. Kinsey; however, she is out of town for the weekend, so on Saturday Dr. Ruffatto admits Aaron to the hospital and checks in on his care. On Monday, when Dr. Kinsey comes back, she goes to see Aaron in the hospital and takes charge of his care.

On Saturday, an initial hospital care visit is reported for Dr. Ruffatto because this is her first time seeing Aaron during this course of treatment at the hospital.

On Sunday, a subsequent hospital care visit is reported for Dr. Ruffatto because this is her second time seeing Aaron during this course of treatment at the hospital.

On Monday, an initial hospital care visit is reported for Dr. Kinsey because this is her first time seeing Aaron during this course of treatment at the hospital, even though it is Aaron's third day in the hospital.

On Tuesday, a subsequent hospital care visit is reported for Dr. Kinsey because this is her second time seeing Aaron during this course of treatment at the hospital.

Read the notes again, and look for the key words that tell you the location of the encounter and the relationship between patient and physician.

The notes state that the doctor went to "her home." That phrase tells us the location of the encounter. Look through the E/M section of the CPT book, and find the group of E/M codes that report this location: Home Services. Next, you need to determine the relationship between Dr. Rodriquez and Margaret. Is Margaret a new patient or an established patient? Margaret has been "a patient of Dr. Rodriquez for several years." Therefore, she is an established patient. Now, you have narrowed down the options to codes 99347–99350.

There are times when the relationship between a patient and a health care provider is expected to be temporary, typically only one visit. In such cases, one physician or health care professional will ask another physician to meet with a patient and evaluate a patient's condition only to offer his or her own professional opinion about the patient's diagnosis and/or treatment options. This temporary relationship is known as a consultation.

EXAMPLE

Dr. Keith reviews Tanya Ruble's lab tests and notices that her lipase level is very high. This may indicate a problem with the patient's pancreas. While Tanya is healthy overall, Dr. Keith does not want to take any chances, so he refers Tanya to Dr. Gail, a gastroenterologist, for a second opinion. Tanya goes to see Dr. Gail, who examines her, reviews the test results, and writes a letter to Dr. Keith agreeing with his assessment. Tanya goes back to Dr. Keith and does not see Dr. Gail again.

The relationship between Dr. Gail and Tanya Ruble is not defined as new or established but as a consultation. Therefore, Dr. Gail's coder will report this one encounter from the Consultations subsection, codes 99241–99255. (More details about coding consultations follow in just a few pages.)

If the patient goes back to see the "consultant" again, this second E/M encounter will be reported as an established patient encounter because this means that the "consultant" has accepted this individual as a patient for continued care. This is the same as when the first physician may refer the patient to another physician for continuing care and not just a second opinion. More commonly known as a referral, the industry term for this is **transfer of care.** Transfer of the care of a patient can be complete, such as when a physician is retiring, or just for one particular portion of a patient's care, such as a primary care physician sending a patient to a specialist for care of just the one issue.

EXAMPLE

Dr. Lerner has been Allen Highter's primary care physician for many years. Today, Allen comes in complaining of a rash all over his legs. Dr. Lerner refers Allen to Dr. Opinheim, a dermatologist, so that she can take over the diagnosis and treatment of this skin condition. Dr. Opinheim agrees to take Allen on as his patient to treat his rash. In this case, there has been a transfer of care for Allen's rash from Dr. Lerner to Dr. Opinheim.

transfer of care
When a physician gives up responsibility for caring for a patient, in whole or with regard to one specific condition, and another physician accepts responsibility for the care of that patient.

Key Components

Once you have found the appropriate subheading with regard to the location and you have determined the relationship between the patient and the physician, there are just a few codes from which to choose.

When E/M services are provided in the locations listed in Box 4-2, you have to determine the level of services that were given.

In the E/M section of the CPT book, look at the key components, identified by bullet points, in the description of each code. Each bullet identifies a different level of work the physician has done and documented, with regard to

1. *Patient history* taken
2. *Physical examination* performed
3. *Medical decision making* required

Go back to the first subheading in the E/M section, and use this as an example. There are only five codes under Office or Other Patient Services: New Patient, codes 99201, 99202, 99203, 99204, and 99205. How do you know which is the correct code? How can you tell them apart? You will notice a difference immediately:

99201 is described as *problem-focused*.

99202 is described as *expanded problem-focused*.

99203 is described as *detailed*.

99204 is described as *comprehensive*.

99205 is described as *comprehensive*.

LO 4.3 **Level of Service** While accurately reporting the level of expertise and knowledge used by the physician during a visit may seem intangible, the coding guidelines give very specific and tangible measurements to recognize an appropriate level of service based on the documentation for the encounter. Let's begin this step of E/M by discussing the elements you need to determine what level of each component has been provided.

Level of Patient History Notice that the first key component (bullet) describes the **level of patient history** taken during this encounter by the physician.

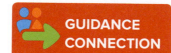

GUIDANCE CONNECTION

Additional explanations can be found in the **Evaluation and Management (E/M) Services Guidelines,** subhead **Instructions for Selecting a Level of E/M Service,** in your CPT book directly in front of the E/M section that lists all the codes.

level of patient history
The amount of detail involved in the documentation of patient history.

BOX 4-2 Service Locations Requiring Key Component Levels

Office and Other Outpatient Services
Hospital Observation Services
Hospital Inpatient Services
Consultations
Emergency Department Services
Nursing Facility Services

Domiciliary, Rest Home (e.g., Boarding Home), or Custodial Care Services
Domiciliary, Rest Home (e.g., Assisted Living Facility), or Home Care Plan Oversight Services
Home Services

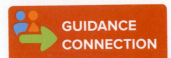

GUIDANCE CONNECTION

Additional explanations can be found in the **Evaluation and Management (E/M) Services Guidelines,** subhead **Determine the Extent of History Obtained,** in your CPT book directly in front of the E/M section that lists all the codes.

There are four levels of patient history. You can measure the level of patient history taken by the physician by reading the notes and matching the documentation to this list. Gathering information from the patient is an important part of the evaluation process for the physician to complete. This is the portion of the visit where the physician asks the patient questions about his or her health and the situations surrounding the health concern that brought him or her to see this doctor.

1. Problem-focused history:
   a. A discussion of the patient's chief complaint.
   b. A brief history of this present illness or concern.

   Taking a problem-focused history from the patient is going to gather information about only the reason the patient came to this physician today. The physician and patient are not discussing anything else—no other concern, just this one aspect.

EXAMPLE

Antonio goes to Dr. Grace because he has a cough. Dr. Grace documents that Antonio explained what type of cough (dry or wet), how long he has been coughing, whether the cough is worse when lying down, and the color of any mucus that may be coughed up.

2. Expanded problem-focused history:
   a. A discussion of the patient's chief complaint.
   b. A brief history of this present illness or concern.
   c. A problem-pertinent system review.

   This means that the physician will expand the scope of the information he or she is gathering to extend through the entire system. The systems included in the CPT definition of a review of systems (ROS) can be seen in Box 4-3.

EXAMPLE

In the visit between Antonio and Dr. Grace, in addition to the questions asked in the problem-focused history, Dr. Grace may also document answers to whether the cough comes from his throat or his chest, whether his throat is sore, and whether he has sinus congestion.

3. Detailed history:
   a. A discussion of the patient's chief complaint.
   b. An extended history of this present illness or concern.

BOX 4-3 Review of Systems

1. Constitutional symptoms, such as fever, weight loss, etc.
2. Eyes
3. Ears, mouth, nose, and throat
4. Cardiovascular
5. Respiratory
6. Gastrointestinal
7. Genitourinary
8. Musculoskeletal
9. Integumentary (skin and/or breast)
10. Neurologic
11. Psychiatric
12. Endocrine
13. Hematologic/lymphatic
14. Allergic/immunologic

c. A problem-pertinent system review extended to include some additional systems.

d. A pertinent past, family, and social history (**PFSH**).

PFSH
An acronym for *past, family,* and *social history.*

Overall components of a PFSH are listed in Box 4-4.

EXAMPLE

In addition to the previous questions for both problem-focused and expanded problem-focused histories, the documentation for the visit between Antonio and Dr. Grace may show information about whether Antonio ever had a cough like this before; whether he has a history of sinus problems, heart problems, respiratory problems, and/or throat problems; whether anyone in his family ever suffered a cough like this; whether he smokes or lives/works/socializes with anyone who does smoke; and in what type of environment he works.

4. Comprehensive history:

   a. A discussion of the patient's chief complaint.

   b. An extended history of this present illness or concern.

   c. A review of systems related to the problem.

   d. A review of all additional body systems.

   e. A complete PFSH.

The table in Figure 4-2 may provide you with help to determine what level of history is documented.

Level of Physical Examination   The second key component (bullet) describes the **level of physical examination** that was performed during this encounter by the physician. There are four levels of physical examination. You can measure the level of examination performed by the physician by reading the notes and matching the documentation to the following list.

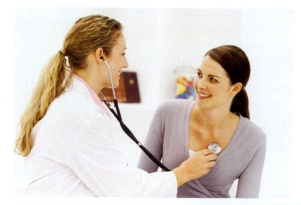

© Stockdisc/PunchStock

level of physical examination
The extent of a physician's clinical assessment and inspection of a patient.

BOX 4-4   PFSH Components

PAST HISTORY [ALSO IDENTIFIED AS PATIENT'S MEDICAL HISTORY (PMH)]

- Prior major illnesses and injuries
- Prior operations
- Prior hospitalizations
- Current medications
- Allergies (e.g., drug, food)
- Age-appropriate immunization status
- Age-appropriate feeding/dietary status

FAMILY HISTORY

- The health status or cause of death of parents, siblings, and children

- Specific diseases related to problems identified in the chief complaint, history of present illness, and/or system review
- Diseases of family members that may be hereditary or place the patient at risk

SOCIAL HISTORY

- Marital status and/or living arrangements
- Current employment
- Occupational history
- Use of drugs, alcohol, and tobacco
- Level of education
- Sexual history
- Other relevant social factors

CPT © 2015 American Medical Association. All rights reserved.

Level of History	Problem Focus (PF)	Expanded PF	Detailed	Comprehensive
Chief complaint	√	√	√	√
HPI (history of present illness)	Brief	Extended	Extended	Extended
System review	None	Problem-pertinent	Extended problem-pertinent	Complete
PFSH (past, family, and social history)	None	None	Pertinent	Complete

FIGURE 4-2 Determine Level of History Documented

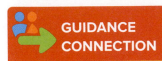

GUIDANCE CONNECTION

Additional explanations can be found in the **Evaluation and Management (E/M) Services** guidelines, subhead **Determine the Extent of Examination Performed,** in your CPT book directly in front of the E/M section that lists all the codes.

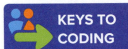

KEYS TO CODING

The CPT book categorizes 7 body areas and 11 organ systems in its determination of the best, most appropriate level of physical examination. See Boxes 4-5 and 4-6.

1. Problem-focused examination:
   a. A limited examination of the affected body area or organ system.

EXAMPLE

Documentation of a problem-focused exam during the visit between Antonio and Dr. Grace may indicate that Dr. Grace looked down Antonio's throat, looked up his nose, and perhaps listened to his lungs.

2. Expanded problem-focused examination:
   a. A limited examination of the affected body area or organ system.
   b. An examination of any other symptomatic or related body area(s) or organ system(s).

EXAMPLE

In addition to looking at Antonio's throat, nose, and lungs, Dr. Grace may also have listened to his heart; manually palpated his lymph nodes and neck; and palpated his abdomen, specifically the upper middle (stomach area).

3. Detailed examination:
   a. An extended examination of the affected body area(s) or organ system(s).
   b. An examination of any other symptomatic or related body area(s) or organ system(s).

EXAMPLE

In addition to all of the above, Dr. Grace may have taken a chest x-ray, done a respiratory efficiency test, and taken a sputum culture and/or throat cultures.

4. Comprehensive examination:
   a. A general, multisystem examination—*or*—
   b. A complete examination of a single organ system
      The CPT definitions of each body area can be seen in Box 4-5, and the list of recognized organ systems is in Box 4-6. The table in Figure 4-3 may provide you with help to determine what level of physical examination is documented.

BOX 4-5 Body Areas

1. Head, including the face
2. Neck
3. Chest, including breasts and axilla
4. Abdomen

5. Genitalia, groin, buttocks
6. Back
7. Each extremity (arms and legs)

Level of Examination Performed	Problem Focus (PF)	Expanded PF	Detailed	Comprehensive
Affected body area or organ system	Limited	Limited	Extended	Complete
Other symptomatic or related organ system	None	√	√	Complete

FIGURE 4-3 Determine Level of Physical Examination Documented

Level of Medical Decision Making The third bullet describes the level of **medical decision making (MDM)** provided by the physician during this encounter. This can be the most challenging component because, in essence, you need to determine from the documentation how hard the physician had to think to determine what to do next to help this patient with this concern. It may be that the physician writes a prescription, recommends a treatment or surgery, or orders some diagnostic tests to provide further information. Your understanding of anatomy and physiology will help you with this portion of determining the most accurate code. The four levels of MDM are

1. Straightforward:
   a. A small number of possible diagnoses.
   b. A small number of treatment or management options.
   c. A low-to-no risk for complications.
   d. Little-to-no data or research to be reviewed.

> **EXAMPLE**
>
> If when Dr. Grace looked down Antonio's throat he observed inflammation of his tonsils, and if Antonio has no problematic history, then Dr. Grace's decision making may be very straightforward. Dr. Grace was trained to recognize tonsillitis and knows exactly what to prescribe to help Antonio heal.

2. Low complexity:
   a. A limited number of possible diagnoses.
   b. A limited number of treatment or management options.
   c. A limited amount of data to be reviewed.
   d. A low risk for complications.

> **EXAMPLE**
>
> If Dr. Grace observed Antonio had a different type of inflammation (other than tonsillitis), such as some indication that his condition might be strep throat, the process of determining what is best to do is slightly more complex.

medical decision making (MDM)
The level of knowledge and experience needed by the provider to determine the diagnosis and/or what to do next.

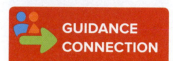

GUIDANCE CONNECTION

Additional explanations can be found in **Evaluation and Management (E/M) Services** guidelines, subhead **Determine the Complexity of Medical Decision Making,** in your CPT book directly in front of the E/M section that lists all the codes.

3. Moderate complexity:

    a. A multiple number of possible diagnoses.

    b. A multiple number of treatment or management options.

    c. A moderate amount of data to be reviewed.

    d. A moderate level of risk for complications, possibly due to other existing diagnoses or medications currently being taken.

EXAMPLE

In addition to the inflammation Dr. Grace observed, he also noted worrisome sounds in Antonio's lungs. This complicates matters because the diagnosis possibilities now extend from tonsillitis to strep throat to asthma, bronchitis, or pneumonia. Or perhaps Antonio has a history of asthma or previous bouts with pneumonia. Or perhaps Antonio has other known current illnesses, such as hypertension or diabetes, which may make diagnosing and treating this condition much more complicated.

4. High complexity:

    a. A large number of possible diagnoses.

    b. A large number of treatment or management options.

    c. A large amount of data and/or research to be reviewed.

    d. A high level of risk for complications, possibly due to other existing diagnoses and/or medications currently being taken.

> **KEYS TO CODING**
>
> Certain terms in the physician's notes may indicate a more complex process of MDM on the physician's part. Orders for several tests with terms such as *rule out, possible,* and *likely* might indicate the physician is looking for evidence of several possible diagnoses.

EXAMPLE

In highly complex cases, the documentation will show issues such as multiple co-morbidities (other conditions or diseases), current multiple medications that may make determining the best treatment for a problem more dangerous for fear of adverse interactions, perhaps allergies to medications under consideration, or other factors that make the determination of the best course of treatment for the patient incredibly complicated.

The table in Figure 4-4 may provide you with help to determine what level of MDM is documented.

EXAMPLE

Carter Allison comes in to his physician's office with a large shard of glass in his hand. You can see that the number of potential diagnoses is very small: a foreign body in his hand. There are a small number of treatment options: remove the shard. There are no real health complications, and the physician should not have to research Carter's condition before deciding what to do. This is a straightforward level of MDM.

	Straightforward	Low Complexity	Moderate Complexity	High Complexity
Number of possible diagnoses	1 or 2	Few	Several	Many
Number of management options	1 or 2	Few	Several	Many
Quantity of information to be obtained, reviewed, analyzed (test results, records, etc.)	None, 1, or 2	Few	Several	Many
Risk of significant complications (morbidity, mortality, interactions, allergies, co-morbidities, systemic underlying conditions, etc.)	None, 1, or 2	Few	Several	Many

FIGURE 4-4 Determine Level of Medical Decision Making Documented

EXAMPLE

Gina Mulvanney comes to see her family physician, Dr. Erickson, and complains of malaise and fatigue. She denies any major changes in her diet or lifestyle prior to the onset of her symptoms. This is a complex situation that will take a lot of investigation and knowledge on the part of the physician to determine Gina's underlying condition. There are numerous possible diagnoses and, therefore, a large number of management options. Dr. Erickson may have to perform several diagnostic tests to help him determine the problem. This is a highly complex case.

Combining Multiple Levels into One Code

Now that you have determined what level of history was taken, what level of physician exam was performed, and what level of MDM was provided by this physician, this all needs to be put together into one code. When all three key components point to the same code, this is a piece of cake.

EXAMPLE

Antonio came to see Dr. Grace in Dr. Grace's office because he had a cough. He had not ever seen Dr. Grace before. After carefully reviewing the documentation, you determine that Dr. Grace took an expanded problem-focused history, he performed an expanded problem-focused physical exam, and the level of MDM was straightforward. All three of these levels of key components point directly to code 99202.

But what about when the three levels point toward different E/M codes? How do you mesh them all into one code? The CPT guidelines state, ". . . must meet or exceed the stated requirements to qualify for a particular level of E/M service." Let's use a scenario to figure this out together.

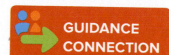

GUIDANCE CONNECTION

Additional explanations can be found in the **Evaluation and Management (E/M) Services Guidelines**, subhead **Select the Appropriate Level of E/M Services Based on the Following**, in your CPT book directly in front of the E/M section that lists all the codes.

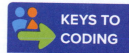

KEYS TO CODING

When the patient history, examination, and MDM are not performed at the same level, the guidelines instruct you to choose the one code that identifies the required key components that have been *met or exceeded* by the physician's documentation.

LET'S CODE IT! SCENARIO

Rebecca Stabler, an 81-year-old female, was admitted today into McGraw Skilled Nursing Facility (SNF) by Dr. Shah for rehabilitation and care. She suffered a stroke 2 weeks ago and was just discharged from the hospital. Dr. Shah documented a comprehensive level of history. She performed a detailed level of physical exam. Due to the patient's advanced age, co-morbidities, and long list of current medications, as well as the late effects of the stroke, Dr. Shah's MDM was of high complexity.

Let's Code It!

First, identify the location where the encounter between Dr. Shah and Rebecca Stabler occurred. The notes state, "admitted into McGraw Skilled Nursing Facility." Turn in the CPT book, E/M section, to Nursing Facility Services. This subsection of E/M is divided into two parts: Initial Nursing Facility Care and Subsequent Nursing Facility Care.

The documentation states that Rebecca was admitted today, so this must be the first time Dr. Shah is caring for Rebecca at this nursing home. Now you know that the correct code for Dr. Shah's evaluation of Rebecca for this visit must be within the Initial Nursing Facility Care 99304–99306 range.

Next, you need to check the requirements for this range of codes. The code descriptions tell you that ALL THREE key components—level of history, exam, and MDM—must be met or exceeded to qualify. In a full case, you will go back and read through the physician's notes to determine the level provided for each of the three components, as you learned earlier in this chapter. This scenario is provided with a shortcut, indicating the levels for you: "comprehensive history . . . detailed exam . . . MDM high complexity."

> *Comprehensive* history meets the descriptions for 99304 and 99305 and 99306.
>
> *Detailed* exam only meets the description of 99304. Codes 99305 and 99306 both require a comprehensive exam to have been performed.
>
> MDM *high* complexity meets the description of 99306 and exceeds (a higher level was actually documented) for codes 99304 and 99305.

You must find the one code that is satisfied by ALL THREE levels of care.

> 99304:
> You have documentation that is equal to this level of history.
> You have documentation that is equal to this level of exam.
> You have documentation that is greater than this level of MDM.
> 99305:
> You have documentation that is equal to this level of history.
> You do **NOT** have documentation that is equal to this level of exam.
> You have documentation that is greater than this level of MDM.
> 99306:
> You have documentation that is equal to this level of history.
> You do **NOT** have documentation that is equal to this level of exam.
> You have documentation that is equal to this level of MDM.

The only code that has ALL THREE levels equal to or greater than is 99304, so this is the code that must be reported.

Now, let's take a look at another scenario that requires only two of the three components.

LET'S CODE IT! SCENARIO

Roger Forshay, a 75-year old male, has been living at Franklin Assisted Living Facility for 6 months. Dr. Henner, his primary physician since he moved in, comes in today to see Roger because of a complaint of leg pain. Dr. Henner documents a problem-focused interval history, an expanded problem-focused exam, and MDM of moderate complexity.

Let's Code It!

Read through the scenario, and identify the location where Dr. Henner provided his evaluation and management services: "assisted living facility."

Let's turn to the Domiciliary, Rest Home or Custodial Care Services subsection of E/M. Why? In the first paragraph under this heading, you will see that CPT directs you to use this category of E/M codes "to report evaluation and management services in an assisted living facility."

This subsection is divided into New Patient and Established Patient, so go back to the scenario. It states, "Dr. Henner, his primary physician since he moved in," meaning that Roger qualifies as an Established Patient. This narrows down the choices to Established Patient 99334–99337.

These codes require TWO of the THREE key components. In a full case, you will go back and read through the physician's notes to determine the level provided for each of the three components, as you learned earlier in this chapter. As we did before, this scenario is provided with a shortcut, indicating the levels for you:

Problem-focused interval history meets the requirement for 99334.

Expanded problem-focused exam meets the requirement for 99335 and exceeds the requirement for 99334.

MDM moderate complexity meets the requirement for 99336 and exceeds the requirements for 99334 and 99335.

You must find the one level that is satisfied by at least TWO of the THREE levels of care.

99334:

You have documentation that is equal to this level of history.

You have documentation that is greater than this level of exam.

You have documentation that is greater than this level of MDM.

99335:

You have documentation that is **NOT** equal to this level of history.

You have documentation that is equal to this level of exam.

You have documentation that is greater than this level of MDM.

99336:

You have documentation that is **NOT** equal to this level of history.

You have documentation that is **NOT** equal to this level of exam.

You have documentation that is equal to this level of MDM.

Now, you must report the highest level of code that has at least TWO levels equal to or greater than its requirements. The only choice is 99335.

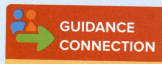

GUIDANCE CONNECTION

The list of these elements, body areas, and organ systems can be found in the **Evaluation and Management (E/M) Services Guidelines**, subhead **Select the Appropriate Level of E/M Services Based on the Following,** in your CPT book directly in front of the E/M section that lists all the codes.

Kenny Wilmington, a 33-year-old male, came to see Dr. Thomas in her office for the first time because of a cough, fever, excessive sputum production, and difficulty in breathing. He had been reasonably well until now. Dr. Thomas did an expanded problem-focused exam of the patient's respiratory system and took Kenny's personal, family, and social history in detail. After a chest x-ray was taken to rule out pneumonia, Dr. Thomas's straightforward MDM led her to diagnose him with bronchitis and prescribe an antibiotic and a steroid.

You Code It!

Go through the steps of E/M coding, and determine the E/M code that should be reported for this encounter between Dr. Thomas and Kenny Wilmington.

Step 1: Read the case completely.

Step 2: Abstract the notes: Which key words can you identify relating to the E/M service performed?

_____

Step 3: What is the location?

_____

Step 4: What is the relationship?

_____

Step 5: What level of patient history was taken?

_____

Step 6: What level of physical examination was performed?

_____

Step 7: What level of MDM was required?

_____

Step 8: What is the most accurate E/M code for this encounter?

_____

Answer:

Did you determine the correct code to be 99202?

You know, from the notes, that Kenny saw the doctor "in her office." This tells you the location. You also can detect that Kenny is a new patient because Dr. Thomas is seeing him "for the first time."

You would need to use code 99203 because the physician documented "history in detail." However, the level of physical examination performed would better match code 99202 because she performed only "an expanded problem-focused exam." Code 99202 is also supported by the "straightforward medical decision-making." So when you examine the requirements to meet or exceed the key components of code 99202, you consider the following:

- Expanded problem-focused history: *Exceeded.*
- Expanded problem-focused exam: *Met.*
- Straightforward decision making: *Met.*

The correct E/M code for this scenario is 99202.

Time Under certain circumstances, the correct E/M code is not determined by the key components of history, physical exam, and MDM but is based on the amount of time the physician spent evaluating the patient's condition and managing his or her care. In these cases, the time shown in the last paragraph of the E/M code description is used as a guide. This detail can be found following the three bullets for the key components. You will see that the last sentence reads something like *Physicians typically spend 20 minutes face-to-face with the patient and/or family* in the last portion of the code 99202 description. This gives you an approximate time frame that may be used instead of the other key components to determine the appropriate level. In order to use this guideline to choose a code, the documentation must contain the appropriate specific information.

Counseling

If the physician spends more than half (51% or more) of the total time *counseling* the patient, then time spent shall be used as the key element in determining the best, most appropriate E/M code. This is not psychological counseling with a therapist (reported with codes 90804–90857) but the physician's discussing diagnosis and treatment with the patient. It might be to review test results or to go over care options with a family member. The CPT guidelines specify

- The results of recommendations for diagnostic tests and/or the review of the results of tests and impressions already gathered.

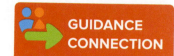

GUIDANCE CONNECTION

Additional explanations of these elements used to determine the most accurate E/M code involving the measurement of time spent with the patient can be found in the **Evaluation and Management (E/M) Services Guidelines,** subhead **Time,** in your CPT book directly in front of the E/M section that lists all the codes.

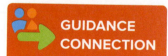

GUIDANCE CONNECTION

Additional explanations can be found in the **Evaluation and Management (E/M) Services** guidelines, subhead **Counseling,** in your CPT book directly in front of the E/M section that lists all the codes.

EXAMPLE

The doctor writes, "*I discussed with the patient that the MRI shows an area of concern . . .*"

- The options of multiple treatments, including risks and benefits.

EXAMPLE

The doctor writes, "*I explained to the patient that his condition can be treated with medication or surgery. The research shows that this new drug has been quite effective; however, there are some side effects . . .*"

- Directions to the patient for treatment and/or follow-up.

EXAMPLE

The doctor writes, "*Prescription provided with instructions to take one tablet three times a day. I want to see you in 1 week.*"

- Emphasizing the importance of compliance with the agreed-upon treatment plan.

> ### EXAMPLE
> The doctor writes, "*I informed the patient that she needs to take all of the pills in this pack. Even if she is feeling better, I instructed her to keep taking them until they are all gone.*"

- Risk factor reduction.

> ### EXAMPLE
> The doctor writes, "*The test was negative this time. However, I discussed with the patient how to prevent possible exposure in the future.*"

- Patient and family education.

> ### EXAMPLE
> The doctor writes, "*I explained to the daughter that her mother is going to need oxygen to treat her respiratory insufficiency. What this means is . . .*"

Face-to-Face (Office and Other Outpatient Visits)

You may have noticed the phrase *face-to-face* in the code description qualification about time. CPT is very specific about what is included in this element of E/M services provided by a physician to a patient, such as the time it takes to collect health care-related history, perform the physician examination, and counsel the patient (as discussed previously).

Everyone understands that most physicians will spend time, before and after their encounters with patients, reviewing records, going over test results, conferencing with other professionals and the patients by writing letters and reports, making phone calls, and performing other non–face-to-face tasks. Officially, these are not included in the time component of the E/M codes.

Unit/Floor Time (Hospital and Other Inpatient Visits)

When a physician attends to a patient in a facility, such as a hospital or nursing home, the aspect of time for purposes of E/M coding is described a bit differently. In addition to the face-to-face time that the physician may spend at bedside examining the patient, meeting with nursing staff and other health care professionals, and speaking with family members, unit/floor time also includes the time the physician spends going over the patient's chart and reviewing notes by other professionals caring for the patient while the physician is still physically present in the hospital unit.

Non–Face-to-Face

Everyone is trying to work more efficiently by using the telephone or the Internet to communicate with an established patient and/or patient's family, coordinate care, discuss test results, or answer a question. This makes good sense.

To report E/M services provided by the physician over the telephone, a code from the range 99441–99443 should be used. The different codes are distinguished by the length of time of the call. However, before you report one of these codes, there are

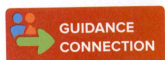

GUIDANCE CONNECTION

Additional explanations can be found in the **Evaluation and Management (E/M) Services** guidelines, subhead **Time,** paragraphs **Face-to-face . . .** and **Unit/floor time . . .,** in your CPT book directly in front of the E/M section that lists all the codes.

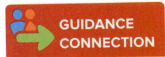

GUIDANCE CONNECTION

Additional explanations can be found in in-section guidelines within the **Evaluation and Management (E/M) Services** section, subhead **Non–Face-to-Face Services,** related to codes 99441–99449 in your CPT book.

restrictions. If the phone call is a follow-up to an E/M service provided for a related problem or concern that occurred within the previous 7 days, none of these codes can be reported because the phone call is considered part of that service. In the same light, if the phone call results in the decision for the patient to come in to see the physician as soon as possible, this phone call is considered a part of that future E/M service, so one of these codes would not be used, either.

Code 99444 is used to report an online E/M service to an established patient, a guardian, or a health care provider as a response to a patient's question. Similar to the restriction on the reporting of a telephone call, code 99444 should not be reported when this e-mail or Internet communication is connected to an E/M service provided for a related concern that occurred within the previous 7 days or within a surgical procedure's postoperative period.

LET'S CODE IT! SCENARIO

Lenore Parker, a 55-year-old female, came to see Dr. Bruce because she had the flu. While she was there, the results of her lab work, ordered by the doctor during her annual physical 2 weeks earlier, came back. Dr. Bruce examined Lenore's eyes, ears, nose, throat, and chest and quickly determined she had the flu. He advised her to rest and drink hot tea with honey. Then Dr. Bruce spent 30 minutes counseling Lenore on her diet and the changes she needed due to her extremely high cholesterol level (as shown in the lab results from the physical exam).

Let's Code It

The fact that Lenore *came to see Dr. Bruce* tells us this encounter occurred at Dr. Bruce's office. The notes document that Lenore had an *annual physical* performed by Dr. Bruce "2 weeks earlier." This means that she is an established patient.

Which levels of history, exam, and MDM were met or exceeded? You will note that established patient office E/M codes require only two key elements to be met. In this case, the physician did not do a history of any kind. However, he did document examining *Lenore's eyes, ears, nose, throat, and chest* (a problem-focused examination) and *quickly determined* (a straightforward MDM).

All these key elements direct us to the code 99212, but the notes also state that Dr. Bruce spent *30 minutes counseling* Lenore on her diet. Code 99212 shows a typical time of 10 minutes. Therefore, using code 99212 would fairly compensate Dr. Bruce for the caring of Lenore's flu but not her high cholesterol. He deserves to be reimbursed for his counseling. Dr. Bruce spent 10 minutes on Lenore's flu plus 30 minutes on Lenore's cholesterol, totaling 40 minutes. Thirty minutes is more than half of 40 minutes, so the guideline regarding counseling time can be applied, and it is correct to use the E/M code 99215 that indicates 40 minutes face-to-face.

LO 4.4 Prolonged Services: 99354–99359

In some cases, patients require greater than the usual amount of attention from a physician, more time than would regularly be spent—either face-to-face or without direct contact—over the course of 1 day.

Prolonged service codes report E/M services that are at least 30 minutes longer than the amount of time represented by standard E/M codes. These codes may be reported in addition to standard E/M codes at any level, as appropriate.

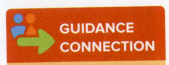
To determine the best, most appropriate code from this subcategory, you have to calculate the total number of minutes that the physician spent with, or on behalf of, the patient, during one date of service. The codes will be calculated as follows:

The first code would be the standard evaluation and management code (such as 99213).

Then, depending upon how long the physician spent with the patient, you would add-on

+ 99354 or 99356 for the time spent lasting at least 30 minutes over the standard evaluation and management service and includes time spent up to 74 minutes.

+ 99355 or 99357 for each 30 minutes additionally spent, over the 74 minutes reported by 99354 or 99356 until the total amount of time spent by the physician is represented.

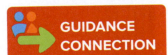
EXAMPLE

Dr. Moro spent a total of 2 hours, in his office, with Gina Fairchild working with her to stabilize her diabetes mellitus. The codes used to report this E/M encounter are

99213	Office visit, established patient, expanded problem-focused	
+99354	Prolonged physician service in the office; first hour	60 min.
+99355	additional 30 minutes	30 min.
+99355	additional 30 minutes	30 min.
		120 min. = 2 hours

LO 4.5 Consultations

As mentioned earlier in this chapter, occasionally a patient will see a physician only for a second opinion and not necessarily to establish a health care relationship. Such encounters are typically identified in the physician's notes as a consultation, so usually you will not have to guess. However, you need to read carefully.

Let's begin with two common terms used and confused: *referral* and *consultation*. As we discussed earlier in this chapter, when one physician *transfers* the care and treatment for a patient (in total or for one particular issue) to another physician, this is a *referral*. The patient is merely being recommended to see another physician and is expected to become a patient of the other physician. These visits are reported using the regular E/M codes, based on the location of the encounter between the new physician (the specialist) and the patient—for example, physician's office 99201–99205, etc.

You will also use the regular E/M codes based on the location of the encounter if the second opinion was sought out by the patient or the patient's family and not another physician. This should be evident in the documentation. For example, the notes may state something like "I am evaluating this patient at the request of the patient's daughter" or "This patient told me that his physician recommended surgery, and he wants a second opinion before agreeing to the procedure."

When a patient goes to a physician for a *consultation* because the first physician is merely seeking a *second opinion* from the consulting physician regarding diagnosis and/or treatment of the patient, it will be reported from the Consultations subsection of E/M. Different than other subsections, the consultation codes 99241–99255 are separated into two parts on the basis of the location of where the consultation took place: *Office and Other Outpatient Consultations* and *Inpatient Consultations.*

EXAMPLE

Loretta Caston, a 47-year-old female, was sent to Dr. Harrington, an oncologist, by her family physician, Dr. Catalane, for a consultation. She had been suffering with moderate pelvic pain and a heavy sensation in her lower pelvis. Upon her arrival at Dr. Harrington's office, she was given a pelvic ultrasound. Dr. Harrington evaluated the test results, spoke with Loretta, and sent a report to Dr. Catalane.

This was a *consultation* that was *requested by another physician* and held in the physician's *office*, leading to the code range 99241–99245.

If Loretta's tests are positive for a malignancy and she decides to have Dr. Harrington treat her cancer, the care for her malignancy will be transferred to Dr. Harrington, she will then become Dr. Harrington's patient, and all future encounters in his office between this doctor and this patient will use E/M codes from 99211–99215 Office or Other Outpatient Services, Established Patient.

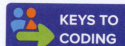

KEYS TO CODING

If it is decided that, after a consulting physician sees a patient, this physician will continue care and/or treatment of the patient, the subsequent encounters will be coded as an *Established Patient*.

YOU CODE IT! CASE STUDY

Dr. Weldon was asked by Dr. Samuels to provide a second opinion on Burton Conner, a 17-year-old male. Burton's pulmonary specialist, Dr. Samuels, wants to perform a lung transplant because of his diagnosis of cystic fibrosis. Dr. Weldon examined Burton's respiratory system in his hospital room, reviewed the x-rays ordered by Dr. Samuels, and wrote a report agreeing that Dr. Samuels should perform the surgery.

You Code It!

Go through the steps of E/M coding, and determine the E/M code that should be reported for this encounter between Dr. Weldon and Burton Conner.

Step 1: Read the case completely.

Step 2: Abstract the notes: Which key words can you identify relating to the E/M service performed?

_____

Step 3: What is the location?

_____

Step 4: What is the relationship?

_____

Step 5: What level of patient history was taken?

_____

Step 6: What level of physical examination was performed?

_____

Step 7: What level of MDM was required?

_____

Step 8:   What is the most accurate E/M code for this encounter?

_____

Answer:

Did you determine the correct code?

99252 Inpatient consultation, expanded problem-focused

LET'S CODE IT! SCENARIO

Harrison Bernardo, a 51-year-old male, was having pain in his lower abdomen, especially when going to the bathroom. His primary care physician, Dr. Mayonni, did a PSA and was not very concerned, so he told Harrison to come back in 6–8 months for a follow-up. Harrison did not feel right about Dr. Mayonni's decision and made an appointment for a second opinion with Dr. Hamilin, a urologist. Dr. Hamilin took a detailed history, he performed a detailed examination, and his documented MDM was moderately complex.

Let's Code It!

The notes indicate that it was Harrison, "the patient," who "requested the consultation" with Dr. Hamilin. Therefore, it is coded as a new patient office visit, and you will find the correct code in the 99201–99205 range.

The documentation reports that Dr. Hamilin completed *a detailed history, he performed a detailed examination, and MDM documented was moderately complex.* Because this subsection of E/M requires all three key components to be met or exceeded, the correct code for this encounter is 99203.

LO 4.6 Reading the Physician's Notes

Sometimes, physicians will actually identify the level of MDM in their notes with a statement such as "MDM was low complexity."

YOU CODE IT! CASE STUDY

Amanda Carter, a 21-year-old female, comes to see Dr. Atwater at his office with complaints of severe pain in her right wrist and forearm. She just moved to the area, and this is the first time Dr. Atwater has seen her. Amanda sees Dr. Atwater for a very specific concern. The doctor asks Amanda about any medical history she may have related to her arm (diagnosed osteoporosis, previous broken bones, etc.). Next, Dr. Atwater examines Amanda's arm. He suspects that the arm is broken and orders an x-ray to be taken. MDM is straightforward.

Go through the steps to determine the E/M code that should be reported for this encounter between Dr. Atwater and Amanda Carter.

Step 1:   Read the case completely.

Step 2:   Abstract the notes: Which key words can you identify relating to the E/M service performed?

_____

Step 3:   What is the location?

_____

Step 4:   What is the relationship?

_____

Step 5:   What level of patient history was taken?

_____

Step 6:   What level of physical examination was performed?

_____

Step 7:   What level of MDM was required?

_____

Step 8:   What is the most accurate E/M code for this encounter?

_____

Answer:

Did you determine the correct code to be 99201 Office or other outpatient visit, new patient?

Let's carefully review the physician's notes.

Where did the encounter occur? Amanda went "to see Dr. Atwater at his office." This will lead us to the first subheading in the E/M section, *Office or Other Outpatient Services.*

What is the relationship? The notes state, *"She just moved to the area, and this is the first time Dr. Atwater has seen her."* This brings us to the category of *New Patient,* and the code range is 99201–99205.

What is the level of history? The notes state, *"The doctor asks Amanda about any medical history she may have related to her arm,"* meaning that all the history he took was *problem-focused.*

What is the level of exam? You will see that *"Dr. Atwater examines Amanda's arm."* This means only one body area (each extremity) or one organ system (musculoskeletal) was examined. That's *problem-focused.*

What is the level of MDM? In this case, the physician actually wrote in his notes that the MDM was *straightforward.* However, you can see that the documentation supports the definition of this level: There is only one diagnosis, the management options are limited (put a cast on it), there are very few complications, and Dr. Atwater didn't really have to do any research to recommend a course of treatment.

This brings you to the best, most appropriate E/M code: 99201.

More often, the physicians will not come right out and use this terminology to describe what occurred during the encounter. Let's inspect various statements from patients' charts and identify the key words that lead to the correct E/M code.

1. Arvin Wasserman, a 65-year-old male, was seen for the first time by Dr. Frieda in the office for a contusion of his hand. Dr. Frieda asked questions about the bruise on Arvin's hand and examined his hand thoroughly.

   a. Location: *Office* tells us where the encounter took place.

   b. Relationship: *First time* tells us this is a new patient.

   c. Key components: *History—problem-focused, physical examination—problem-focused, medical decision making—straightforward.* Therefore, the correct code is 99201.

2. Dr. Pratt performed an initial observation at the hospital of Gerda Illianni, a 27-year-old female. After asking about her personal medical history, including pertinent history of stomach problems, digestive problems, and pertinent family and social history directly relating to her complaints, he examined Gerda's abdomen, chest, neck, and back, which revealed lower right quadrant pain accompanied by nausea, vomiting, and a low-grade fever. Dr. Pratt made the straightforward decision to admit Gerda overnight to the hospital to rule out appendicitis.

   a. Location: *Initial observation at the hospital* tells us this code is in the Hospital Observation Services section.

   b. Relationship: *Observation at the hospital* codes are the same for both new and established patients.

   c. Key components: *History—detailed, physical examination—detailed, medical decision making—straightforward,* and *overnight admission to the hospital* all lead us to the correct code of 99218.

3. Dr. Sierra, a general surgeon, saw Carolina Hommen, a 37-year-old female, in her office for a second opinion requested by Carolina's gynecologist, Dr. Keller, regarding a lump in her right breast. Dr. Sierra took a brief history of Carolina's present illness and a personal and family medical history relating to her hematologic and lymphatic system, which was positive for breast cancer on her maternal side. After reviewing the mammogram and performing a limited physical exam of her breasts and chest area, the physician made the straightforward decision to advise a lumpectomy.

   a. Location: *In her office* tells us where the encounter took place.

   b. Relationship: *Second opinion requested by a physician* tells us this is a consultation.

   c. Key components: *History—expanded problem-focused, physical examination—expanded problem-focused,* and *medical decision-making—straightforward* lead us directly to the correct code of 99242.

4. Matthew Claussen, a 15-year-old male, presented at the ED with a painful, swollen wrist. The patient stated he had been hurt at a softball game. Dr. Alexander took a brief history and asked some key questions about Matthew's arm/hand. He then examined Matthew's wrist and arm, checked his musculoskeletal system, and ordered x-rays to be taken. It was rather simple to determine that Matthew's diagnosis was a sprained wrist.

   a. Location: *ED* tells you the location.

   b. Relationship: Codes in the Emergency Department Services section do not differentiate between new and established patients.

   c. Key components: *History—expanded problem-focused, physical examination—expanded problem-focused,* and *medical decision-making low complexity* tell us the extent of the encounter. The correct code is 99282.

Dr. Abbanni arrived at the Denton Nursing Facility to do an annual assessment of her patient, Hannah Swannson, an 80-year-old female. Dr. Abbanni reviews the latest test results in Hannah's chart, takes a comprehensive interval history, and performs a comprehensive physical examination. Decision making is extremely complex because the patient has senile dementia, hypertension, and hypothyroidism. A new treatment plan is created due to changes in the patient's condition.

Let's Code It!

"Nursing Facility" tells us the location, and *"her patient"* tells us that this is an established patient. Comprehensive interval history, comprehensive physical examination, and highly complex decision making lead us directly to the correct code of 99310.

Chapter Summary

Evaluation and management (E/M) codes report the energy and knowledge a health care professional puts into gathering information, reviewing data, and determining the best course of treatment for the patient's current condition. Many health information management professionals find these difficult to correctly determine due to the complex formula of such codes. Don't become overwhelmed. Once you get a job, you will find that a particular portion of this section will become your main focus.

EXAMPLE

- If you work for a provider in a private medical office, most of your E/M codes will be found under the Office heading on the first two pages of the section.
- If you work for a physician who cares for patients at a skilled nursing facility, you will use codes from under the Nursing Facility Services heading.

So in the real world, most of the time, you will be using the same small set of codes over and over again. But because you don't know where you will be working in the future, you should learn the entire section.

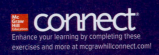

Using Terminology

Match each key term to the appropriate definition.

_____ 1. LO 4.2 The level of familiarity between provider and patient.

_____ 2. LO 4.2/4.5 An encounter for purposes of a second physician's opinion or advice, requested by another physician, regarding the management of a patient's specific health concern. A consultation is planned to be a short-term relationship between a health care professional and a patient.

_____ 3. LO 4.3 The extent of a physician's clinical assessment and inspection of a patient.

_____ 4. LO 4.3 The level of knowledge and experience needed by the provider to determine the diagnosis and/or what to do next.

_____ 5. LO 4.2 When a physician gives up responsibility for caring for a patient, in whole or with regard to one specific condition, and another physician accepts responsibility for the care of that patient.

_____ 6. LO 4.3 The amount of detail involved in the documentation of patient history.

_____ 7. LO 4.3 An acronym for past, family, and social history.

_____ 8. LO 4.2 A person who has received professional services within the last 3 years from either this provider or another provider of the same specialty belonging to the same group practice.

_____ 9. LO 4.2 A person who has not received any professional services within the past 3 years from either the provider or another provider of the same specialty who belongs to the same group practice.

_____ 10. LO 4.1 Specific characteristics of a face-to-face meeting between a health care professional and a patient.

A. Consultation

B. Established patient

C. Evaluation and management (E/M)

D. Level of patient history

E. Level of physical examination

F. Medical decision making (MDM)

G. New patient

H. PFSH

I. Relationship

J. Transfer of care

Checking Your Understanding

Choose the most appropriate answer for each of the following questions.

1. LO 4.1 E/M codes enable the physician to be reimbursed for all of these services except

   a. talking with the patient and his or her family.
   b. taking continuing education classes.
   c. consulting with other health care professionals.
   d. reviewing data such as test results.

2. LO 4.1 Often, finding the correct E/M code begins with knowing

   a. where the patient met with the physician.
   b. which credential is held by the provider.
   c. what type of insurance policy is held by the patient.
   d. what the patient does for an occupation.

3. LO 4.2 A patient who has not seen a particular physician in the last 3 years is categorized as

   a. an established patient.
   b. a referral.
   c. a consultation.
   d. a new patient.

4. LO 4.2 The three key components of many E/M codes include all of these *except*

   a. history.
   b. exam.
   c. chief complaint.
   d. MDM.

5. LO 4.3 Levels of patient history include all *except*

   a. expanded problem-focused.
   b. comprehensive.
   c. detailed.
   d. high complexity.

6. LO 4.3 Body areas that might be included in a physical examination include

   a. eyes.
   b. each extremity.
   c. respiratory.
   d. neurologic.

7. LO 4.3 When services are provided at different levels, the guidelines state you should code to a level of

   a. at least one of three key components achieved.
   b. all key components met or exceeded.
   c. the number of minutes face-to-face.
   d. the number of diagnosis codes.

8. LO 4.3 If _____ of the time with the patient is spent counseling, you should use time rather than key components to determine the level of service code.

   a. 51% or more.
   b. 45% or more.
   c. 50% or less.
   d. 25% or more.

9. LO 4.2/4.5 A consultation is expected to be a(n) _____ relationship with the patient.

   a. extended.
   b. transferred.
   c. temporary.
   d. continuing.

10. LO 4.1 A patient seen in the office and then admitted to the hospital the same day should be coded with E/M codes from subsection(s)

   a. Office Visit only.
   b. Office Visit and Initial Hospital Care.
   c. Initial Hospital Care only.
   d. Emergency Department.

Applying Your Knowledge

1. LO 4.1 What is an E/M code, and what does it report? _____

   _____

2. LO 4.2 Explain the difference between a new patient and an established patient. _____

   _____

3. LO 4.1 List the location-specific headings in the E/M section. _____

   _____

4. LO 4.2 List the three types of relationships used to determine the most appropriate E/M code. _____

   _____

5. LO 4.2 List the three components of an E/M code. _____

   _____

6. LO 4.3 List the four levels of patient history. _____

   _____

7. LO 4.3 Explain the level of physical examination. _____

   _____

8. LO 4.3 List the seven body areas. _____

   _____

and endocrine body systems. Dr. Harrington noted that her past medical history was noncontributory to the present problem. The detailed physical examination centered on her gastrointestinal and genitourinary systems with a complete pelvic exam. Dr. Harrington ordered lab tests and a pelvic ultrasound in order to consider uterine fibroids, endometritis, or other internal gynecologic pathology. MDM complexity was moderate.

_____

7. Martin Mazzenthorp decided to see Dr. Appleton for a second opinion regarding his own physician's recommendation for surgical repair of a hernia. After a brief problem-focused history of present illness and a problem-focused exam of the affected body area and organ system, Dr. Appleton made a straightforward medical decision to support the original recommendation for surgery.

_____

8. Carolina Tanner came into the ED with a what appeared to be a wrist sprain that she sustained during a baseball game when she slid into home base. She was in obvious pain, and the wrist was swollen and too painful upon attempts to flex. Dr. Ramada performed an expanded problem-focused history and exam before he ordered x-rays. Reports confirmed a simple fracture of the distal radius. MDM was low.

_____

9. Bernard Kristenson, an 82-year-old male, was diagnosed with advanced Alzheimer's disease about 1 year ago. He was seen by the nursing facility's physician, Dr. Mintz, over concern of the development of urinary and fecal incontinence, as well as a number of other medical problems that have appeared to increase in severity. In addition to the detailed interval history, the physician spoke with family members and the nursing staff. Then, Dr. Mintz reviewed the patient's record to create an extended history necessary for an extended review of systems (ROS). Dr. Mintz performed a comprehensive physical exam to assess all body systems. Afterward, he wrote all new orders due to the dramatic change in the patient's physical and mental condition. A new treatment plan was created. The MDM complexity was high.

_____

10. Verniece Dantini, a 61-year-old female, sees Dr. Smallerman for the first time for a variety of medical problems. She was diagnosed 5 years ago with insulin-dependent diabetes mellitus with complicating eye and renal problems. In addition, she suffers from hypertensive heart disease with episodes of congestive heart failure. Her peripheral vascular disease has worsened, and she can walk only a block before being crippled with extreme leg pain. The patient reports that a new problem has surfaced: throbbing headaches with radiating neck pain. In order to manage and investigate the multiplicity of problems, Dr. Smallerman performs a comprehensive history and physical exam. A complete ROS is performed, and her complete PFSH is updated. Dr. Smallerman has to take a multitude of factors into consideration, as the patient's problems are highly complex.

_____

11. Maribelle Johannsen, a 75-year-old female, lives in Barton Assisted Living Center, where she is seen by Dr. Modesta as a part of her annual assessment. Dr. Modesta completes a detailed interval history with a comprehensive head-to-toe physical exam. He reviews and affirms the medical plan of care developed by the multidisciplinary care team at Barton. Maribelle's condition is stable, her hypertension and diabetes (type II) are in good control, and she has no new problems. There is minimal data for Dr. Modesta to review and several diagnoses to consider. The MDM is moderate.

_____

12. George Carter, a 17-month-old male, is admitted to the hospital by his pediatrician, Dr. Mitchell, after confirming via chest x-ray that the child has pneumonia. The initial hospital care includes a detailed history and detailed physical exam with an extended problem-focused ROS completed with Petula Carter, the child's mother. The course of treatment planned by Dr. Mitchell is straightforward as the child's condition is of low severity. MDM is of low complexity.

_____

13. Tricia Thornwell, a 27-year-old female, is admitted to the hospital for observation after falling from the roof of her carport (approximately 8 feet high). Tricia has complaints of pain in multiple areas, and numerous x-rays are ordered. Dr. Dijohn performs a comprehensive history and physical exam. The possibility of multiple fractures makes the MDM moderately complex.

_____

14. Ellen Onoton, a 45-year-old female, recently diagnosed with asthma, comes to see her family physician, Dr. Pashma, with a complaint of severe headaches. He performs a comprehensive history and exam, with highly complex MDM.

_____

15. Raymond Catertell, a 20-year-old male, was admitted into the hospital 2 days ago for bronchitis. While in the hospital, Raymond requested that his family physician, Dr. Kaminsky, perform a circumcision, so Dr. Kaminsky called in Dr. Longwell, a urologist, for a consultation. Dr. Longwell performed a problem-focused history and problem-focused physical exam and made the straightforward decision to recommend that Raymond have the surgical procedure done as an outpatient at a later date. Code for Dr. Longwell's services.

_____

The following exercises provide practice in the application of abstracting the physicians' notes and learning to work with SOAP notes from our health care facility, Cipher, Victors & Associates. These case studies (SOAP notes) are modeled on real patient encounters. Using the techniques described in this chapter, carefully read through the case studies and determine the most accurate E/M code(s) for each case study.

CIPHER, VICTORS & ASSOCIATES
A Complete Health Care Facility
234 MAIN STREET • ANYTOWN, FL 32711 • 407-555-1234

PATIENT: OATES, MARLENE
ACCOUNT/EHR #:   OATEMA001
DATE: 09/16/18

Attending Physician: James I. Cipher, MD

S: This new Pt is a 29-year-old female who was involved in a two-car motor vehicle accident (MVA) while driving on the job. She is complaining about some neck pain. She has tingling in her left hand and both feet. She states that her left arm hurts when she tries to pull it overhead. She apparently was told by a friend that she should likely need to see a spine doctor, but somehow she came to see me first. PMH is remarkable for kidney trouble. Past bronchoscopy, laparoscopy, and kidney stone surgery, otherwise noncontributory as per the medical history form completed by the patient and reviewed at this visit.

O: Ht 5′5″ Wt 179 lb. R 16. Pt presented in a sling. She was told to use it by the same friend. She states if she does not use it, her arm does not feel any different, so I had her remove it. She states that she has not had any prior injury to this area and has no previous problems with her musculoskeletal system. On exam, HEENT is unremarkable. Neck muscles are taut, particularly on the left side. The left shoulder demonstrates full passive motion, with normal strength testing. No deformity is observable. Pt states there is some tenderness over the left trapezius area. The reflexes are brisk and symmetric. X-rays of her chest two views and C spine AP/LAT are relatively benign, as are complete x-rays of the shoulder.

A: Contusion of upper left arm and left shoulder

P: 1. MRI to rule out torn ligament
   2. Rx Naprosyn
   3. Referral to PT
   4. Referral to orthopedist

James I. Cipher, MD

JIC/mg   D: 09/16/18 09:50:16   T: 09/18/18 12:55:01

Determine the most accurate E/M code(s).

_____

_____

_____

CIPHER, VICTORS & ASSOCIATES
A Complete Health Care Facility
234 MAIN STREET • ANYTOWN, FL 32711 • 407-555-1234

PATIENT: KATTMAN, PHILLIP
ACCOUNT/EHR #:   KATTPH001
DATE: 10/01/18

Attending Physician: Valerie R. Victors, MD

S: This 31-year-old male was brought to the ED by ambulance after he was found unconscious on the living room floor this morning. He regained consciousness within several minutes, but complained of a severe headache and nausea. Pt states that the last thing he remembers he was on a ladder, changing the bulb in the track lighting. He believes he lost his balance trying to reach too far to take out the next light on the track and fell, hitting his head on the coffee table.

O: Ht 5'10" Wt 195 lb. R 16. Head: Scalp laceration on the right posterior parietal bone. Bruise indicates trauma to this area. Eyes: PERL. Neck: Neck muscles are tense; there is minor pain upon rotation of the head. Musculoskeletal: All other aspects of the shoulders, arms, and legs are unremarkable. X-rays of skull, two views, and soft tissue of the neck are all benign.

A: Concussion

P: 1. MRI to rule/out subdural hematoma
    2. Repair laceration and bandage

_____

Valerie R. Victors, MD

VRV/mg   D: 10/01/18 09:50:16   T: 10/05/18 12:55:01

Determine the most accurate E/M code(s).

_____

_____

_____

CIPHER, VICTORS & ASSOCIATES
A Complete Health Care Facility
234 MAIN STREET • ANYTOWN, FL 32711 • 407-555-1234

PATIENT: MADISON, MATTHEW
ACCOUNT/EHR #:   MADIMA001
DATE: 10/18/18

Attending Physician: James I. Cipher, MD

S: Matthew is an 11-month-old male brought in today by his mother. I last saw this patient at his regular 6-month checkup. He has been waking up at night and is irritable. Mother states that he has been tugging at his right ear and has been running a low-grade fever since yesterday. There has been no cough. Pt has a history of problems with his ears and sinuses. Pt is teething.

O: Ht 2′1″ Wt 25 lb. R 20. T 101.3 HEENT: Purulent nasal discharge, yellow-green in color, is noted. Right TM is erythematous unilaterally, bulging, and with purulent effusions. Oropharynx is nonerythematous without lesions. One tooth on the bottom. Tonsils are unremarkable. Neck: Neck is supple with good range of motion (ROM). Positive cervical adenopathy. Lungs: Clear. Heart: Regular rate and rhythm without murmurs.

A: Acute suppurative otitis media, right side

P: 1. Rx Augmentin 40 mg/kg divided tid 10 days
    2. Bed rest, lots of fluids
    3. Follow-up prn or if no improvement in 10 days

James I. Cipher, MD

JIC/mg   D: 10/18/18 09:50:16   T: 10/23/18 12:55:01

Determine the most accurate E/M code(s).

_____

_____

_____

CIPHER, VICTORS & ASSOCIATES
A Complete Health Care Facility
234 MAIN STREET • ANYTOWN, FL 32711 • 407-555-1234

PATIENT: TRIVETTE, FRANCIS
ACCOUNT/EHR #: TRIVFR001
DATE: 09/29/18

Attending Physician: Benjamin L. Johnston, MD
Referring Physician: James I. Cipher, MD

S: Pt is a 39-year-old male, referred by Dr. Cipher for a consultation regarding a sore on his left temple, at the hairline. Pt states he is very involved in beach and water sports. He knows the importance of sunscreen; however, he does not always remember to put it on. He has not had any dermatologic concerns prior to this. Patient states that his skin is very dry occasionally and that he has adult onset acne.

O: Ht 6′1″ Wt 225 lb. R 17. T 98.6 After an examination of the skin along the hairline, as well as the rest of the face and neck, a culture is taken of the lesion. The pathology report confirms a malignant melanoma of the skin of the scalp.

A: Malignant melanoma, scalp

P: 1. Discuss surgical and pharmaceutical options for treatment
   2. Report sent to Dr. Cipher

_____

Benjamin L. Johnston, MD

BLJ/mg   D: 09/29/18 09:50:16   T: 10/01/18 12:55:01

Determine the most accurate E/M code(s).

_____

_____

_____

CIPHER, VICTORS & ASSOCIATES
A Complete Health Care Facility
234 MAIN STREET • ANYTOWN, FL 32711 • 407-555-1234

PATIENT: STEIGLE, RALPH
ACCOUNT/EHR #:   STEIRA001
DATE: 09/29/18

Attending Physician: James I. Cipher, MD

S: Pt is a 77-year-old male requesting a second opinion. His current ophthalmologist, Dr. Quinones, diagnosed him with bilateral senile cataracts 3 weeks ago. According to the patient, Dr. Quinones is recommending surgical removal of the cataracts and implantation of lens. Pt is concerned about having surgery. He states he has always had excellent vision, but has noticed a decrease in his ability to see clearly over the last year or two. He denies any trauma to the area. Pt has no personal medical history that reveals an unusual risk for this type of surgical procedure. Pt is a social drinker. He denies smoking cigarettes but states he enjoys a cigar "on occasion." I reviewed the complete medical history form filled out by the patient at the beginning of this visit.

O: Ht 5′9″ Wt 225 lb. R 18. T 98.6. A detailed examination of the patient's eyes and visual acuity confirmed the original diagnosis made by Dr. Quinones. Examination of patient's chest reveals no arrhythmia. It appears to be a case of low complexity.

A: Bilateral senile cataracts

P: I told the patient that I confirmed the diagnosis and agreed with Dr. Quinones's recommendation for surgery.

_____

Benjamin L. Johnston, MD

BLJ/mg   D: 09/29/18 09:50:16   T: 10/01/18 12:55:01

Determine the most accurate E/M code(s).

_____

_____

_____

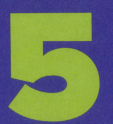

5 EVALUATION AND MANAGEMENT CODES, PART 2

Key Terms

Anticipatory guidance

Basic personal services

Care plan oversight services

Critical care services

Global surgery package

Hospice

Interval

Nursing home

Preventive

Risk factor reduction
    intervention

Evaluation and management (E/M) services go beyond those included in the typical office or hospital visit. **Preventive** medicine assessments— more commonly called annual physicals or wellness visits, evaluations of patients in short-term and long-term care facilities, counseling, and critical care—are just some of the areas of focus that might be required of the attending physician. This chapter reviews these subcategories of E/M codes.

LO 5.1 Preventive Medicine

There may be times when the physician's notes do not clearly identify all the individual components (for instance, history, exam, and medical decision making [MDM]) of an encounter, such as when a patient comes in for an annual physical. In these cases, you should be careful not to force the components or make them up. Instead, you should look at other areas of the E/M section. For example, the Preventive Medicine section, codes 99381–99429, may be more appropriate.

When provided at the same time as a comprehensive preventive medical examination, preventive medicine service codes 99381–99397 include

- Counseling.
- Anticipatory guidance.
- Risk factor reduction interventions.

From your own personal experience, you may be familiar with discussions with your physician during your annual physical. The talks cover everything from quitting smoking to exercising more and perhaps having a better diet. These are all examples of counseling.

Anticipatory guidance refers to the physician's offering suggestions for behavior modification or other preventive measures related to a patient's high risk for a condition. The concern may be based on specifics in a patient's condition or history (or perhaps a family history or an occupational hazard).

EXAMPLE

Dr. Darby provides anticipatory guidance to Randolph Muldoon with regard to being careful about protecting his respiratory health. Randolph works at an automobile paint shop, and the fumes are very dangerous if a breathing mask is not worn.

A physician prescribing a patch to help a patient quit smoking or referring a patient to a registered dietician to help him or her with a new diet—each of these is considered a **risk factor reduction intervention.** It means the physician is taking action to intervene with, or help stop, patient behaviors that put the patient at a higher risk for certain illnesses or conditions.

If such elements such as risk factor reduction intervention or counseling occur during a separate visit (not at the same time as the physical examination), you have to code them separately with a code from the 99401–99412 range.

If during the course of the preventive medicine examination, the physician finds something of concern that warrants special and extra attention involving the key components of a problem-oriented E/M service, the extra work should be coded with a separate E/M code appended with modifier 25. It is applicable only when the same physician does the extra service on the same date.

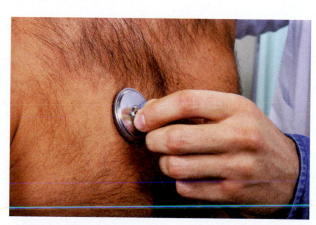

© PhotoLink/Getty Images

preventive
A type of action or service that stops something from happening or from getting worse.

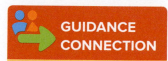

GUIDANCE CONNECTION

Additional explanations can be found in in-section guidelines located within the **Evaluation and Management (E/M)** section, subhead **Preventive Medicine Services,** directly above code 99381 in the E/M section.

anticipatory guidance
Recommendations for behavior modification and/or other preventive measures.

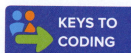

KEYS TO CODING

In regard to these preventive evaluations, the term *counseling* does not refer to a formalized relationship between a mental health counselor, psychologist, or psychiatrist but to the advice and guidance provided by a health care professional to his or her patient.

risk factor reduction intervention
Action taken by the attending physician to stop or reduce a behavior or lifestyle that is predicted to have a negative affect on the individual's health.

LET'S CODE IT! SCENARIO

Arlene Barry, a 47-year-old female, comes to see her regular physician, Dr. Fermat, for her annual physical. During the examination, Dr. Fermat finds a mass in her abdomen that concerns him. After the exam, he sits and talks with Arlene about past or current problems with her abdomen, including pain, discomfort, and other details regarding her abdominal issue. He asks whether any family members have had problems in that area, as well as about her alcohol consumption and sexual history as they relate to this concern. Dr. Fermat then goes into his office to analyze the multiple possibilities of diagnoses, evaluates the information in Arlene's chart, and reviews the moderate risk of complications that might occur due to her current list of medications. He orders an abdominal CT scan, blood work, and a UA for further input.

According to the notes, Dr. Fermat performed an "annual physical exam," also known as a preventive medicine exam, on Arlene, a "47-year-old" female. Go to the alphabetic index and look up *Evaluation and Management, Preventive Services,* or go directly to the E/M section and look for the Preventive Medicine Services subheading. The phrase "her regular physician," reveals that Arlene is an established patient, helping you to determine to report code

99396 Periodic comprehensive preventive medicine, 40–64 years

Dr. Fermat's notes also reveal that during the exam he found a mass in Arlene's abdomen that he felt needed further investigation. He spent additional time getting details about her personal, family, and social history regarding abdominal problems; he reviewed concerns about multiple possible diagnoses, complications, and treatments. As per the guidelines, this is extra work done on Dr. Fermat's part, and therefore he is entitled to additional reimbursement, reported with a separate E/M code. As you review the notes, you should be able to determine the best, most appropriate E/M code for the additional service. Dr. Fermat did a comprehensive examination, and his MDM was certainly at a high level of complexity, leading you to the code

99215 Office or other outpatient visit with comprehensive exam and medical decision-making of high complexity

Plus the modifier:

–25 Significant, separately identifiable evaluation and management service

The claim form for Dr. Fermat's encounter with Arlene Barry will show 99396, 99215-25. Good job!

99396 will reimburse Dr. Fermat for his time and services for the annual physical, and 99215 will reimburse him for the extra work he did regarding the abdominal mass. The modifier -25 explains that, while unusual, Dr. Fermat did both of these services at the same encounter.

(Note: More information on E/M modifiers is given later in this chapter.)

Counseling and/or Risk Factor Reduction Intervention

When a physician sees a patient at a visit, separate from the annual preventive medicine evaluation, for the purposes of helping the patient learn about, understand, and/or adopt better health practices, including

- Preventing injury or illness, such as the proper way to lift or the importance of testing one's blood glucose levels regularly.
- Encouraging good health, such as nutritional counseling or a new exercise regime.

Services, such as these, are reported with codes from:

99401–99404 Preventive medicine, individual counseling
99411–99412 Preventive medicine, group counseling
99420–99429 Other preventive medicine services

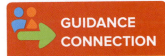

GUIDANCE CONNECTION

Additional explanations can be found in in-section guidelines located within the **Evaluation and Management (E/M)** section, subhead **Counseling Risk Factor Reduction and Behavior Change Intervention,** directly above code 99401 in the E/M section.

Home Services

If a physician provides E/M services to a patient at his or her private residence, use codes 99341–99350. Determine the most appropriate code by using the same key components as those for E/M services provided in the physician's office. (You learned about these in Chap. 4 of this textbook.)

Some home health agencies employ physicians, some physicians may volunteer to see homebound patients, while others visit only established patients who are homebound.

Physicians use different methods and tools to assess a patient's status and to create and/or update an appropriate treatment plan for the ongoing care of the individual. Such methods and tools include

Resident assessment instrument (RAI)

Minimum data set (MDS)

Resident assessment protocols (RAP)

When a health care professional other than the physician—such as a nurse or respiratory therapist—cares for a patient at the patient's home, report these services with a code from the range 99500–99602.

LET'S CODE IT! SCENARIO

Morgan Garrison, a 45-year-old male, suffers from agoraphobia and cannot leave his home. Dr. Lavattney went to the house to examine Morgan because he was complaining of chest congestion. Dr. Lavattney took a problem-focused history, as this was the first time he had seen Morgan. The doctor examined Morgan's HEENT and chest and concluded that Morgan had a chest cold. He told Morgan to get some over-the-counter cold medicine and to call if the symptoms did not go away within a week.

Let's Code It!

You need to find the appropriate code to reimburse Dr. Lavattney for his E/M services to Morgan Garrison. You know that "Dr. Lavattney went to the house," so the location section is titled Home Services. The notes say that "this was the first time he had seen Morgan," meaning that Morgan is a new patient, narrowing the choices to codes 99341–99345. The book tells us that a new patient home visit requires three key components: history, examination, and MDM. According to the notes, Dr. Lavattney

1. Took a *problem-focused history*.
2. Examined the patient's head, ears, eyes, nose, throat (HEENT), and chest: *expanded problem-focused* because the doctor examined the affected body system and other related organ systems.
3. Concluded, without tests or additional resources: *straightforward*.

When you assess the levels and use the meet or exceed rule, the most accurate code for the visit is 99341. Good job!

nursing home
A facility that provides skilled nursing treatment and attention along with limited medical care for its (usually long-term) residents, who do not require acute care services (hospitalization).

basic personal services
Services that include washing/bathing, dressing and undressing, assistance in taking medications, and getting in and out of bed.

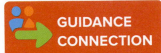

GUIDANCE CONNECTION

Additional explanations can be found in in-section guidelines located within the **Evaluation and Management (E/M)** section, subhead **Nursing Facility Services,** directly above code 99304 in the E/M section.

care plan oversight services
E/M of a patient, reported in 30-day periods, including infrequent supervision along with preencounter and postencounter work, such as reading test results and assessment of notes.

hospice
An organization that provides services to terminally ill patients and their families.

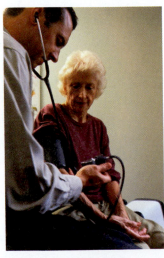

© Keith Brofsky/Getty Images

LO 5.2 Long-Term Care Services

Specific codes are used to report E/M services provided to patients in residential care facilities.

Use 99304–99318 and 99379–99380 for reporting services to patients in the following places:

NURSING HOMES

Skilled nursing facilities (SNF)

Intermediate care facilities (ICF)

Long-term care facilities (LTCF)

Psychiatric residential treatment centers

Use 99324–99340 for reporting services to patients in locations where room, meals, and **basic personal services** are provided but medical services are not included:

Assisted living facilities

Domiciliaries

Rest homes

Custodial care settings

Alzheimer's facilities

EXAMPLE

Dr. Sanders goes to see William Karlson at the halfway house where William resides. William is autistic, and Dr. Sanders wants to examine him and adjust his medication for asthma. You should report Dr. Sanders's visit to William with code 99334.

Care Plan Oversight Services

When a physician provides **care plan oversight services,** you have to use the appropriate code determined by the length of time involved and the type of facility in which the patient is located.

99339–99340 for patients in assisted living or domiciliary facility.

99374–99375 for home health care patients.

99377–99378 for **hospice** patients.

99379–99380 for residents in a nursing facility—but only if the management of the patient involves repeated direction of therapy by the attending physician.

Admission to the Nursing Facility: 99304–99306

When a patient is admitted into a nursing facility as a continued part of an encounter at the physician's office or the emergency department (ED) (on the same day by the same physician), you report only one code (from the Nursing Facility section of the E/M codes) that will include all the services provided from all the locations on that day. You may remember from Chap. 4 that admission to the hospital from the physician's office or ED is reported all in the one hospital admission E/M code. The same rule also applies to admission to a nursing facility.

However, if the patient has been discharged from inpatient status on the same day as being admitted to a nursing facility, you code the physician's discharge services separately from the admission.

Three key components, similar to other E/M codes, are used to determine the appropriate level of E/M service provided by the attending physician to a patient on the first day at a nursing facility. There is no differentiation made in this section of codes between a new patient and an established patient.

Subsequent Nursing Facility Care

Once the patient is in the facility, it is expected that the physician will continue to review the patient's chart, as well as assess test results and changes in the patient's health status. Notice that the code description for the history key component includes the term **interval**. The physician needs to evaluate the patient's history only back to the last visit to gain a complete, up-to-date picture of the individual's health. The continuing care type of assessment is reported with the most appropriate code from the 99307–99310 range.

If the physician does only an annual assessment of the patient in the nursing facility (typically in cases where the patient is stable, progressing as expected, or recovering), you use code

> 99318 Evaluation and management of a patient involving an annual nursing facility assessment

interval
The time measured between one point and another, such as between physician visits.

LET'S CODE IT! SCENARIO

Rita Anne Brigham, a 59-year-old female, was diagnosed with advanced pancreatic cancer and is being cared for at her home by her family, with the help of a home health agency. Dr. Brosseau is providing care plan oversight services for the first month of care. The plan includes home oxygen, IV medications for pain control management, and diuretics for edema and ascites control. Dr. Brosseau also discusses end-of-life issues, living will directive, and other concerns with the family, the nurse, and the social worker. Dr. Brosseau includes documentation of his 45-minute assessment, as well as notes on modifications to the care plan. Certifications of care from the nursing staff, the social worker, the pharmacy, and the company supplying the durable medical equipment for support are also in the record.

Let's Code It!

Dr. Brosseau documented that he provided "care plan oversight services" for Rita Anne Brigham. Turn to the alphabetic index, and look up *Care Plan Oversight Services.* The index instructs you to see *Physician Services.* Turn to *Physician Services,* and you will see *Care Plan Oversight Services.*

As you look at the indented list below that phrase, note that you have to identify the location at which the patient is being cared for. Rita Anne Brigham is being cared for at home by a home health agency. This index entry suggests code 99374.

Physician services

Care plan oversight services

    Home health agency care. 99374

Now, let's turn to code 99374 to read the entire code description:

> 99374 Physician supervision of a patient under care of home health agency (patient not present) in home, domiciliary or equivalent environment requiring complex and multidisciplinary care modalities involving regular physician development and/or revision of care plans; 15–29 minutes
>
> 99375　　30 minutes or more

Dr. Brosseau's notes report that he spent 45 minutes. Therefore, the correct code is 99375.

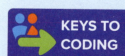

KEYS TO CODING

Note that code 99375 was not listed in the alphabetic index. You had to go to the numerical listing to find that 99375 is the most accurate code for the encounter. This instance is a reminder to *never, never, never* code from the alphabetic index, even when there is only one code shown.

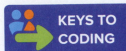
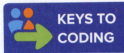
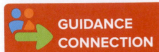
LO 5.3 Critical Care Codes

The management and care of severely ill patients take a great deal of skill, knowledge, and time. Critically ill or injured patients have a high likelihood of a deteriorating life-threatening condition. E/M services reported include

- Highly complex decision making to assess, manipulate, and support vital system function.
- Treatment of single or multiple vital organ system failure.
- Efforts to avoid additional life-threatening decline of the patient's condition.
- Interpretation of various vital function factors.
- Evaluation of advantages and disadvantages of using advanced technology.

The health care provider must document the amount of time spent so that you will know how to code the encounter. The physician may spend his or her time

- Reviewing test results and films at the nurses' station.
- Discussing the patient's treatment and care with the other members of the medical team.
- Charting (writing in the patient's chart).
- Attending to the patient at bedside.

All such activities are a part of the time spent providing critical care.

Critical care services can be, but do not have to be, provided in a coronary care unit (CCU), an intensive care unit (ICU), a respiratory care unit (RCU), or an emergency care facility.

The codes you choose to report critical care services are determined by the services provided for the critically ill or injured patient and the total length of unit/floor time of the encounter. Use the following for coding physician services for the critically ill or injured patient:

> **99291** Critical care, evaluation and management of a critically ill or critically injured patient; first 30–74 minutes
>
> **+99292** each additional 30 minutes

(Note: If the physician spends less than 30 minutes of unit/floor E/M time with a critically ill or critically injured patient, regular E/M inpatient codes should be reported. Critical care codes do not become applicable until the 30th minute.)

LET'S CODE IT! SCENARIO

Jason Howard, an 18-year-old male, was brought into the ED by ambulance after being involved in a motorcycle accident. He was not wearing a helmet, and his head hit a brick wall. After initial evaluation and testing by the ED physician, Jason was sent to the CCU and Dr. Oppenheim spent 2 hours reviewing test results, performing a complete physical exam of Jason, and discussing a care management plan with the rest of the medical team.

Let's Code It!

Dr. Oppenheim spent "2 hours" managing the care of Jason Howard in the "critical care unit." Turn to the Critical Care codes, and let's look at the chart. Two hours *equals* 2 *times* 60 minutes, or 120 minutes. When you look at the chart, you will see that 105–134 minutes (120 minutes is right in the middle of this range) is coded with 99291×1 and 99292×2 (read ×2 as reported twice). Look at the following complete description:

99291 Critical care, evaluation and management of the critically ill or critically injured patient; first 30–74 minutes

+99292 each additional 30 minutes

You know that Dr. Oppenheim spent 120 minutes and that 120 minutes *minus* 74 minutes (which is represented by code 99291) leaves 46 minutes unreported. Therefore, you must add 99292 to report an additional 30 minutes. However, 16 minutes still remains. So you must include 99292 again to account for the leftover minutes. The claim form that you complete will show 99291, 99292, 99292 or 99291, 99292×2. Great job!

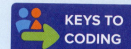

KEYS TO CODING

If the same physician provides critical care services to the same patient on the same date as other E/M services, codes from both subheadings may be reported.

LO 5.4 Case Management Services

If a patient has several or complex health issues or diagnoses, a team of health care professionals may have to work together to provide proper management and treatment. The team may involve several physicians or the attending physician and a physical therapist, for example, conferencing together. To properly reimburse the health care professional for the time and expertise spent on the patient's behalf with other professionals, you report such services using codes from ranges

99363–99364	Anticoagulant management
99366–99368	Medical team conferences
99441–99443	Telephone services
99444	On-line medical evaluation

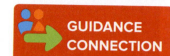

GUIDANCE CONNECTION

Additional explanations can be found in in-section guidelines located within the **Evaluation and Management (E/M)** section, subhead **Case Management Services**, directly above code 99363, and subhead **Medical Team Conferences**, directly above code 99366 in the E/M section.

YOU CODE IT! CASE STUDY

Arthur Unger, a 73-year-old male, is still having pain and swelling in his hands. Dr. Hertzwell calls Roger Bowen, a physical therapist, to adjust the therapy plan based on current test results. The call is brief.

You Code It!

Go through the steps of coding, and determine the E/M code that should be reported for the encounter between Dr. Hertzwell and Roger Bowen.

Step 1: Read the case completely.

Step 2: Abstract the notes: Which key words can you identify relating to the E/M service performed?

_____

Step 3: What is the most accurate E/M code for this encounter?

_____

LO 5.5 E/M in the Global Surgical Package

global surgery package
A group of services already included in the code for the operation and not reported separately.

As a part of the standard of care, there are certain E/M encounters that are already included in the code for a surgical procedure. This is called the **global surgery package.** You are probably familiar with this: A patient is being discharged after a procedure, and the doctors says, "I want to see you in the office in a week." A physician gets paid for performing surgery *and* for the time spent checking on the patient after the surgery to make certain the body is healing correctly. When the follow-up visit in the office (or wherever) occurs, you will not report this by using a regular E/M code because the physician will not be paid separately. However, you do need to report that this encounter occurred. Therefore, you will report a special services code from the Medicine section of the CPT book. Take a look at

99024 Postoperative follow-up visit, normally included in the surgical package to indicate that an evaluation and management service was performed during a postoperative period for a reason(s) related to the original procedure

You will learn more about the global period and surgical package in Chap. 7.

YOU CODE IT! CASE STUDY

Ten days after Dr. Tamara performed a carpal tunnel revision on Andrea Sorenson's left hand, Andrea, a 23-year-old female, came to see him in his office, as instructed when he discharged her. He asked how she was feeling, checked the flexibility of the wrist, removed the stitches, and checked the healing of the incision. She was doing fine, so Dr. Tamara told her to come in only if she needed anything.

You Code It!

Go through the steps of coding, and determine the E/M code that should be reported for the encounter between Dr. Tamara and Andrea Sorenson.

Step 1: Read the case completely.

Step 2: Abstract the notes: Which key words can you identify relating to the E/M service performed?

_____

Step 3: What is the most accurate E/M code for this encounter?

_____

Answer:

Did you determine the correct code to be 99024? I knew you could do it!

LO 5.6 Evaluation and Management Modifiers

Several modifiers may be used in conjunction with an E/M code to provide additional information about an encounter. Each modifier specifically explains an unusual circumstance that may justify the payment to the provider and helps you avoid having to appeal a denied claim later on. CPT Level I modifiers are two-digit codes that are listed in Appendix A of the CPT book. You first learned about these modifiers in Chap. 3 in this textbook.

24 **Unrelated evaluation and management service by the same physician during a postoperative period.** The physician may need to indicate that an evaluation and management service was performed during a postoperative period for a reason(s) unrelated to the original procedure. This circumstance may be reported by adding modifier 24 to the appropriate level of E/M service.

As a part of the standard of care and the global surgery package, a physician gets paid for performing surgery and for the time spent checking on the patient after the surgery to make certain the body is healing correctly. Modifier 24 would explain that the physician had to see the patient about a *totally different concern* during this time period.

YOU CODE IT! CASE STUDY

Dr. Longenstein removed Mark Katzman's gallbladder (cholecystectomy) on February 27. The global period for this surgical procedure is 90 days. On March 15, Mark came to see Dr. Longenstein because he had been out in his garden and developed a rash on his arms. The physician examined Mark's arms and gave him an ointment for the rash.

You Code It!

Go through the steps of coding, and determine the E/M code that should be reported for the encounter between Dr. Longenstein and Mark Katzman.

Step 1: Read the case completely.

Step 2: Abstract the notes: Which key words can you identify relating to the E/M service performed?

_____

Step 3: What is the most accurate E/M code for this encounter?

_____

Answer:

Did you determine the correct code to be 99212-24? Good for you!

Mark *came to see Dr. Longenstein,* meaning the encounter happened at the doctor's office. Considering that Dr. Longenstein *just performed surgery on Mark* 2 weeks ago, it is very reasonable to consider Mark an established patient. Dr. Longenstein did a *problem-focused examination* (limited exam of the problem area) and his *decision making was straightforward.* This directs us to code 99212.

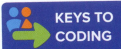

KEYS TO CODING

In order for modifier 25 to be used correctly, it is best if the E/M code links or relates to a different diagnosis from the procedure performed that day. So there would be at least two diagnosis codes on the same claim form before you consider using this modifier. Although different diagnoses are not required, there is concern in the industry about overuse of modifier 25, so this may trigger an audit without a separately identifiable diagnosis.

25   Significant, separately identifiable evaluation and management service by the same physician on the same day of the procedure of other service. It may be necessary to indicate that on the day a procedure or service identified by a CPT code was performed, the patient's condition required a significant, separately identifiable E/M service above and beyond the other service provided or beyond the usual preoperative and postoperative care associated with the procedure that was performed. A significant, separately identifiable E/M service is defined or substantiated by documentation that satisfies the relevant criteria for the respective E/M service to be reported. The E/M service may be prompted by the symptom or condition for which the procedure and/or service was provided. As such, different diagnoses are not required for reporting of the E/M services on the same date. This circumstance may be reported by adding modifier 25 to the appropriate level of E/M service. Note: This modifier is not used to report an E/M service that resulted in a decision to perform surgery. See modifier 57.

Certainly this happens quite frequently: A patient goes to see the doctor for a minor procedure in the office. Then the patient says, "Oh, Doc, while I'm here, I want to talk to you about so-and-so." Should that happen, you have to append the E/M code with modifier 25 to explain that there were two visits in one at this encounter.

LET'S CODE IT! SCENARIO

Harriet Robertson goes to see her dermatologist for a scheduled appointment to have a 1.5-cm mole removed from her cheek. Once Dr. Guilley completes the procedure, Harriet asks the doctor to look at a cyst that has developed under her arm. Dr. Guilley discusses the presence of the cyst with her (how long has it been there? Does it hurt? etc.), and then he examines her underarm area and determines that the best course of action is to wait and see what happens with the cyst. He advises Harriet to keep the area clean and to come back in 3 weeks if the cyst has not gone away.

Let's Code It!

Harriet met with *her dermatologist* (documenting that she is an established patient), Dr. Guilley, *at* his office (identifying an outpatient location). The notes document that Dr. Guilley did a *problem-focused history* (because they discussed nothing else other than the cyst) and a *problem-focused examination* (because Dr. Guilley examined only the area where the cyst is located), and his *decision making was straightforward* (because he is very knowledgeable about cysts and Harriet has no other conditions or medications that would cause more evaluation). This directs you to code 99212.

But wait! The claim for this encounter is going to include the code for the surgical removal of the mole—a totally different concern from the reason prompting the E/M of the patient. In essence, there were two encounters in one: the first for the removal of the mole and the second for the concern about the cyst. Therefore, the correct code would be 99212-25 (plus the procedure code for the excision of the mole: 11312).

32 **Mandated services:** Services related to mandated consultation and/or related services (e.g., third-party payer, governmental, legislative, or regulatory requirement) may be identified by adding modifier 32 to the basic procedure.

Modifier 32 indicates that a third-party payer, a governmental agency, or other regulatory or legislative action required the encounter, consultation, and/or procedure(s).

LET'S CODE IT! SCENARIO

Elaine Geller, a 53-year-old female, went to see Dr. Overton for a comprehensive physical assessment, as a requirement for her application for life insurance. The insurance carrier would not consider the policy without the examination. She had never seen Dr. Overton before today's visit.

Let's Code It!

Elaine met with the physician at his office and had never seen Dr. Overton before meaning that she is a new patient. According to the notes, Dr. Overton did an initial comprehensive preventive medicine E/M of a 53-year-old female. That directs you to code 99386.

Notice that the insurance carrier, a third-party payer, mandated the evaluation. Therefore, you must add the modifier to the E/M code to get 99386-32 to explain this fact.

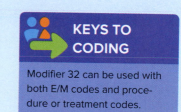

KEYS TO CODING

Modifier 32 can be used with both E/M codes and procedure or treatment codes.

57 **Decision for surgery.** An evaluation and management service that resulted in the initial decision to perform the surgery may be identified by adding modifier 57 to the appropriate level of E/M service.

If a physician meets a patient in order to determine whether the patient should have a surgical procedure and the decision is to go ahead and perform the surgery, then the E/M code should be appended with modifier 57.

LET'S CODE IT! SCENARIO

Dr. Matson referred Gary Matlin, a 35-year-old male, to Dr. Angelli for a consultation to determine whether he needs a prostatectomy. After taking a comprehensive history, performing a comprehensive examination, and reviewing all the previous test results, Dr. Angelli informs Gary that he recommends the procedure. Gary agrees, and they select a date for the surgery to be performed.

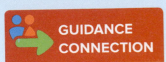

GUIDANCE CONNECTION

Additional explanations can be found in in-section guidelines located within the **Evaluation and Management (E/M)** section, subhead **Newborn Care Services**, directly above code 99460, and subhead **Inpatient Neonatal Intensive Care Services**, directly above code 99466 in the E/M section.

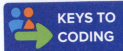

KEYS TO CODING

A newborn is described as a baby aged 28 days old or younger.

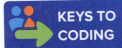

KEYS TO CODING

When a physician sees a newborn at an office visit after seeing the baby initially at the hospital or other birth location, the visit is coded as an established patient visit (as long as it is within 3 years, of course).

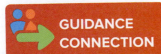

GUIDANCE CONNECTION

Additional explanations can be found in in-section guidelines located within the **Evaluation and Management (E/M)** section, subhead **Initial and Continuing Intensive Care Services**, directly above code 99477 in the E/M section.

Gary met with Dr. Angelli at his office at the request of Dr. Matson for a *consultation*. According to the documentation, Dr. Angelli did a *comprehensive history* and a *comprehensive examination*. His medical decision making was of moderate complexity. This directs you to code 99244. BUT this encounter ended in Gary's decision to have Dr. Angelli perform the surgery. As you learned in Chap. 4, this means there has been a transfer of care in addition to the decision for surgery. Therefore, you must add the modifier 57 to the E/M code for a new patient, office visit: 99204-57.

Newborn and Pediatric Evaluation and Management Care

The E/M for a newborn or child may be performed by a neonatologist, pediatrician, or other physician. This portion of the E/M section is divided into several parts:

Newborn Care Services: 99460–99463

Determining the most accurate code in this subsection will require you to have two essential pieces of information:

- Location: Hospital or birthing center, or other location.
- Initial or subsequent: Was this the first day of care for this newborn or second/additional day of care by this physician for this newborn?

Note that these code descriptions report a day of E/M service, not just history/exam/MDM or even time spent.

Delivery/Birthing Room Attendance and Resuscitation Services: 99464–99465

When requested by the delivering physician (most often the obstetrician), a neonatologist or pediatrician may need to be there in the delivery room to resuscitate and/or stabilize a baby immediately upon his or her birth.

EXAMPLE

Dr. Bryce is a neonatologist. Dr. Opell, an obstetrician, asked Dr. Bryce to be in attendance during the delivery of Cybil Thyme's baby because of a concern over her excessive alcohol consumption during pregnancy. Dr. Bryce was there and stabilized the baby after birth. You would report Dr. Bryce's service with code 99464.

Inpatient Neonatal and Pediatric Critical Care 99468–99476

These services will most often be provided in sections of a hospital known as a neonatal intensive care unit (NICU) or pediatric intensive care unit (PICU), but these codes are not exclusive to those designated areas. The guidelines included in the CPT directly above code 99468 contain a great deal of detail on the specific services that are included in these codes and not reported separately.

Determining the most accurate code in this subsection will require you to have two essential pieces of information:

- Age: Is the patient 28 days or younger, 29 days to 24 months, or 2 to 5 years of age?
- Initial or subsequent: Was this the first day of care for this baby or second/additional day of care by this physician for this newborn?

Note that these code descriptions report a day of E/M service, not just history/exam/MDM or even time spent.

Intensive Care Services—Child: 99477–99480

There is a difference between a patient who is critically ill and one who requires intensive care services, such as intensive observation, cardiac and respiratory monitoring, vital sign monitoring, and other services detailed in the guidelines for this subsection (shown above code 99477).

Determining the most accurate code in this subsection will require you to have two essential pieces of information:

- 99477 reports the initial hospital care for a neonate, 28 days of age or younger, who requires intensive care, as per those services identified in the guidelines.
- Subsequent intensive care codes 99478–99480 are distinguished by the present weight of the neonate.

Note that these code descriptions report a day of E/M service, not just history/exam/MDM or even time spent.

Special Evaluation Services

In cases when a patient is about to have a life insurance or disability certificate issued, the insurer often requires the attending physician to provide an evaluation to establish a baseline of data. The visit does not involve any actual treatment or management of the patient's condition—it accounts for the time to create the appropriate documentation. The codes in range 99450–99456 apply to both new and established patients.

Complex Chronic Care Coordination Services

Patients with chronic illnesses, such as diabetes mellitus or hypertension, need more attention from their health care team. Code 99487 represents the first hour of clinical staff time for complex chronic care coordination directed by a physician or other qualified health care professional with no face-to-face time. Code 99488 is used for a face-to-face visit, and code 99489 is an add-on code for each additional 30 minutes of complex chronic care coordination.

Numerous studies prove that patients with chronic illnesses and conditions benefit from coordinated care across the many disciplines of physicians and other members of the clinical staff in addition to community service agencies. This specific subset of E/M codes focuses on support services and management of care provided to patients who are living in their own homes, domiciliary, rest homes, or assisted living facilities.

These services are provided to patients who

- Require repeated hospital admissions or ED visits.
- Are diagnosed with one or more chronic continuous or episodic medical and/or psychiatric conditions lasting at least 1 year (12 months).
- Are at significant risk of death, acute exacerbation, decompensation, and/or functional decline.
- Require continuing care from multiple health care specialties that need to be coordinated for efficacy and efficiency of medical conditions, psychosocial conditions, and activities of daily living (ADL).
- Require moderate or highly complex medical decision making during treatment.

Physicians and other qualified health care professionals must implement a documented care plan to coordinate multiple disciplines and agencies, which is shared with the patient and/or family or caregiver.

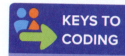

KEYS TO CODING

Be aware of codes 99000–99091 in the Special Services, Procedures and Reports subsection of the Medicine section of CPT—most specifically 99080. Read the notes carefully, as well as the descriptions of the codes, to choose the most accurate.

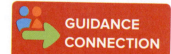

GUIDANCE CONNECTION

Additional explanations can be found in in-section guidelines located within the **Evaluation and Management (E/M)** section, subhead **Complex Chronic Care Coordination Services,** directly above code 99487 in the E/M section.

With all of the services and activities involved with the care of a chronically ill patient, CPT has specifically identified those services characteristically reported by these codes, including

- Developing and maintaining a comprehensive care plan.
- Facilitating access to care and services needed by the patient and/or family.
- Assessing and supporting patient compliance with the treatment plan, including schedule of medication.
- Educating the patient, family, and/or caregiver to enable and support self-management, independent living, and ADL.
- Identifying community and health care resources available to the patient and/or family.
- Communicating with home health agencies and other community services available and used by the patient.
- Communicating aspects of care to the patient, family, and/or caregiver.
- Collecting health outcomes data and registry documentation.

Services identified by codes 99487 and 99488 overlap longstanding E/M codes. Therefore, when reporting 99487 or 99488, do not separately report the following:

- Care plan oversight services (CPT codes 99339, 99340, 99374–99378).
- Prolonged services without direct patient contact (99358, 99359).
- Anticoagulant management (99363, 99364).
- Medical team conferences (99366–99368).
- Education and training (98966–98968, 99441–99443).
- On-line medical evaluation (98969, 99444).
- Preparation of special reports (99080).
- Analysis of data (99090, 99091).
- Transitional care management services (99495, 99496).
- Medication therapy management services (99605–99607).

Codes 99487 and 99488 should not be reported separately, nor should they include the time spent when reporting the following:

- End-stage renal disease services (ESRD) (90951–90970) during the same month.
- Postoperative care services during the global period.
- E/M services (99211–99215, 99334–99337, 99347–99350).
- E/M services while patient is an inpatient or in observation (99217–99239, 99241–99255, 99291–99318).
- Transitional care management services (99495, 99496).

As you can see, either 99487 or 99488 would be reported only once per month by the physician or health care professional who has taken on the role of coordinator for this patient for the first 31 to 75 minutes of services. The difference between the two codes is whether this health care professional participated in a face-to-face encounter with this patient during that month.

Add-on code 99489 can be reported in conjunction with either 99487 or 99488 to represent time greater than 75 minutes during the month.

Transitional Care Management Services

It can be a complex event to transfer the care and management of a patient's ongoing condition from one facility to another, especially when the new location will involve a new care team. Code 99495 (transitional care management services) requires the physician to document the following elements:

- Communication (direct contact, telephone, electronic) with the patient and/or caregiver within 2 business days of discharge.

- Medical decision making of at least moderate complexity during the service period.
- Face-to-face visit within 14 calendar days of discharge.

Code 99496 (transitional care management services) requires the following elements:

- Communication (direct contact, telephone, electronic) with the patient and/or caregiver within 2 business days of discharge.
- Medical decision making of high complexity during the service period.
- Face-to-face visit within 7 calendar days of discharge.

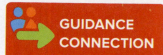

GUIDANCE CONNECTION

Additional explanations can be found in in-section guidelines located within the **Evaluation and Management (E/M)** section, subhead **Transitional Care Management Services**, directly above code 99495 in the E/M section.

Providers are often concerned that patients with multiple medical and/or psychosocial issues may "slip through the cracks" when transferred from inpatient status to the care of an assisted living facility, a domiciliary, or the patient's own home. These two codes provide an effective way to report the provision of these services to an established patient by the physician or other qualified health care professional or licensed clinical staff member under direction of the physician.

Transitional care management (TCM) includes one episode of face-to-face contact along with non–face-to-face services provided by the physician and clinical staff. The period of TCM service begins on the date of discharge and runs for 29 consecutive days.

Within 48 hours (2 days) after discharge, the first TCM interactive contact between the reporting physician and the patient must occur. This contact may be face-to-face, over the telephone, or by use of electronic communication. The contact must encompass the professional's ability to promptly act upon patient needs and go beyond simply scheduling follow-up care.

When the provider documents two or more attempts contact within the prescribed time period and is unable to connect with the patient, family, and/or caregiver, the provider may still report TCM services as long as the other transitional care management criteria have been met.

Reporting either of the two TCM codes requires at least one face-to-face visit, as well as reconciliation of prescribed medication, with the patient. For patients requiring highly complex medical decision-making services, the provider must meet with the patient face-to-face within the first 7 calendar days after the patient is discharged from inpatient status.

For patients requiring a moderate level of medical decision making, the first face-to-face visit must occur during the first 14 calendar days of discharge. This first patient contact is included in the TCM code and not reported separately. However, any additional E/M services provided afterwards may be reported with a separate E/M code accordingly.

The CPT guidelines include specific services by the physician or other health care professional included in TCM, as well as services provided by clinical staff under the direction of that physician.

Services provided by the physician or other qualified health care professional include

- Obtaining and reviewing the discharge information.
- Reviewing the need for or follow-up on pending diagnostic tests and treatments.
- Educating the patient, family, and/or caregiver.
- Establishing (or reestablishing) referrals.
- Arranging for required community resources.
- Assisting in scheduling any required follow-up with community providers and services.
- Interacting with other qualified health care professionals who will assume (or reassume) care of the patient's system-specific problems.

Services provided by clinical staff under the direction of the physician include

- Communicating about various aspects of care with the patient, family, caregiver, and/or other professionals.
- Identifying available community and health resources.

- Assessing and supporting compliance with the treatment plan, including medication management.
- Communicating with home health agencies and other community services used by the patient.
- Educating the patient, family, and/or caregiver to support self-management, independent living, and ADL.
- Facilitating access to care and services required by the patient, family, and/or caregiver.

When reporting 99495 or 99496, do *not* separately report the following

- Care plan oversight services (CPT codes 99339, 99340, 99374–99380).
- Prolonged services without direct patient contact (99358, 99359).
- Anticoagulant management (99363, 99364).
- Medical team conferences (99366–99368).
- Education and training (98960–98962, 99071, 99078).
- Telephone services (98966–98968, 99441–99443).
- ESRD services (90951–90970).
- On-line medical evaluation (98969, 99444).
- Preparation of special reports (99080).
- Analysis of data (99090, 99091).
- Complex chronic care coordination services (99487–99489).
- Medication therapy management services (99605–99607).

KEYS TO CODING

ESRD stands for end-stage renal disease.

TCM may be reported only once within 30 days of discharge by only one health care professional, even if there is a subsequent discharge within that time. This professional is permitted to report hospital or observation discharge services concurrently with TCM services, but not within the global period of postoperative care.

Chapter Summary

In this chapter you learned that, for the key components of coding for services rendered in a nursing home, a long-term care facility, or the patient's home, you use a different set of codes from those reporting physician services in an office or a hospital.

Understand that the elements of the distinct types of encounters, such as annual physicals (preventive medical assessments) and case management services, also use varying sets of parameters.

Your job as a professional coding specialist is to understand the variety of essentials involved in coding E/M services properly and to report those services accurately.

CHAPTER **5** REVIEW
Evaluation and Management Codes, Part 2

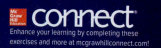
Enhance your learning by completing these
exercises and more at mcgrawhillconnect.com!

Using Terminology

Match each key term to the appropriate definition.

_____ **1.** LO 5.5 A group of services already included in the code for the operation and not reported separately.

_____ **2.** LO 5.1 Action taken by the attending physician to stop or reduce a behavior or lifestyle that is predicted to have a negative effect on the individual's health.

_____ **3.** LO 5.2 An organization that provides services to terminally ill patients and their families.

_____ **4.** LO 5.2 Services that include washing/bathing, dressing and undressing, assistance in taking medications, and getting in and out of bed.

_____ **5.** LO 5.1 A type of action or service that stops something from happening or from getting worse.

_____ **6.** LO 5.2 A facility that provides skilled nursing treatment and attention along with limited medical care for its (usually long-term) residents, who do not require acute care services (hospitalization).

_____ **7.** LO 5.2 The time measured between one point and another, such as between physician visits.

_____ **8.** LO 5.3 Services for a patient who has a life-threatening condition expected to worsen.

_____ **9.** LO 5.2 E/M of a patient, reported in 30-day periods, including infrequent supervision along with pre-encounter and post-encounter work, such as reading test results and assessment of notes.

_____ **10.** LO 5.1 Recommendations for behavior modification and/or other preventive measures.

A. Anticipatory guidance
B. Basic personal services
C. Care plan oversight services
D. Critical care services
E. Global surgery package
F. Hospice
G. Interval
H. Nursing home
I. Preventive
J. Risk factor reduction intervention

Checking Your Understanding

Choose the most appropriate answer for each of the following questions.

1. LO 5.1 A preventive medical E/M encounter may include any of these services *except*

   a. counseling.
   b. admission into the hospital.
   c. anticipatory guidance.
   d. risk factor reduction intervention.

2. LO 5.1 If the physician finds a health concern during a preventive medicine examination requiring additional E/M services and the extra service is performed by the same physician on the same day, then the extra service should be coded with

   a. the preventive medicine code only.
   b. the additional E/M code.
   c. whichever code is reimbursable at a higher rate.
   d. a separate E/M code appended with modifier 25.

3. LO 5.2 E/M services provided to a patient in an assisted living facility are reported from the subsection

   a. Nursing Facility.
   b. Home Services.
   c. Domiciliary, Rest Homes, and Custodial Care Settings.
   d. Care Plan Oversight Services.

4. LO 5.2 If a patient is discharged from the hospital and admitted into an SNF on the same day by the same physician, report the E/M services with

   a. an admission to the nursing facility E/M code only.
   b. a hospital discharge code and an admission to the nursing facility code.
   c. one outpatient E/M services code.
   d. a subsequent nursing facility E/M code.

5. LO 5.2 Care plan oversight services provided for a patient in a hospice setting are coded from the

   a. 99339–99340 range.
   b. 99374–99375 range.
   c. 99377–99378 range.
   d. 99379–99380 range.

6. LO 5.2 Mary Suppano goes to Dr. Wisabbi's office for an appointment. After a full history, an exam, and comprehensive MDM, Dr. Wisabbi recommends that she be admitted into a psychiatric residential treatment center. He takes her over and admits her into the facility that afternoon. You will code the E/M services with

   a. one office visit code.
   b. an admission to nursing facility code.
   c. both an office visit code and an admission to nursing facility code.
   d. a domiciliary, rest home, custodial care center code only.

7. LO 5.3 Jacob Brassman, a 3-day-old male, was admitted into the NICU for complications of his low birthweight status. Dr. Dakota saw him yesterday and is in again today. You will code today's E/M services from the

   a. 99468–99469 range.
   b. 99478–99479 range.
   c. 99307–99310 range.
   d. 99210–99215 range.

8. LO 5.3 Critical care codes are determined by

   a. length of time.
   b. inpatient or outpatient status.
   c. level of history, exam, and MDM.
   d. new or established patient.

9. LO 5.4 Conferencing with other health care professionals regarding management and/or treatment of a patient is

   a. included in all E/M codes.
   b. coded as a consultation E/M code.
   c. coded from 99366–99368.
   d. coded from 99201–99205.

10. LO 5.6 A modifier

   a. explains an unusual circumstance.
   b. has five digits.
   c. begins with the letter *M*.
   d. explains how a patient became injured.

Applying Your Knowledge

1. LO 5.1 Explain anticipatory guidelines. _____

_____

2. LO 5.2 What is a nursing home? _____

_____

3. LO 5.2 What is considered part of basic personal services? _____

_____

4. LO 5.3 List three of the most common places where critical care services are provided. _____

_____

5. LO 5.4 Explain case management terms/services. _____

_____

6. LO 5.5 Explain a global surgery package. _____

_____

7. LO 5.6 What are mandated services, and how are they identified on a claim? _____

_____

8. LO 5.6 What modifier is appended when the patient makes a decision for surgery? _____

_____

9. LO 5.6 What code range identifies intensive care services: child? _____

_____

10. LO 5.6 When transferring care and management of a patient to another facility, code 99495 requires the physician to document what elements? _____

_____

Using the techniques described in this chapter, carefully read through the case studies and determine the most accurate E/M code(s) and modifier(s), if appropriate, for each case study.

1. Dr. Anthony spends approximately 1 hour on a conference call talking with an oncologist in Texas and a reconstructive specialist in California. The three professionals discuss treatments and options for Zena Johnson, a 37-year-old female, who was recently diagnosed with parosteal osteogenic sarcoma. This one could be a little tricky, since consultations can be billed as well. Code the conference call.

   _____

2. Frank Childers, a 72-year-old male in good health, came to see his regular family physician, Dr. Rappoport, for his yearly physical exam.

   _____

3. Premier Life & Health Insurance Company required Tom Cavellini, a 31-year-old male, to get Dr. Louisman, his regular physician, to complete a certificate confirming that Tom's current disability prevents him from working at his regular job and makes him eligible for disability insurance.

   _____

4. Oscar Unger, a 27-year-old male, goes to his family physician, Dr. Carter, for a tetanus shot after stepping on a rusty nail at the beach. While there, he asks Dr. Carter to look at a cut on his left hand. Dr. Carter examines the wound and tells him to keep the wound clean and bandaged. Dr. Carter documents a problem-focused history and exam and straightforward MDM. Code only the E/M.

   _____

5. Catalina King, a 15-month-old female, is admitted today by Dr. Ervin into the pediatric critical care unit because of severe respiratory distress.

   _____

6. Dr. Lunden spent 2½ hours evaluating Byron Curtis upon his admission into the ICU.

   _____

7. Owen Stabler has been living in the Barton Nursing Center for the last 12 months. Dr. Gilman comes in to do his annual assessment, including a detailed interval history, comprehensive exam, and MDM of moderate complexity.

   _____

8. Howard Shires moved into the Barton Assisted Living Center today. Dr. Bowyer, the center's resident physician, introduced himself to Howard and then took a detailed history, performed a comprehensive examination, and found the MDM to be moderate.

_____

9. Reisa Haven is at home recuperating from surgery on her left hip with the help of Barton Home Health Services. Her attending physician, Dr. Alfaya, comes to her house do a problem-focused interval history and exam. MDM is straightforward.

_____

10. David Magruder was discharged today from the Barton Nursing Center after Dr. Fanelli spent 25 minutes performing a final examination, discussing David's stay, and providing instructions to David's wife for continuing care.

_____

11. Dr. Servina provided care plan oversight services for Raymond Johnston, one of her patients at the Barton Assisted Living Center. It took her 20 minutes.

_____

12. Ronald Lassier, an 18-year-old male, is the son of two alcoholics. Dr. Foller spends 40 minutes with him providing risk factor reduction behavior modification techniques to help him avoid becoming an alcoholic himself.

_____

13. Makayla Sorensen, a 3-day-old female, currently weighs 2,000 grams and requires intensive cardiac and respiratory monitoring. This is her third day in the NICU, and Dr. Pitassin comes in to do his E/M of her condition.

_____

14. Dr. Dodge works in a very small town in Ohio and travels up to 200 miles to see his patients in the surrounding rural areas. His patient, Sarah Matthews, gave birth at her home the previous day to a 6-lb, 3-oz baby girl, Amelia Rose. Dr. Dodge sees Amelia Rose for the first time today, does a complete history and exam, and prepares her medical chart. Amelia Rose is a healthy newborn.

_____

15. George Terazzo's legs have finally healed to the point that he can be discharged from the nursing facility, where he has been for the last 6 weeks. Before he can go home, Dr. Horatio comes in for the final examination and to provide continuing care instructions to George's wife, who will be caring for George at home. Dr. Horatio prepares the discharge records and gives a prescription to George for pain medication. This whole process takes Dr. Horatio about 45 minutes to complete.

_____

The following exercises provide practice in the application of abstracting the physicians' notes and learning to work with SOAP notes from our health care facility, Cipher, Victors & Associates. These case studies (SOAP notes) are modeled on real patient encounters. Using the techniques described in this chapter, carefully read through the case studies and determine the most accurate E/M code(s) and modifier(s), if appropriate, for each case study.

CIPHER, VICTORS & ASSOCIATES
A Complete Health Care Facility
234 MAIN STREET • ANYTOWN, FL 32711 • 407-555-1234

PATIENT: CHERONE, SALENE
ACCOUNT/EHR #:   CHERSA001
DATE: 10/17/18

Attending Physician: Valerie R. Victors, MD

S: This 53-year-old female came for her routine physical exam. Pt does not smoke, drinks alcohol occasionally, and exercises three times per week. Pt states she has no specific health concerns at this time.

O: Ht 5′3″ Wt 145 lb. R 20. HEENT: unremarkable; Respiratory: unremarkable; Musculoskeletal: age appropriate. No sign of osteoporosis. Bone density appropriate. Discussed the importance of keeping up her exercise regimen.

A: Pt is in good health.

P: 1. Follow-up prn
    2. Schedule blood work: comprehensive metabolic panel
    3. Schedule screening mammogram

Valerie R. Victors, MD

VRV/mg   D: 10/17/18 09:50:16   T: 10/23/18 12:55:01

Determine the most accurate E/M code(s) and modifier(s), if appropriate.

_____

_____

_____

CIPHER, VICTORS & ASSOCIATES
A Complete Health Care Facility
234 MAIN STREET • ANYTOWN, FL 32711 • 407-555-1234

PATIENT: MCTRAVIS, COLIN
ACCOUNT/EHR #:   MCTRCO001
DATE: 10/25/18

Attending Physician: Valerie R. Victors, MD

S: This 85-year-old male is seen this day at Barton Assisted Living Center, where he has been living for the last 6 months. The last time I saw this patient was right before he moved into the center. Nurse Thomas states that he has been complaining of mild abdominal pain and some discomfort upon urination. Other than this issue, he has been well and stable.

O: Ht 5'2.5". Wt 145 lb. R 18. Abdomen is unremarkable. No masses or rigidity noted.

A: Suspected bladder infection

P: Order written for UA to rule out bladder infection.

_____

Valerie R. Victors, MD

VRV/mg   D: 10/25/18 09:50:16   T: 10/28/18 12:55:01

Determine the most accurate E/M code(s) and modifier(s), if appropriate.

_____

_____

_____

CIPHER, VICTORS & ASSOCIATES
A Complete Health Care Facility
234 MAIN STREET • ANYTOWN, FL 32711 • 407-555-1234

PATIENT: PALLER, ELLYN
ACCOUNT/EHR #:   PALLEL001
DATE: 11/21/18

Attending Physician: Valerie R. Victors, MD

S: This 41-year-old female is seen at her home, where she is on complete bed rest due to complications of her pregnancy. She has hypertension and gestational diabetes. She is at 27 weeks gestation. She states that she has had no problems since my last visit 6 days ago. She states that she has had no instances of lightheadedness and has had no sense of weakness.

O: Ht 5′5″. Wt 151 lb. R 22. G1 P0. Abdomen is unremarkable. No masses or rigidity noted. B/P 140/97, nonfasting glucose stick 110.

A: Patient improving nicely

P: 1. Continue bed rest
    2. Revisit 1 week

Valerie R. Victors, MD

VRV/mg   D: 11/21/18 09:50:16   T: 11/23/18 12:55:01

Determine the most accurate E/M code(s) and modifier(s), if appropriate.

_____

_____

_____

CIPHER, VICTORS & ASSOCIATES
A Complete Health Care Facility
234 MAIN STREET • ANYTOWN, FL 32711 • 407-555-1234

PATIENT: JACOBS, LEAH
ACCOUNT/EHR #:   JACOLE001
DATE: 10/01/18

Attending Physician: Valerie R. Victors, MD

This 17-month-old female is being admitted to the pediatric critical care unit today. Mother claims that onset of symptoms was sudden. She states that she rushed the child to the ED immediately.
    Respiration is shallow. Child is unresponsive. PERL. B/P low. T 102.
    Complete blood workup ordered: CBC with diff, tox screen, bilirubin, and basic metabolic panel.
    IV fluids to keep hydrated.
    Await test results.

_____

Valerie R. Victors, MD

VRV/mg   D: 10/01/18 09:50:16   T: 10/03/18 12:55:01

Determine the most accurate E/M code(s) and modifier(s), if appropriate.

_____

_____

_____

CIPHER, VICTORS & ASSOCIATES
A Complete Health Care Facility
234 MAIN STREET • ANYTOWN, FL 32711 • 407-555-1234

PATIENT: GORMANN, BLAISE
ACCOUNT/EHR #:   GOREBL001
DATE: 11/15/18

Attending Physician: Valerie R. Victors, MD

Infant was born this morning at 0710 to a healthy 27-year-old female in the delivery room of Barton Hospital.
   Full examination of normal newborn; perinatal history; complete notes in medical record created for baby.
   Baby discharged home today 16:30.
   Office visit follow-up 10 days.

Valerie R. Victors, MD

VRV/mg   D: 11/15/18 09:50:16   T: 11/17/18 12:55:01

Determine the most accurate E/M code(s) and modifier(s), if appropriate.

_____

_____

_____

ANESTHESIA CODING

6

The procedure codes for identifying the administration of anesthetics are in the second section of the main part of the CPT book, directly after evaluation and management (E/M) codes. The anesthesiology codes range from 00100 to 01999 and 99100 to 99140.

As a professional coder, you will typically use codes from this section only if you work for an anesthesiologist, in his or her office, or for a billing company that codes and files claims for **anesthesiologists.** Generally, anesthesiologists have their own practices. While almost all their services occur in a hospital or an ambulatory surgical center setting, they are not employees of the hospital, and they must submit their own claim forms to the insurance carrier for their services.

LO 6.1 Types of Anesthesia

Anesthesia is defined as the suppression of nerve sensations to relieve or prevent the feeling of pain, usually by the use of pharmaceuticals. Essentially, it is more commonly described as the administration of drugs to enable a patient to avoid the feeling of pain. While there are many types of anesthesia, they are all primarily divided into three preliminary categories: topical/local, regional, and general.

1. Topical and/or local anesthesia. **Topical anesthesia** refers to the numbing of surface nerves, whereas **local anesthesia** refers to the dulling of feeling in a limited area of the body.

EXAMPLE

Dr. Dentmann, a general dentist, rubbed a *topical anesthetic* onto Bernard's gum to prevent him from feeling any pain from the injection of the *local anesthetic.* The local anesthetic will prevent him from feeling pain while the doctor drills the cavity that Bernard has in his left, lower molar.

Key Terms

Anesthesia

Anesthesiologists

Certified registered nurse anesthetist (CRNA)

Conscious sedation

General anesthesia

Local anesthesia

Monitored anesthesia care (MAC)

Regional anesthesia

Topical anesthesia

anesthesiologists
Physicians specializing in the administration of anesthesia.

anesthesia
The loss of sensation, with or without consciousness, generally induced by the administration of a particular drug.

topical anesthesia
The application of a drug to the skin to reduce or prevent sensation in a specific area temporarily.

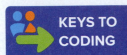
KEYS TO CODING

Topical: Think *top* for the top layer.

local anesthesia
The injection of a drug to prevent sensation in a specific portion of the body; includes local infiltration anesthesia, digital blocks, and pudendal blocks.

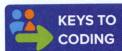
KEYS TO CODING

Local: The effect of the anesthesia stays close to the injection site.

regional anesthesia
The administration of a drug in order to interrupt the nerve impulses without loss of consciousness.

general anesthesia
The administration of a drug in order to induce a loss of consciousness in the patient, who is unable to be aroused even by painful stimulation.

conscious sedation
The use of a drug to reduce stress and/or anxiety.

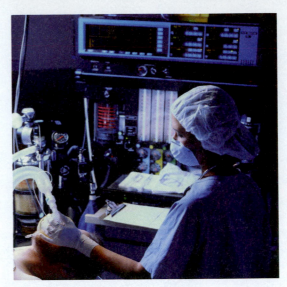

2. **Regional anesthesia.** Regional anesthesia prevents a section of the body from transmitting pain and includes epidural, caudal, spinal, axillary, stellate ganglion blocks, regional blocks, and brachial anesthesia.

EXAMPLE

Dr. Siestaman, an anesthesiologist, was paged to come to the maternity ward to administer *epidural anesthesia* for Robyn Caldwell. After the epidural was given, Robyn was able to proceed with the birth of her baby without the pain of childbirth. The loss of sensation was only from the waist down. She was otherwise awake and alert.

3. **General anesthesia.** Also called *surgical anesthesia,* general anesthesia creates a total loss of consciousness and sensation. General anesthesia is given to the patient by inhalation, intravenous (IV) injection, or, on rare occasions, intramuscular (IM) injection.

EXAMPLE

Dr. Jacobs, an anesthesiologist, administered *general anesthesia* to Jamal Johnson after he was brought into the operating room (OR) and positioned on the table. Dr. Haverhill was preparing to remove Jamal's gallbladder because of the collection of stones in that organ, and everyone wanted to be certain that Jamal would not feel anything during the surgical procedure.

One additional type of anesthesia that you should know about when coding anesthetic and surgical services is called **conscious sedation.** It is a form of ultralight general anesthesia because it affects the entire body.

With conscious sedation, the physician gives the patient medication to reduce anxiety and stress. The patient remains awake and aware of his or her surroundings and what is going on. He or she can answer questions and respond to verbal commands.

Most often, conscious sedation is used for procedures that will not typically cause pain but may be worrisome to patients, causing them to be nervous and frightened. The services of an anesthesiologist are not required for the provision of conscious sedation, so the physician performing the procedure, or a member of the nursing staff, may administer this before the patient goes into the procedure room. This is one of the reasons the codes for this service are not found in the Anesthesia section of CPT, but in the Medicine section.

LET'S CODE IT! SCENARIO

*Eunice Harrah, a 37-year-old female, came into Dr. Mancini's office to have a hemorrhoidopexy by stapling. She was very nervous because she had never had this procedure before. Dr. Mancini gave Eunice an IV of Versed, a sedative to relieve her anxiety. The procedure is not really painful, so there was no need for a full anesthetic or painkiller. Raymond Elvers, a **certified registered nurse anesthetist (CRNA),** sat with Eunice throughout the procedure to ensure her safety and comfort level. Dr. Mancini accomplished the procedure in one stage, taking 30 minutes.*

certified registered nurse anesthetist (CRNA)
A registered nurse (RN) who has taken additional, specialized training in the administration of anesthesia.

Let's Code It!

Dr. Mancini administered Versed, a mild "sedative," to Eunice before the procedure. When you look at the procedure code for a *"hemorrhoidopexy by stapling"* (46947), you will notice that there is no symbol ⊙ next to the code. The absence of this symbol indicates that conscious sedation is not already included and must be coded separately. Let's go to the alphabetic index and find *conscious sedation.*

Note that the CPT book tells you to *see Sedation.* Under *Sedation,* you find

Moderate	**99143–99150**
With independent observation	**99143–99145**

When you read the complete description of these codes in the numerical section of the CPT book, you will see that code 99144 is the most accurate. This identifies *moderate sedation, administered by the same physician who performed the procedure* (Dr. Mancini), *and includes the presence of an independent trained observer* (Raymond Elvers, CRNA) *to monitor the patient, age 5 years or older, first 30 minutes intra-service.* So in addition to the code for the *hemorrhoidopexy* (46947), you need to include the code for the *conscious sedation* (99144) on the report and claim form.

In some instances, when conscious sedation is administered, health care professionals prefer that an anesthesiologist be present and monitoring the patient's vital signs throughout the procedure. This is referred to as **monitored anesthesia care (MAC).** Code MAC services from the main anesthesia code section 00100–01999.

LO 6.2 Coding Anesthesia Services

When coding anesthetic services, you should follow these steps to find the best, most appropriate code.

1. *Confirm* that the physician who performed the procedure for which the anesthesia is necessary is a different professional from the person who administered the anesthesia.

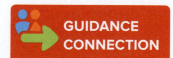

GUIDANCE CONNECTION

Additional explanations can be found in in-section guidelines located within the **Medicine** section, subhead **Moderate (Conscious) Sedation,** directly above code 99143 in the E/M section.

monitored anesthesia care (MAC)
The administration of sedatives, anesthetic agents, or other medications to relax but not render the patient unconscious while under the constant observation of a trained anesthesiologist; also known as "twilight" sedation.

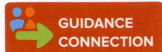

On those occasions when the same physician who performs the procedure also administers regional or general anesthesia, you must append modifier 47 Anesthesia by Surgeon to the appropriate procedure code. The modifier is not attached to an anesthesia procedure code; it is added to the basic procedure code. No additional code from the Anesthesia section will be used.

2. *Identify* the anatomical site of the patient's body upon which the surgical procedure was performed.

3. *Confirm* the exact surgical procedure performed, as documented in the physician's notes.

4. *Consult* the alphabetic index of the CPT book, look under the heading of Anesthesia, and read down the list to find the anatomical site shown below that heading. Identify the suggested code or codes for this site.

EXAMPLE

Anesthesia
Skull 00190

5. *Turn* to the numerical portion of the CPT book, Anesthesia section, and find the subsection identifying that anatomical site.

EXAMPLE

00190 Anesthesia for procedures on facial bones or skull; not otherwise specified

00192   radical surgery (including prognathism)

6. *Read* the descriptions written next to each code option suggested in the alphabetic index carefully. Then compare them with the terms used by the physician in his or her notes documenting the procedure. This will lead you to the best, most appropriate code available.

LET'S CODE IT! SCENARIO

Dr. Jacobs is called in to administer general anesthesia to Miriam Delveccio, a 6-month-old female, diagnosed with congenital tracheal stenosis. Dr. Quartermain performs a surgical repair of her trachea.

Let's Code It!

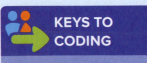

The notes indicate that Dr. Jacobs administered the anesthesia and Dr. Quartermain performed a "surgical repair of her trachea." Remember, this means that an anesthesia code will be used, not a modifier appended to the procedure code. So let's go ahead and find the best code for the anesthesia service.

Turn to the alphabetic index and look up *anesthesia*. Going down the alphabetic listing of the sites beneath this heading, look for more than a page until you get to the correct anatomical site: *Trachea*.

Trachea   00320, 00326, 00542
Reconstruction 00539

The physician's notes state that Dr. Quartermain performed a *"repair,"* not a reconstruction, so focus on the codes shown next to *Trachea*. Turn to the numerical listings of the CPT book to find the codes: 00320, 00326, and 00542. Read the descriptions written next to each code, as well as the others found in the subsection, in order to determine the best, most appropriate code available.

Neck

00320 Anesthesia for all procedures on esophagus, thyroid, larynx, trachea and lymphatic system of neck; not otherwise specified, age 1 year or older

00322 Anesthesia for all procedures on esophagus, thyroid, larynx, trachea and lymphatic system of neck; needle biopsy of thyroid

00326 Anesthesia for all procedures on the larynx and trachea in children less than 1 year of age

00542 Anesthesia for thoracotomy procedures involving lungs, pleura, diaphragm, and mediastinum (including surgical thoracoscopy); decortication

As you review the code descriptions, you can identify which terms or words are most important in matching the code to the physician's documentation of the procedure. Look at the physician's notes one more time and identify the key terms.

Dr. Jacobs is called in to administer *general anesthesia* to Miriam Delveccio, a *6-month-old* female *diagnosed with congenital tracheal stenosis*. Dr. Quartermain performs *a surgical repair* of her trachea.

The combination of all these terms matches only one of our available code descriptions, doesn't it?

00326 <u>Anesthesia</u> for all procedures on the larynx and <u>trachea</u> in children <u>younger than 1 year</u> of age

You found the best, most appropriate code for the administration of general anesthesia for Miriam Delveccio's surgery.

Anesthesia Guidelines

The official guidelines specifically intended for coding anesthesia services (general and regional anesthesia) are shown at length on the pages at the beginning of the Anesthesia section of the CPT book. Go through these guidelines and review how they might help you determine the best, most appropriate anesthesia code.

All the codes within the Anesthesia section of the CPT book include activities that are most often performed by anesthesiologists when they are preparing to administer anesthesia to a patient. The following services are included in the *anesthesia code package* and are not coded separately.

1. *Usual preoperative visits.* Most of the time, the anesthesiologist will stop in to interview the patient, in addition to taking the time to thoroughly read the chart and patient history, before administering the anesthesia. It gives the physician the opportunity to discuss any potential reactions or other considerations with the patient.

2. *Anesthesia care during the procedure.* The time and expertise the anesthesiologist uses not only to administer the actual anesthetic but also to observe the patient throughout the procedure are very important parts of his or her job responsibilities.

3. *Administration of fluids.* The anesthesiologist gives the patient fluids, as well as analgesics (liquid form), as needed during the procedure.

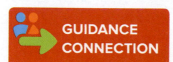

GUIDANCE CONNECTION

Additional explanations can be found in the **Anesthesia** guidelines in your CPT book directly in front of the **Anesthesia** section.

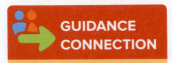
4. *Usual monitoring services* (such as ECG [electrocardiogram], temperature, BP [blood pressure]). As a part of the natural course of the anesthesiologist's duties, he or she must monitor the patient's vital signs throughout the procedure and make certain that there are no unexpected effects from the anesthesia.

5. *Usual postoperative visits.* The anesthesiologist normally visits the patient while he or she is in recovery to ensure that there are no lingering affects of the anesthesia and there are no other concerns as a result of the anesthesia.

When multiple procedures are performed during the same operative session, the anesthesia should be coded for the most complicated procedure only.

LO 6.3 Time Reporting

Time reporting may be used for billing general anesthesia services in certain areas or by certain third-party payers instead of CPT codes. If this is the custom in your local area, the clock begins when the anesthesiologist starts to prepare the patient for the administration of the anesthetic drug in the OR and is typically measured in 15-minute increments. The time ends when the anesthesiologist is no longer required to be present, once the patient has been safely transferred to postoperative supervision. When multiple procedures are completed during the same operative session, the time calculated should be the total time for all the procedures performed. A formula is used to calculate the amount of compensation the anesthesiologist will receive. The formula is

$$\text{Compensation} = (B + T + M) \times CF$$

where B = base unit
T = time spent by the anesthesiologist with the patient
M = modifying factors
CF = conversion factor

The base unit is assigned by the American Society of Anesthesiologists (ASA), as published in the annual *Relative Value Guide.* The unit includes reimbursement for the usual time and services performed by the anesthesiologist preoperatively and postoperatively. Modifying factors are any adjustments made to allow for the additional challenges presented by the physical status of the patient at the time anesthesia is administered. The conversion factor is the number used to translate units into dollars.

Figure 6-1 is an example of an anesthesiologist's sedation record showing the time log of service.

LO 6.4 Qualifying Circumstances

Sometimes special circumstances, also called qualifying circumstances, cause the anesthetic process to be more complicated than usual. In these cases, a second—or add-on—code is used to identify that circumstance.

The available add-on codes for qualifying circumstances are

+99100 Patient of extreme age . . . younger than 1 year or older than 70 years. This add-on code is not to be used when the code description already includes an age definition, such as code 00326, 00834, or 00836.

+99116 Anesthesia complicated by total body hypothermia. Hypothermia is defined as *extremely low body temperature,* below 36.1°C (97°F). Because monitoring vital signs, including body temperature, is an important part of the anesthesia process, a very low body temperature would make the safe administration of anesthesia more complex.

+99135 Anesthesia complicated by controlled hypotension. Hypotension is defined as *abnormally low blood pressure.* The critical connection between blood pressure and heart rate makes this situation very intricate for the anesthesiologist.

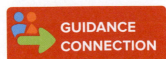

Monitoring	Time	*Level of Sedation	Pulse	Resp	B/P	O2 sat	**Skin	ecg/rhythm as ordered	Medications
Pre Sedation	1300	I	51	17	142/43	98	WD	SR	
During Sedation Procedure	1400	I	61	18	149/72	92	WD	SR	Demerol 25 mg Versed 2
	1403	II	66	17	109/53	97	WD	SR	TEE Probe In
	1406	II	70	19	156/64	100	WD	SR	
	1409	II	72	18	154/71	100	WD	SR	
	1412	II	73	18	146/46	100	WD	SR	10cc NSXI contrast
	1415	II	72	18	152/45	100	WD	SR	TEE done
Post Sedation	1420	I	59	18	153/59	97	WD	SR	
	1425	I	57	18	143/58	96	WD	SR	
	1430	I	56	15	124/5	96	WD	SB	
	1435	I	5	16	115/48	96	WD	SR	

Notify physician immediately if any symptomatic change in heart rate, resp status or O2 sat. < 92%
(if patient had a baseline O2 sat < 92% physician must set acceptable post sedation O2 sat. level)

**Skin   W/D = Warm/Dry, D = Diaphoretic, C - Cool   Color   1 - Pink 2 - Pale 3 - Cyanotic 4 - Mottled

Level 1 Awake, verbalizes, cooperative	Observe & record Q 15 min: level of sedation.
Level 2 Drowsy but awake, eyes closed or open, verbalizes	Observe & record Q 15 min: level of sedation, cont pulse ox, resp, pulse, BP.
Level 3 Eyes closed, mimics sleep, arouses with minimal to moderate stimulation.	Continuous observation. Record Q5 min: Level of sedation, cont pulse oximeter, resp, pulse, BP.
Level 4 Sleep, arousable with moderate to intense stimulation May have potential for loss of protective reflexes.	Continuous observation. Record Q5 min: Level of sedation, cont Level of sedation, cont pulse oximeter, resp, pulse, BP.

* CAUTION: Asleep and nonarousable, temporary loss of protective reflexes: patient has progressed beyond Level IV and now falls under the guidelines of anesthesia.

NARRATIVE NOTES   NPO until 1700; check gag reflex before feed. Pt. tol. well. No c/o of sore throat, pt alert x3, trans to room. Report given to

Signature: _Philomena Nobler_   RN

FIGURE 6-1 Anesthesiologist's Sedation Record

+99140 Anesthesia complicated by emergency conditions. An emergency is characterized as a situation in which the patient's life, or an individual body part, would be threatened if there were any delay in providing treatment. In such a case, the anesthesiologist may not have the time to get the patient history or other information necessary to do his or her job most efficiently or effectively.

LO 6.5 Moderate (Conscious) Sedation

Codes 99143–99150 report the administration of moderate (conscious) sedation and include

- Assessing the patient.
- Establishing IV access and fluids to maintain patency, when performed.
- Administration of the drug.
- Maintaining the sedated level.
- Monitoring oxygen saturation, heart rate, and blood pressure.
- Observation and assessment during recovery.

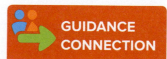

GUIDANCE CONNECTION

Additional explanations can be found in in-section guidelines located within the **Medicine** section, subhead **Moderate (Conscious) Sedation**, directly above code 99143 in the E/M section.

Coding for the administration of conscious sedation also has a few guidelines to help you determine the best, most appropriate code:

1. If the physician performing the procedure also administers the conscious sedation, use a code from the 99143–99145 range (located in the Medicine section of the CPT book).

2. If conscious sedation is administered by a physician other than the physician performing a procedure listed in Appendix G, in a facility (hospital, ambulatory surgical center, or skilled nursing facility), use the appropriate code(s) from 99148–99150. However, if this second professional provides the service in a physician's office or freestanding imaging center, the conscious sedation service is not separately reported. If a procedure is performed but not listed in Appendix G and a second physician administers conscious sedation, use the appropriate code from the main anesthesia section, 00100–01999.

3. Note that some CPT codes already include the administration of conscious sedation in the procedure code. In such cases, you are not permitted to use a separate sedation code. The CPT codes that include conscious sedation are identified in the numerical listing of the CPT book with the symbol ⊙ (a circle with a dot in the center) in front of the code and are listed in Appendix G.

4. The time spent with the patient under conscious sedation determines the correct code or codes. Intraservice time is measured in an initial 30-minute segment, followed by 15-minute segments. The clock starts when the physician administers the sedative and stops when the patient is discharged and the physician is no longer required to supervise the patient. Total time is calculated only for the minutes the physician continuously spends face-to-face with the patient.

EXAMPLES

⊙ 33010 Pericardiocentesis; initial

⊙ 92953 Temporary transcutaneous pacing

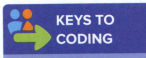

KEYS TO CODING

Read the entire description of modifier 23 in your CPT book, Appendix A.

Unusual Anesthesia

Unusual circumstances might require the administration of general anesthesia for a procedure that typically requires either local anesthesia or no anesthesia. In these cases, the modifier 23 Unusual Anesthesia must be appended to the procedure code for that basic service (not to the anesthesia code); you will not assign a code from the Anesthesia section of CPT.

LET'S CODE IT! SCENARIO

Margaret Cabaña, a 68-year-old female, arrived for the insertion of a permanent pacemaker, atrial with transvenous electrodes. Dr. Fowler noticed that Margaret has been diagnosed with Parkinson's disease, causing her to have uncontrollable tremors. Dr. Fowler decided that conscious sedation (which is included with the procedure code) was insufficient to ensure the patient's safety. He believed that general anesthesia would be more appropriate and administered the anesthesia himself.

Let's Code It!

Dr. Fowler decided that Margaret needed general anesthesia for this procedure, even though it is not the standard, because her Parkinson's disease made the procedure unsafe without it. He was inserting *a permanent pacemaker, atrial with transvenous electrodes.*

The alphabetic index shows

Insertion

Pacemaker

Fluoroscopy/Radiography 71090

Heart   33206–33208, 33212–33213

Look through the descriptions for the codes in the first range, 33200–33208. Do any of the descriptions match the notes?

⊙ **33206 Insertion or replacement of permanent pacemaker with transvenous electrode(s); atrial**

Before you move on to the next section, remember that Dr. Fowler administered general anesthesia. You can tell from the symbol ⊙ next to procedure code 33206 that conscious sedation is included with the code. It indicates that general anesthesia is unusual. How will you ensure Dr. Fowler gets reimbursed for the administration of the anesthesia? This is what modifiers do—identify unusual circumstances. Modifier 23 is specifically for a case when unusual anesthesia is used.

In this case, the correct code is 33206-23.

Same Provider

If the physician performing the procedure also administers either regional or general anesthesia, the modifier 47 Anesthesia by Surgeon must be appended to the procedure code for that basic service (not to the anesthesia code). In such cases, an anesthesia code would not be reported. However, it is permissible to report a code for the injection of the anesthetic drug.

So to completely and accurately report Dr. Fowler's care of Margaret, the correct code is 33206-23-47. This tells the third-party payer that Dr. Fowler inserted a permanent atrial pacemaker with transvenous electrodes with unusual anesthesia that he administered himself. This one code with two modifiers tells the whole story of this encounter. (Of course, you should include a letter explaining why the unusual anesthesia had to be administered in the first place.)

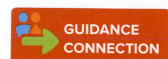

GUIDANCE CONNECTION

Additional explanation can be found in the **Anesthesia** guidelines, first column, last paragraph, in your CPT book directly in front of the **Anesthesia** section, and read the entire description of modifier 47 in **Appendix A** of your CPT book.

YOU CODE IT! CASE STUDY

Marshall Levine, a 27-year-old male, came to see Dr. Houghton for a repair of his extensor tendon in his right wrist. Dr. Houghton administered a regional nerve block and then performed the repair.

You Code It!

Go through the steps and determine the procedure code(s) that should be reported for this encounter between Dr. Houghton and Marshall Levine.

Step 1:   Read the case completely.

Step 2:   Abstract the notes: Which key words can you identify relating to the procedures performed?

Step 3: Query the provider, if necessary.

Step 4: Diagnosis: Torn tendon, wrist.

Step 5: Code the procedure(s).

Step 6: Link the procedure codes to at least one diagnosis code.

Step 7: Back code to double-check your choices.

Answer:

Did you determine the correct codes?

25270-47 Repair, tendon or muscle, extensor, forearm and/or wrist; primary, single, each tendon or muscle, regional anesthesia administered by surgeon

64450 Injection, anesthetic agent; other peripheral nerve or branch

Excellent!

LO 6.6 Physical Status Modifiers

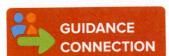

GUIDANCE CONNECTION

Additional explanation can be found in the **Anesthesia** guidelines, subsection **Anesthesia Modifiers,** in your CPT book directly in front of the **Anesthesia** section, and read the entire descriptions in **Anesthesia Physical Status Modifiers** in **Appendix A** of your CPT book.

The American Society of Anesthesiologists (ASA) established six levels of measuring the physical condition of a patient with regard to the administration of anesthesia. Each level, identified by the letter *P* and a number from 1 to 6, denotes issues that may increase the complexity of delivering anesthetic services and are measured at the time the anesthetic is about to be administered. The anesthesiologist is the professional who determines the correct physical status modifier. However, you, as the coding specialist, must be certain to look for the information and include it on the claim form.

Physical status modifiers are mandatory with every code from the Anesthesia section of the CPT book and are placed directly after the five-digit CPT code (with a hyphen between the two). (Note: Physical status modifiers are different from the regular CPT and HCPCS modifiers.)

Following are the physical status modifiers that are to be used only with anesthesia codes:

P1 (*a normal healthy patient*). Modifier P1 indicates that the patient to whom the anesthetic was given had no medical concerns that would interfere with the anesthesiologist's responsibilities for keeping the patient sedated and safe.

EXAMPLE

Dr. Tomberg administered general anesthesia to Sarah Robbins, a 17-year-old otherwise healthy female gymnast, before Dr. Navarro performed an arthroscopic extensive debridement of her shoulder joint. The correct code is 01630–P1.

P2 (*a patient with mild systemic disease*). When a patient has a disease that may affect the general workings of his or her body, it must be taken into consideration with regard to administering anesthesia. However, if the disease is under control, then its involvement is less of a concern.

EXAMPLE

Dr. Geller administered general anesthesia to Roberta Ferrara, a 37-year-old female with controlled type I diabetes mellitus, for her radical mastectomy with internal mammary node dissection, to be performed by Dr. Jackson. The correct code is 00406–P2.

P3 (*a patient with severe systemic disease*). In this case, the patient's disease is serious throughout his or her body and is an important factor for the anesthesiologist to contend with, in addition to the reason for the procedure.

EXAMPLE

Dr. Holloran administered general anesthesia to Vern Amberdeen, a 59-year-old male with benign hypertension due to Cushing's disease. Vern came today for Dr. Colombo to perform a laparoscopic cholecystectomy with cholangiography for acute cholecystitis. The correct code is 00790–P3.

P4 (*a patient with severe systemic disease that is a constant threat to life*). Modifier P4 describes any patient having medical problems that have invaded or affected multiple systems of the body. The large number of issues regarding the effects of the disease, along with existing medications and treatments that have been ongoing in the patient's system, and the potential interactions with the anesthetic make it a very complex case.

EXAMPLE

Dr. Ellerbee administers general anesthesia to Carl Umber, a 61-year-old male. Carl has advanced esophageal cancer that has metastasized throughout his body. Dr. Torres will be performing a partial esophagectomy. The correct code is 00500–P4.

P5 (*a moribund patient who is not expected to survive without the operation*). This is a life or death situation, but not necessarily an emergency. In such cases, the patient is in critical condition, and there are serious medical complications that make administering anesthesia more challenging.

EXAMPLE

Dr. Spinosa administered general anesthesia to Debra Ann Brodsky, a 41-year-old female with acute arteriosclerosis. Dr. Chesterfield was called back in from vacation to perform a heart/lung transplant this morning. The correct code is 00580–P5.

P6 (*a declared brain-dead patient whose organs are being removed for donor purposes*). This modifier is provided by the ASA for use with brain-dead patients. Individuals in this condition need to have anesthesia administered to slow bodily functions and give the transplant team time to harvest the viable organs.

Elba Carter, an 83-year-old female, comes to see Dr. Jacobs for a total knee arthroplasty due to acute arthritis. Dr. Sinonna is called in to administer the general anesthesia for the procedure. Elba is in otherwise good health.

You Code It!

Go through the steps and determine the code(s) that should be reported for the anesthesia provided by Dr. Sinonna to Elba Carter.

Step 1: Read the case completely.

Step 2: Abstract the notes: Which key words can you identify relating to the procedures performed?

_____

Step 3: Query the provider, if necessary.

Step 4: Diagnosis: acute arthritis.

Step 5: Code the procedure(s): The administration of the anesthesia.

_____

Step 6: Link the procedure codes to at least one diagnosis code.

Step 7: Back code to double-check your choices.

Answer:

Did you determine the correct codes?

01402-P1 Anesthesia for open or surgical arthroscopic procedures on knee joint; total knee arthroplasty; a normal healthy patient

99100 Anesthesia for patient of extreme age, younger than 1 year and older than 70

HCPCS Level II Modifiers

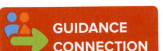

GUIDANCE CONNECTION

Additional explanation can be found in the HCPCS Level II codebook, subsection **Level II National Modifiers.**

Specific HCPCS Level II modifiers are designated for use with anesthesia service codes. These modifiers are used only if the insurance carrier, such as Medicare, accepts HCPCS Level II codes and modifiers. It is your responsibility, as a professional coder, to know the rules for the different third-party payers with which you will work.

AA Anesthesia services performed personally by the anesthesiologist

AD Medical supervision by a physician: *more than four concurrent anesthesia procedures*

G8 Monitored anesthesia care (MAC) for deep complex, complicated, or markedly invasive surgical procedure

G9 Monitored anesthesia care (MAC) for a patient who has a history of a severe cardiopulmonary condition

QK Medical direction of *two, three, or four concurrent anesthesia procedures* involving qualified individuals

QS	Monitored anesthesia care (MAC) service
QY	Medical direction of one certified registered nurse anesthetist (CRNA) by an anesthesiologist

The QY modifier would be used to indicate that an anesthesiologist was available and oversaw the administration of anesthesia services provided by someone else, such as a CRNA. The QY modifier is for the supervision of one case at a time. QK is used for two to four cases at one time, and AD is for more than four cases at one time.

If your office uses a CRNA to provide anesthesia services, there are two additional modifiers that might be used with the codes for the services they provide.

QX	CRNA service: with medical direction by a physician
QZ	CRNA service: without medical direction by a physician

Appendix B (in this textbook), "HCPCS Level II Modifiers," reviews the guidelines and rules that apply to the usage of HCPCS Level II modifiers in general.

Chapter Summary

For the most part, anesthesia coding is for the purposes of submitting health insurance claim forms on behalf of the anesthesiologist or a member of his or her staff, such as a CRNA.

To find the best, most appropriate code that accurately represents the anesthesia services administered, you must first know which type of anesthesia was used. Then you must determine the anatomical site upon which the procedure was performed and exactly which procedure was provided to the patient. In addition, you must know who administered the anesthesia to the patient: Was it the physician who also performed that procedure, or was it a different health care professional? When using HCPCS Level II modifiers, you also need to know whether the physician who administered the anesthetic was an anesthesiologist.

Once you determine the best, most appropriate code for the dispensation of the anesthesia, you also have to append the correct modifiers, when applicable.

CHAPTER 6 REVIEW
Anesthesia Coding

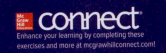

Enhance your learning by completing these
exercises and more at mcgrawhillconnect.com!

Using Terminology

Match each key term to the appropriate definition.

_____ 1. LO 6.1 The administration of sedatives, anesthetic agents, or other medications to relax but not render the patient unconscious while under the constant observation of a trained anesthesiologist; also known as "twilight" sedation.

_____ 2. LO 6.1 The loss of sensation, with or without consciousness, generally induced by the administration of a particular drug.

_____ 3. LO 6.1 The application of a drug to the skin to reduce or prevent sensation in a specific area temporarily.

_____ 4. LO 6.1 The administration of a drug in order to interrupt the nerve impulses without loss of consciousness.

_____ 5. LO 6.1 The administration of a drug in order to induce a loss of consciousness in the patient, who is unable to be aroused even by painful stimulation.

_____ 6. LO 6.1 The use of a drug to reduce stress and/or anxiety.

_____ 7. LO 6.1 Physicians specializing in the administration of anesthesia.

_____ 8. LO 6.1 A registered nurse (RN) who has taken additional, specialized training in the administration of anesthesia.

_____ 9. LO 6.1 The injection of a drug to prevent sensation in a specific portion of the body; includes local infiltration anesthesia, digital blocks, and pudendal blocks.

_____ 10. LO 6.1 Near the hind part, or tail, of the body; the sacrum and coccyx areas.

A. Anesthesia
B. Anesthesiologists
C. Caudal
D. Certified registered nurse anesthetist (CRNA)
E. Conscious sedation
F. General anesthesia
G. Local anesthesia
H. Monitored anesthesia care (MAC)
I. Regional anesthesia
J. Topical anesthesia

Checking Your Understanding

Choose the most appropriate answer for each of the following questions.

1. LO 6.1 Health care professionals permitted to administer anesthetics include
   a. anesthesiologists.
   b. certified registered nurse anesthetists.
   c. surgeons.
   d. all of these.

2. LO 6.1 The categories of anesthesia include all *except*
   a. topical/local.
   b. conscious sedation.
   c. regional.
   d. general.

3. LO 6.1 Topical anesthesia is administered
   a. to the skin.
   b. intravenously.
   c. intramuscularly.
   d. via inhalation.

4. LO 6.1 MAC is an acronym that stands for
   a. medically administered care.
   b. mutually accessible care.
   c. monitored anesthesia care.
   d. medical anesthetic characters.

5. LO 6.1/6.5 Conscious sedation is provided in order to
   a. eliminate pain.
   b. reduce anxiety.
   c. render the patient unconscious.
   d. block the nerve sensations to an extremity.

6. LO 6.2 When the physician performing the procedure also administers regional or general anesthesia, modifier 47 should be appended to
   a. the correct anesthesia code.
   b. the correct procedure code.
   c. either the correct anesthesia code or the correct procedure code.
   d. Modifier 47 should not be used in this circumstance.

7. LO 6.2 The anesthesia code package includes all *except*
   a. preoperative visits.
   b. postoperative visits.
   c. usual monitoring services.
   d. home health follow-up.

8. LO 6.3 When reporting anesthesia services using time reporting, the formula used is
   a. $(B + T + M) \times CF$.
   b. $(B + Q + CF) \times T$.
   c. $(Q + T + CF) \times B$.
   d. $(CF + B + T) \times M$.

9. LO 6.4 Qualifying circumstances are conditions that might require more work on the part of the anesthesiologist, including all *except*
   a. extreme age.
   b. emergency conditions.
   c. severe systemic disease.
   d. total body hypothermia.

10. LO 6.6 A physical status modifier describes issues that may increase the complexity of delivering anesthetic services, including
   a. emergency situations.
   b. mild systemic disease.
   c. extreme age.
   d. controlled hypotension.

Applying Your Knowledge

1. LO 6.1 List the three preliminary categories of anesthesia. _____
   _____

2. LO 6.2 List the six steps to coding anesthesia. _____
   _____

3. LO 6.2 What is included in the anesthesia code package? _____
   _____

4. LO 6.3 Why is time important to coding anesthesia? When does the clock start and stop? _____
   _____

5. LO 6.3 What is the formula used to calculate the amount of compensation the anesthesiologist will receive? _____
   _____

6. LO 6.4 List the qualifying circumstances add-on codes. _____
   _____

7. LO 6.6 List the physical status modifiers. _____
   _____

8. LO 6.6 What modifier would be appended when the anesthesia services were performed personally by the anesthesiologist? _____
   _____

9. LO 6.6 What does modifier AD identify? _____
   _____

10. LO 6.6 CRNA service with medical direction by a physician would be identified with what modifier? _____
    _____

YOU CODE IT! Practice
Chapter 6: Anesthesia Coding

Using the techniques described in this chapter, carefully read through the case studies and determine the most accurate anesthesia code(s) and modifier(s), if appropriate, for each case study.

1. Tammy Mirandosa, a healthy 31-year-old female, received anesthesia before delivering her daughter at the hospital. It was a vaginal delivery. The patient is otherwise healthy.

   _____

2. Dr. Adams administered general anesthesia to Manny Perez, an otherwise healthy 29-year-old firefighter. Dr. Zelmono performed a third-degree burn excision, followed by a skin grafting on Manny's chest where 9% of his body surface was burned while he was rescuing a little boy from a house fire.

   _____

3. Karen Walkins, a 41-year-old female, was previously diagnosed with benign hypertension due to morbid obesity. Dr. Masters administers general anesthesia so that Dr. Morgenstern can perform a direct venous thrombectomy on her lower left leg.

   _____

4. Dr. Beaumont administered anesthesia to Annalee McDonald, a 37-year-old female, diagnosed with a malignant neoplasm of the uterus. Her gynecologist, Dr. Billingsley, performed a vaginal hysterectomy.

   _____

5. Dr. Alexander administered anesthesia to Thomas Valentine, a 9-month-old male requiring a hernia repair in the lower abdomen. Dr. Georges, the neonatologist, noted that, without the surgery, Thomas was not expected to survive.

   _____

6. Miriam Worshille, a 71-year-old female with a history of hypertension and diabetes mellitus, is brought into the OR for Dr. Auerbach to perform a corneal transplant. Dr. Yankovich, the anesthesiologist, administers the anesthesia.

   _____

7. Dr. Quanarian is preparing to perform a ventriculography with burr holes on Benjamin Elliston, a 10-year-old male, who fell off the monkey bars onto a cement floor yesterday. Dr. Yorkshire administers the anesthesia. Benjamin is otherwise healthy.

   _____

8. Dr. Frankfurt administers anesthesia so that Dr. Clausson can perform a diagnostic lumbar puncture on Franklin Keiths, a 45-year-old male. Over the course of the last year, Franklin, a construction worker, has developed essential hypertension, which is currently controlled by diet. This lumbar puncture is to confirm the suspected diagnosis of bacterial meningitis.

_____

9. John Kinekopsi, a 23-year-old male, plays professional basketball and is given anesthesia by Dr. O'Neill before having a diagnostic arthroscopy of his right knee by Dr. Malone.

_____

10. Peter Siskowsky, a 15-year-old male, was in a go-kart accident and fractured his upper arm 3 months ago. Today, Dr. Longine operated on him to repair the malunion of his humerus. Dr. Carole administered the anesthesia. Peter is otherwise healthy.

_____

11. Juana Ramirez brought her 4-year-old daughter, Sasha, into the emergency room with a deep laceration of her scalp above her right ear, measuring 2.25 cm. Sasha was distraught, crying, and combative, kicking at the physician and the nurse as they attempted to clean the wound. At the recommendation of Dr. Ferrara, Juana held Sasha in her lap while the physician administered 10 mg of Versed intranasally. Once the sedation took effect, Dr. Ferrara was able to perform a layered repair of the laceration while the nurse monitored Sasha's vital signs. The entire procedure took 25 minutes.

_____

12. Suzanna St. James, a healthy 31-year-old female, was given an epidural during labor, with the expectations of a vaginal delivery. After a time, Dr. Wolfe, her obstetrician, determined that the labor was obstructed and notified the hospital staff that they would have to do a cesarean (C-section).

_____

13. Dr. Reddington administered anesthesia to Carla Corderez, a 47-year-old female, in preparation for the breast reconstruction with TRAM flap to be performed by Dr. Shapiro. Carla has a history of breast cancer and is postmastectomy.

_____

14. Dr. Harrison brought Jared Johannson, a 9-month-old male, into the OR for repair of his complete transposition of the great arteries under cardiopulmonary bypass. Pump oxygenation was used. Jared was not expected to survive without the surgery. Dr. Leistner, the anesthesiologist, administered the anesthesia.

_____

15. Sharita Solington, a 76-year-old female, was given anesthesia by Dr. Welbill, the anesthesiologist, in preparation for the repair of her ventral hernia in her lower abdomen, to be performed by Dr. Chen. Sharita has uncontrolled diabetes mellitus and essential hypertension.

_____

YOU CODE IT! Application
Chapter 6: Anesthesia Coding

The following exercises provide practice in the application of abstracting the physicians' notes and learning to work with SOAP notes from our health care facility, Cipher, Victors & Associates. These case studies (SOAP notes) are modeled on real patient encounters. Using the techniques described in this chapter, carefully read through the case studies and determine the most accurate anesthesia code(s) and modifier(s), if appropriate, for each case study.

CIPHER, VICTORS & ASSOCIATES
A Complete Health Care Facility
234 MAIN STREET • ANYTOWN, FL 32711 • 407-555-1234

PATIENT:	HUAN, ANNA
ACCOUNT/EHR #:	HUANAN001
DATE:	10/15/18

Preoperative DX: Locked right knee, rule out medial meniscus tear
Postoperative DX: 1. Grade 2 Tear, anterior, cruciate ligament
2. Medial meniscus tear, anterior, horn
3. Grade 2 Chondrosis, medial femoral condyle

Procedure: 1. Arthroscopy
2. Partial anterior cruciate ligament debridement
3. Partial medial meniscectomy

Attending Physician: James I. Cipher, MD
Anesthesia: General
Anesthesiologist: Richard Kastor, MD

INDICATIONS: The patient is a 33-year-old female who was in her usual state of good health until about 10 days ago when she sustained a twisting injury to the right knee with inability to fully extend the knee, with pain and swelling.

PROCEDURE: Estimated blood loss: None. Complications: None. Tourniquet time: See anesthesia notes. Specimens: None. Drains: None. Disposition: To the recovery room in stable condition.

Pt taken to surgery and was placed on the OR table in the supine position. After adequate general anesthesia was administered, she received a gram of intravenous Kefzol preoperatively. A proximal thigh tourniquet was applied. Examination revealed no significant Lachman or drawer and a moderate effusion. No varus or valgus instability. Distal pulses intact. The right lower extremity was placed in the arthroscopic leg holder; shaved, prepped, and draped in the usual meticulously sterile fashion for lower extremity surgery. Esmarch exsanguinations of the limb were performed, and the tourniquet was inflated. Proximal medial, anteromedial, and anterolateral portals were fashioned. A systematic evaluation of the knee was performed. The undersurface of the patella demonstrated normal tracking with no chondrosis.

The suprapatellar pouch, medial, and lateral gutters were well within normal limits, and in the notch a grade 2 tear of the anterior cruciate ligament was identified. There were some bloody fragments of the ACL that seemed to be impinging in the medial compartment. This was meticulously debrided. Approximately 50% of the ACL appeared to be intact. Attention was turned to the lateral compartment. The articular surface of the meniscus was normal. On the medial side, a grade 2 lesion in medial femoral condyle, lateral side, was noted. This was not debrided. Also, an anterior tear of the medial meniscus, which was frayed and torn, was another potential source of impingement. This was meticulously debrided to a smooth, stable mechanical limb, and the wound was irrigated and closed with 4-0 nylon simple interrupted sutures. Xeroform, 4 × 4s, Webril and Ace bandage from the tips of the toes to the groin completed the sterile dressing. There were no intraoperative or immediate postoperative complications. The prognosis is good, although it may be limited by potential for arthritis and instability in the future.

Richard Kastor, MD

RK/mg   D: 10/15/18 09:50:16   T: 10/23/18 12:55:01

Determine the most accurate anesthesia code(s) and modifier(s), if appropriate.

CIPHER, VICTORS & ASSOCIATES
A Complete Health Care Facility
234 MAIN STREET • ANYTOWN, FL 32711 • 407-555-1234

PATIENT:	FRIEDLE, VERNON
ACCOUNT/EHR #:	FRIEVE001
DATE:	10/21/18

Preoperative DX:	C5–C6 and C6–C7 herniated nucleus pulposus
Postoperative DX:	Same

Procedure:	C5–C6 and C6–C7 anterior cervical diskectomy and fusion with cadaver bone and plate

Attending Physician:	James I. Cipher, MD
Anesthesia:	General endotracheal
Anesthesiologist:	Richard Kastor, MD

INDICATIONS: The patient is a 35-year-old male with a history of neck and arm pain. MRI scan showed disk herniation at C5–C6 and C6–C7. The patient failed conservative measures and was subsequently set up for surgery. The patient is otherwise healthy.

PROCEDURE: The patient was taken to the OR. The patient was induced, and an endotracheal tube was placed. A Foley catheter was placed. The patient was given preoperative antibiotics. The patient was placed in slight extension. The left neck was prepped and draped in the usual manner. A linear incision was made above the C6 vertebral body. The platysma was divided. Dissection was continued medial to the sternocleidomastoid to the prevertebral fascia. The longus colli were cauterized and elevated. The C5–C6 disk space was addressed first. A retractor was placed. A large anterior osteophyte was removed with a large Leksell and drill. Distraction pins were then placed. The disk space was drilled out. Large bone spurs were drilled posteriorly. The posterior longitudinal ligament was removed. A free fragment was removed from beneath the ligament. The dura was visualized. A piece of bank bone was measured and slightly countersunk. The C6–C7 disk space was then addressed. Distraction pins were placed. A large anterior osteophyte was removed with a large Leksell and drill. The disk space was drilled out. Large bone spurs were drilled posteriorly. The Kerrison punch was used to remove the posterior longitudinal ligament. The dura was visualized. One piece of bank bone was in the C5, one in the C6, and two in the C7 vertebral bodies. The locking screws were tightened. The wound was irrigated. A drain was placed. The platysma was approximated with simple interrupted Vicryl. The dressing was applied. The patient was placed in a soft collar. The patient tolerated the procedure without difficulty. All counts were correct at the end of the case. The patient was extubated and transferred to recovery.

___

Richard Kastor, MD

RK/mg   D: 10/21/18 09:50:16   T: 10/23/18 12:55:01

___

Determine the most accurate anesthesia code(s) and modifier(s), if appropriate.

___

___

___

CIPHER, VICTORS & ASSOCIATES
A Complete Health Care Facility
234 MAIN STREET • ANYTOWN, FL 32711 • 407-555-1234

PATIENT: WESCOTT, PALMER
ACCOUNT/EHR #:   WESCPA001
DATE: 11/07/18

Preoperative DX: Inguinal hernia, right
Postoperative DX: Inguinal hernia, right, direct and indirect

Procedure: Repair of right inguinal hernia with mesh

Attending Physician: James I. Cipher, MD
Anesthesia: General
Anesthesiologist: Richard Kastor, MD

PROCEDURE: The patient is a 41-year-old male who was taken to the OR and prepped in the usual sterile fashion. After satisfactory anesthesia, a transverse incision was made above the inguinal ligament and carried down to the fascia of the external oblique, which was then opened, and the cord was mobilized. The ilioinguinal nerve was identified and protected. A relatively large indirect hernia was found. However, there was an extension of the hernia, such that one could definitely tell there had been a long-standing hernia here that probably had enlarged fairly recently. The posterior wall, however, was quite dilated and without a great deal of tone and bulging as well, and probably fit the criteria for a hernia by itself. Nonetheless, the hernia sac was separated from the cord structures, and a high ligation was done with a purse string suture of 2-0 silk and a suture ligature of the same material prior to amputating the sac. The posterior wall was repaired with Marlex mesh, which was sewn in place in the usual manner, anchoring two sutures at the pubic tubercle tissue, taking one lateral up the rectus sheath and one lateral along the shelving border of Poupart's ligament past the internal ring. The mesh had been incised laterally to accommodate the internal ring. Several sutures were used to tack the mesh down superiorly and laterally to the transversalis fascia. Then the two limbs of the mesh were brought together lateral to the internal ring and secured to the shelving border of Poupart's ligament. The mesh was irrigated with Gentamicin solution. The subcutaneous tissue was closed with fine Vicryl, as was the internal oblique. Marcaine was infiltrated in the subcutaneous tissue and skin. The wound was closed with fine nylon. The patient tolerated the procedure well.

Richard Kastor, MD

RK/mg   D: 11/07/18 09:50:16   T: 11/11/18 12:55:01

Determine the most accurate anesthesia code(s) and modifier(s), if appropriate.

_____

_____

_____

CIPHER, VICTORS & ASSOCIATES
A Complete Health Care Facility
234 MAIN STREET • ANYTOWN, FL 32711 • 407-555-1234

PATIENT:	NEWLAND, STACEY
ACCOUNT/EHR #:	NEWLST001
DATE:	11/15/18

Preoperative DX:	Chronic cholelithiasis
Postoperative DX:	Chronic cholelithiasis; subacute cholecystitis
Procedure:	Laparoscopic cholecystectomy; intraoperative cholangiogram

Attending Physician:	Valerie R. Victors, MD
Anesthesia:	General endotracheal
Anesthesiologist:	Richard Kastor, MD

PROCEDURE: The patient, a 57-year-old female, was taken to the OR. The patient was induced and an endotracheal tube was placed. The patient was then placed in the supine position. The abdomen was prepped and draped in the usual fashion. The patient had several previous lower midline incisions and right flank incision; therefore, the pneumoperitoneum was created via epigastric incision to the left of the midline with a Verres needle. After adequate pneumoperitoneum, the 11-mm trocar was placed through the extended incision in the left epigastrium just to the left of the midline, and the laparoscope and camera were in place. Inspection of the peritoneal cavity revealed it to be free of adhesions, and another 11-mm trocar was then placed under direct vision through a small infraumbilical incision. The scope and camera were then moved to this position, and the gallbladder was easily visualized. The gallbladder was elevated, and Hartmann's pouch was grasped. Using a combination of sharp and blunt dissection, the cystic artery was identified. The gallbladder was somewhat tense and subacutely inflamed. Therefore, a needle was passed through the abdominal wall into the gallbladder, and the gallbladder was aspirated free until it collapsed. One of the graspers was held over this region to prevent any further leakage of bile. Again, direction was turned to the area of the triangle of Calot. The cystic duct was dissected free with sharp and blunt dissection. A small opening was made in the duct, and the cholangiogram catheter was passed. The cholangiogram revealed no stones or filling defects in the bile duct system. The biliary tree was normal. There was good flow into the duodenum, and the catheter was definitely in the cystic duct. The catheter was removed, and the cystic duct was ligated between clips, as was the cystic artery. The gallbladder was then dissected free from the hepatic bed using electrocautery dissection, and it was removed from the abdomen through the umbilical port. Inspection of the hepatic bed noted that hemostasis was meticulous. The region of dissection was irrigated and aspirated dry. The trocars were removed, and the pneumoperitoneum was released. The incisions were closed with Steri-Strips, and the umbilical fascial incision was closed with 2-0 Maxon. The patient tolerated the procedure well; there were no complications. She was returned to the recovery room awake and alert.

Richard Kastor, MD

RK/mg   D: 11/15/18 09:50:16   T: 11/19/18 12:55:01

Determine the most accurate anesthesia code(s) and modifier(s), if appropriate.

_____

_____

_____

CIPHER, VICTORS & ASSOCIATES
A Complete Health Care Facility
234 MAIN STREET • ANYTOWN, FL 32711 • 407-555-1234

PATIENT: ZEMBOWER, ROGER
ACCOUNT/EHR #:   ZEMBRO001
DATE: 12/01/18

Preoperative DX: Sensory deficit of common digital nerve; tendon laceration
Postoperative DX: Same

Procedure: Repair of digital nerve, right hand; repair of tendon laceration

Attending Physician: Valerie R. Victors, MD
Anesthesia: General
Anesthesiologist: Richard Kastor, MD

INDICATIONS: The patient is a 23-year-old male who was stabbed in the right hand during a street fight. Examination showed a sensory deficit of the thumb and index finger due to an injury to the common digital nerve and a tendon laceration involving the abductor pollicis and first dorsal interosseous. He was taken immediately to the OR for repair.

PROCEDURE: The patient was taken to the OR. General anesthesia was administered, a tourniquet was applied, and the wound was explored. The common digital nerve to the thumb was identified and found to be divided at the level just proximal to the first metacarpal. The digital nerve to the radial aspect of the index finger was also divided. The abductor pollicis and the first dorsal interosseous tendons were then repaired with 3-0 Vicryl to the fascia.

Following this, both digital nerves were repaired by using interrupted 9-0 Nylon, suturing epineurium to epineurium. When completed, the wound was thoroughly irrigated with saline solution and the skin was closed with interrupted Ethilon. A dorsal splint was applied to the thumb and remains in IP flexion at about 30 degrees and slight adduction. Tourniquet time totaled 190 minutes.

Richard Kastor, MD

RK/mg   D: 12/01/18 09:50:16   T: 12/04/18 12:55:01

Determine the most accurate anesthesia code(s) and modifier(s), if appropriate.

_____

_____

_____

SURGERY CODING, PART 1

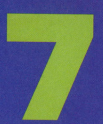

Learning Outcomes *After completing this chapter, the student should be able to:*

LO 7.1 Distinguish among the types of surgical procedures.

LO 7.2 Determine which services are included in the global surgical package.

LO 7.3 Interpret the impact on coding of the global time frames.

LO 7.4 Identify unusual services and treatments and report them accurately.

LO 7.5 Apply the guidelines to determine the meaning of a separate procedure.

LO 7.6 Abstract physician documentation of procedures on the integumentary system.

Typically, a surgical procedure can be performed in any one of several locations: the physician's office, an ambulatory care center, or a hospital. Of course, the location will most often be determined by the intensity or complexity of the procedure. You certainly would not expect an entire operating room (OR) at the hospital to be used for a physician repairing a simple laceration (cut), and no one could imagine agreeing to have a heart transplant performed in a physician's office. As a coding specialist, your responsibilities will vary, depending upon where you work, when it comes to coding surgical procedures. In addition, there may be more than one coding specialist involved with reporting one procedure.

EXAMPLE

For a surgical procedure performed in a hospital OR, there may be as many as three coders involved:

1. The hospital's coder codes for the support personnel, facilities, and supplies.

2. The surgeon's coder codes for his or her professional services.

3. The anesthesiologist's coder codes for his or her professional services.

Coding operative reports and procedure notes becomes easier with experience because the longer you work for a physician or facility the more you will learn about the procedures and services. Experience will train you to decipher which services are included in procedures and which are not. Throughout this chapter and the next, the guidelines and specifications for coding the various types of surgical and nonsurgical procedures are reviewed.

Key Terms

Complex closure

Donor area (site)

Excision

Full-thickness

Global period

Harvesting

Intermediate closure

Recipient area

Simple closure

Standard of care

Surgical approach

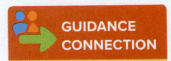
LO 7.1 Types of Surgical Procedures

When hearing the word *surgery,* most people picture an all-white room with health care professionals dressed in masks, gowns, and gloves and a patient under general anesthesia. However, this is a very narrow perspective on surgical procedures. You, as a professional coding specialist, need to understand the various types of surgical processes because this detail may be important for determining the most accurate code.

Prophylactic, Diagnostic, and Therapeutic Procedures

In certain circumstances, the purpose of the procedure will affect the code you use to report the service. Three key terms to watch for are *prophylactic, diagnostic,* and *therapeutic.*

A *prophylactic* treatment is one that is performed to prevent a condition from developing. This may be a surgical procedure, a series of injections, or a prescription.

A *diagnostic* procedure or test is performed so that the physician can gather more details about the condition or concern at issue. In other words, the reason for performing the test or procedure is to get closer to an accurate diagnosis.

A *therapeutic* procedure is provided, most often, to correct or fix a problem.

EXAMPLES

27187 Prophylactic treatment (nailing, pinning, plating or wiring) with or without methylmethacrylate, femoral neck and proximal femur

49320 Laparoscopy, abdomen, peritoneum and omentum, diagnostic, with or without collection of specimen(s) by brushing or washing (separate procedure).

50541 Laparoscopy, surgical; ablation of renal cysts

There are times when, for the safety of the patient, a procedure begins as a diagnostic examination and turns into a therapeutic procedure. Generally, a therapeutic, or surgical, procedure will include the diagnostic portion, thereby requiring only one code when both are done at the same encounter.

Above both of the two laparoscopic codes (49320 and 50541), CPT includes the guideline "Surgical laparoscopy always includes diagnostic laparoscopy." Therefore, if the physician performed a diagnostic laparoscopy solely to determine what was wrong with the patient, the correct code might be 49320. However, if while the physician was performing the diagnostic laparoscopy, he observed a renal cyst and decided to ablate the cyst at the same time, this would mean that the diagnostic procedure (to discover the cyst) and a therapeutic procedure (ablation of the cyst) were done at the same time. In that case, only 50541 might be reported, as it is one code that includes both the diagnostic and therapeutic portions of the procedure.

Surgical Approaches

surgical approach
The methodology or technique used by the physician to perform the procedure, service, or treatment.

Procedure coding requires that you understand the various **surgical approaches** a physician can take to provide care for a patient:

- A *noninvasive,* or *external,* procedure is one that does not enter the patient's body; these are procedures that are applied or performed directly to the skin without physical entry into the visceral (internal) part of the body. An example of a noninvasive procedure is a shave biopsy, a technique to acquire pathology specimens of an elevated growth on the skin by razor.

- *Minimally invasive* procedures are becoming more and more available as health care researchers continue to find methods to diagnose and correct problems with the least amount of trauma to the patient. Although there is a big difference in our perception between a patient being stabbed by a mugger and a patient being cut open by a physician during a surgical procedure, the human body knows only that it is being invaded by a sharp piece of metal. It is traumatic, and healing must occur at the point of the incision as well as to whatever was done to internal organs.

- *The percutaneous approach* uses instruments inserted into the body by way of a puncture or small incision to access the intended anatomical site. Example: needle biopsy.

- *The percutaneous endoscopic approach* uses instruments inserted into the body by way of a puncture or small incision to access and visualize the intended anatomical site. Example: diagnostic anoscopy.

- *The via natural or artificial opening approach* involves instrumentation entered into the body through a natural opening (such as the vagina) or an artificial opening (such as a stoma) to visualize the intended anatomical site. Example: flexible esophagoscopy.

- *The via natural or artificial opening endoscopic approach* involves insertion of a scope through a natural opening (such as the mouth) or an artificial opening (such as a stoma) to visualize and aid in the performance of a procedure on the intended anatomical site. Example: colonoscopy with polyp removal.

- *Open approach* procedures are fully invasive, as the surgeon cuts the body open to enable access to internal tissues and organs. These procedures involve using a scalpel or laser to cut through the skin, membranes, and body layers to access the intended anatomical site.

EXAMPLES

Surgical procedures on a woman's uterus can be performed using

- The vaginal canal as the entry point (endoscopic using a natural opening) to avoid surgical entry through the abdomen, reported with 58262 *Vaginal hysterectomy, for uterus 250g or less; with removal of tube(s) and/or ovary(s).*

- Laparoscopy (a minimally invasive procedure through the abdominal cavity) using small incisions into the patient's skin and muscle, reported with 58542 *Laparoscopy, surgical, supracervical hysterectomy, for uterus 250g or less; with removal of tube(s) and/or ovary(s).*

- Open procedure with a longer incision through the abdominal wall, reported with 58150 *Total abdominal hysterectomy, (corpus and cervix) with or without removal of tube(s), with or without removal of ovary(s).*

You can see that all three of these codes accurately report a hysterectomy (the surgical removal of the uterus) with the removal of the fallopian tubes and ovaries. The difference between these codes is the surgical technique reported: 58150 reports an open abdominal procedure using an incision through the patient's abdominal wall, 58262 reports a procedure using a natural orifice (the vagina) so that no surgical incision was required, and 58542 reports a laparoscopic procedure that uses three tiny incisions in the patient's abdomen. The information provided by the reporting of these different versions of this procedure includes not only the level of work required by the physician to perform the procedure but also the level of postoperative care that the patient will require.

LO 7.2 The Surgical Package

One of the trickiest portions of coding surgical events is distinguishing between which services and procedures are included in the code and which services and procedures might need to be coded separately for additional reimbursement. Whereas the services

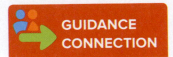
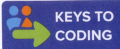
standard of care
The accepted principles of conduct, services, or treatments that are established as the expected behavior.

global period
The length of time allotted for postoperative care included in the surgical package, which is generally accepted to be 90 days for major surgical procedures and up to 10 days for minor procedures.

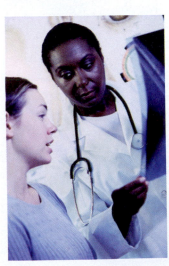

© Photodisc/Getty Images

included in each surgical protocol may vary with the procedure itself, some elements are already integrated in most CPT codes.

Services Always Included

Let's begin by reviewing services that are *always included* in the CPT surgical procedure code.

Once the physician and patient agree to move forward with the operation or procedure, the surgical package includes the following elements:

1. *Evaluation and management (E/M) encounters provided after the decision to have surgery.* These visits may begin the day before the surgical procedure (for more complex procedures) or the day of the procedure (for minor procedures), as needed.

2. *Local infiltration, metacarpal/metatarsal/digital block, or topical anesthesia.* You learned about the different types of anesthesia in Chap. 6. The surgical package includes specific types of local and regional anesthesia services, only when they are provided by the surgeon (the same professional who will be performing the procedure).

3. *The operation itself, along with any services normally considered a part of the procedure being performed.* This would include supplies, as well as applying sutures, bandages, casts, and so on to enable the patient to leave the OR safely after the procedure.

4. *Immediate postoperative care.* This includes assessing the patient in the recovery area; attending to any complications exhibited by the patient (not including any additional trips to the OR); dictating or writing the operative notes; talking with the patient, the patient's family, and other health care professionals; and writing orders.

5. *Follow-up care.* This care includes postoperative visits; care for complications following surgery; pain management; dressing changes; removal of sutures, staples, tubes, casts, and so on; and any other services considered to be the **standard of care,** during the **global period** for the specific surgical procedure. However, be careful. Some procedures may require a longer period of postoperative care by the surgeon. The period is determined by the accepted standard of care guidelines for each specific procedure and the details regarding the particular patient's health.

6. *Supplies provided in a physician's office.* With a few specific exceptions, included supplies are determined by the insurance carrier.

Services Not Included

Some functions that are commonly performed when a patient is going to have, or has had, surgery are *not included* in the surgical package. When such services and/or procedures are performed, you must code them separately.

1. *Diagnostic tests and procedures.* Tests or procedures that the physician needs to confirm the medical necessity for the surgery or investigate other issues related to the surgery are coded separately.

EXAMPLE

Diagnostic tests and procedures include biopsies, blood tests, and x-rays.

2. *Postoperative therapies.* Examples of postoperative therapies include immunosuppressive therapy after an organ transplant and chemotherapy after surgery to remove a malignancy.

3. *A more comprehensive version of the original procedure.* If the physician attempted to use a less extensive procedure first that was not sufficient to treat the patient, the

second, more extensive procedure would be coded separately, with its own surgical package; it is not an extension of the first procedure. Also, the CPT code for the second event would be appended with modifier 58.

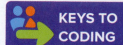

EXAMPLE

Dr. Jeppapai performed a lumpectomy on Sandra Wattell's left breast. The biopsy of the tissue removed during the lumpectomy showed that the malignancy had spread farther through the breast. Dr. Jeppapai had to take Sandra back into the OR for a simple, complete mastectomy. The code for the mastectomy is appended with modifier 58.

19301 Mastectomy, partial (e.g., lumpectomy, tylectomy, quadrantectomy, segmentectomy)

19303 Mastectomy, simple, complete

4. *Staged or multipart procedures.* Each stage or operation has its own surgical package and global period for aftercare. You must add modifier 58 to the second procedure code and all additional procedure codes reported for the same encounter.

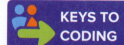

58 Staged or Related Procedure or Service by the Same Physician During the Postoperative Period. It may be necessary to indicate that the performance of a procedure or service during the postoperative period was: (a) planned or anticipated (staged); (b) more extensive than the original procedure; or (c) for therapy following a surgical procedure. This circumstance may be reported by adding modifier 58 to the staged or related procedure.

EXAMPLE

Jacob Simmons, a 29-year-old male, suffered a fracture to his upper arm that severely damaged the shaft of his right humerus. Dr. Bearmann decides to first do a bone graft to support the healing process of the fracture and follow that with a second surgical procedure—an osteotomy. This is a staged, or multipart, surgical procedure.

24516 Treatment of humeral shaft fracture, with insertion of intramedullary implant, with or without cerclage and/or locking screws

24400–58 Osteotomy, humerus, with or without internal fixation, staged procedure by the same physician during the postoperative period

5. *Management of postoperative complications that require additional surgery.* As you may remember about the surgical package from Services Always Included #4, the physician's attention to any postoperative complications is included in the original package *unless* those complications require the patient to return to the operating room. In such cases, you must use a modifier with the CPT code for the procedure performed.

76 Repeat Procedure by the Same Physician. It may be necessary to indicate that a procedure or service was repeated subsequent to the original procedure or service. This circumstance may be reported by adding modifier 76 to the repeated procedure or service.

78 **Unplanned Return to the Operating/Procedure Room by the Same Physician Following Initial Procedure for a Related Procedure During the Postoperative Period.** It may be necessary to indicate that another procedure was performed during the postoperative period of the initial procedure (unplanned procedure following initial procedure). When this procedure is related to the first, and requires the use of an operating/procedure room, it may be reported by adding modifier 78 to the related procedure.

77 **Repeat Procedure by Another Physician.** The physician may need to indicate that a basic procedure or service performed by another physician had to be repeated. This situation may be reported by adding modifier 77 to the repeated procedure/ service.

6. *Unrelated surgical procedure during the postoperative period.* If the same physician must perform an unrelated surgical procedure during the postoperative period, you have to include a modifier to explain that this procedure has nothing to do with the first.

79 **Unrelated Procedure or Service by the Same Physician During the Postoperative Period.** The physician may need to indicate that the performance of a procedure or service during the postoperative period was unrelated to the original procedure. This circumstance may be reported by using modifier 79.

7. *Supplies.* In certain cases, for certain procedures performed in a physician's office, a separate code is permitted for supplies, such as a surgical tray, casting supplies, splints, and drugs. You have to check the reimbursement rules for the specific third-party payer.

LO 7.3 Global Period Time Frames

Essentially, all procedures have assigned global period time frames based on the standard of care for a treatment or service. These range from 0 (zero) [the global period for providing cardiopulmonary resuscitation (CPR)] or 1 day for a very simple procedure (removing a splinter from a finger) to 10 days for a minor procedure to 90 days for major surgery. Endoscopies, most often, are considered minor procedures and will normally run a 10-day global period.

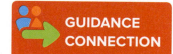

GUIDANCE CONNECTION

Refer to the *Global Surgery Fact Sheet* from CMS: www.cms.gov/Outreach-and-Education/Medicare-Learning-Network-MLN/MLNProducts/downloads/GlobalSurgery-ICN907166.pdf.

Most often, major surgeries will include 1 day in the preoperative period plus the date of surgery plus 90 days postoperatively.

Services Provided by More Than One Physician

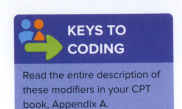
It is expected that the same physician will provide all of the surgical package's elements. This is an umbrella that covers only one health care professional.

Occasionally, however, more than one physician will be involved in providing all the necessary services for one patient having one operation. In such cases, modifiers explain to the third-party payer who did what and when.

54 **Surgical Care Only.** You must add this modifier to the correct CPT surgical procedure code when your physician is only going to perform the procedure itself, and not provide or be involved in any preoperative or postoperative care of the patient.

55 **Postoperative Management Only.** This modifier is added to the CPT code for the surgical procedure included on a claim from the physician who only cares for the patient after the operation.

56 **Preoperative Management Only.** When a physician, other than the surgeon who performed the procedure, cares for the patient from the decision to have surgery up to but not including the operation itself, modifier 56 is appended to the CPT code for the procedure.

LET'S CODE IT! SCENARIO

Rahima Gonzalez, a 43-year-old female, was on vacation, hiking through the mountains, when she fell over a log and wrenched her knee very badly. She was flown to the nearest hospital and placed under the care of Dr. Peterman. After the diagnostic tests were completed, Dr. Peterman recommended arthroscopic surgery to treat the knee. Dr. Peterman called in Dr. Mathews, an orthopedic surgeon, to perform the procedure. Dr. Mathews performed a surgical arthroscopy and repaired the medial meniscus. Immediately after the surgery, Rahima flew home, and she went to her family physician, Dr. Donaldson, for the follow-up appointments.

Let's Code It!

The notes indicate that Dr. Peterman, Dr. Matthews, and Dr. Donaldson were all involved, to some extent, in caring for Rahima during the procedure—*surgical arthroscopy* and *repair of the medial meniscus*. Let's go to the Alphabetic Index and look up the procedure.

Find *arthroscopy*. As you go down the list, you will see the subcategories: Diagnostic and Surgical. You know from the notes that this was surgical. Continue down and find the anatomical site for this procedure: Knee . . . 29871–29889. Indented under knee, you will find additional listings that don't really match, so let's look at the suggested codes:

29871 Arthroscopy, knee, surgical; for infection, lavage and drainage

The description is correct, up to the semicolon. So continue down the page to find any additional information that might be applicable to the case, according to our documentation. (Remember: Read up to the semicolon on the code, because it is at the margin, and then finish the description with each indented description.)

Continue reading until you see

29882   with meniscus repair (medial OR lateral)

The complete description of this code is

> **29882** Arthroscopy, knee, surgical; with meniscus repair (medial OR lateral)

This matches the notes exactly, doesn't it? It does! Good job!

As you have learned, the surgical package for this procedure includes all the services and treatments that Rahima received. However, instead of just one physician, Rahima actually had three doctors caring for her throughout. Each physician will send his or her own claim form in an effort to get paid for the services he or she provided. You need to supply some explanation to the third-party payer so that it can understand receiving three claim forms for one procedure provided to the one patient.

- **Dr. Peterman will have the 29882–56 modifier to indicate he only provided the preoperative care.**
- **Dr. Mathews will have the 29882–54 modifier to indicate he only performed the surgery.**
- **Dr. Donaldson will have the 29882–55 modifier to indicate she only provided the postoperative care.**

LO 7.4 Unusual Services and Treatments

Every service and treatment or procedure has an industry standard of care. Included in the assessment of each service is a calculation of how much work is involved and how long it will take to complete the procedure. It is all part of the formula used by third-party payers to determine how much to pay the health care professional. As you might expect, though, particularly in health care, things do not always go exactly as planned. There may be an issue with a patient that requires more work on the physician's part. When this happens, the physician should receive additional compensation. Therefore, you have to attach the modifier 22 to the procedure code to identify an unusual circumstance. You also have to attach documentation that fully explains the circumstances.

> **22** **Increased Procedural Services.** When the work required to provide a service is substantially greater than typically required, it may be identified by adding modifier 22 to the usual procedure code. Documentation must support the substantial additional work and the reason for the additional work (i.e., increased intensity, time, technical difficulty of procedure, severity of patient's condition, physical, and mental effort required). Note: The modifier should not be appended to an E/M service.

YOU CODE IT! CASE STUDY

Douglas Bamberger, a 15-year-old male, is 5 ft. 6 in., 365 lb. Dr. Oswald performs a partial colectomy with anastomosis. The procedure, however, takes several hours longer than usual due to the fact that Douglas is morbidly obese.

You Code It!

Go through the steps and determine the procedure code(s) that should be reported for this encounter between Dr. Oswald and Douglas Bamberger.

Step 1:   Read the case completely.

Step 2:   Abstract the notes: Which key words can you identify relating to the procedures performed?

_____

Step 3:   Query the provider, if necessary.

Step 4:   Diagnosis: Ulcerative colitis; morbid obesity.

Step 5:   Code the procedure(s).

_____

Step 6:   Link the procedure codes to at least one diagnosis code.

Step 7:   Back code to double-check your choices.

Answer:

Did you determine the correct code?

44140-22 Colectomy, partial; with anastomosis, increased procedural service

In addition to the code, you should attach a letter with the claim to explain the circumstance that complicated the procedure.

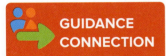

GUIDANCE CONNECTION

Additional explanation can be found in the guidelines pages directly before the **Surgery** section, subhead **Separate Procedure,** in your CPT book.

LO 7.5 Surgery Guidelines

Separate Procedure

Throughout the CPT book, you will see code descriptions that include the notation "separate procedure." Such services and treatments are generally performed along with a group of other procedures. When this happens, you will be able to find a combination, or bundled, code that includes all the treatments together. However, this particular procedure can also be performed alone. If so, you would use the code for the "separate procedure."

LET'S CODE IT! SCENARIO

Dr. Torres performed a repair of the secondary tendon flexor in Bobby Morton's right foot. He first performed an open tenotomy and then did the repair with a free graft.

Let's Code It!

The *repair* that Dr. Torres performed on Bobby Morton actually includes the *tenotomy.* Therefore, we will use the one combination code for the entire procedure.

Go to the Alphabetic Index, and look up the procedure: *repair.* Under repair, let's find the anatomical site: *foot.* Under foot, let's find the part of the foot that was treated: *tendon.* The index suggests the code range 28200–28226, 28238. Let's go to the first one.

28200 Repair, tendon, flexor, foot; primary or secondary, without free graft, each tendon

28202   secondary with free graft, each tendon (includes
              obtaining graft)

It seems we have found the code description that matches the physician's notes.

**28202 Repair, tendon, flexor, foot; secondary with free graft, each
        tendon (includes obtaining graft)**

Great job!
Had Dr. Torres performed the tenotomy only, the correct code would be

**28230 Tenotomy, open, tendon flexor; foot, single or multiple
        tendon(s) (separate procedure)**

On occasion, you may find that the "separate procedure" is performed along with other procedures, not those in the bundle. Should this be the situation, you have to add the modifier 59 to the "separate procedure" code. Documentation must support these facts, as always.

**59 Distinct Procedural Service. When the physician performs
    a procedure or service that is not normally performed with the
    other procedures or services, modifier 59 should be added to
    the second procedure.**

LET'S CODE IT! SCENARIO

Barbara Bracken brought her daughter, Darlene, a 5-year-old female, to her pediatrician's office after they had attended a friend's birthday party in the park. After a cursory examination, Dr. Jackson removed a jellybean from Darlene's nose. Then Dr. Jackson removed a splinter from Darlene's hand.

Let's Code It!

Dr. Jackson *removed a jellybean* and a *splinter*. Let's go to the alphabetic index and look up the first procedure: *removal*. Check the list of terms below Removal. Dr. Jackson removed a jellybean—a foreign body from Darlene's nose, so find *foreign body*. Under foreign body, find the anatomical site: *nose*. The index suggests code 30300. Check it out:

30300 Removal foreign body, intranasal; office type procedure

Good. Now let's find the code for the second procedure. Let's look up the second procedure, also a *removal*. Dr. Jackson removed a *foreign body* (the splinter) from Darlene's *hand*. Code 26070 is suggested.

**26070 Arthrotomy, with exploration, drainage, or removal of loose or
        foreign body; carpometacarpal joint**

This does not match the notes. Let's go back to the list under *removal* and find the true anatomical site: *subcutaneous tissue*. Remember, the splinter is actually in her tissue. The index suggests the code range 10120–10121. Go to these codes in the numerical listing and read the descriptions.

**10120 Incision and removal of foreign body, subcutaneous tissues;
        simple**

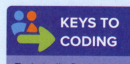

KEYS TO CODING

Technically, Dr. Jackson did not remove the splinter from Darlene's hand; he removed it from her subcutaneous tissue (underneath her skin).

Great! There is one more point to address—the removal of the splinter actually had nothing to do with the removal of the jellybean. Without an explanation, the third-party payer may think that these two procedures might have been reported in error. To confirm that this is not an error and that these two procedures were actually performed on the same patient at the same encounter, you have to add the modifier 59. The second code will be reported as

10120-59 Incision and removal of foreign body, subcutaneous tissues; simple; distinct procedural service

The claim form you prepare for Dr. Jackson's services to Darlene Bracken for this encounter will include two codes: 30300 and 10120-59.

LO 7.6 Integumentary System

The largest organ of the human body, the skin, formally known as the integumentary system, is taken for granted by the average person. Yet this is the body's protective layer, the first line of defense for the anatomical organs and systems within.

Incision and Drainage (I&D)

A cyst, an abscess, a furuncle (boil), or a paronychia (infected skin around a fingernail or toenail) can harbor infection. When this happens, most often a physician will perform an incision (cut into the tissue) and drainage (I&D) to extract the infectious material.

Debridement

The process of carefully cleaning out a wound to encourage the healing process is called *debridement*. The basis of this term comes from the word *debris,* meaning wreckage or rubble, and relates to the process of taking away necrotic (dead or dying) tissue that can impede the creation of new, healthy tissue. This may be necessary for burn patients, for victims of penetrating wounds, and sometimes for patients with complex wounds such as an open, penetrating fracture.

Biopsies

Although a specimen of tissue may be excised, shave removed, or lased and then sent to pathology for testing, this does not automatically indicate the need for a separate biopsy code. The guidelines state that you should use a biopsy procedure code only when the procedure is conducted individually, or distinctly separate, from any other procedure or service performed at the same time.

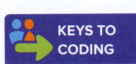

KEYS TO CODING

Remember there is a difference between incision and excision. Incision means *cut into,* while excision means *cut out.*

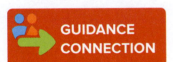

GUIDANCE CONNECTION

Additional explanation can be found in the **Surgery** section, directly beneath the subhead **Biopsy,** in your CPT book.

EXAMPLE

Carole had a rash that would not go away. So she went to see Dr. Michaels, a dermatologist, who took a biopsy of one of the pustules in an effort to diagnose the cause of her rash. Dr. Michaels closed the small defect with one stitch. Dr. Michaels's coder would report

11100 Biopsy of skin, subcutaneous tissue and/or mucous membrane (including simple closure), unless otherwise listed; single lesion

Ethan Monahan, a 73-year-old male, came to see Dr. Greenberg get rid of some skin tags on his left cheek. After applying a local anesthetic, Dr. Greenberg removed nine tags and sent them to the lab.

Let's Code It!

Let's go to the alphabetic index and find the key term for the procedure: *removal*. Now, what did the physician remove? *Skin tags.* Find the term "skin tags" indented under Removal . . . skin tags . . . : the codes suggested are 11200–11201. Turn to the numerical listing of the book, in the Surgery section, and look for those codes. You will see

11200 Removal of skin tags, multiple fibrocutaneous tags, any area; up to and including 15 lesions

+11201 each additional 10 lesions or part thereof (list separately in addition to code for primary procedure)

(Use 11201 in conjunction with 11200)

The next question is . . . How many skin tags (lesions) did the physician remove from Ethan's face? When you reread the notes, you will see that he removed *nine tags.* This confirms the correct code is 11200.

The notes also indicate that the lesions were sent to pathology, meaning a biopsy. Should we add another code for the biopsy? Remember that the guidelines state that a separate code for the biopsy is used only when the biopsy is a procedure distinctly separate from other procedures and not a part of another service. In this case, the biopsy is a part of the removal of the skin tags and does not require a second code.

Excisions

When the physician removes a lesion from a patient, you must code the **excision** of each lesion separately. Codes for the excision, or **full-thickness** removal, of a lesion are determined first by the anatomical site from where the lesion was removed and then by the size of the lesion removed. The code for the excision includes the administration of a local anesthetic and a **simple closure** of the excision site, as mentioned in the definition.

excision
The full-thickness removal of a lesion, including margins; includes (for coding purposes) a simple closure.

full-thickness
A measure that extends from the epidermis to the connective tissue layer of the skin.

simple closure
A method of sealing an opening in the skin (epidermis or dermis), involving only one layer. It includes the administration of local anesthesia and/or chemical or electro-cauterization of a wound not closed.

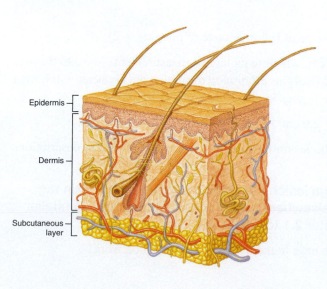

To correctly measure what was excised, you must look at the dimensions of the lesion itself *plus* a proper margin around the lesion. That will give you the total amount actually excised by the physician and lead you to the correct code. In order to find the correct size of the lesion excised, we must do the following: Add the size of the lesion to the size of the margin doubled (margins *all around* mean that the diameter will have a margin on each side).

The formula is

$$\text{Coded size of lesion} = \text{size of lesion} + (\text{size of margins} \times 2)$$

LET'S CODE IT! SCENARIO

Dr. Vitali excised a lesion that measured 2.0 cm by 1.0 cm, with 0.2-cm margins all around, from Benita Corraldo's neck. The pathology report confirmed that the lesion was benign.

Let's Code It!

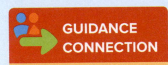

GUIDANCE CONNECTION

Additional explanation can be found in the guidelines within the **Surgery** section, directly under the subheads **Excision—Benign Lesions** and **Excision—Malignant Lesions** and **Excision** (above code 19100) in your CPT book.

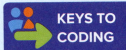

KEYS TO CODING

Some surgeons include the measurement of the margins in their operative notes. In other cases, you may need to review the pathologist's report to determine an accurate measurement.

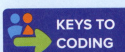

KEYS TO CODING

1 centimeter (cm) = 10 millimeters (mm) = 0.4 inch (in.)

1 millimeter (mm) = 0.1 centimeter (cm) = 0.04 inch (in.)

1 inch (in.) = 2.54 cm

Let's go to the Alphabetic Index and find the suggested code or codes. Look up *excision* for the procedure and then *neck* for the anatomical site, right? Well, you will see that there is no listing for *neck* under *excision*. What should you do now? Analyze what you see in the physician's notes. Where exactly is the lesion? It isn't really on her *neck;* it is on her *skin.* So look at *excision, skin.* Aha! Under *skin,* you will see *lesion.* Good. And now, look for *benign,* as per the notes, to find suggested codes 11400–11471.

When you go to the numerical listing, you will see the description for the first code in our range:

11400 Excision, benign lesion including margins, except skin tag (unless listed elsewhere), trunk, arms or legs; excised diameter 0.5 cm or less

The description for code 11400 matches our physician's notes except for the mention of the anatomical sites: trunk, arms, or legs. Our patient had the lesion on her neck. Continue looking down the listings, and take a look at the description for code 11420.

11420 Excision, benign lesion including margins, except skin tag (unless listed elsewhere), scalp, neck, hands, feet, genitalia; excised diameter 0.5 cm or less

This matches our physician's notes! Next, you must determine the size of the lesion. Remember the formula:

$$\text{Coded size of lesion} = \text{size of lesion} + (\text{size of margins} \times 2)$$

To the size of the lesion (2.0 cm, which is its largest measurement), we add the size of the margin (0.2 cm) times 2 (margins *all around* mean that the diameter will have a margin on each side). With the figures in place, our formula becomes

$$\text{Coded size of lesion} = 2.0\ \text{cm} + (0.2\ \text{cm} \times 2) = 2.4\ \text{cm}$$

Therefore, the total size of the lesion excised is 2.4 cm. Now find the descriptions indented underneath 11420.

11423 Excision, benign lesion including margins, except skin tag (unless listed elsewhere), scalp, neck, hands, feet, genitalia; excised diameter 2.1 to 3.0 cm

This matches exactly. You have found the code: 11423. Good work!

You may find that the physician's notes indicate that the excision of the lesion was complicated or unusual in some way. Should this be the situation, remember to add modifier 22 to the procedure code. The difficulty is related to the process of excising the lesion, not the closure.

Simple closure is included in the excision code. However, if the closure of the excision site becomes more involved and is described as an **intermediate closure** or a **complex closure,** the repair is no longer included in the code for the excision procedure. You need to report an additional code.

As you read the procedure notes or operative report, pay close attention to the description documented as to how deep into the skin the physician worked. When you see a layered closure that involves the deeper layers of the subcutaneous tissue, the superficial fascia, and the epidermal and dermal layers of the skin, you will report an intermediate repair. Also reported as an intermediate repair is a single-layer closure that first requires extensive cleaning or particulate matter removal before closing.

When a complex repair has been performed, the documentation will include more than just a layered enclosure: Scar revision, traumatic laceration debridement, avulsions, extensive undermining, stent insertion, or retention suture(s) all describe this more involved level of repair.

intermediate closure
A multilevel method of sealing an opening in the skin involving one or more of the deeper layers of the skin. Single-layer closure of heavily contaminated wounds that required extensive cleaning or removal of particulate matter also constitutes intermediate closure.

complex closure
A method of sealing an opening in the skin involving a multilayered closure and a reconstructive procedure such as scar revision, debridement, or retention sutures.

LET'S CODE IT! SCENARIO

Dr. Simmons excised a lesion measuring 3.1 by 3.0 cm, with 0.3-cm margins on each side, from Raymond Fulbright's left forearm. Due to the lesion's proximity to the wrist bone, performing the excision took more exactness than the typical procedure. Finally, the lesion was successfully removed. The pathology report confirmed that the lesion was benign.

Let's Code It!

The notes tell you that Dr. Simmons performed an *excision; skin; lesion; benign.* The Alphabetic Index suggests the code range of 11400–11471. When you go to the numerical listing, you will need to look for the code that identifies the correct anatomical site of the lesion that was excised: *forearm.* You find the following:

11400 Excision, benign lesion including margins, except skin tag (unless listed elsewhere), trunk, arms or legs; excised diameter 0.5 cm or less

The first code matches perfectly. Now, you must determine the exact size of the lesion plus margins that was excised. The largest measurement of the lesion is 3.1 cm, and the margins are 0.3 cm. Fit the numbers into the formula:

Coded size of lesion = 3.1 cm + (0.3 cm × 2) = 3.7 cm

The coded size will direct you to the correct code for the procedure:

11404 Excision, benign lesion including margins, except skin tag (unless listed elsewhere), trunk, arms or legs; excised diameter 3.1 to 4.0 cm

Excellent! However, there is one other thing mentioned in the notes. The physician wrote that the *excision took more exactness than the typical procedure.* The documentation indicates that this was an *unusual procedure,* meaning that you must add the appropriate modifier. The final correct code is 11404-22.

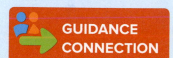

GUIDANCE CONNECTION

Additional explanation can be found in the guidelines within the **Surgery** section, directly under the subhead **Repair (Closure),** in your CPT book.

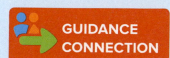

GUIDANCE CONNECTION

Additional explanations can be found in in-section guidelines located within the **Surgery** section, subhead **Repair (Closure), Definitions,** directly above code 12001.

Dr. Burgoud excised a lesion that measured 2.1 by 3.0 cm, with 0.5-cm margins on each side, from Wanda Wainright's abdomen. Wanda is diagnosed clinically obese and the excess fatty tissue around the lesion required a complex closure of the excision site. The pathology report confirmed that the lesion was malignant.

Let's Code It!

The Alphabetic Index will direct you to a slightly different group of codes—*excision, skin, lesion, malignant*—suggesting a code within the range of 11600–11646. Just as before, you will need to find the code in this range that identifies the correct anatomical location of the lesion:

11600 Excision, malignant lesion including margins, trunk, arms or legs; excised diameter 0.5 cm or less

The abdomen is a part of the trunk, so this code is OK. Next, you will need to add up the size of the lesion.

$$\text{Coded size of lesion} = 3.0 \text{ cm} + (0.5 \text{ cm} \times 2) = 4.0 \text{ cm}$$

The answer 4.0 cm leads to the code

11604 Excision, malignant lesion including margins, trunk, arms or legs; excised diameter 3.1 to 4.0 cm

Excellent! Wanda's case was not as complicated as Raymond's, so modifier 22 will not be required. However, Dr. Burgoud did note that Wanda's procedure "required a complex closure of the excision site." The guidelines tell you that only a simple closure is included in the excision code. A complex closure, just like an intermediate closure, is coded in addition to the code for the excision. So let's code it!

Let's go back to the Alphabetic Index and find the key term *closure*. None of the indented descriptors seem to match, so you should investigate the code range shown next to the word *closure:* 12001–13160.

You will notice the heading immediately above the first code in the range: 12001. It reads "Repair–Simple." But you are looking for a complex closure, so continue down the page. The next section, above code 12031, is "Repair–Intermediate." This is closer to what you need, but not exactly. Above code 13100 you find the heading you have been looking for: "Repair–Complex."

Remember that Wanda's lesion was located on her abdomen (trunk). Look at the codes in this section, and find the best code for the *complex closure* of her excision site.

13100 Repair, complex, trunk; 1.1 cm to 2.5 cm

Excellent! You have found the correct level of closure (repair) for the correct anatomical site (trunk). Now, you must find the correct size of the excision site. Your calculation totaled 4.0 cm, which brings you to the correct code:

13101 Repair, complex, trunk; 2.6 cm to 7.5 cm

Excellent! You now know that, for this one procedure on Wanda, the claim form will include the codes

11604 Excision, malignant lesion including margins, trunk, arms or legs; excised diameter 3.1 to 4.0 cm

13101 Repair, complex, trunk; 2.6 cm to 7.5 cm

Good job!

Reexcision

When the pathology report indicates that the physician did not excise around the lesion (the margins) widely enough to get all the malignancy, an additional excision procedure may be needed.

If the reexcision is performed during the same operative session, adjust the total size of the lesion being coded to include the new total measurement. Report just the one code, with the largest measurement shown in the operative or procedure notes.

If the reexcision is performed during a subsequent encounter during the postoperative period, you should attach modifier 58 Staged Procedure to the procedure code for that second excision. The reexcision to remove additional tissue around the original site during the postoperative period would directly apply to modifier 58's description: (b) *more extensive than the original procedure.*

Wound Repair

When multiple wounds are repaired with the same complexity on the same anatomical site(s) as indicated by the code descriptor, add all the lengths together to use one code for the total repair. You may sometimes have more than one code to report repairs performed at this encounter. In these cases, the codes should be listed in order from the most complex to the simplest, then from head to toe. All procedure codes, after the first, should have the modifier 59 Distinct Procedural Service appended.

Debridement or decontamination of a wound is included in the code for the repair of that wound. However, if the contamination is so extensive that it requires extra time and effort, it should be coded separately. Also, if the debridement is performed and the wound is not closed or repaired during the same session, code the debridement separately.

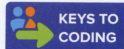

KEYS TO CODING

The multiple wound repair guideline is different from the guideline for multiple lesions. Remember that, with lesions, each lesion is coded separately. With wounds, you will report one code for the total length of all wounds being repaired on the same anatomical site.

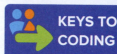

KEYS TO CODING

Modifier 59 is used to report multiple procedures that are performed at the same encounter by the same provider. This modifier is appended to the codes reporting the second and additional services, not the primary procedure code.

LET'S CODE IT! SCENARIO

Quentin Alexander, a 22-year-old male, got into a bar fight and sustained multiple wounds to his hand and arm. Dr. Havilland performed intermediate repair of a 5- by 2-cm wound and a 3.1- by 1-cm wound on Quentin's right hand and a simple repair to a 3.2- by 1-cm wound to his right forearm.

Let's Code It!

You can see by Dr. Havilland's notes that Quentin had two wounds, treated with intermediate closures, both on his right hand, and one wound, with a simple repair, on his right forearm. Let's go to the Alphabetic Index and find *repair, wound, intermediate* (suggesting 12031–12057) and *repair, wound, simple* (suggesting 12001–12021).

The intermediate repairs were done to the right *hand,* so let's turn to the numerical listing for the code range 12031–12057 and find the best code for this anatomical site.

12041 Repair, intermediate, wounds of neck, hands, feet and/or external genitalia; 2.5 cm or less

There were two wounds on Quentin's right hand (the first is 5 × 2 cm and the second 3.1 × 1 cm). The guidelines state that, because the wounds are on the same anatomical site as per the code description (*hands*) and received the same level of repair (*intermediate*), you must add them together. Let's add the two longest measurements together (5 cm + 3.1 cm) for a total of 8.1 cm. This brings us to the correct code:

12044 Repair, intermediate, wounds of neck, hands, feet and/or external genitalia; 7.6 cm to 12.5 cm

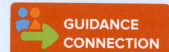

GUIDANCE CONNECTION

Additional explanations can be found in in-section guidelines located within the **Surgery** section, subhead **Repair (Closure), Definitions,** directly above code 12001.

Good job! Now, the last wound on Quentin's forearm is different. It is a simple repair rather than an intermediate repair, and the wound is on his arm, not his hand. Therefore, this wound repair will have its own code. Follow the code descriptions, and see if you can come up with the most accurate code. Did you determine the correct code to be

> **12002 Simple repair of superficial wounds of scalp, neck, axillae, external genitalia, trunk and/or extremities (including hands and feet); 2.6 cm to 7.5 cm**

Now that you know the guideline regarding multiple wound repairs, do you think any adjustments should be made to the claim form you are preparing for Dr. Havilland to be reimbursed for his work on Quentin? You need to report them in the correct sequence and append a modifier:

> **12044 (The intermediate repair tells us this was the more severe or complicated procedure. Therefore, this code is reported first.)**

> **12002–51 (This was the simple repair of a smaller wound. This was less complicated and, therefore, the code is listed second and appended with the modifier 51.)**

That's great! You did excellent work!

YOU CODE IT! CASE STUDY

A woman was screaming in a parking lot and calling for help. She had accidentally locked her keys in the car, along with her infant son. It was a hot day, and she was quite concerned about her child. Martin Hendry came along and used a rock to break a window on the other side of the car, reached in through the broken glass, and unlocked the door. Without question, Martin is a hero, but he also cut his wrist on the broken glass. At the ED, Dr. Albertson discovered that the subcutaneous tissue at the laceration site was littered with tiny shards of glass. Dr. Albertson administered a local anesthetic. It took Dr. Albertson quite a long time to debride the 5.3- by 1.6-cm wound of all the glass before he was able to suture it.

You Code It!

Go through the steps and determine the procedure code(s) that should be reported for this encounter between Dr. Albertson and Martin Hendry.

Step 1: Read the case completely.

Step 2: Abstract the notes: Which key words can you identify relating to the procedures performed?

_____

Step 3: Query the provider, if necessary.

Step 4: Diagnosis: Laceration.

Step 5: Code the procedure(s).

_____

Step 6:   Link the procedure codes to at least one diagnosis code.

Step 7:   Back code to double-check your choices.

Answer:

Did you determine the correct codes?

11042 Debridement, subcutaneous tissue (includes, epidermis and dermis, if performed); first 20 sq. cm or less

12002-51 Simple repair of superficial wounds of scalp, neck, axillae, external genitalia, trunk and/or extremities (including hands and feet); 2.6 cm to 7.5 cm; multiple procedures

Excellent! You are really learning how to code!

Adjacent Tissue Transfer and/or Rearrangement

When an excision is repaired with an adjacent tissue transfer or rearrangement, you will see several terms in the procedure notes that are included in this code subcategory.

- Z-plasty is a double transposition flap, most often used to correct a skin web or perform a scar revision.
- W-plasty uses several small, triangular-shaped flaps, alternating inversion, just like the letter "W," to break up a long scar.
- V-Y plasty uses a V-shaped flap that is next to the defect with surrounding skin raised up and brought into the wound.
- Rotation flap is a raised subdermal plane, semicircular in shape, pivoted around into the defect.
- Random island flap is a section of skin moved into the defect with its blood supply.
- Advancement flap involves a subdermal place of skin, longitudinally moved to the defect.

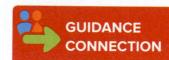

GUIDANCE CONNECTION

Additional explanations can be found in in-section guidelines located within the **Surgery** section, subhead **Adjacent Tissue Transfer or Rearrangement,** directly above code 14000.

The correct code to report a tissue transfer or rearrangement requires two elements from the physician's notes:

- Anatomical site: The anatomical location of the primary defect—the skin opening that needs to be repaired, as well as the location of the secondary defect—the skin area from where the surgeon took the skin being transferred.
- Size of the defect: Add together the sizes of the primary defect and the secondary defect.
- For all defects over 30 sq. cm, all anatomical sites are reported with the same codes—code 14301 with code 14302, depending upon the total size.

LET'S CODE IT! SCENARIO

Lillah Claire had a 2.5 cm × 1 cm contracted scar on the back of her hand, making it difficult to use her fingers completely. Dr. Lafferty performed a Z-plasty tissue transfer to disrupt the scar tissue and elongate the transferred tissues. He notes that the secondary defect was 3 sq. cm.

Let's Code It!

Dr. Lafferty did a "Z-plasty tissue transfer" on Lillah. However, when you look in the CPT alphabetic index for *Z-plasty,* you will find nothing. Take a look at the Alphabetic

Index for *transfer*. There are a few items listed below, but none of these seem to relate to the procedure on Lillah. So let's take a look at the CPT Alphabetic Index listings for *tissue*. Below this you will see:

Tissue

  Transfer

    Adjacent

      Skin 14000–14350

As you review the guidelines in this subsection, shown above code 14000, you can see that Z-plasty is included in this section, confirming that you are in the right area. Next, you can see that the code descriptions require you to know the anatomical location of the procedure.

14000 Adjacent tissue transfer or rearrangement, trunk

14020 Adjacent tissue transfer or rearrangement, scalp, arms, and/ or legs

14040 Adjacent tissue transfer or rearrangement, forehead, cheeks, chin, mouth, neck, axillae, genitalia, hands and/or feet

14060 Adjacent tissue transfer or rearrangement, eyelids, nose, ears, and/or lips

Go back to the scenario and identify the anatomical site: "on the back of her hand." This leads you to code 14040. You must now choose between the following two codes determined by the size of the defects:

14040 Adjacent tissue transfer or rearrangement, forehead, cheeks, chin, mouth, neck, axillae, genitalia, hands and/or feet; defect 10 sq. cm or less

14041 Adjacent tissue transfer or rearrangement, forehead, cheeks, chin, mouth, neck, axillae, genitalia, hands and/or feet; defect 10.1 sq. cm to 30.0 sq. cm

How big was the defect? In the guidelines above code 14000, it says "The primary defect resulting from the excision and the secondary defect resulting from flap design to perform the reconstruction are measured together to determine the code."

Lilliah's original scar—the primary defect—is noted to be 2.5 cm × 1. Multiply these two numbers to get 2.5 sq. cm. The secondary defect, the source of the tissue transfer, is noted to be 3 sq. cm. Add 2.5 sq. cm to 3 sq. cm and get a total of 5.5 sq. cm. Compare this measurement to the measurements included in the code descriptions for tissue transfers done on the hands. This confirms the correct code for the procedure Dr. Lafferty did for Lillah is

14040 Adjacent tissue transfer or rearrangement, forehead, cheeks, chin, mouth, neck, axillae, genitalia, hands and/or feet; defect 10 sq. cm or less

Good job!

Skin Replacement Surgery and Flaps

The codes for skin grafts are determined by three things:

1. The size of the **recipient area** (the size of the wound to be grafted).
2. The location of the recipient area (the anatomical site).
3. The type of graft (pinch graft, split graft, full-thickness graft, and so on).

recipient area
The area, or site, of the body receiving a graft of skin or tissue.

The codes include a simple debridement, or avulsion, of the recipient site. Through **harvesting,** grafts can be taken from another part of the patient's body, from another body (a live donor), a cadaver (a deceased person), skin substitutes (such as neodermis, synthetic skin), or another species (for instance, a porcine graft). You have to know where the graft came from in order to determine the best, most appropriate code.

It is not uncommon for skin grafts to be planned, from the beginning, to be done in stages. When this is the case, the second and subsequent portions of the staged procedure should be appended with modifier 58. This is directly described in CPT's modifier 58 description: *(a) planned or anticipated (staged).*

If the **donor area (site)** requires a skin graft or a local flap to repair it, it should be coded as an additional procedure. When evaluating the size of the wound that has been grafted, the measurement of *100 sq. cm* is used with patients aged 10 and older. The code descriptor referring to a *percentage of the body area* applies only to patients under the age of 10.

harvesting
The process of taking skin or tissue (on the same body or another).

donor area (site)
The area or part of the body from which skin or tissue is removed with the intention of placing that skin or tissue in another area or body.

EXAMPLE

15002 Surgical preparation or creation of recipient site by excision of open wounds, burn eschar, or scar (including subcutaneous tissues), or incisional release of scar contracture, trunk, arms, legs; first *100 sq cm or 1% of body area of infants and children*

In the subheading relating to flaps and grafts, when the physician attaches a flap, either in transfer or to the final site, the anatomical site identified in the code's description is the *recipient* site, not the donor site.

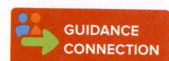

GUIDANCE CONNECTION

Additional explanation can be found in the guidelines within the **Surgery** section, directly under the subhead **Skin Replacement Surgery,** in your CPT book.

EXAMPLE

15732 Muscle, myocutaneous, or fasciocutaneous flap; head and neck (e.g., temporalis, masseter muscle, sternocleidomastoid, levator scapulae)

When a tube is formed to be used later, or when "delay" of flap is done before the transfer, the anatomical sites indicated in the code description refer to the *donor* site, not the recipient site.

GUIDANCE CONNECTION

Additional explanation can be found in the guidelines within the **Surgery** section, directly under the subhead **Flaps (Skin and/or Deep Tissues),** in your CPT book.

EXAMPLE

15620 Delay of flap or sectioning of flap (division and inset); at forehead, cheeks, chin, mouth, neck, axillae, genitalia, hands or feet

When extensive immobilization is performed, such as large plaster casts or traction, the application of the immobilization device should be coded as a separate procedure. However, make note that the procedure codes in the range 15570–15738 already include small or standard immobilization, such as a sling or splint.

YOU CODE IT! CASE STUDY

Rudy Fetland, an 11-year-old male, had burn eschar on his face from an accident. Dr. Imatione performed a surgical preparation of the area. Two days later, Dr. Imatione applied a dermal autograft to the 30-sq.-cm area.

Based on the notes, find the best, most appropriate procedure code(s) to report all of Dr. Imatione's work for Rudy's injury.

Step 1: Read the case completely.

Step 2: Abstract the notes: Which key words can you identify relating to the procedures performed?

_____

Step 3: Query the provider, if necessary.

Step 4: Diagnosis: Burn eschar.

Step 5: Code the procedure(s).

_____

Step 6: Link the procedure codes to at least one diagnosis code.

Step 7: Back code to double-check your choices.

Answer:

Did you determine the following codes?

15004 Surgical preparation or creation of recipient site by excision of open wounds, burn eschar, or scar (including subcutaneous tissues), or incisional release of scar contracture, face, scalp, eyelids, mouth, neck, ears, orbits, genitalia, hands, feet, and/or multiple digits; first 100 sq cm or 1% of body area of infants and children

15135-58 Dermal autograft, face, scalp, eyelids, mouth, neck, ears, orbits, genitalia, hands, feet, and/or multiple digits; first 100 sq cm or less, or 1% of body area of infants and children; staged procedure

Great work!

Destruction

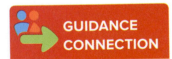

GUIDANCE CONNECTION

Additional explanations can be found in in-section guidelines located within the **Surgery** section, subhead **Destruction,** directly above code 17000.

Destruction is the term used for the removal of diseased or unwanted tissue from the body by surgical or other means, such as surgical curettement (also known as curettage), laser treatment, electrosurgery, chemical treatment, or cryosurgery. Ablation is the surgical destruction of tissue or a body part. When the tissue is destroyed rather than excised, there is nothing left. Therefore, there will be no specimens sent to pathology for analysis. The codes in the destruction subheading of the surgical section include the administration of local anesthesia.

There are several methods that a physician can use to destroy tissue.

- *Cauterization* is the process of destroying tissue with the use of a chemical or electricity to seal a wound and stop bleeding. Some cauterizations can be accomplished with extreme heat or cold. For example, you might see physician's notes document the removal of an internal polyp with the use of hot forceps.

- *Cryosurgical* techniques use liquid nitrogen or freezing carbon dioxide to destroy the tissue of concern.

- *Curettage* is the method of using a special surgical tool, called a curette, to scrape an organ, a muscle, or other anatomical site.

- *Electrosurgical* methods use high-frequency electrical current instead of a scalpel to separate and destroy tissue. One example of this is electrolysis, which removes hair by using electricity to destroy the hair follicle.
- *Laser* surgery uses light to cut, separate, or destroy tissue. The term *laser* is actually an acronym for light amplification by stimulated emission of radiation.

LET'S CODE IT! SCENARIO

Frank Mulrooney, a 43-year-old male, came to see Dr. Johnston, his podiatrist, for the removal of a benign plantar wart from the sole of his left foot. Dr. Johnston administered a local anesthetic and then destroyed the wart using a chemosurgical technique. A protective bandage was applied to the foot, and Frank was sent home with an appointment to return in 1 week for a follow-up check.

Let's Code It!

The notes indicate that Frank had a *benign plantar wart* that Dr. Johnston *destroyed* using *chemosurgery*.

Let's go to the Alphabetic Index and look up *destruction*.

Under *destruction*, you will see an alphabetical list that includes both anatomical sites as well as skin conditions, such as cysts and lesions. You know from the notes that Dr. Johnston destroyed a wart on Frank's foot. There are no listings for foot or sole of foot. However, there is a listing for Warts, flat . . . 17110–17111. Do you know if a plantar wart is a flat wart? Because this is the only choice here, let's go to the codes suggested and see if the numerical listing can provide more information.

The code descriptions read

17110 Destruction (e.g., laser surgery, electrosurgery, cryosurgery, chemosurgery, surgical curettement), of benign lesions other than skin tags or cutaneous vascular proliferative lesions; up to 14 lesions

17111 15 or more lesions

These descriptions do not really answer our question about whether a plantar wart is a flat wart or a benign lesion. But before you query the doctor, go to the beginning of this subsection and read down. Directly below the description for code 17003 is a notation:

(For destruction of common or plantar warts, see 17110, 17111.)

This is an excellent example of how you must investigate all possibilities and really give the CPT book a chance to point you toward the correct code.

Dr. Johnston destroyed with chemosurgery Frank's benign lesion that was not a skin tag or a cutaneous vascular proliferative lesion, and he only had one. 17110 is perfect!

Mohs Micrographic Surgery

The group of codes for Mohs micrographic surgery (17311–17315) will be used only when you are coding for a physician who is specially trained in this type of procedure because it requires one doctor to act as *both* surgeon and pathologist. If two different professionals perform these functions, these codes cannot be used.

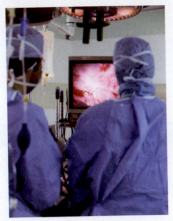

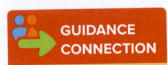

GUIDANCE CONNECTION

Additional explanation can be found in the guidelines within the **Surgery** section, directly under the subhead **Mohs Micrographic Surgery,** in your CPT book.

If a repair is performed during the same session, the repair procedures should be coded separately.

If a biopsy is performed on the same day as the Mohs surgery because the physician suspects that the patient has skin cancer, it should be reported separately, as well, appended with modifier 59 Distinct Procedural Service.

Chapter Summary

When coding surgical procedures, you have the challenge of determining which services are included in the procedure code, which services are part of the global package, and which services must be coded separately.

In addition, it is important to remember that the Surgery section of the CPT book not only includes codes for reporting services provided in an operating room under general anesthesia but also includes codes for reporting simple and small procedures such as removing a splinter.

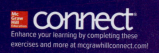

Using Terminology

Match each key term to the appropriate definition.

_____ 1. LO 7.2 The length of time allotted for postoperative care included in the surgical package, which is generally accepted to be 90 days for major surgical procedures and up to 10 days for minor procedures.

_____ 2. LO 7.6 The process of taking skin or tissue (on the same body or another).

_____ 3. LO 7.6 The area or part of the body from which skin or tissue is removed with the intention of placing that skin or tissue in another area or body.

_____ 4. LO 7.1 The methodology or technique used by the physician to perform the procedure, service, or treatment.

_____ 5. LO 7.2 The accepted principles of conduct, services, or treatments that are established as the expected behavior.

_____ 6. LO 7.6 A method of sealing an opening in the skin involving a multilayered closure and a reconstructive procedure such as scar revision, debridement, or retention sutures.

_____ 7. LO 7.6 The full-thickness removal of a lesion, including margins; includes (for coding purposes) a simple closure.

_____ 8. LO 7.6 The area, or site, of the body receiving a graft of skin or tissue.

_____ 9. LO 7.6 A multilevel method of sealing an opening in the skin involving one or more of the deeper layers of the skin.

_____ 10. LO 7.6 A method of sealing an opening in the skin (epidermis or dermis), involving only one layer. It includes the administration of a local anesthesia and/or chemical or electrocauterization of a wound not closed.

_____ 11. LO 7.6 A measure that extends from the epidermis to the connective tissue layer of the skin.

A. Complex closure
B. Donor area
C. Excision
D. Full-thickness
E. Global period
F. Harvesting
G. Intermediate closure
H. Recipient area
I. Simple closure
J. Standard of care
K. Surgical approach

Checking Your Understanding

Choose the most appropriate answer for each of the following questions.

1. LO 7.2 The global surgical package includes all *except*

    a. preprocedure evaluation and management.
    b. general anesthesia.
    c. the procedure.
    d. follow-up care.

2. LO 7.3 The global period is determined by

    a. the type of anesthesia provided.
    b. the size of the excision.
    c. the location of the donor site.
    d. the standard of care.

3. LO 7.2 Which of the following is an example of a diagnostic test not included in the global package?

    a. closure.
    b. local infiltration.
    c. biopsy.
    d. metacarpal block.

4. LO 7.2 When a procedure is planned as a series of procedures, each service after the first should be appended with the modifier

    a. 76.
    b. 79.
    c. 58.
    d. 59.

5. LO 7.3 When a surgeon does not provide preoperative or postoperative care to the patient upon whom he or she operates, the procedure code should be appended with modifier

    a. 54.
    b. 55.
    c. 56.
    d. 77.

6. LO 7.6 Excision of lesions is reported

    a. with total measurement of all lesions removed in one code.
    b. with only the largest lesion coded.
    c. with each lesion coded separately.
    d. as a part of the total surgical procedure.

7. LO 7.6 The code for excision includes this type of repair.

    a. intermediate.
    b. complex.
    c. none.
    d. simple.

8. LO 7.6 If the surgeon performs a reexcision of a lesion during a later encounter with the patient, append the procedure code with modifier

    a. 58.
    b. 59.
    c. 51.
    d. 77.

9. LO 7.6 If multiple wounds located on the same anatomical site are repaired with the same complexity, report this procedure by

    a. coding each wound separately.
    b. coding only the largest wound.
    c. adding all the lengths together and coding the total.
    d. coding the average of all the wounds repaired.

10. LO 7.6 The elements of determining the most accurate code for a skin graft include all *except*

    a. the size of the recipient area.
    b. the type of donor.
    c. the location of the recipient area.
    d. the type of graft.

Applying Your Knowledge

1. **LO 7.1** List the three key terms to watch for when coding a procedure. _____
   _____

2. **LO 7.1** Differentiate among prophylactic, diagnostic, and therapeutic treatments. _____
   _____

3. **LO 7.2** What elements are included in the surgical package? _____
   _____

4. **LO 7.3** What are the global period time frames? _____
   _____

5. **LO 7.4** What are "Unusual Services and Treatments," and how are they identified? _____
   _____

6. **LO 7.5** What does the notation "Separate Procedure" tell a professional coder? _____
   _____

7. **LO 7.6** What is the largest organ in the human body? What is its function? _____
   _____

8. **LO 7.6** What is the formula to find the correct coded size of an excised lesion? _____
   _____

9. **LO 7.6** Differentiate between intermediate closure and complex closure. _____
   _____

10. **LO 7.6** List the three things that determine the most accurate codes for skin grafts. _____
    _____

Using the techniques described in this chapter, carefully read through the case studies and determine the most accurate surgery CPT code(s) and modifier(s), if appropriate, for each case study.

1. Dr. Quartermain performed a rhinoplasty to correct the nasal deformity on Frank Chestnut, a 3-year-old male born with a cleft palate. The tip, septum, and osteotomies were all treated.

   _____

2. Roger Appleton, a 27-year-old male, cut his thumb at work on a construction site 3 weeks ago. He did not get any treatment for the wound, which became infected. Today, Dr. Kenny will amputate the thumb. The procedure is made more complicated by the spread of the infection to the surrounding tissues, as Dr. Kenny fights to save as much of the hand as possible.

   _____

3. One week ago, Dr. Sweetzer performed a ureteroneocystostomy with cystoscopy and ureteral stent placement laparoscopically on Patricia Worster. However, today he must perform an open procedure on her to drain a renal abscess that was discovered. Code the drainage of Patricia's renal abscess.

   _____

4. On May 1, Dr. Monmouth performed a percutaneous core needle biopsy on Stephan English. Two days later, after reviewing the results of the biopsy, Dr. Monmouth performed a complete thyroidectomy on Stephan. Code both procedures.

   _____

5. Dr. Macintosh performed a lumbar laminectomy on Rick Greenlaw on September 15. One month later, as originally planned, Dr. Macintosh took Rick back into the OR to implant an epidural drug infusor with a subcutaneous reservoir. Code both procedures.

   _____

6. Warren Samuels, a 47-year-old male, owns a landscaping business. While he was reviewing some property to write a proposal, a toy poodle belonging to the property owners bit him on the leg. While the 12-cm wound was not severe, Warren wanted Dr. Dawson to check it out. Dr. Dawson performed a simple closure and applied a bandage.

   _____

7. Jackie Thurman, a 35-year-old female, was seen by her regular physician, Dr. Callman, after she spilled a pot of boiling water on her stomach and legs. Thankfully, her apron and corduroy dress absorbed most of the heat, and she had only first-degree burns. Dr. Callman performed initial local treatment and sent her home.

_____

8. Colleen Sizmauski, a 59-year-old female, came to Dr. Lafferty's office to have an epidermal facial chemical peel performed.

_____

9. Mark Matthews, a 32-year-old male, was seen by Dr. Rothstein, his regular physician, because Mark smashed his finger with a hammer while installing wallboard. Dr. Rothstein performed an evacuation of a subungual hematoma.

_____

10. Cletus Jones, a 23-year-old male, was in a fight at a hockey game and was hit in the head with a bottle, which caused some deep lacerations in his scalp. Dr. Fairchild performed a layered closure of the wounds: one 2.0 cm, one 4.5 cm, and two that were each 1.0 cm in length.

_____

11. Cassandra Twillinger, a 29-year-old female, is postmastectomy and comes in today so that Dr. Edwin can perform a breast reconstruction with free flap.

_____

12. Jason McCall, a 51-year-old male, has a pilonidal cyst. Dr. Bonneti performs an I&D.

_____

13. Denita Tauber found a sore on her neck. The lab test identified it as a malignant lesion, and Dr. Capp excised the lesion, which measured 2.9 cm with margins.

_____

14. Hannah Lopez, a 63-year-old female, is bedridden with two broken legs in traction. Dr. Quinn excised an ischial pressure ulcer with a primary suture.

_____

15. Ruth Ann Marcelle, a 9-year-old female, had a partial thickness burn on her hand. Dr. Assiss performed a debridement and dressing of the injury.

_____

The following exercises provide practice in the application of abstracting the physicians' notes and learning to work with SOAP notes from our health care facility, Cipher, Victors & Associates. These case studies (SOAP notes) are modeled on real patient encounters. Using the techniques described in this chapter, carefully read through the case studies and determine the most accurate surgery CPT code(s) and modifier(s), if appropriate, for each case study.

CIPHER, VICTORS & ASSOCIATES
A Complete Health Care Facility
234 MAIN STREET • ANYTOWN, FL 32711 • 407-555-1234

PATIENT: FORESTER, ASA
ACCOUNT/EHR #: FOREAS01
Admission Date: 10/09/18
Discharge Date: 10/09/18

DATE: 10/09/18
Preoperative DX: Lacerations of arm, hand, and leg
Postoperative DX: Same
Procedure: Layered closure of leg laceration; simple closure of arm and hand lacerations

Surgeon: Geoff Conner, MD
Assistant: None
Anesthesia: General

INDICATIONS: The patient is a 4-year-old male brought to the emergency room by his father. He was helping his father install a new window when the window fell and shattered. The boy suffered lacerations on his left hand, left arm, and left leg.

PROCEDURE: The patient was placed on the table in supine position. Satisfactory anesthesia was obtained. The area was prepped, and attention to the deeper laceration of the left thigh, right above the patella, was first. A layered closure was performed, and the 5.1-cm laceration was closed successfully with sutures. The lacerations on the upper extremity, a 2-cm laceration on the left hand at the base of the fifth metacarpal, and the 3-cm laceration on the left arm, just below the joint capsule in the posterior position, were successfully closed with 4-0 Vicryl, as well. The patient tolerated the procedures well and was transported to the recovery room.

Geoff Conner, MD

GC/mg D: 10/09/18 09:50:16 T: 10/09/18 12:55:01

Determine the most accurate surgery CPT code(s) and modifier(s), if appropriate.

_____

_____

_____

CIPHER, VICTORS & ASSOCIATES
A Complete Health Care Facility
234 MAIN STREET • ANYTOWN, FL 32711 • 407-555-1234

PATIENT: UNGER, SOPHIE
ACCOUNT/EHR #:   UNGESO01
Admission Date: 10/15/18
Discharge Date: 10/15/18

DATE: 10/15/18
Preoperative DX: Augmentation of lips
Postoperative DX: Same
Procedure: Collagen injections

Surgeon: Wayne Fleeter, MD
Assistant: None
Anesthesia: Local

INDICATIONS: The patient is a 41-year-old female with a low self-image. She presents today for enhancement of her lips.

PROCEDURE: The patient was placed on the table in supine position. Local anesthesia was administered. As soon as patient stated a complete loss of feeling in the area, the injections were given subcutaneously—a total of 2.3 cc.

Wayne Fleeter, MD

WF/mg D: 10/09/18 09:50:16 T: 10/09/18 12:55:01

Determine the most accurate surgery CPT code(s) and modifier(s), if appropriate.

_____

_____

_____

CIPHER, VICTORS & ASSOCIATES
A Complete Health Care Facility
234 MAIN STREET • ANYTOWN, FL 32711 • 407-555-1234

PATIENT: FREMONT, CASSIE
ACCOUNT/EHR #:   FREMCA01
Admission Date: 11/01/18
Discharge Date: 11/01/18

DATE: 11/01/18
Preoperative DX: Toxic epidermal necrolysis
Postoperative DX: Same
Procedure: Xenogaft

Surgeon: Wayne Fleeter, MD
Assistant: None
Anesthesia: Local

INDICATIONS: The patient is a 26-year-old female with a diagnosis of toxic epidermal necrolysis as a result of a reaction to procainamide, previously prescribed by a physician no longer in attendance.

PROCEDURE: The patient was placed on the table in supine position. Local anesthesia was administered. As soon as patient stated a complete loss of feeling in the left forearm, the dermal xenograft proceeded. Procedure was repeated for right forearm.

 A total of 150 sq. cm of grafting was successfully completed.
 Bandages were applied. A prescription for Darvocet N100 po q4-6h prn was given to the patient before discharge.

 Follow-up appointment in office scheduled for 10 days.

Wayne Fleeter, MD

WF/mg D: 11/01/18 09:50:16 T: 11/01/18 12:55:01

Determine the most accurate surgery CPT code(s) and modifier(s), if appropriate.

_____

_____

_____

CIPHER, VICTORS & ASSOCIATES
A Complete Health Care Facility
234 MAIN STREET • ANYTOWN, FL 32711 • 407-555-1234

PATIENT: TOMLINSON, MARINA
ACCOUNT/EHR #:   TOMLMA01
DATE: 11/01/18

Attending Physician: James I. Cipher, MD

A 9 year-old girl is brought to our pediatric clinic today with the chief complaint of a large, red, circular rash on her right thigh. The rash has been present for 2 weeks and has been enlarging. Her mother states that 3 weeks ago, the family was visiting relatives at a rural farm in Iowa and one day after playing outside in the woods, the girl was found to have a tick attached to her thigh. Her father removed the tick with tweezers; however, a red macule remained at the site where the tick had been attached. One week after the tick was removed, a red ring developed around the macule, and then the ring appeared to grow larger by expanding outward, leaving an area of central clearing. The girl has had a mild headache and myalgia but has been afebrile.

EXAM: VS T 37.1, P 90, RR 20, BP 100/70. Pt is alert, active, in no distress, and is nontoxic. Over the anterior surface of her right thigh, there is a red ring, 20 cm in diameter, with central clearing, and a central brownish-red macule that is 3 mm in diameter. The thigh is nontender. All joints are nontender and nonswollen. Her neck is supple without lymphadenopathy. The remainder of her exam is unremarkable.

No laboratory tests are performed. The skin lesion is biopsied and diagnosed as erythema migrans (EM), and a diagnosis of Lyme disease is made. She is judged to have early localized infection.

RX: Amoxicillin, 50 mg/kg/day po divided tid for 21 days.

Follow-up if headache and myalgia do not resolve within 1 week.

James I. Cipher, MD

JIC/mg D: 11/01/18 09:50:16 T: 11/01/18 12:55:01

Determine the most accurate surgery CPT code(s) and modifier(s), if appropriate.

_____

_____

_____

CIPHER, VICTORS & ASSOCIATES
A Complete Health Care Facility
234 MAIN STREET • ANYTOWN, FL 32711 • 407-555-1234

PATIENT:	VIANCE, ELLIOT
ACCOUNT/EHR #:	VIANEL01
Admission Date:	09/23/18
Discharge Date:	09/23/18
DATE:	09/23/18
Preoperative DX:	Third-degree burns, palm of right hand
Postoperative DX:	Same
Procedure:	Allograft
Surgeon:	Wayne Fleeter, MD
Assistant:	None
Anesthesia:	General

INDICATIONS: The patient is a 19-year-old male with electrical burns on the palm of his right hand.

PROCEDURE: The patient was placed on the table in supine position. Anesthesia was administered. Skin grafted from a healthy cadaveric donor was prepared and applied to resurface the palm of the hand. Total of 75 sq. cm used.

    Sterile bandage was applied with instructions to patient for care and replacement.

    A prescription for Darvocet N100 po q4h prn was given to the patient before discharge.

Follow-up appointment recommended for 1 week.

_____

Wayne Fleeter, MD

WF/mg D: 09/23/18 09:50:16 T: 09/23/18 12:55:01

Determine the most accurate surgery CPT code(s) and modifier(s), if appropriate.

_____

_____

_____

SURGERY CODING, PART 2

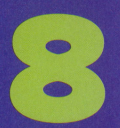

Learning Outcomes *After completing this chapter, the student should be able to:*

LO 8.1 Correctly apply the guidelines for coding procedures on the musculoskeletal system.

LO 8.2 Recognize the details required to accurately report procedures on the respiratory system.

LO 8.3 Identify guidelines to direct reporting services to the cardiovascular system.

LO 8.4 Distinguish the various procedures on the digestive system.

LO 8.5 Ascertain the elements of coding services to the urinary system.

LO 8.6 Determine how to accurately report procedures to the male genital system.

LO 8.7 Apply the guidelines to report procedures to the female genital system.

LO 8.8 Interpret documentation to accurately report procedures on the nervous system.

LO 8.9 Recognize the necessary details to report procedures on the eye and ocular adnexa.

LO 8.10 Report accurately procedures on the auditory system.

In CPT, the term *surgery* is not limited to only those services and treatments performed in an operating room (OR) or even in a hospital. Within this section of the CPT book, codes are listed that report

- Incision and drainage of a cyst.
- Debridement.
- Simple repair of a superficial wound.

All these services can easily be performed in a physician's office. In addition, many procedures are now performed at an ambulatory surgical center or outpatient department.

In Chap. 7, you began learning about coding surgical procedures involving the integumentary system. This chapter continues from that point through the balance of the Surgery section of the CPT.

LO 8.1 Musculoskeletal System

The musculoskeletal system subsection of codes reports procedures and treatments performed on the bones, ligaments, cartilage, muscles, and tendons in the human body.

Key Terms

Allotransplantation

Arthrodesis

Closed treatment

Laminectomy

Manipulation

Open treatment

Percutaneous skeletal fixation

Saphenous vein

Transplantation

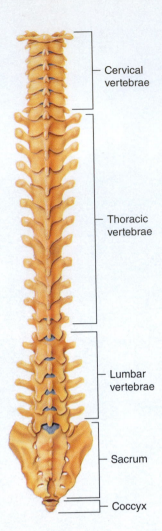

Cervical vertebrae

Thoracic vertebrae

Lumbar vertebrae

Sacrum

Coccyx

The Code Package

Codes in this subsection already include the application and removal of a cast or traction device as a part of the procedure performed.

Open or Closed Treatment

Procedures and services can be provided for various sites of the musculoskeletal system as an open treatment or a closed treatment. These two words, *open* and *closed*, are used for both the description of the fracture itself (in the diagnostic statement) and the description of the procedure. Be careful not to confuse these identifiers because they are NOT interrelated—that is, a compound (open) fracture is not automatically treated with an open procedure. Be certain to differentiate the description of the fracture from the description of the procedure. Let's begin with understanding what CPT means by open treatment or closed treatment.

Open Treatment CPT defines **open treatment** as a procedure provided to treat a fractured bone that is either

> Surgically opened, so that the fracture can be visualized and internal fixation may be applied.
>
> or
>
> The fractured site is not opened surgically, but the fractured bone is opened remotely from the site to enable the surgeon to insert an intramedullary nail.

Closed Treatment According to CPT, the **closed treatment** of a fracture is performed:

- With or without manipulation.
- With or without traction.
- Without the fracture being opened and visualized.

Penetrating Trauma Wounds

The CPT book distinguishes between wounds and penetrating trauma wounds. A penetrating trauma wound requires

1. Surgery to explore the wound.
2. Determination of the depth and complexity of the wound.
3. Identification of any damage created by the penetrating object (such as the stabbing from a knife or the wound from a bullet).
4. Debridement of the wound to remove any particles, dirt, and foreign fragments.
5. Ligation or coagulation of minor subcutaneous tissue, muscle fascia, and/or muscle (not severe enough to require a thoracotomy or laparotomy).

You will use codes 20100–20103 to report the exploration of such wounds. Then, code whichever repair the physician actually performs, as documented in the notes.

Bone Grafts and Implants

Medical science and technology have progressed amazingly. Be certain to differentiate between skin grafts (as reviewed in Chap. 7) and bone, cartilage, tendon, and fascia lata grafts that are coded from the musculoskeletal subsection.

If the code description does not specifically reference the harvesting of the graft or implant (for example, code 20936 "includes harvesting the graft"), then the procedure for obtaining autogenous bone, cartilage, tendon, fascia lata grafts, or other tissues should be reported separately.

open treatment
Surgically opening the fracture site, or another site in the body nearby, in order to treat the fractured bone.

closed treatment
The treatment of a fracture without surgically opening the affected area.

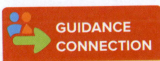

GUIDANCE CONNECTION

Additional explanation can be found in the guidelines within the **Surgery** section, directly under the subhead **Musculoskeletal System,** subsection **Wound Exploration—Trauma (e.g., Penetrating Gunshot, Stab Wound),** in your CPT book.

Spine

As you may remember from anatomy class, the human spine is referred to in sections: cervical (at or near the neck), thoracic (the chest area), lumbar (at the waist and lower back), and sacral. References to the individual vertebrae are most often identified by their alphanumeric identifiers, such as C1 (cervical vertebra number 1), L5 (lumbar vertebra number 5), or S3 (sacral vertebra number 3).

Arthrodesis   **Arthrodesis** is the surgical immobilization of a joint so that the bones can heal, or grow solidly, together. When coding arthrodesis, you will need to identify the approach technique used by the physician, such as

- Lateral extracavitary technique.
- Anterior transoral or extraoral technique.
- Anterior interbody technique.
- Posterior technique: craniocervical or atlas-axis.
- Posterior or posterolateral technique.
- Posterior interbody technique with number of interspaces treated.

Arthrodesis can be performed alone or in combination with other procedures such as bone grafting, osteotomy, fracture care, vertebral corpectomy, or **laminectomy.** When arthrodesis is done at the same time as another procedure, modifier 51 Multiple Procedures should be appended to the code for the arthrodesis. This applies to almost all procedures, with the exception of bone grafting and instrumentation. Modifier 51 Multiple Procedures is not used in those cases because bone grafts and instrumentation are never performed without arthrodesis.

Laminotomy   A laminotomy is a partial laminectomy used to treat lumbar disc herniation. Removing a portion of the lamina is often sufficient to access the affected nerve root. Then, the disc herniation can be visualized and accessed from beneath the nerve root. This procedure should be reported with the most accurate code, based on the details in the documentation:

> **63020** Laminotomy (hemilaminectomy), with decompression of nerve root(s), including partial facetectomy, foraminotomy and/or excision of herniated intervertebral disc, including open or endoscopically-assisted approach; one interspace, cervical
>
> **63030** Laminotomy (hemilaminectomy), with decompression of nerve root(s), including partial facetectomy, foraminotomy and/or excision of herniated intervertebral disc, including open or endoscopically-assisted approach; one interspace, lumbar

What's the difference between these two codes? Let's compare them:

63020	63030
Laminotomy (hemilaminectomy)	Laminotomy (hemilaminectomy),
With decompression of nerve root(s),	With decompression of nerve root(s),
Including partial facetectomy, foraminotomy and/or excision of herniated intervertebral disc, including open or endoscopically-assisted approach;	Including partial facetectomy, foraminotomy and/or excision of herniated intervertebral disc, including open or endoscopically-assisted approach;
One interspace, cervical	One interspace, lumbar

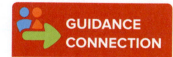

GUIDANCE CONNECTION

Additional explanation can be found in the guidelines within the **Surgery** section, directly under the subhead **Spine (Vertebral Column),** in your CPT book.

arthrodesis
The immobilization of a joint using a surgical technique.

laminectomy
The surgical removal of a vertebral posterior arch.

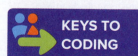

KEYS TO CODING

CPT describes a vertebral interspace as the non-bony compartment between two adjacent vertebral bodies. This space houses the intervertebral disc and includes the nucleus pulposus, the annulus fibrosus, and two cartilaginous endplates.

You can see that the only difference between the two code descriptions is the location of the vertebra being treated. This is a piece of information you will need to determine the correct code.

Then, depending upon how many discs were involved, you might add

+63035 each additional interspace, cervical or lumbar

LET'S CODE IT! SCENARIO

Jamica Jones, a 51-year-old female, was diagnosed with degenerative disc disease 3 months ago. She is admitted today for Dr. Veronic to perform a posterior arthrodesis of L5–S1 (transverse process), utilizing a morselized autogenous iliac bone graft harvested through a separate fascial incision. Jamica tolerates the procedure well and is returned to her hospital room after 2 hours in recovery.

Let's Code It!

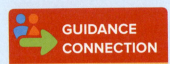

GUIDANCE CONNECTION

Additional explanation can be found in the guidelines within the **Surgery** section, directly under the subhead **Spine**, subsection **Arthrodesis**, in your CPT book.

GUIDANCE CONNECTION

Additional explanation can be found in the guidelines within the **Surgery** section, directly under the subhead **Spine (Vertebral Column)**, subsection **Fracture and/or Dislocation**, in your CPT book.

percutaneous skeletal fixation
The insertion of fixation instruments (such as pins) placed across the fracture site. It may be done under x-ray imaging for guidance purposes.

Pull out the description of the procedures that Dr. Veronic performed. First, note the "posterior arthrodesis of L5–S1" and then the "morselized autogenous iliac bone graft harvested through a separate fascial incision."

Let's begin in the alphabetic index with the listing for arthrodesis. The designation of L5–S1 tells you this was done to Jamica's spine. However, *spine* isn't listed under arthrodesis. Keep reading and you will see *vertebra* listed, *lumbar* underneath that, and *posterior* beneath that. However, the physician noted "transverse process," which is listed here as well. Let's investigate code 22612, as suggested by the index.

22612 Arthrodesis, posterior or posterolateral technique, single level; lumbar (with or without lateral transverse technique)

This matches the physician's notes.

Now, let's move to the next procedure performed. Look in the alphabetic index under *bone graft*. Read through the list until you reach the item that reflects what was done for Jamica: *spine surgery*. Indented below that you will see *autograft* (the same as *autogenous*) and then *morselized*. The index suggests code 20937. Turn to the numerical list and take a look at the code's description:

+20937 Autograft for spine surgery only (includes harvesting the graft); morselized (through separate skin or fascial incision)

Notice the symbol to the left of code 20937: +. The plus sign means this is an add-on code and it cannot be used alone. However, the notation below 20937 indicates that you are permitted to use this code along with 22612.

In addition, the guidelines state that when arthrodesis is performed with another procedure, you need to add modifier 51 to the arthrodesis code *except* when the other procedure is a bone graft. This is the case in Jamica's record, so the claim form for Jamica Jones's surgery will show procedure codes 22612 and 20937—with no modifiers. Great job!

Fractures and Dislocations

Many different types of treatments may be provided for a fracture and/or dislocation. Be careful not to confuse the diagnosed state of the fracture (closed, open, or compound) with the description of the treatment (for instance, **percutaneous skeletal fixation** or manipulation) provided by the physician.

Fracture Treatments Needless to say, the treatment plan for the patient will be determined by the type and location of the fracture.

Reduction or **manipulation** may be necessary to realign the bone pieces so that union can occur properly. This may be done externally (closed reduction, known as manipulation) or surgically (open reduction).

Whether the fracture is open or closed, it may require fixation. *Internal fixation* is the process of placing plates and screws, or pins, or other devices directly onto or around the bone, inside of the patient. When *external fixation* is used, a device—such as a brace, cast, or halo—prevents motion in a certain area of the body. The care for a facture may also include the external application of traction.

manipulation
The attempted return of a fracture or dislocation to its normal alignment manually by the physician.

LET'S CODE IT! CASE SCENARIO

Benjamin Zabine, a 17-year-old male, plays basketball on his high school team. While practicing in his driveway, he fell and fractured the shaft of his tibia. Dr. Casson, the orthopedist on duty at the emergency room, is able to use a percutaneous fixation using pins.

Let's Code It!

Let's turn to the Alphabetic Index. This time, we won't look up the procedure by the type of treatment (*percutaneous*), but we will look at the condition that was treated: *fracture*. Under *fracture*, find the anatomical site of the fracture—*tibia*—and then the *percutaneous fixation*. The index suggests code 27756. Let's check the description in the numerical listing:

> 27756 Percutaneous skeletal fixation of tibial shaft fracture (with or without fibular fracture)(e.g., pins or screws)

That's exactly what Dr. Casson did. Great job!

Spinal Procedures There are several procedures often performed on patients with spinal concerns:

- *Arthrodesis* is the surgical immobilization of a joint.
- *Arthroplasty* is the insertion of an artificial disc.
- *Discectomy* is the surgical removal of an intervertebral disc, either a portion of the disc or the entire component.
- *Laminectomy* is the surgical removal of the lamina (posterior arch) of the vertebra.
- *Osteotomy* is performed to remove, or cut out, a portion of a bone.
- *Vertebroplasty* and *kyphoplasty* may be performed surgically or percutaneously for the purpose of repairing a vertebra that has been compromised by a compression fracture.

Spinal Fusion Spinal fusion permanently locks two or more spinal vertebrae together so that they move as a single unit utilizing bone grafts, with or without screws, plates, cages, or other devices. The bone grafts are placed around the problem area of the spine during surgery. As the body heals itself, the graft helps join the bones together.

Performed under general anesthesia, fusion of lumbar vertebrae is generally done using a posterior lumbar approach, whereas cervical vertebrae are accessed using an anterior cervical approach. An anterior thoracic approach is normally used for fusion of thoracic vertebrae.

Spinal fusion is known to diminish mobility because of the connections made between the individual vertebrae involved in the procedure. This is one of the primary

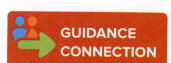

GUIDANCE CONNECTION

Additional explanation can be found in the guidelines within the **Surgery** section, directly under the subhead **Spine (Vertebral Column,** subsection **Spinal Instrumentation,** in your CPT book.

reasons health care technology has been working diligently on an artificial intervertebral disc that can continue to permit individual vertebral motion. Artificial discs have been evidenced to allow for six degrees of freedom.

After removing the ineffective or damaged disc, two metal plates are pressed into the bony endplates above and below the interspace and held into place by metal spikes. A plastic spacer, usually made of a polyethylene core, is inserted between the plates. The patient's own body weight compresses the spacer after the surgery is complete.

YOU CODE IT! CASE STUDY

Hannah Rosensweig, a 71-year-old female, fell and sustained a fracture to the C4 vertebral process. Due to the position of the fracture, Dr. Plant was able to use a closed treatment without having to put her through a surgical procedure.

You Code It!

Go through the steps and determine what procedure code(s) should be reported for this encounter between Dr. Plant and Hannah Rosensweig.

Step 1: Read the case completely.

Step 2: Abstract the notes: What key words can you identify relating to the procedures performed?

_____

Step 3: Query the provider, if necessary:

Step 4: Diagnosis: Fracture, vertebral process.

Step 5: Code the procedure(s).

_____

Step 6: Link the procedure codes to at least one diagnosis code.

Step 7: Back code to double-check your choices.

Answer:

Did you find the correct code?

22305 Closed treatment of vertebral process fracture(s)

Great job!

Lumbar Puncture (Spinal Tap)

When a patient exhibits certain signs and symptoms, the physician may decide to perform a lumbar puncture, commonly known as a spinal tap. In this procedure, a needle is inserted into the spinal canal between two lumbar vertebrae to collect cerebrospinal fluid (CSF).

The two key procedure codes are differentiated by the reason the procedure is performed—diagnostic or therapeutic.

62270 Spinal puncture, lumbar, diagnostic

62272 Spinal puncture, therapeutic, for drainage of cerebrospinal fluid (by needle or catheter)

LO 8.2 Respiratory System

The organs and tissues involved with bringing oxygen into the body and discharging gases make up the respiratory system. Procedures and treatments affecting this sector are coded from the Respiratory System subsection.

Sinus Endoscopy

The upper respiratory system includes the nasal passages and sinus cavities. The standard for a nasal/sinus endoscopic procedure, performed for diagnostic purposes, includes assessment of the interior nasal cavity, the middle and superior meatus, the turbinates, and the sphenoethmoid recess. Therefore, the inspection of all of these areas is included in the diagnostic sinus endoscopy procedure code.

When a surgical sinus endoscopy is provided, the code descriptions include both the sinusotomy and a diagnostic endoscopy.

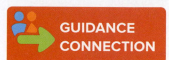

GUIDANCE CONNECTION

Additional explanation can be found in the guidelines within the **Surgery** section, directly under the subhead **Respiratory System**, subsection **Endoscopy**, in your CPT book.

LET'S CODE IT! SCENARIO

Gregory Paulson, a 39-year old male, had been diagnosed with chronic sinusitis many years ago and has tried everything. He told Dr. Kittleson that no medication has worked and the inflammation just won't go away. Dr. Kittleson performed a nasal/sinus diagnostic endoscopy via the inferior meatus, with a maxillary sinusoscopy.

Let's Code It!

The documentation explains that Dr. Kittleson performed a "diagnostic endoscopy via the inferior meatus, with a maxillary sinusoscopy," so let's turn to the CPT Alphabetic Index and find Endoscopy. You can see a long list of anatomical sites beneath. On what anatomical site did Dr. Kittleson perform this endoscopy? The notes state "nasal/sinus." Find the term nose under Endoscopy and you will see there are three choices: diagnostic, surgical, and unlisted services and procedures. Let's go back to the notes and find out which of these is most appropriate. The notes state specifically "diagnostic endoscopy." The index suggests a range of codes: 31231–31235. Let's turn to the main portion of CPT to read the complete code descriptions.

31231 Nasal endoscopy, diagnostic, unilateral or bilateral (separate procedure)

31233 Nasal/sinus endoscopy, diagnostic with maxillary sinusoscopy (via inferior meatus or canine fossa puncture)

31235 Nasal/sinus endoscopy, diagnostic with sphenoid sinusoscopy (via puncture of sphenoidal face or cannulation of ostium)

Let's go back to the physician's notes to confirm exactly what was done for Mr. Paulson.

. . . diagnostic endoscopy . . . all three code choices include this term

. . . via the inferior meatus . . . only code 31233 mentions the inferior meatus specifically

. . . with a maxillary sinusoscopy . . . only code 31233 mentions the maxillary sinusoscopy

The code description for 31233 matches the notes and is our most accurate code to report.

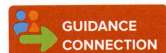

GUIDANCE CONNECTION

Additional explanation can be found in the guidelines within the **Surgery** section, directly under the subhead **Respiratory System**, subsection **Lung Transplantation**, in your CPT book.

Lung Transplantation

Special guidelines help you report any lung transplant. However, as soon as you begin to read the notation shown before codes 32850–32856, you will see that the editors of the CPT book use the term lung **allotransplantation** in addition to **transplantation.** These words have a very similar meaning.

A lung transplant requires three steps, which can be performed by a single physician or a team of physicians, with each physician submitting his or her own claim. Each step has its own code.

Cadaver Donor Pneumonectomy Because a human cannot live without lungs, the donor has to be deceased (a cadaver) prior to the harvesting of the organ. This portion of the transplant, or allotransplantation, procedure should be identified with the code

> 32850 Donor pneumonectomy(s) (including cold preservation), from cadaver donor

Backbench Work The actual preparation of the cadaver lung allograft prior to the transplant procedure is known as *backbench work*. The actual preparation of the cadaver donor lung allograft prior to the transplant procedure is coded by using either of the following:

> 32855 Backbench stand preparation of cadaver donor lung allograft prior to transplantation . . . ; unilateral

or

> 32856 Backbench stand preparation of cadaver donor lung allograft prior to transplantation . . . ; bilateral

Recipient Lung Allotransplantation The final code for the entire operation identifies the placement of the allograft in the patient (the recipient). The selection of a code from the range 32851–32854 is determined by whether the procedure is performed unilaterally or bilaterally and with or without a cardiopulmonary bypass.

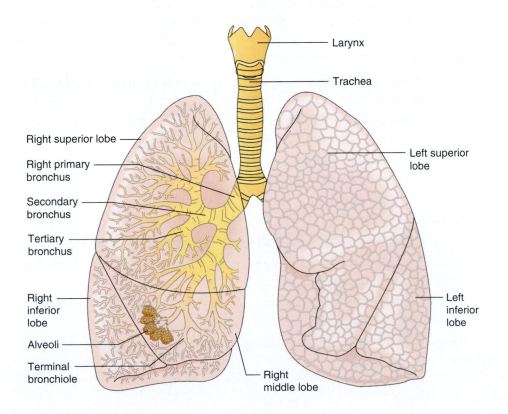

Ilonia Gonzalez, a 15-year-old female, was diagnosed 3 years ago with idiopathic pulmonary fibrosis, a chronic interstitial pulmonary disease. Corticosteroid therapy has not improved her condition, so Dr. Lancer admitted her today for a double-lung transplantation. The harvesting of the allograft and the preparation of the cadaver donor double-lung allograft was done by Dr. Cannon. Dr. Lancer only performed the actual lung transplant, en bloc, along with a cardiopulmonary bypass, Ilonia tolerated the procedure well and has an excellent prognosis.

Let's Code It!

The notes indicate that Dr. Lancer performed only one of the three steps. Therefore, you will have only one code on his claim form for Ilonia's surgery.

Let's go to the Alphabetic Index and look for *transplant*. Read down until you find *lung*. You know that Ilonia received a *double-lung* transplant, *en bloc, with a bypass*. That information leads to the suggested code 32854. Now go to the numerical listing to check the complete code description.

> **32854** Lung transplant, double (bilateral sequential or en bloc); with cardiopulmonary bypass

Terrific! This code matches the notes.

LO 8.3 Cardiovascular System

Treatments and procedures on the heart as well as the entire network of veins, arteries, and capillaries are coded from the Cardiovascular System subsection.

Pacemakers

When a physician inserts a single-chamber pacemaker system into a patient, it includes the pulse generator and one electrode inserted into *either* the atrium or the ventricle.

When a dual-chamber pacemaker system is placed, the system includes the pulse generator and one electrode into *both* the right atrium and the right ventricle.

Occasionally, the physician will insert an additional electrode into the left ventricle, as well as the dual-chamber insertion. This is called *biventricular pacing*. The insertion of the pacing electrode is coded separately, with code 33224 and possibly 33225.

> **33224** Insertion of pacing electrode, cardiac venous system, for left ventricular pacing, with attachment to previously placed pacemaker or pacing cardioverter-defibrillator pulse generator (including revision of pocket, removal, insertion and/or replacement of generator)
>
> **+ 33225** Insertion of pacing electrode, cardiac venous system, for left ventricular pacing, at time of insertion of pacing cardioverter-defibrillator or pacemaker pulse generator (including upgrade to dual chamber system) (List separately in addition to code for primary procedure.)

Pacing Cardioverter-Defibrillators

Pacing cardioverter-defibrillator systems are similar to pacemaker systems. While they also consist of a pulse generator and electrodes, the units may use several leads inserted into a single chamber (ventricle) or into dual chambers (atrium and ventricle). The system is actually a combination of antitachycardia pacing, low-energy

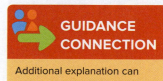

GUIDANCE CONNECTION

Additional explanation can be found in the guidelines within the **Surgery** section, directly under the subhead **Cardiovascular System**, subsection **Pacemaker or Pacing Cardioverter-Defibrillator,** in your CPT book.

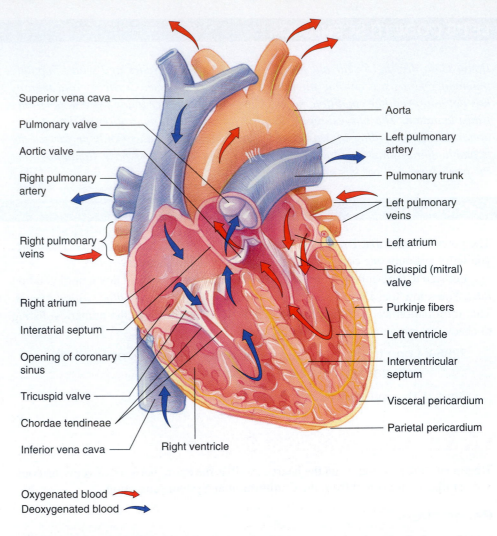

Superior vena cava
Pulmonary valve
Aortic valve
Right pulmonary artery
Right pulmonary veins
Right atrium
Interatrial septum
Opening of coronary sinus
Tricuspid valve
Chordae tendineae
Inferior vena cava
Right ventricle

Aorta
Left pulmonary artery
Pulmonary trunk
Left pulmonary veins
Left atrium
Bicuspid (mitral) valve
Purkinje fibers
Left ventricle
Interventricular septum
Visceral pericardium
Parietal pericardium

Oxygenated blood
Deoxygenated blood

cardioversion, and/or defibrillating shocks to address a patient's ventricular tachycardia or ventricular fibrillation.

In some cases, an additional electrode may be needed to regulate the pacing of the left ventricle, called *biventricular pacing*. When this occurs, the placement of the electrode transvenously should be coded separately, just as the pacemaker is coded, with either 33224 or 33225.

Battery Replacement

Commonly referred to as replacing the battery in the pacemaker or cardioverter-defibrillator, this procedure involves the removal of the old pulse generator and the insertion of a new pulse generator. These two actions should be coded individually—one code for the removal of the old and another code for the insertion of the new.

Bypass Grafting

Venous Grafts When a venous graft is performed, use codes from the range 33510–33516. All these codes include a **saphenous vein** graft.

However, if the graft is harvested from an upper extremity (arm) vein, you need to code this separately, using code 35500, in addition to the code for the bypass procedure itself.

+35500 Harvest of upper extremity vein, one segment for lower extremity or coronary artery bypass procedure (List separately in addition to code for primary procedure.)

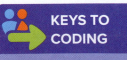

KEYS TO CODING

If the graft comes from a femoropopliteal vein, use code 35572 in addition to the bypass procedure code.

saphenous vein
Either of the two major veins in the leg that run from the foot to the thigh near the surface of the skin.

+35572 Harvest of femoropopliteal vein, one segment, for vascular reconstruction procedure (e.g., aortic, vena caval, coronary, peripheral artery) (List separately in addition to code for primary procedure.)

Combined Arterial-Venous Grafts When both venous grafts and arterial grafts are used during the same procedure, you will use two codes. First, code the combined arterial-venous graft from the range 33517–33523. Just like the codes for the venous grafts, these include getting the graft from the saphenous vein. Second, code the appropriate arterial graft from the range 33533–33536. Harvesting the arterial vein section is included in those codes.

Arterial Grafts When an arterial graft is performed, use codes from the range 33533–33545. All these codes include the use of grafts from the internal mammary artery, gastroepiploic artery, epigastric artery, radial artery, and arterial conduits harvested from other sites. For example, examine the following code description:

33533 Coronary artery bypass, using arterial graft(s); single arterial graft

Use one of the following codes (in addition to the code for the bypass procedure) if the graft is harvested from another site:

- From an upper extremity artery, add code 35600.
- From an upper extremity vein, add code 35500.
- From the femoropopliteal vein, use code 35572.

Composite Grafts When two or more vein segments are harvested from a limb other than that part of the body undergoing the bypass, you must use the best, most appropriate code from the range 35682–35683 to report the harvesting and anastomosis of the multiple vein segments.

+35682 Bypass graft; autogenous composite, two segments of veins from two locations (List separately in addition to code for primary procedure.)

+35683 Bypass graft; autogenous composite, three or more segments of vein from two or more locations (List separately in addition to code for primary procedure.)

A little confusing? Hopefully, Table 8-1 will help you organize all the rules for coding bypass grafts.

Heart/Lung Transplantation

Similar to the components of the lung transplantation that we reviewed earlier in this chapter, a heart transplant, with or without a lung allotransplantation, requires three steps to be performed by a single physician or a team of physicians. Each step has its own codes.

Cadaver Donor Cardiectomy with or without a Pneumonectomy A human cannot live without a heart or lungs, so the donor has to be deceased (a cadaver) prior to any organ harvesting. This portion of the transplant or allotransplantation procedure is identified with the code 33930 (heart and lungs) or 33940 (heart alone):

33930 Donor cardiectomy-pneumonectomy (including cold preservation)

or

33940 Donor cardiectomy (including cold preservation)

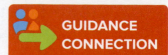

GUIDANCE CONNECTION

Additional explanation can be found in the guidelines within the **Surgery** section, directly under the subhead **Cardiovascular System**, subsection **Venous Grafting Only for Coronary Artery Bypass**, in your CPT book.

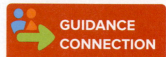

GUIDANCE CONNECTION

Additional explanation can be found in the guidelines within the **Surgery** section, directly under the subhead **Cardiovascular System**, subsection **Combined Arterial-Venous Grafting for Coronary Bypass**, in your CPT book.

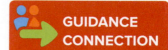

GUIDANCE CONNECTION

Additional explanation can be found in the guidelines within the **Surgery** section, directly under the subhead **Cardiovascular System**, subsection **Arterial Grafting for Coronary Artery Bypass**, in your CPT book.

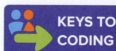

KEYS TO CODING

The same exceptions apply as before: If the graft is harvested from an upper extremity artery, code it separately from the bypass procedure, using code 35600. And if the graft is obtained from the femoropopliteal vein, code it with 35572 in addition to the code for the bypass procedure.

TABLE 8-1 Bypass Grafts

Graft	Harvested From	Use Code(s)
Venous graft	Saphenous vein	Choose from 33510–33516
Venous graft	Upper extremity vein	Choose from 33510–33516; + 35500
Venous graft	Femoropopliteal vein	Choose from 33510–33516; + 35572
Arterial-venous	Saphenous vein	Choose from 33517–33523; + choose from 33533–33536
Arterial-venous	Upper extremity vein	Choose from 33510–33516; + choose from 33533–33536 + 35500
Arterial-venous	Upper extremity artery	Choose from 33510–33516; + choose from 33533–33536 + 35600
Arterial-venous	Femoropopliteal vein	Choose from 33510–33516; + choose from 33533–33536 + 35572
Arterial graft	Internal mammary artery Gastroepiploic artery Epigastric artery Radial artery Arterial conduits from other sites	Choose from 33533–33545
Arterial graft	Upper extremity vein	Choose from 33533–33545; + 35500
Arterial graft	Upper extremity artery	Choose from 33533–33545; + 35600
Arterial graft	Femoropopliteal vein	Choose from 33533–33545; + 35572
Composite graft	Two or more segments from another part of body	+ 35682 or 35683

Backbench Work The actual preparation of the cadaver donor heart, or heart and lung, allograft prior to the transplant procedure is known as *backbench work*. The second portion of the transplant is coded by using either of the following:

> **33933** Backbench standard preparation of cadaver donor heart/lung allograft

> or

> **33944** Backbench standard preparation of cadaver donor heart allograft

Recipient Heart with or without Lung Allotransplantation The third code for the entire operation identifies the placement of the allograft into the patient (the recipient). Select the code from either of the following:

> **33935** Heart-lung transplant with recipient cardiectomy-pneumonectomy

> or

> **33945** Heart transplant with or without recipient cardiectomy

The codes for the insertion of the transplanted organs include the removal of the damaged or diseased organs.

Arteries and Veins

The primary vascular procedure codes 34001–37799 include

1. Ensuring both the inflow and the outflow of the arteries and/or veins involved.
2. The operative arteriogram that is performed by the surgeon during the procedure.
3. Sympathectomy for aortic procedures.

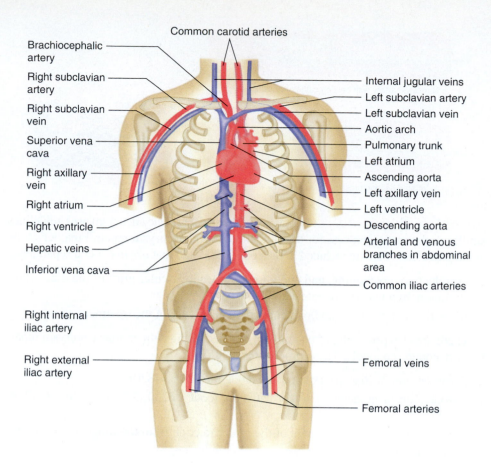

Common carotid arteries
Brachiocephalic artery
Right subclavian artery
Right subclavian vein
Superior vena cava
Right axillary vein
Right atrium
Right ventricle
Hepatic veins
Inferior vena cava
Right internal iliac artery
Right external iliac artery

Internal jugular veins
Left subclavian artery
Left subclavian vein
Aortic arch
Pulmonary trunk
Left atrium
Ascending aorta
Left axillary vein
Left ventricle
Descending aorta
Arterial and venous branches in abdominal area
Common iliac arteries
Femoral veins
Femoral arteries

Repair of Abdominal Aortic Aneurysm The repair of an abdominal aortic aneurysm, codes 34800–34826, includes several procedures, such as:

1. Placement of an endovascular graft for an abdominal aortic aneurysm repair.
2. Open femoral or iliac artery exposure.
3. Manipulation and deployment of the device used.
4. Closure of the arteriotomy site(s).
5. Balloon angioplasty and/or stent deployment, as long as it is within the target treatment area for the endoprosthesis.

When the notes indicate that any or all of these procedures were done at the same time as the abdominal aortic repair, they *are not* coded separately. However, several other procedures may be performed at the same time and are coded separately (in addition to the code for the repair itself):

1. The introduction of guidewires and/or catheters (36140, 36200, 36245–36248).
2. Extensive repair or replacement of an artery (35226 or 35286).
3. Renal transluminal angioplasty (the enlargement of the renal artery when it has become narrowed, using a balloon-tip catheter).
4. Arterial embolization (blocking an artery with a material such as gelatin or sponge, to stop uncontrollable internal bleeding).
5. Intravascular ultrasound.
6. Balloon angioplasty (reconstruction of a blood vessel).
7. Stenting of the native artery outside of the endoprosthesis area (when done before or after deployment of a graft).
8. Fluoroscopic guidance in conjunction with the repair (75952 or 75953).

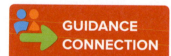

GUIDANCE CONNECTION

Additional explanation can be found in the guidelines within the **Surgery** section, directly under the subhead **Cardiovascular System,** subsection **Endovascular Repair of Abdominal Aortic Aneurysm,** in your CPT book.

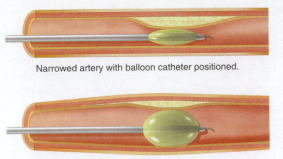

Narrowed artery with balloon catheter positioned.

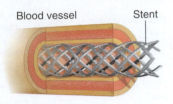

Blood vessel   Stent

Inflated balloon presses against arterial wall.

Repair of Iliac Aneurysm Endovascular repair of an iliac aneurysm uses guidelines similar to the coding process for the abdominal aortic aneurysm repair. First, let's look at the procedures that are included in the code 34900 and that *are not* coded separately:

1. Introduction, positioning, and operation of an endovascular graft of the iliac artery (common, hypogastric, or external).
2. All balloon angioplasty and/or stent deployments within the treatment area.

There are also procedures frequently performed along with an iliac aneurysm repair that *are* coded separately. These procedures include

1. Open femoral or iliac artery exposure (code 34812 or 34820).
2. Introduction of guidewires and/or catheters (code 36200, 36215, 36216, 36217, or 36218).
3. Extensive repair or replacement of the artery (a code from the range 35201–35286, as appropriate).
4. Transluminal angioplasty outside the aneurysm area.
5. Arterial embolization.
6. Intravascular ultrasound.
7. Fluoroscopic guidance in conjunction with the iliac aneurysm repair. (Use code 75954.)

Catheterizations and Vascular Families Understanding the vascular families can be useful to coders when reporting the provision of a catheterization. Tables 8-2, 8-3, and 8-4 show some examples of the vascular orders when reporting

TABLE 8-2 Vascular Families: Superior Mesenteric

First Order	Second Order Branch	Third Order Branch
	Middle colic	
		Posterior inferior pancreaticoduodenal
	Interior pancreaticoduodenal	Anterior inferior pancreaticoduodenal
Superior mesenteric	Jejunal	
	Ileocolic	
	Appendicular	
	Posterior cecal	
	Anterior cecal	
	Marginal	
	Right colic	

GUIDANCE CONNECTION

Additional explanation can be found in the guidelines within the **Surgery** section, directly under the subhead **Cardiovascular System,** subsection **Endovascular Repair of Iliac Aneurysm,** in your CPT book.

TABLE 8-3 Vascular Families: Left Common Carotid

First Order	Second Order Branch	Third Order Branch
Left common carotid	Left internal carotid	Left ophthalmic
		Left posterior communicating
		Left middle cerebral
		Left anterior cerebral
		Left superior thyroid
	Left external carotid	Left ascending pharyngeal
		Left facial
		Left lingual
		Left occipital
		Left posterior auricular
		Left superficial temporal
		Left internal maxillary

the catheterization of the aorta. The catheterization of the femoral or carotid arteries would have their own families, of course. A full listing can be found in your CPT code book, Appendix L, Vascular Families.

A vascular family begins with the vessel that branches off from the aorta, femoral, or carotid artery and continues to track all vessels that branch from that. For example, in Table 8-2, in the first order (first column) you see that the superior mesenteric is one of the arteries that branch off the aorta (see Table 8-3, in the center, about where the kidneys are shown). The middle colic, interior pancreaticoduodenal, jejunal, ileocolic, appendicular, posterior cecal, anterior cecal, marginal, and right colic arteries all branch off the superior mesenteric. From this point, only the interior pancreaticoduodenal has additional vessels branching off it—the posterior inferior pancreaticoduodenal and the anterior inferior pancreaticoduodenal.

LET'S CODE IT! SCENARIO

Zena Quinones, a 15-week-old female, was diagnosed with ventricular septal defect (VSD) after her pediatrician, Dr. Osterman, ordered an echocardiography. A large VSD was identified in the septum. Due to the size of the defect, Dr. Osterman admitted Zena into the hospital today to close the defect with a patch graft.

Let's Code It!

Review the notes and abstract the key terms. Let's go to the Alphabetic Index and look up *closure*, the procedure being performed. Under the word *closure*, you will find *septal defect*, which suggests the code 33615.

While we are in the Alphabetic Index, let's try one other way to look up the code. Let's go to *heart*, the anatomical site where the procedure is being performed. When you read the column below *heart*, you will see *closure, septal defect*, which again suggests code 33615. However, just out of curiosity, continue reading down the columns until you get to *repair* (another word for the procedure being done). As you read everything listed under *repair,* keep going past *septal defect* all the way to *ventricular septum*—33545, 33647, 33681–33688, 33692–33697, 93581. *Ventricular septum* is a much better match to the physician's notes than *septal defect,* isn't it? Not certain? That's great, because you need to let the actual code descriptions in the numerical listing give you more details before you make a decision.

This is where time and patience are important to the coding process. Read carefully through the description of each code suggested by the alphabetic index. You will probably agree that the best, most appropriate code is

33681 Closure of single ventricular septal defect, with or without patch

Great job!

TABLE 8-4 Vascular Families: Common Iliac

First Order	Second Order Branch	Third Order Branch	Beyond Third Order Branches
Common iliac	Internal iliac	Iliolumbar	
		Lateral sacral	
		Umbilical	
		Superior vesical	
		Obturator	
		Inferior vesical	
		Middle rectal	
		Inferior rectal	
		Internal pudendal	
		Inferior gluteal	
	External iliac	Inferior epigastric	Cremasteric
		Deep circumflex iliac	Pubic
			Ascending deep circumflex iliac
			Medial descending
			Perforating branches
			Lateral descending
		Profunda femoris	Lateral circumflex
	Common femoral	Deep external pudendal	
		Superficial external pudendal	
		Ascending lateral circumflex femoral	
		Descending lateral circumflex femoral	
		Transverse lateral circumflex femoral	
		Superficial femoral	Geniculate
			Popliteal
			Anterior tibial
			Peroneal
			Posterior tibial

Central Venous Access Procedures Venous access devices (VAD) can be challenging to report because of the various types of procedures involved with their insertion as well as the multitude of purposes for the procedure itself. According to the CPT guidelines, the tip of the VAD or catheter must come to an end in the subclavian vein, brachiocephalic (innominate) vein, iliac vein, superior or inferior vena cava, or right atrium of the heart to be considered a *central* VAD or catheter.

Catheter or Device   A catheter is a tube that is used for various medical reasons. It may be inserted to withdraw bodily fluids, as a urinary catheter collects urine from the bladder. Catheters can also be used to deliver medications, such as an intravenous (IV) injection of drugs directly into the patient's veins. In addition, catheters can be used as a vehicle to enable the insertion of a device such as a stent.

In this usage, a device is most often a subcutaneous pump or a subcutaneous port designed to achieve ongoing access internally without the need to repeatedly obtain a new entry site.

Entry Site: Centrally Inserted or Peripherally Inserted   For these procedures, it is important to the coding process that you read the physician's notes carefully to determine exactly where on the patient's body the VAD or catheter was inserted. A centrally inserted device enters the body at the jugular, subclavian, or femoral vein or the inferior vena cava. A VAD or catheter that enters the body at either the basilic vein or the cephalic vein is called a peripherally inserted central catheter, often referred to by its initials—a PICC line.

Nontunneled or Tunneled   A tunneled catheter does exactly as its name describes—it tunnels under the skin. These tubes are more flexible; they are inserted into a vein at one location, such as the neck, chest, or groin, and wended through beneath the skin to emerge at a separate site in the body. A nontunneled catheter is inserted directly into the vein by venipuncture.

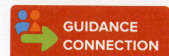

GUIDANCE CONNECTION

Additional explanation can be found in the guidelines within the **Surgery** section, directly under the subhead **Cardiovascular System**, subsection **Central Venous Access Procedures,** in your CPT book.

LO 8.4 Digestive System

Beginning at the mouth and traveling through the body all the way to the anus is the digestive tract. The organs along the pathway process food and nourishment, so cells can absorb nutrients and eliminate waste. The digestive tract is also referred to as the alimentary canal or the gastrointestinal (GI) tract.

Endoscopic Procedures

There are times when a physician needs to visually examine and/or obtain a specimen for pathologic testing of the interior of an organ, such as the throat, stomach, or bladder, in order to make a more accurate diagnosis. In these cases, an endoscope may be used.

An esophagogastroduodenoscopy (EGD), more commonly known as an upper endoscopy, enables the physician to view the patient's esophagus, stomach, and duodenum without a surgical invasion of the body.

Endoscopic retrograde cholangiopancreatography (ERCP) uses a combination of x-rays and the endoscope to enable visualization of the patient's stomach, the duodenum, and the bile ducts in the biliary tree and pancreas.

Sigmoidoscopy and colonoscopy are endoscopic procedures used to examine the internal aspects of the lower digestive system. A sigmoidoscopy permits the physician to visually investigate a patient's anus, rectum, and sigmoid colon. A colonoscopy permits the physician to look at the entire large intestine: the anus, the rectum, the descending (sigmoid) colon, the transverse colon, the ascending colon, and the cecum.

Endoscopy can be used for therapeutic procedures as well, as when Dr. Sanger had to remove a penny (foreign body) from little Billy's esophagus after he tried to swallow the coin, code 43247.

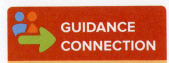

GUIDANCE CONNECTION

Additional explanation can be found in the guidelines within the **Surgery** section, directly under the subhead **Digestive System**, subsection **Bariatric Surgery**, in your CPT book.

Bariatric Surgery

Bariatric surgical procedures may be performed on the stomach, the duodenum, the jejunum, and/or the ileum and are most often provided to patients who have been diagnosed as morbidly obese. Consideration for performing this surgery may include the physician's evaluation of the candidate's eating behaviors as well as the patient's predisposition for serious obesity-related co-morbidities such as coronary heart disease, type 2 diabetes mellitus, and/or acute sleep apnea.

These surgeries may be performed as an open procedure or laparoscopically, and this detail will affect the determination of the correct code. The four most common versions of this surgery are

- Adjustable gastric band (AGB). See codes 43770–43774.

AGB is a procedure that places a small, adjustable band to create a proximal pouch, thereby limiting the passage of food. The attending physician can increase or decrease the size of the passage using saline solution to inflate or deflate as needed for the patient's situation.

- Roux-en-Y gastric bypass (RYGB). See codes 43846, 43847, 43644.

RYGB limits food intake by use of a small pouch that is similar in size to the adjustable gastric band. In addition, absorption of food in the digestive tract is reduced by excluding most of the stomach, duodenum, and upper intestine from contact with food by routing food directly from the pouch into the small intestine.

- Biliopancreatic diversion with a duodenal switch (BPD-DS). See codes 43775 and 43843.

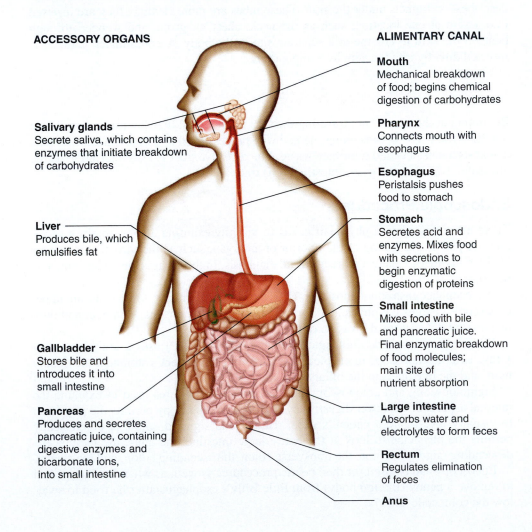

ACCESSORY ORGANS

Salivary glands
Secrete saliva, which contains enzymes that initiate breakdown of carbohydrates

Liver
Produces bile, which emulsifies fat

Gallbladder
Stores bile and introduces it into small intestine

Pancreas
Produces and secretes pancreatic juice, containing digestive enzymes and bicarbonate ions, into small intestine

ALIMENTARY CANAL

Mouth
Mechanical breakdown of food; begins chemical digestion of carbohydrates

Pharynx
Connects mouth with esophagus

Esophagus
Peristalsis pushes food to stomach

Stomach
Secretes acid and enzymes. Mixes food with secretions to begin enzymatic digestion of proteins

Small intestine
Mixes food with bile and pancreatic juice. Final enzymatic breakdown of food molecules; main site of nutrient absorption

Large intestine
Absorbs water and electrolytes to form feces

Rectum
Regulates elimination of feces

Anus

BPD-DS, most often referred to as a "duodenal switch," includes transection of the stomach, a bypass to route digested material away from the small intestine, as well as re-routing bile and other digestive juices that impair digestion.

A vertical sleeve gastrectomy (VSG) is performed and connected to a very short segment of the duodenum, which is then directly connected to a lower part of the small intestine. A small portion of the duodenum is untouched to provide passage for food and absorption of some vitamins and minerals. The distance between the stomach and colon is made much shorter after this operation, resulting in malabsorption.

- Vertical sleeve gastrectomy (VSG). See code 43775.

A VSG procedure includes the resectioning of the stomach and is most often performed solely as the first stage of the multistaged BPD-DS on those patients determined to be unable to go through such a long procedure at one encounter. VSG is not without benefits, as research has shown that some VSG patients report significant weight loss. Should a second-stage procedure be performed, that second procedure and any others in the sequence would be reported with the appropriate procedure code appended by modifier 58 Staged Procedure.

During the postoperative period, adjustments of an adjustable gastric restrictive device is included in the global surgical package and therefore not coded separately.

Liver Transplantation

Again, the components that we have reviewed for the other organ transplants are involved with a liver allotransplantation.

Donor Hepatectomy A human can live without a portion of the liver, so the donor can be either deceased (a cadaver) or living. The best code for this portion of the transplant process is determined by whether or not the donor is living, and if living, what percentage or portion of the liver is donated.

47133 Donor hepatectomy (including cold preservation), from cadaver donor

or

47140 Donor hepatectomy (including cold preservation), from living donor; left lateral segment only

or

47141 Donor hepatectomy (including cold preservation), from living donor; total left lobectomy

or

47142 Donor hepatectomy (including cold preservation), from living donor; total right lobectomy

Backbench Work The actual preparation of the whole liver graft prior to the transplant procedure is coded with

47143 Backbench standard preparation of cadaver donor whole liver graft

In certain cases, and almost always if the donor is living, some reconstruction of the liver will be required prior to the transplantation. If the notes indicate that a venous and/or arterial anastomosis was also performed, then you will need to use

47146 Backbench reconstruction of cadaver or living donor liver graft prior to allotransplantation; venous anastomosis, each

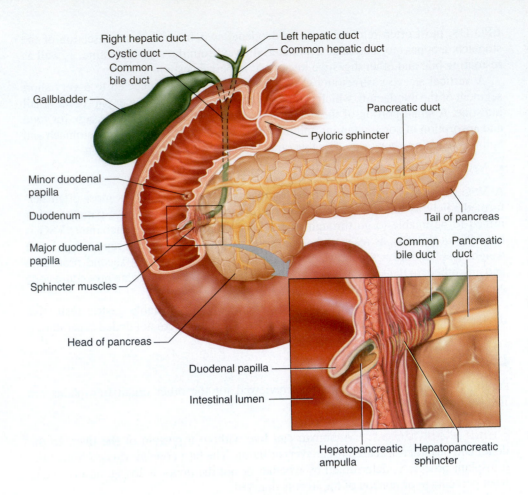

Right hepatic duct — — Left hepatic duct
Cystic duct — — Common hepatic duct
Common bile duct
Gallbladder — Pancreatic duct
Pyloric sphincter
Minor duodenal papilla
Duodenum — Tail of pancreas
Major duodenal papilla
Common bile duct   Pancreatic duct
Sphincter muscles
Head of pancreas —
Duodenal papilla
Intestinal lumen
Hepatopancreatic ampulla   Hepatopancreatic sphincter

Recipient Liver Allotransplantation The third code for the entire operation identifies the placement of the allograft in the patient (the recipient): orthotopic (normal position) or heterotopic (other than normal position).

> **47135** Liver allotransplantation; orthotopic, partial or whole, from cadaver or living donor, any age
>
> or
>
> **47136** Liver allotransplantation; heterotopic, partial or whole, from cadaver or living donor, any age

Pancreas Transplantation

Again, the components that we have reviewed for the other organ transplants are involved with a pancreatic allotransplantation.

Cadaver Donor Pancreatectomy A pancreas graft has to come from a deceased (a cadaver) donor.

> **48550** Donor pancreatectomy (including cold preservation), with or without duodenal segment for transplantation

Backbench Work When the preparation of the pancreas graft prior to the transplant procedure is routine, you use the following code:

> **48551** Backbench standard preparation of cadaver donor pancreas allograft

However, in certain cases, some reconstruction of the pancreas will be required prior to the transplantation. If the notes indicate that a venous and/or arterial anastomosis was performed, then you have to use

48552 Backbench reconstruction of cadaver donor pancreas allograft prior to allotransplantation; venous anastomosis, each

Recipient Pancreatic Allotransplantation The final code for the entire operation identifies the placement of the allograft in the patient (the recipient). For this, use the following code:

48554 Transplantation of pancreatic allograft

LET'S CODE IT! SCENARIO

Paul Williamson, a 57-year-old male, was suffering from fecal incontinence, diarrhea, and constipation. He came to the Ambulatory Care Center so that his gastroenterologist, Dr. Apterman, could perform a colonoscopy. Demerol and Versed were given IV, and the patient was brought into the examination room. The variable flexion Olympus colonoscope was introduced into the rectum and advanced to the cecum. In the midsigmoid colon, a 3-mm sessile polyp was destroyed. Paul tolerated the procedure well.

Let's Code It!

We know that the main procedure was a *colonoscopy,* so let's look that up in the alphabetic index. When you refer to the notes, what else was done for Paul in conjunction with the colonoscopy? *A polyp was destroyed.*

Find *destruction* beneath *colonoscopy.* Do you know whether a polyp is a lesion or a tumor? It happens to be a lesion; however, you don't have to know this because the index suggests the same code for both: 45383. Let's look at the complete description in the numerical listing.

45383 Colonoscopy, flexible, proximal to splenic flexure; with ablation of tumor(s), polyp(s), or other lesion(s) not amenable to removal by hot biopsy forceps, bipolar cautery, or snare technique

You might think about also coding the moderate sedation that was given to Paul (the Demerol and Versed). However, look at the bull's-eye symbol next to 45383—the sedation is included in this code. So you are not to code the moderate sedation separately. Great job!

LO 8.5 Urinary System

The urinary system is responsible for maintaining the proper level and composition of fluids in the body.

Renal (Kidney) Transplantation

The same three components exist for renal transplantation as for the other organ transplants.

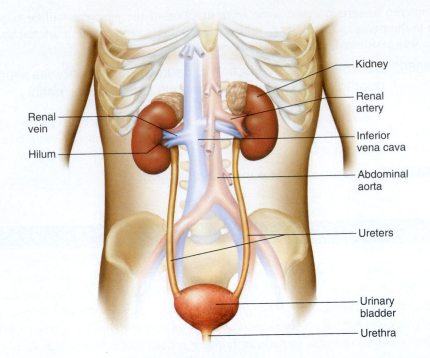

Kidney

Renal artery

Inferior vena cava

Abdominal aorta

Ureters

Urinary bladder

Urethra

Renal vein

Hilum

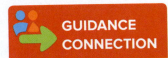

GUIDANCE CONNECTION

Additional explanation can be found in the guidelines within the **Surgery** section, directly under the subhead **Urinary System,** subsection **Renal Transplantation,** in your CPT book.

Donor Nephrectomy A human can live without one kidney, so the donor can be either deceased (a cadaver) or living.

50300 Donor nephrectomy (including cold preservation); from cadaver donor, unilateral or bilateral

or

50320 Donor nephrectomy (including cold preservation); open, from living donor

or

50547 Laparoscopy, surgical; donor nephrectomy (including cold preservation), from living donor

Backbench Work Performing the routine preparation of the allograft is coded differently, depending upon whether the donor is living or a cadaver.

50323 Backbench standard preparation of cadaver donor renal allograft

or

50325 Backbench standard preparation of living donor renal allograft

In certain cases, some reconstruction of the kidney will be required prior to the transplantation. If the notes indicate that a venous, arterial, and/or ureteral anastomosis was performed, then you have to use one of the following codes:

50327 Backbench reconstruction of cadaver or living donor renal allograft prior to allotransplantation; venous anastomosis, each

or

50328 Backbench reconstruction of cadaver or living donor renal allograft prior to allotransplantation; arterial anastomosis, each

or

50329 Backbench reconstruction of cadaver or living donor renal allograft prior to allotransplantation; ureteral anastomosis, each

Recipient Renal Allotransplantation The final code for the entire operation identifies the placement of the allograft in the patient (the recipient). Choose the code by whether or not a recipient nephrectomy (the removal of the organ being replaced) is performed at the same time by the same physician:

> 50360 Renal allotransplantation; implantation of graft; without recipient nephrectomy

> or

> 50365 Renal allotransplantation; implantation of graft; with recipient nephrectomy

Urodynamics

The codes listed for the procedures in the Urodynamics section, 51725–51798, include the services of the physician to perform the procedure (or directly supervise the performance of the procedure), as well as the use of all instruments, equipment, fluids, gases, probes, catheters, technician's fees, medications, gloves, trays, tubing, and other sterile supplies.

If the physician for whom you are coding did not actually perform the procedure but only interpreted the results, then the appropriate procedure code from this section should be appended with modifier 26 Professional Component.

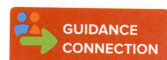

GUIDANCE CONNECTION

Additional explanation can be found in the guidelines within the **Surgery** section, directly under the subhead **Urinary System,** subsection **Urodynamics,** in your CPT book.

YOU CODE IT! CASE STUDY

Barbara Barnette, a 45-year-old female, G3 P3, states she has been dealing with stress incontinence increasingly over the last several years. She had three vaginal deliveries, with the largest infant weighing 7.5 lb. Barbara states that her leakage frequency, volume, timing, and associated symptoms (urgency, stress, urinary frequency, nocturia, enuresis, incomplete emptying, straining to empty, leakage without warning) have become bothersome and she wants to do something about it.

Today she presents for a complex cystometrogram with voiding pressure study to confirm or deny the diagnosis of stress urinary incontinence prior to the scheduling of surgery.

You Code It!

Go through the steps and determine what procedure code(s) should be reported for the encounter with Barbara.

Step 1: Read the case completely.

Step 2: Abstract the notes: What key words can you identify relating to the procedures performed?

_____

Step 3: Query the provider, if necessary.

Step 4: Diagnosis: Urinary frequency.

Transurethral Surgery

When a diagnostic or therapeutic cystourethroscopic intervention is performed, the appropriate codes, 52320–52356, include the insertion and removal of a temporary stent. Therefore, those services are not reported separately—when done at the same time as the cystourethroscopy.

If the physician, however, inserts a self-retaining, indwelling stent during the diagnostic or therapeutic cystourethroscopic intervention, use either of the following:

1. Code 52332 with the modifier 51, along with the code for the cystourethroscopy for a unilateral procedure.
2. Code 52332 with modifiers 50 and 51, along with the code for the cystourethroscopy for a bilateral procedure.

Note that when the physician removes the self-retaining, indwelling ureteral stent, use either 52310 or 52315 with modifier 58.

LET'S CODE IT! SCENARIO

Anita Jullianni, a 37-year-old female, is admitted today for the surgical removal of a kidney stone. The stone was too big for her to pass, so Dr. Hernandez decided to remove it surgically. The nephrolithotomy, with complete removal of the calculus, went as planned, and Anita tolerated the entire procedure well.

Let's Code It!

Dr. Hernandez performed a *nephrolithotomy*, involving the *removal of a kidney stone*, also known as *calculus*. Let's try something direct and look up *nephrolithotomy* in the Alphabetic Index.

The index suggests the code range 50060–50075. Let's go to the numerical listing and read the different code descriptions.

Do you agree that, according to the physician's notes, the best, most appropriate code available is the following?

50060 Nephrolithotomy; removal of calculus

You are getting very good at this.

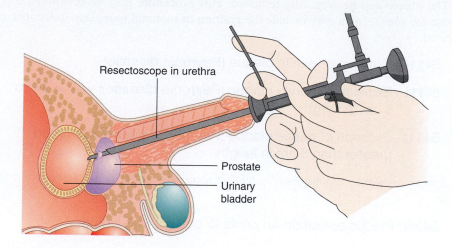

Resectoscope in urethra

Prostate

Urinary bladder

LO 8.6 Male Genital System

The male genital system is closely situated with the urinary bladder, so a urologist may be the specialist most often performing procedures on this area of the male anatomy.

Penile Plaque

This type of plaque is a flat layer of scar tissue that can form on the inside of a thick membrane called the tunica albuginea, which envelopes the erectile tissues, and is known as Peyronie disease. This is believed to begin as an inflammation, and the plaque is benign, not contagious, and not sexually transmitted. However, it can cause discomfort and pain in men with this condition. There are several ways to treat the problem.

Injections of steroids and chemotherapy agents, such as interferon, can be directly delivered to the site of the plaque to work to reduce the effect. These procedures may be reported with

54200 Injection procedure for Peyronie disease

54205 Injection procedure for Peyronie disease; with surgical exposure of plaque

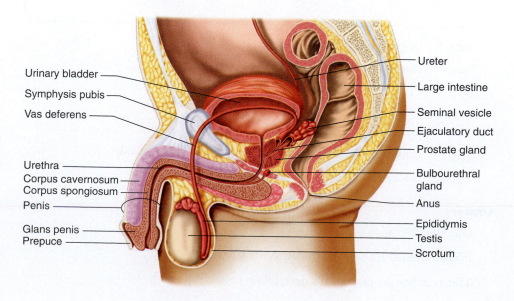

The plaque can be surgically removed. This procedure may be performed just to excise the plaque, or it may include the grafting of material to replace tissue that was excised.

54110 Excision of penile plaque (Peyronie disease)

54111 Excision of penile plaque (Peyronie disease); with graft to 5 cm in length

54112 Excision of penile plaque (Peyronie disease); with graft greater than 5 cm in length

Severe cases may require more extensive reconstruction and will be reported with code

54360 Plastic operation on penis to correct angulation

YOU CODE IT! CASE STUDY

Doug Daniels, a 17-year-old male, came to see his regular physician, Dr. Bomgarden, for help. Doug and his friends were fooling around at his father's construction company, and a staple gun went off, projecting a staple into his scrotum. Dr. Bomgarden carefully removed the staple and applied some antibiotic ointment to prevent infection until the two small wounds healed.

You Code It!

Go through the steps and determine the procedure code(s) that should be reported for this encounter between Dr. Bomgarden and Doug Daniels.

Step 1: Read the case completely.

Step 2: Abstract the notes: Which key words can you identify relating to the procedures performed?

_____

Step 3: Query the provider, if necessary.

Step 4: Diagnosis: Foreign body in scrotum.

Step 5: Code the procedure(s).

_____

Step 6: Link the procedure codes to at least one diagnosis code.

Step 7: Back code to double-check your choices.

Answer:

Did you determine the correct code?

55120 Removal of foreign body in scrotum

This matches the physician's description perfectly!

LO 8.7 Female Genital System

Vulvectomy

Sometimes physicians use direct terms in their notes, such as *simple, partial, radical,* or *complete*. Such terms make finding the best code easier. However, other physicians may be more descriptive in their notes regarding the procedure. Therefore, you have to know what these terms mean. The CPT book defines them as follows:

Simple: The removal of skin and *superficial* subcutaneous tissues.
Radical: The removal of skin and *deep* subcutaneous tissues.
Partial: The removal of *less than* 80% of the vulvar area.
Complete: The removal of *more than* 80% of the vulvar area.

EXAMPLES

56620 Vulvectomy, simple; partial

The description of this code represents a physician's statement that he or she removed less than 80% of the skin and superficial subcutaneous tissues of the vulvar area.

56633 Vulvectomy, radical; complete

The description of this code represents a physician's statement that he or she removed more than 80% of the skin and deep subcutaneous tissues of the vulvar area.

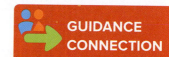

GUIDANCE CONNECTION

Additional explanation can be found in the guidelines within the **Surgery** section, directly under the subhead **Female Genital System,** subsection **Vulva, Perineum, and Introitus,** in your CPT book.

Maternity Care and Delivery

The complete package of services provided to a woman for uncomplicated maternity care includes the antepartum (prenatal) care, the delivery of the baby, and the post-partum care of the mother. Similar to working with the services already provided in the global surgical package, you must know the components of the maternity care

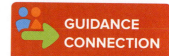

GUIDANCE CONNECTION

Additional explanation can be found in the guidelines within the **Surgery** section, directly under the subhead **Maternity Care and Delivery,** in your CPT book.

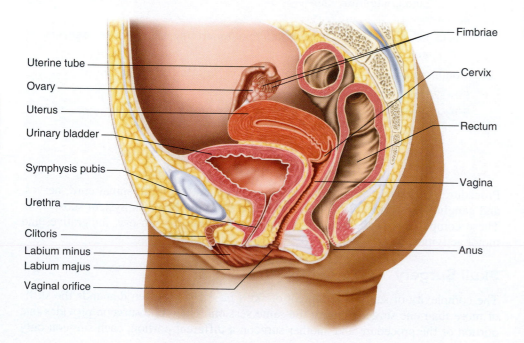

Uterine tube — Ovary — Uterus — Urinary bladder — Symphysis pubis — Urethra — Clitoris — Labium minus — Labium majus — Vaginal orifice — Fimbriae — Cervix — Rectum — Vagina — Anus

package. This is the only way you can determine what is already included and what services should be reported separately.

Antepartum care includes

- Initial patient history.
- Subsequent patient history.
- Physical examinations.
- Documentation of weight, blood pressure, fetal heart tones, routine chemical urinalysis.
- Monthly visits from conception up to 28 weeks gestation.
- Bi-weekly visits from 28 weeks to 36 weeks gestation.
- Weekly visits from 36 weeks gestation to delivery.

Delivery services include

- Admission to the hospital.
- Admission history and physical examination (H&P).
- Management of uncomplicated labor.
- Delivery: Vaginal (with or without episiotomy, with or without forceps) or Cesarean section.

Postpartum care includes

- Hospital and office visits following the delivery.

Should a physician provide one portion of the services, but not all, this will affect the determination of the correct code.

EXAMPLE

Dr. Sophina provided antepartum care for Lorraine DeAngelo. While on vacation in Europe, Lorraine suffered a miscarriage (spontaneous abortion) and lost the baby. Dr. Sophina provided postpartum care for Lorraine, when she returned home. Therefore, instead of reporting

59400 Routine obstetric care including antepartum care, vaginal delivery, and postpartum care

or

59510 Routine obstetric care including antepartum care, cesarean delivery, and postpartum care

Dr. Sophina's complete care for Lorraine will be reported with two codes:

59425 Antepartum care only; 4–6 visits
59430 Postpartum care only (separate procedure)

LO 8.8 Nervous System

Procedures performed on the nervous system organs (the brain, spinal cord, nerves, and ganglia) and connective tissues are coded from the Nervous System subsection. These components of the human body are responsible for sensory, integrative, and motor activities.

Skull Surgery

The complexity of surgical treatment of skull base lesions often demands the skills of more than one surgeon during the same session. When one surgeon provides one portion of the procedure and another surgeon a different portion, each surgeon only

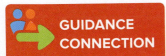

GUIDANCE CONNECTION

Additional explanation can be found in the guidelines within the **Surgery** section, directly under the subhead **Nervous System**, subsection **Surgery of Skull Base**, in your CPT book.

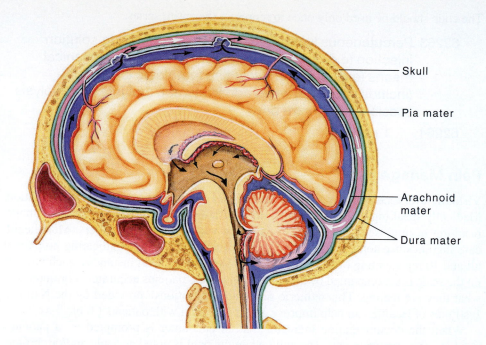

Skull

Pia mater

Arachnoid mater

Dura mater

uses the code for the surgical procedure he or she performed. Typically, the segments include the following:

1. The *approach* describes the tactic of the procedure, such as craniofacial, orbitocranial, or trancochlear:
   a. Anterior cranial fossa, 61580–61586.
   b. Middle cranial fossa, 61590–61592.
   c. Posterior cranial fossa, 61595–61598.

2. The *definitive* describes the procedure itself, such as resection, excision, repair, biopsy, or transection:
   a. Base of anterior cranial fossa, 61600–61601.
   b. Base of middle cranial fossa, 61605–61613.
   c. Base of posterior cranial fossa, 61615–61616.

3. The *repair/reconstruction* identifies a secondary repair, such as
   a. Extensive dural grafting.
   b. Cranioplasty.
   c. Local or regional myocutaneous pedicle flaps.
   d. Extensive skin grafts.

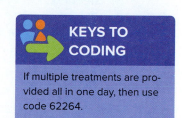

KEYS TO CODING

If multiple treatments are provided all in one day, then use code 62264.

If one surgeon performs more than one of the procedures, each segment should be reported separately, with the second (and third, if applicable) appended with modifier 51 to indicate that multiple procedures were performed at the same session by the same physician.

When a surgeon embeds a neurostimulator electrode array and performs microelectrode recording, the recording is included in the implantation code and shouldn't be coded separately.

Code 62263 includes the following:

- Percutaneous insertion of an epidural catheter.
- Removal of the catheter several days later.
- Procedure injections.
- Fluoroscopic guidance and localization.
- Multiple adhesiolysis sessions over the course of 2 or more days.

The code should be used only once to represent the entire series.

62263 Percutaneous lysis of epidural adhesions using solution injection (e.g., hypertonic saline, enzyme) or mechanical means (e.g., catheter) including radiologic localization (includes contrast when administered), multiple adhesiolysis sessions; 2 or more days

62264 1 day

Pain Management

Virtually everyone knows what pain feels like, and this is a very personal evaluation. Medically speaking, pain is an unpleasant sensation often initiated by tissue damage, resulting in impulses transmitted to the brain via specific nerve fibers. Most health care facilities use some type of pain scale from 0 to 10, with 0 indicating no pain at all and 10 representing excruciating, intolerable pain. In most instances, each number on the scale is accompanied by an illustration to help patients accurately communicate what they are feeling. This numeric scale (no illustrations), provided by the National Institutes of Health, can help improve communication with patients (Table 8-5).

When the documentation indicates that an encounter is prompted by a patient's need for pain management, especially when the pain is noted as acute and/or chronic, there are several options for treatment.

Electrical Reprocessing Researchers are consistently searching for new ways to help patients manage their pain. Transcutaneous electrical modulation pain reprocessing (TEMPR), also referred to as scrambler therapy, administers electrical impulses designed to interrupt pain signals. Although this experimental procedure uses a type of transcutaneous electrical nerve stimulation (TENS), it is not the same procedure. Each session lasts about an hour, with the physician making adjustments approximately every 10 minutes. Each treatment session is reported with category III code 0278T.

Epidural/Intrathecal Medication Administration Medication administered intrathecally (directly into the cerebrospinal fluid via the subarachnoid space in the spinal cord) may be used for chronic pain management. This methodology typically uses pumps, devices that can provide continual delivery of the drug, biologicals, or genetically engineered encapsulated cells. This route of administration has been found to be less invasive for the patient and enables treatment of a larger portion of the central nervous system utilizing the cerebrospinal fluid circulation pathways. Epidural administration tenders the medication into the dura mater of the spinal cord rather than the subarachnoid space.

EXAMPLES

62350 Implantation, revision, or repositioning of tunneled intrathecal or epidural catheter, for long-term medication administration via an external pump or implantable reservoir/infusion pump; without laminectomy

62360 Implantation or replacement of device for intrathecal or epidural drug infusion; subcutaneous reservoir

62362 Implantation or replacement of device for intrathecal or epidural drug infusion; nonprogrammable pump

99601 Home infusion/specialty drug administration, per visit (up to 2 hours)

TABLE 8-5 Numeric Rating Scale for Pain

0	= No pain
1–3	= Mild pain (nagging, annoying, interfering little with ADL*)
4–6	= Moderate pain (interferes significantly with ADL*)
7–10	= Severe pain (disabling; unable to perform ADL*)

*ADL = activities of daily living

Source: National Institutes of Health.

Intravenous Therapy This may be the administration route with which you are most familiar. The medication enters the body via the patient's vein, most often using a point inside the patient's antecubital fossa (elbow). If the condition is chronic, a peripherally inserted central catheter (PICC) line may be inserted and used for the administration of the medication for the duration of the therapy.

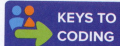

KEYS TO CODING

Whenever you report the administration of a drug, you will need the code for the administration, such as implantation of a pump or infusion, as well as a code to report the specific drug that is administered. Most often, the codes used to report the specific drug come from the HCPCS Level II code set. See Part 2, Chaps. 13 and 14, in this textbook for more information on these codes.

EXAMPLES

96365   Intravenous infusion, for therapy, prophylaxis, or diagnosis; initial, up to 1 hour

36568   Insertion of peripherally inserted central venous catheter (PICC), without subcutaneous port or pump; younger than 5 years of age

36569   Insertion of peripherally inserted central venous catheter (PICC), without subcutaneous port or pump; 5 years or older

LET'S CODE IT! SCENARIO

Barry Gauchier, a 63-year-old male, was admitted for the implantation of a cerebral cortical neurostimulator. Dr. Jackson performed a craniotomy and then successfully implanted the electrodes.

Let's Code It!

Dr. Jackson first performed a *craniotomy.* Let's go to the Alphabetic Index and look. Below *craniotomy,* you will see the listing *for implant of neurostimulators.* That matches our notes, so let's go to the numerical listing and check the descriptions for 61850–61875, as suggested. Read through the codes and their descriptions in this section. Do you agree that the following matches our notes the best?

61860   Craniectomy or craniotomy for implantation of neurostimulator electrodes, cerebral, cortical

It does!

LO 8.9 Eye and Ocular Adnexa

Ophthalmologists diagnose and treat problems and concerns of the eye and ocular adnexa (anatomical parts and sites adjacent to an organ). Most commonly, cataracts are corrected and foreign materials are removed.

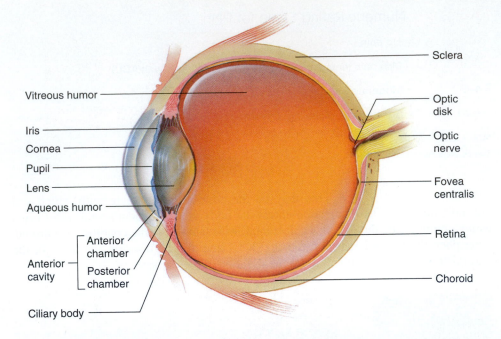

Sclera

Vitreous humor

Optic disk

Optic nerve

Iris

Cornea

Pupil

Lens

Aqueous humor

Fovea centralis

Retina

Anterior chamber

Anterior cavity

Posterior chamber

Choroid

Ciliary body

LET'S CODE IT! SCENARIO

Dianna Marshant was diagnosed with a herniated orbital mass, OD (right inferior orbit). Dr. Deleon performed an excision of the mass and repair. From his notes, "The lower lid was everted and the inferior fornix examined. The herniating mass was viewed and measured at 0.81 cm in diameter. Westcott scissors were used to incise the conjunctival fornices. The herniating mass was then clamped, excised, and cauterized. It appeared to contain mostly fat tissue, which was sent to pathology. The inferior fornix was repaired using running suture of 6-0 plain gut. Bacitracin ointment was applied to the eye followed by an eye pad."

Let's Code It!

The procedure performed was "excision of mass and repair, right inferior orbit."

In the CPT Alphabetic Index, turn to Excision, and review the long list of anatomical sites below. What did Dr. Deleon excise? Not the eye (that would be removal of the eyeball). He removed a "*mass from the eye orbit*" and then "*repaired the orbit.*"

There is no listing for *mass,* but you should remember from medical terminology class (or look it up in a medical dictionary) that another term for *mass* is *lesion.* In the Alphabetic Index, find:

Excision. . . . Lesion . . . another long list. On your scratch pad, write down the code suggested next to the word *Orbit*—61333 so that you can check it out. However, while you are here, also write down the codes suggested for *Conjunctiva*—68110–68130. Why? Because in the body of the notes, it states "incise the conjunctival fornices." This is why it is so important to read the complete notes and not just code from the procedure statement at the top.

Now, let's turn to the main portion of the CPT and find the complete code descriptions:

61333 Exploration of orbit (transcranial approach); with removal of lesion

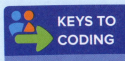

KEYS TO CODING

The conjunctival fornices are the area between the eyelid and the eyeball. The superior fornix is between the upper lid and eyeball; the inferior fornix is between the lower lid and the eyeball.

68110 Excision of lesion, conjunctiva; up to 1 cm

68115 Excision of lesion, conjunctiva; over 1 cm

68130 Excision of lesion, conjunctiva; with adjacent sclera

Which code description matches the physician's notes accurately? 68110.

YOU CODE IT! CASE STUDY

Edward Yankovic, a 53-year-old male, was working in a metal shop. As he was trimming a steel bar, some metal splinters got into his eye. Fortunately, Dr. Madison found that the metal pieces presented superficial damage and had not embedded themselves in Edward's conjunctiva. Dr. Madison removed all the metal pieces and placed a patch over Edward's eye.

You Code It!

Go through the steps and determine the procedure code(s) that should be reported for this encounter between Dr. Madison and Edward Yankovic.

Step 1: Read the case completely.

Step 2: Abstract the notes: Which key words can you identify relating to the procedures performed?

_____

Step 3: Query the provider, if necessary.

Step 4: Diagnosis: Foreign body, conjunctiva, superficial.

Step 5: Code the procedure(s).

_____

Step 6: Link the procedure codes to at least one diagnosis code.

Step 7: Back code to double-check your choices.

Answer:

Did you determine the correct code?

65205 Removal of foreign body, external eye; conjunctival superficial

Good for you!

LO 8.10 Auditory System

The auditory system of the human body is referenced in three sections:

THE OUTER EAR

- Auricle (pinna).
- External acoustic meatus (also known as the external auditory canal).
- Eardrum (the tympanic membrane).

THE MIDDLE EAR

- Auditory ossicles: malleus, incus, and stapes.
- Oval window.
- Eustachian tube (auditory tube) connects the middle ear to the nasopharynx (throat).

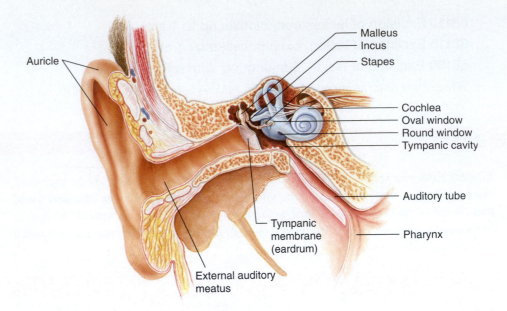

Auricle
Malleus
Incus
Stapes
Cochlea
Oval window
Round window
Tympanic cavity
Auditory tube
Pharynx
Tympanic membrane (eardrum)
External auditory meatus

THE INNER EAR

- Semicircular canals.
- Cochlea.

Tympanostomy

When a patient has a middle ear infection (otitis media), pressure caused by the build-up of fluid or pus in the middle ear compresses the eardrum, causing pain and decreasing the patient's ability to hear. Tympanostomy (ear tube surgery) is a relatively common procedure performed on about 2 million children each year in the United States. It involves the insertion of a ventilating tube into the opening of the tympanum to relieve the pressure.

When reporting a tympanostomy, you need to know what type of anesthesia was provided to the patient: local or general anesthesia.

69433 Tympanostomy (requiring insertion of ventilating tube), local or topical anesthesia

69436 Tympanostomy (requiring insertion of ventilating tube), general anesthesia

These codes report the insertion of the tube into one ear only. When the physician performs this for both ears at the same encounter, you will need to append modifier 50 Bilateral procedure to the correct procedure code.

Sometimes, over a period of time, the tubes naturally fall out. However, when the physician must go in and surgically remove the tubes under general anesthesia, this procedure will be reported separately:

69424 Ventilating tube removal requiring general anesthesia

YOU CODE IT! CASE STUDY

Rochelle McMillian, a 31-year-old female, has been deaf since she was 12. She is admitted today for Dr. Donaldson to put a cochlear implant in her left ear. It is expected that Rochelle will gain back much of her hearing.

Go through the steps and determine the procedure code(s) that should be reported for this encounter between Dr. Donaldson and Rochelle McMillian.

Step 1: Read the case completely.

Step 2: Abstract the notes: Which key words can you identify relating to the procedures performed?

_____

Step 3: Query the provider, if necessary.

Step 4: Diagnosis: Deafness, acquired.

Step 5: Code the procedure(s).

_____

Step 6: Link the procedure codes to at least one diagnosis code.

Step 7: Back code to double-check your choices.

Answer:

Did you determine the correct code?

69930 Cochlear device implantation, with or without mastoidectomy

Operating Microscope

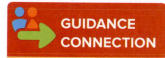

GUIDANCE CONNECTION

Additional explanation can be found in the guidelines within the **Surgery** section, directly under the subhead **Operating Microscope,** in your CPT book.

When a surgeon performs microsurgery, he or she has to use an operating microscope. In such cases, you must code the use of the microscope (69990) in addition to the procedure in which the microscope is used.

+**69990** **Microsurgical techniques, requiring use of operating microscope (List separately in addition to code for primary procedure.)**

There are two guidelines with regard to this add-on code:

1. Do not append modifier 51 Multiple Procedures to the code for the microscope. It is not an additional procedure. Code 69990 indicates the use of a special technique or tool, making modifier 51 incorrect.

2. There are some codes that already include the use of the operating microscope. Therefore, adding code 69990 is redundant. The tough part here is that none of the codes that already include use of the operating microscope include this information in their description. Following, and in many CPT books above the code description, is the list of codes to which you are *not* permitted to add code 69990 because it is already included:

15756–15758	31526	49906
15842	31531	61548
19364	31536	63075–63078
19368	31541	64727
20955–20962	31561	64820–64823
20969–20973	31571	65091–68850
26551–26554	43116	0184T
26556	43496	0226T
		0227T
		0308T

> ### EXAMPLE
>
> 19364 Breast reconstruction with free flap
> (Do not report code 69990 in addition to code 19364.)

As you can see, the codes involved are throughout the Surgery section of the CPT. You might want to go through and mark or highlight the codes, should you be coding for a physician who works with an operating microscope.

Chapter Summary

When reporting surgical procedures, it is important to (1) identify the components of the operation and (2) determine which services are included in the code's description and which services require a separate code. The Surgery section of the CPT book is divided into subsections identified by the body system upon which the technique was performed.

CHAPTER **8** REVIEW
Surgery Coding, Part 2

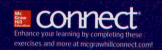

Enhance your learning by completing these
exercises and more at mcgrawhillconnect.com!

Using Terminology

Match each key term to the appropriate definition.

_____ **1.** LO 8.1 Surgically opening the fracture site, or another site in the body nearby, in order to treat the fractured bone.

_____ **2.** LO 8.1 The treatment of a fracture without surgically opening the affected area.

_____ **3.** LO 8.1 The insertion of fixation instruments (such as, pins) placed across the fracture site. It may be done under x-ray imaging for guidance purposes.

_____ **4.** LO 8.1 The surgical removal of a vertebral posterior arch.

_____ **5.** LO 8.3 Either of the two major veins in the leg that run from the foot to the thigh near the surface of the skin.

_____ **6.** LO 8.2 The relocation of tissue from one individual to another (both of the same species) without an identical genetic match.

_____ **7.** LO 8.2 The transfer of tissue from one site to another.

_____ **8.** LO 8.1 The immobilization of a joint using a surgical technique.

_____ **9.** LO 8.1 The attempted return of the fracture or dislocation to its normal alignment manually by the physician.

A. Allotransplantation
B. Arthrodesis
C. Closed treatment
D. Laminectomy
E. Manipulation
F. Open treatment
G. Percutaneous skeletal fixation
H. Saphenous vein
I. Transplantation

Checking Your Understanding

Choose the most appropriate answer for each of the following questions.

1. LO 8.1 Codes within the musculoskeletal subsection include

    a. x-rays.
    b. cast.
    c. medications.
    d. shoes.

2. LO 8.1 Arthrodesis is performed

    a. alone.
    b. in combination with other procedures.
    c. alone and in combination with other procedures.
    d. none of these.

3. LO 8.1 An open treatment of a fracture is performed

    a. only on a compound fracture.
    b. after the cast is applied.
    c. surgically.
    d. in the radiology department.

4. LO 8.2/8.3 Backbench work during a transplant process is

   a. the harvesting of an organ from a donor.
   b. the implantation of the new organ.
   c. the documentation of the surgery.
   d. the preparation of the organ.

5. LO 8.3 The cardiovascular system includes all *except*

   a. heart.
   b. veins.
   c. lungs.
   d. arteries.

6. LO 8.3 Venous grafts harvested from the saphenous vein

   a. are included in the graft code.
   b. require an add-on code.
   c. are coded with a modifier.
   d. are coded separately.

7. LO 8.3 The code for an endovascular repair of an iliac aneurysm includes all *except*

   a. introduction of graft.
   b. stent deployment.
   c. balloon angioplasty.
   d. pacemaker.

8. LO 8.4 An enterectomy is the harvesting of a donor's

   a. lung.
   b. liver.
   c. intestine.
   d. artery.

9. LO 8.4 A pancreatic donor must be

   a. living.
   b. deceased.
   c. either living or deceased.
   d. a relative.

10. LO 8.5 A physician who only interprets the results of a urodynamic procedure must be coded with

   a. modifier 32.
   b. modifier 26.
   c. modifier 53.
   d. modifier 51.

Applying Your Knowledge

1. LO 8.1 Differentiate between an open treatment and a closed treatment. _____

   _____

2. LO 8.1 List the requirements of a penetrating trauma wound. _____

   _____

3. LO 8.1 List five of the approach techniques a coder may need to identify when coding an arthrodesis. _____

   _____

4. LO 8.1 What is a laminotomy? _____

   _____

5. LO 8.2 What are the three steps required in a lung transplant? _____

   _____

6. LO 8.3 What code range do you use for arterial grafts? What do these codes include? _____

   _____

7. LO 8.3 What codes do you have to choose from when coding a venous graft harvested from the femoropopliteal vein? _____

   _____

8. LO 8.4 What is the difference between an EGD and an ERCP? What are their functions? _____

   _____

9. LO 8.5 When a diagnostic or therapeutic cystourethroscopic intervention is performed, including the insertion and removal of a temporary stent, what is the appropriate code range? _____

   _____

10. LO 8.7 What does antepartum care include? _____

_____

11. LO 8.7 What do delivery services include? _____

_____

12. LO 8.7 What does postpartum care include? _____

_____

13. LO 8.8 List the activities the nervous system is responsible for. _____

_____

14. LO 8.9 What problems and concerns does an ophthalmologist treat? _____

_____

15. LO 8.10 What are the sections of the auditory system of the human body? _____

_____

16. LO 8.10 When a surgeon performs microsurgery, he or she has to use an operating microscope. What code identifies the use of the microscope? _____

_____

Using the techniques described in this chapter, carefully read through the case studies and determine the most accurate surgery CPT code(s) and modifier(s), if appropriate, for each case study.

1. Peter Lynch, a 15-year-old male, came to see Dr. Ferguson for the first time. He was in a fight at school and got punched in the jaw, dislocating his temporomandibular joint. Dr. Ferguson performed a closed treatment of the temporomandibular dislocation. The dislocation did not require any wiring or fixation.

   _____

2. Bobby Sherman, a 13-year-old male, was brought to the emergency room by his camp counselor. Two weeks prior, Bobby had broken his arm and had a short-arm cast applied. While walking by the pool, his friends pushed him in, getting the cast wet. Bobby was brought here to have his cast reapplied.

   _____

3. Brad Vitalli, a 49-year-old male, was admitted to the hospital so that Dr. Alden could remove a tumor found on his larynx. Brad tolerated the laryngotomy and the removal of the tumor well.

   _____

4. Dr. Unger ordered a catheter aspiration of Marion Gerstein's tracheobronchial tree. Marion was given some Versed (conscious sedation), and the procedure was performed at her bedside in her hospital room.

   _____

5. Dr. Albertson performed the backbench preparation of a cadaver donor heart allograft prior to Dr. Contini's performing the transplantation. Code for Dr. Albertson's work.

   _____

6. Dr. Eldersten performed an endovascular graft on Wanda Popu, a 45-year-old female, diagnosed with an arteriovenous malformation of the iliac artery.

   _____

7. George Jaden, a 59-year-old male, is admitted for a partial colectomy. Dr. Issacson resected a segment of George's colon and performed an anastomosis between the remaining ends of the colon. George tolerated the procedure well.

   _____

8. Patricia Morrison, a morbidly obese 37-year-old female, was admitted for a gastric restrictive procedure. In addition to the gastric bypass performed by Dr. Wattel, Patricia's small intestine was reconstructed to limit absorption.

_____

9. Israel Ortega, a 51-year-old male, is admitted to the hospital today so that Dr. Warren can perform a total urethrectomy and a cystostomy.

_____

10. Jan Springer, a 51-year-old male with multiple sclerosis, has been diagnosed with Peyronie disease. He is admitted today so that Dr. Rudner can excise the penile plaque that has developed.

_____

11. Jack Friedman, an 83-year-old male, had a programmable cerebrospinal fluid (CSF) shunt inserted 6 weeks ago by Dr. Girald. Today, Jack comes to the office so that Dr. Girald can reprogram the shunt and make the adjustments as shown necessary by the computed tomography (CT) scan taken last week.

_____

12. Bridgette Smith, a 17-year-old female, was taken to the OR so that Dr. Payas could perform a twist drill hole in order to evacuate and drain a subdural hematoma that formed after she banged her head on an overhead bar while on a roller coaster at an amusement park.

_____

13. Donna Travellina, a 33-year-old female, noticed a lesion on her left eyelid. Over the period of a few months, it not only bothered but also worried her. She was admitted today so that Dr. Charne could excise the lesion. He used a simple, direct closure. Donna's prognosis is excellent.

_____

14. Jay Ericson, a 41-year-old male, hurt his eye in an accident. Dr. Lucas examined him and noticed that his cornea was scratched. It was not a perforating laceration. Dr. Lucas repaired the laceration of the cornea in the office.

_____

15. Having trouble hearing, Rodney Loman, a 61-year-old male, came to see Dr. Beariman, an audiologist. After examination, Dr. Beariman removed the impacted earwax from both ears. Rodney was amazed at the improvement in his hearing and left the office feeling much better.

_____

The following exercises provide practice in the application of abstracting the physicians' notes and learning to work with SOAP notes from our health care facility, Cipher, Victors & Associates. These case studies (SOAP notes) are modeled on real patient encounters. Using the techniques described in this chapter, carefully read through the case studies and determine the most accurate surgery CPT code(s) and modifier(s), if appropriate, for each case study.

CIPHER, VICTORS & ASSOCIATES
A Complete Health Care Facility
234 MAIN STREET • ANYTOWN, FL 32711 • 407-555-1234

PATIENT: WALLERSTEIN, KARIN
ACCOUNT/EHR #:   WALLKA01
DATE: 09/23/18

Procedure performed: Colonoscopy

Physician: Matthew Appellet, MD

INDICATIONS: History of inflammatory bowel disease

PROCEDURE: The patient was given no premedication at her request, and the Olympus PCF-130 colonoscope was used. The mucosa of the rectum was essentially normal apart from some mild nonspecific edema. Photographs and biopsies were obtained. The remainder of the rectum was normal. The sigmoid was normal as was the descending colon, splenic flexure, transverse colon, hepatic flexure, right colon, and cecum. No evidence of polyps, tumors, masses, or inflammation. The scope was then withdrawn, and these findings were confirmed. The procedure was terminated, and the patient tolerated it well.

IMPRESSION: Normal colonic mucosa through the cecum.
PLAN: Await results of rectal biopsies.

Matthew Appellet, MD

MA/mg   D: 09/23/18 09:50:16   T: 09/25/18 12:55:01

Determine the accurate surgery CPT code(s) and modifier(s), if appropriate.

_____

_____

_____

CIPHER, VICTORS & ASSOCIATES
A Complete Health Care Facility
234 MAIN STREET • ANYTOWN, FL 32711 • 407-555-1234

PATIENT: PEONIE, RONALD
ACCOUNT/EHR #:   PEONRO002

Date of Operation: 06/17/18
Preoperative Diagnosis: Orbital mass, OD
Postoperative Diagnosis: Herniated orbital fat pad, OD
Operation: Excision of mass and repair, right superior orbit

Surgeon: Mark C. Warren, MD
Assistant: None
Anesthesia: Local

DESCRIPTION OF OPERATIVE PROCEDURE:

After proparacaine was instilled in the eye, it was prepped and draped in the usual sterile manner and 2% Lidocaine with 1:200,000 epinephrine was injected into the superior aspect of the right orbit.

A corneal protective shield was placed in the eye. The eye was placed in down-gaze. The upper lid was everted and the fornix examined. The herniating mass was viewed and measured at 0.75 cm in diameter. Westcott scissors were used to incise the fornix conjunctiva. The herniating mass was then clamped, excised, and cauterized. It appeared to contain mostly fat tissue, which was sent to pathology. The superior fornix was repaired using running suture of 6-0 plain gut. Bacitracin ointment was applied to the eye followed by an eye pad. The patient tolerated the procedure well and left the OR in good condition.

Mark C. Warren, MD

MCW/mg   D: 06/17/18 09:50:16   T: 06/19/18 12:55:01

Determine the accurate surgery CPT code(s) and modifier(s), if appropriate.

_____

_____

_____

CIPHER, VICTORS & ASSOCIATES
A Complete Health Care Facility
234 MAIN STREET • ANYTOWN, FL 32711 • 407-555-1234

PATIENT: VINOMAKKER, ANTONIA
ACCOUNT/EHR #:   VINOAN001
DATE: 09/23/18

Attending Physician: James Healer, MD

Preoperative Diagnosis: C5 compression fracture
Postoperative Diagnosis: same
Procedure: C5 corpectomy and fusion fixation with fibular strut graft and Atlantis plate
Anesthesia: General endotracheal

This is a 25-year-old female status post assault. The patient sustained a C5 compression fracture. MRI scan showed compression with evidence of posterior ligamentous injury. The patient was subsequently set up for the surgical procedure. The procedure was described in detail, including the risks. The risks included but not limited to bleeding, infection, stroke, paralysis, death, CSF leak, loss of bladder and bowel control, hoarse voice, paralyzed vocal cord, death, and damage to adjacent nerves and tissues. The patient understood the risks. The patient also understood that bank bone instrumentation would be used and that the bank bone could collapse and the instrumentation could fail, break, or the screws could pull out. The patient provided consent.

    The patient was taken to the OR. The patient was induced. An endotracheal tube was placed. A Foley was placed. The patient was given preoperative antibiotics. The patient was placed in slight extension. The right neck was prepped and draped in the usual manner. A linear incision was made over the C5 vertebral body. The platysma was divided. Dissection was continued medial to the sternocleidomastoid to the prevertebral fascia. This was cauterized and divided. The longus colli was cauterized and elevated. The fracture was visualized. A spinal needle was used to verify the location using fluoroscopy. The C5 vertebral body was drilled out. The bone was saved. The disks above and below were removed. The posterior longitudinal ligament was removed. The bone was quite collapsed and fragmented. Distraction pins were then packed with bone removed from the C5 vertebral body prior to implantation. A plate was then placed with screws in the C4 and C6 vertebral bodies. The locking screws were tightened. The wound was irrigated. Bleeding was helped with the bipolar. The retractors were removed. The incision was approximated with simple interrupted Vicryl. The subcutaneous tissue was approximated, and skin edges were approximated subcuticularly. Steri-Strips were applied. A dressing was applied. The patient was placed back in an Aspen collar. The patient was extubated and transferred to recovery.

___

James Healer, MD

JH/mgr   D: 09/23/18 12:33:08 PM   T: 09/25/18 3:22:54 PM

Determine the accurate surgery CPT code(s) and modifier(s), if appropriate.

___

___

___

CIPHER, VICTORS & ASSOCIATES
A Complete Health Care Facility
234 MAIN STREET • ANYTOWN, FL 32711 • 407-555-1234

PATIENT:	MINNEON, CHARLISE
ACCOUNT/EHR #:	MINNCH01
Admission Date:	09/18/18
Discharge Date:	09/18/18
DATE:	09/18/18
Preoperative DX:	High-grade squamous intraepithelial lesion of the cervix
Postoperative DX:	same
Operation:	Loop electrosurgical excision procedure (LEEP) and ECC (endocervical curettage)
Surgeon:	Rodney L. Cohen, MD
Assistant:	None
Anesthesia:	General by LMA
Findings:	Large ectropion, large non-staining active cervix essentially encompassing the entire active cervix
Specimens:	To pathology
Disposition:	Stable to recovery room

PROCEDURE: The patient was taken to the OR where she was placed in the supine position and administered general anesthesia. She was then placed in cane stirrups and prepped and draped in the usual fashion. Her vaginal vault was not prepped. The coated speculum was then placed and the cervix exposed. It was then painted with Lugol and the entire active cervix was nonstaining with the clearly defined margins where the stain began to be picked up. The cervix was injected with approximately 7 cc of lidocaine with 1% epinephrine. Using a large loop, the anterior cervix was excised, and then the posterior loop was excised in separate specimens. Because of the size of the lesion one piece in total was not accomplished. Prior to the excision, the endocervical curettage was performed, and specimens were collected. All specimens were sent to pathology. The remaining cervical bed was cauterized and then painted with Monsel for hemostasis. The case was concluded with this. Instruments were removed. The patient was taken down from candy cane stirrups, awakened from the anesthesia, and taken to the recovery room in stable condition.

Rodney L. Cohen, MD

RLC/mgr D: 09/23/18 12:33:08 PM T: 09/25/18 3:22:54 PM

Determine the accurate surgery CPT code(s) and modifier(s), if appropriate.

_____

_____

_____

CIPHER, VICTORS & ASSOCIATES
A Complete Health Care Facility
234 MAIN STREET • ANYTOWN, FL 32711 • 407-555-1234

PATIENT: EMPANNY, CAROLINE
ACCOUNT/EHR #:   EMPACA01
DATE: 09/25/18

Diagnosis: Medulloblastoma
Procedure: Central Venous Access Device (CVAD) insertion

Physician: Frank Vincent, MD
Anesthesia: Conscious sedation

PROCEDURE: Patient is a 4-year-old female, with a recent diagnosis of malignancy. Due to an upcoming course of chemotherapy, the CVAD is being inserted to ease administration of the drugs. The patient was placed on the table in supine position. The patient was given Versed to achieve conscious sedation. The incision was made to insert a central venous catheter, centrally. During the placement of the catheter, a short tract (nontunneled) was made as the catheter was advanced from the skin entry site to the point of venous cannulation. The catheter tip was set to reside in the subclavian vein. The patient was gently aroused from the sedation and was awake when transported to the recovery room.

_____

Frank Vincent, MD

FV/mg   D: 09/25/18 09:50:16   T: 09/25/18 12:55:01

Determine the accurate surgery CPT code(s) and modifier(s), if appropriate.

_____

_____

_____

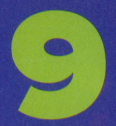

RADIOLOGY CODING

Key Terms

Angiography

Arthrography

Computed tomography (CT)

Computed tomography angiography (CTA)

Fluoroscope

Magnetic resonance arthrography (MRA)

Magnetic resonance imaging (MRI)

Nuclear medicine

Radiation

Sonogram

Venography

Health care professionals use radiologic imaging to see inside the body. Radiologic services, also known as *interventional radiology,* can be used to investigate a potential condition (diagnostically), measure the progress of a disease or condition, or aid in the actual reduction or prevention of disease or other condition (therapeutically).

Many, many years ago, radiology was simply known as x-ray, because this was the extent of the equipment. Now, technology has made tremendous advancements in the science of imaging, and health care professionals can screen, diagnose, monitor, and treat patients much more effectively and efficiently. As you read through this chapter, you will learn about the various types of imaging: x-rays, computed tomography (CT) scans, magnetic resonance imaging (MRI), positron emission tomography (PET), ultrasound, arthrography, and more.

LO 9.1 Technical vs. Professional

Essentially, there are two primary components of any radiologic procedure: the technical and the professional (referred to as supervision and interpretation in the CPT). This is not to say that radiologic technicians are not professionals. The designation is merely to divide the services provided so that it can be determined which facility or practitioner should be paid for what.

EXAMPLE

Meredith Atkins, a 33-year-old female, was sent to the Diagnostic Imaging Center to get an x-ray, three views, of her skull after she was hit in the head by a bat at a softball game.

The x-ray equipment is owned by the facility. Sarah Carter, the x-ray technician who will operate the equipment, is a member of the facility's staff, and Dr. Rivers, a board-certified radiologist who will interpret the films and send a report of this evaluation to Meredith's physician, is also a staff member of the center. Therefore, Diagnostic Imaging's coding specialist will ask the insurance company for reimbursement for both the technical procedure (the use of the equipment, materials, and the staff to work and maintain that equipment) and the professional aspect (the cost and work to supervise and interpret the films).

For Meredith's case, the code to be reported is 70250.

Purchasing (or leasing) and maintaining imaging equipment is very expensive and cannot be supported by every health care facility. In addition, physicians who are specially trained radiologists are not necessarily staff members of all health care facilities with the equipment. Therefore, circumstances may arise when the technical procedure and the professional service must be billed separately. In those cases, the coder who is responsible for charging for the professional services must use modifier 26 to identify the separation of the components.

> **26 Professional Component:** Certain procedures are a combination of a physician component and a technical component. When the physician component is reported separately, the service may be identified by adding modifier 26 to the usual procedure number.

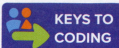

Clifford Sienna, a 27-year-old male, was brought into the emergency department of a small hospital near his farm after he fell off a ladder onto his back while working in the barn. The physician sent Clifford to radiology for an entire spine survey study. The hospital does not have a staff radiologist, so Dr. Chen is brought over to evaluate the x-rays and write the report for the physician.

The hospital, which owns the equipment and pays the salary of the technician, will bill the insurance carrier for the technical portion of the examination, using code 72010-TC.

Dr. Chen's coding specialist will send in a claim for Dr. Chen's interpretation only, the professional services he provided. In order to make this clear on the claim form, the modifier 26 Professional Component will be appended to the code for the radiologic examination; the code that will be reported on his claim form will be 72010-26.

As you have already learned, sometimes the CPT book will save you work. Certain radiologic examination codes distinguish the technical component and professional component of services for you. One of the easiest ways to identify such cases is by the notation within the code's description that specifies the code is for radiologic supervision and interpretation only.

EXAMPLE

70015 Cisternography, positive contrast, radiological supervision and interpretation

From the example, you can see that code 70015 excludes the technical component. If you are coding for the physician's services only, that makes it easy. If you are coding for the facility for the technical aspect, you need to add modifier TC Technical Component. After a while, you will learn the details about the procedures performed by all of the professionals in your health care facility, and you will be able to identify the components easily. It just takes some practice.

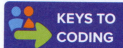

KEYS TO CODING

You learned in medical terminology class that the suffix -graphy means the recording of an image and the suffix -scopy means to look or view. We tend to think of all these procedures and services as radiology. However, not all of them are coded from the Radiology section of the CPT book. For example, cardiography is listed in the Medicine section. Therefore, always use the alphabetic index to help point you toward the correct area of the book. It will save you time in the long run.

KEYS TO CODING

Technical component: Coded to gain reimbursement for the facility that owns and maintains the equipment used; amortized cost of the machine, supplies, maintenance, overhead (electricity and so on), and the technician.

Professional component: Coded to gain reimbursement for the health care professional, radiologist, or physician who supervises and interprets the images taken.

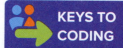

KEYS TO CODING

If the third-party payer accepts HCPCS Level II, append modifier TC Technical Component to the CPT code, when appropriate.

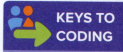

KEYS TO CODING

Some third-party payers will determine the TC and PC components for payment without the modifier by the place of service code shown on the claim form.

Derick Norton, an 8-year-old male, is brought into the emergency department by ambulance. He was skateboarding off a homemade ramp and fell on his neck and shoulder. Dr. Defeaux suspects a broken clavicle and orders a complete radiologic exam of the area. The staff radiologist, Dr. Grace, reads the films and sends a report to Dr. Defeaux confirming the fracture.

Let's Code It!

The physician's notes state that a *radiologic exam* of Derick's *clavicle* was performed. Let's turn to the Alphabetic Index under *radiology.* Note that the choices are not going to satisfy our needs. Therefore, let's try an alternate term for radiology: x-ray. Turn to *x-ray,* and you find a long list of anatomical sites. Next to the word *clavicle* you see only one suggested code. Let's go to the numerical listing and read the complete description:

73000 Radiologic examination; clavicle, complete

This is exactly what Dr. Defeaux ordered for Derick.
Good job!

sonogram
The use of sound waves to record images of internal organs and tissues; also called an *ultrasound.*

Marisol Martinez, a 31-year-old female, is 10 weeks pregnant. This is her first pregnancy, and twins run in her family. In order to determine how many fetuses there are, Dr. Phillips orders a **sonogram.** Brenda Hughes is the technician at the imaging center next door to Dr. Phillips's office. The Imaging Center performs Marisol's real-time transabdominal exam and sends the documentation to Dr. Phillips so that he can read and interpret the results. A single fetus was observed.

Let's Code It!

You are Dr. Phillips's coder, and his notes state that a sonogram of Marisol was performed at the imaging center. We know that she is pregnant, and this is why she is having the test done, so the anatomical site of the examination is her *pregnant uterus.* Turn to the Alphabetic Index under *sonography,* and the CPT book tells you to *see echography,* which is the type of technology that sonograms use. Turn to *echography* (caution—not echo*cardio*graphy; this is not of Marisol's heart), and find a list of anatomical sites. Looking for *pregnant uterus,* you see a range of suggested codes. Let's go to the numerical listing and read the complete description of the first one.

76801 Ultrasound, pregnant uterus, real time with image documentation, fetal and maternal evaluation, first trimester (<14 weeks 0 days), transabdominal approach; single or first gestation

Great! The very first code seems to match the notes perfectly. However, to make certain you are using the best, most appropriate code, you will want to read through all the suggested codes.

Remember, you are coding for Dr. Phillips. With regard to Marisol's radiologic exam, he provided the interpretation—the professional component only. Therefore, the claim form you prepare should show this code as 76801-26.

LO 9.2 Screening vs. Diagnostic

Identifying whether an imaging service is performed as a screening or a diagnostic tool can be important to determining the correct code for the procedure. This designation refers to the reason the physician ordered the test.

A screening image is one done as part of a regular preventive checkup. This is ordered because the standard of care and the calendar have matched up. For example, a screening mammogram will be ordered the same time every year for a woman over the age of 50. There are no signs or symptoms that would prompt the test. It is just the wise thing to do to make certain all is fine.

A diagnostic image is one that is taken to assist in the identification and/or confirmation of a suspected condition or diagnosis. In these cases, the physician would identify specific signs or symptoms that led him or her to decide this test was needed.

There are times when an imaging session for a patient begins as a screening test and becomes a diagnostic test while the patient is still there. With technology providing instant imaging, the radiologist can review the images almost immediately after they have been taken, while the patient is still on the premises. This eliminates a patient's needing to come back at another time to retake an image that was not clear or the technician's having to take additional views because the radiologist identified a suspicious element. When a screening test turns into a diagnostic test, report only the diagnostic imaging service because that will include the screening aspect of the procedure.

EXAMPLES

74261 Computed tomography (CT) colonography, diagnostic
74263 Computed tomography (CT) colonography, screening

Views

Throughout the Radiology section of the CPT book, radiologic examinations are often described by the number of views taken by the technician.

EXAMPLE

73060 Radiologic examination, humerus, minimum of two views

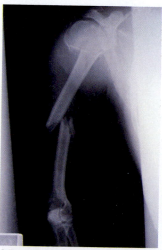
© David Frazier/Corbis

The "two views" refers to the number of angles, or perceptions, from which the images were taken, such as anterior and posterior. Such codes represent the norm, or standard, in imaging when it comes to these certain anatomical sites.

The most common angles, or pathways, of imaging include

- AP *Anteroposterior:* Front to back.
- PA *Posteroanterior:* Back to front.
- O *Oblique:* At an angle.
- RAO *Right anterior oblique:* At an angle from the right front.
- RPO *Right posterior oblique:* At an angle from the right back.
- LAO *Left anterior oblique:* At an angle from the left front.
- LPO *Left posterior oblique:* At an angle from the left back.
- Lat *Lateral (lat):* From one side to the other side.

In those cases when the radiologist takes fewer than the minimum number of views included in the description, you have to append the radiologic code with modifier 52 Reduced Services.

52 **Reduced Services:** Under certain circumstances a service or procedure is partially reduced or eliminated at the physician's discretion. Under these circumstances, the service provided can be identified by its usual procedure number and the addition of modifier 52, signifying that the service is reduced. This provides a means of reporting reduced services without disturbing the identification of the basic service.

YOU CODE IT! CASE STUDY

Caroline Stephens, an 18-month-old female, is brought into the office of her pediatrician, Dr. Katzman. She fell off the couch onto a hard tile floor and it appears that her hip is painful to her. Dr. Katzman has his staff take an x-ray of the pelvis and hip to determine if there is a fracture. He orders only the anteroposterior view to be taken. He does not subject his patients to radiology exposure unnecessarily, and he believes that the one view will tell him what he needs to know. The x-ray confirms a hairline fracture, and he applies a cast.

You Code It!

Go through the steps and determine the code(s) that should be reported for radiologic service Dr. Katzman provided to Caroline Stephens.

Step 1: Read the case completely.

Step 2: Abstract the notes: Which key words can you identify relating to the procedures performed?

_____

Step 3: Query the provider, if necessary.

Step 4: Diagnosis: Fracture, hip.

Step 5: Code the procedure(s).

_____

Step 6: Link the procedure codes to at least one diagnosis code.

Step 7: Back code to double-check your choices.

Answer:

Did you determine the correct code?

73540-52 Radiologic examination, pelvis and hips, infant or child, minimum of two views, reduced service

Good job!

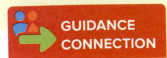

GUIDANCE CONNECTION

Additional explanation can be found in the guidelines pages directly before the **Radiology** section, subhead **Administration of Contrast Material(s),** in your CPT book.

LO 9.3 Procedures With or Without Contrast

Some imaging examinations use contrast materials to gain a clearer picture of an organ or anatomical site. The phrase "with contrast" means that the technician or physician gave the patient a substance to enhance the image. For example, arthrography is used to identify abnormalities that may be present within a joint (wrist, hip, shoulder, knee). Gadolinium is injected into the joint that is to be visualized to provide better-quality images of the patient's condition. In other procedures, different substances are injected. For example, when myelography is done to examine a patient's spinal cord and nerves, an injection of x-ray dye may be used to more clearly visualize a patient's disc herniation, bone spurs, or vertebral stenosis.

1. When radiographic **arthrography** is performed, use an additional code for the supervision and interpretation of the appropriate joint. This includes the use of a **fluoroscope.**

EXAMPLE

Dr. Goldtree, a radiologist, supervised a radiographic arthrography of Conrad Douglas's ankle; later the interpreted results were reported with code 73615.

2. Imaging "with contrast" has some guidelines that you have to know in order to code accurately.

   a. If the code description includes the term "with contrast," such as **computed tomography (CT)** with contrast, **computed tomography angiography (CTA)** with contrast, **magnetic resonance arthrography (MRA)** with contrast, or **magnetic resonance imaging (MRI)** with contrast, the injection of the contrast materials, when administered intravenously, is already included in the code and should *not* be reported separately.

   b. If the contrast material is injected intra-articularly (into a joint) or intrathecally (into a tendon or sheath), an additional code is reported for the appropriate injection.

   c. Providing contrast materials orally and/or rectally alone does not constitute an exam "with contrast."

EXAMPLE

Dr. Holmes injected David Rogers's elbow intrathecally with contrast materials to do a radiographic arthrography for his tennis elbow. This is reported with codes 24220, and 73085.

3. When a CT or MR arthrography is performed without radiographic arthrography, you will need three different codes:

   a. A code for the imaging guidance (fluoroscopy) of the placement of the needle to inject the contrast material.

   b. A code for the injection of the contrast material into the specific joint.

   c. A code for the appropriate CT or MR.

EXAMPLE

Bernadette Hughes is experiencing pain in her pelvic region. Dr. Mateo orders an MRA of her hip/pelvis with contrast. The material is injected intra-articularly. This is reported using codes 77002, 27093, and 72198.

Other types of radiologic procedures include

Positron emission tomography (PET): Uses a variety of radiopharmaceuticals that mimic natural sugars, water, proteins, and oxygen and collect in various tissues and organs. It is a time-exposure picture of cellular biologic activities.

arthrography
The recording of a picture of an anatomical joint after the administration of contrast material into the joint capsule.

fluoroscope
A piece of equipment that emits x-rays through a part of the patient's body onto a fluorescent screen, causing the image to identify various aspects of the anatomy by density.

computed tomography (CT)
A specialized computer scanner with very fine detail that records imaging of internal anatomical sites; also known as computerized axial tomography (CAT).

computed tomography angiography (CTA)
A CT scan using contrast materials to visualize arteries and veins all over the body.

magnetic resonance arthrography (MRA)
MR imaging of an anatomical joint after the administration of contrast material into the joint capsule.

magnetic resonance imaging (MRI)
A three-dimensional radiologic technique that uses nuclear technology to record pictures of internal anatomical sites.

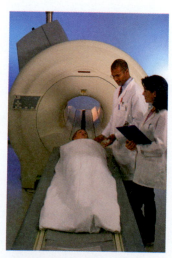
© Pete Saloutos/Corbis

Bone density scan (DEXA): Used most often for osteoporosis screenings; enables assessment of bone minerals in spine, hip, and other skeletal sites.

Nuclear medicine scan: Used to assess organ system function.

LET'S CODE IT! SCENARIO

Jason Tennison, a 75-year-old male, has been having problems with his memory and his walking. After an extensive examination, his neurologist, Dr. Grunion, orders an MRI, brain, with and without contrast, to determine if Jason is suffering from hydrocephalus.

Let's Code It!

This is very straightforward. Jason had an *MRI* of his *brain* taken. Let's go to the Alphabetic Index and look this up. Under *magnetic resonance imaging (MRI)*, you see the list of anatomical sites, including *brain,* which suggests code range 70551–70553. (Note: *Intraoperative,* indented below *brain,* means that the MRI was performed during surgery. This was not the case for Jason, according to the physician's notes.) Let's go to the numerical listing and read the descriptions.

70551 Magnetic resonance (e.g., proton) imaging, brain (including brain stem); without contrast material

70552 with contrast material(s)

70553 without contrast material, followed by contrast material(s) and further sequences

Dr. Grunion's notes state that the MRI is *with and without contrast.* That means both types of imaging were done. Code 70551 describes without contrast, and code 70552 includes the contrast. When you keep reading, you see that code 70553 is the correct code because, as the notes state, it includes both sequences: without the contrast followed by with contrast materials. Of course, you will also add the appropriate HCPCS Level II codes to report the contrast materials used.

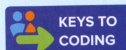 **KEYS TO CODING**

Appropriate HCPCS Level II codes from the range Q9951–Q9969 based on the number of units, should be assigned to report the contrast materials supplied.

LO 9.4 Diagnostic Radiology

Diagnostic Angiography

The coding of the process of imaging the body's blood vessels, diagnostic **angiography,** carries certain guidelines affecting the use of the codes.

angiography
The imaging of blood vessels after the injection of contrast material.

1. In some cases, interventional coding guidelines don't permit you to report a diagnostic angiography when it is performed at the same time as a therapeutic interventional procedure. This rule applies when the patient has already been diagnosed and has scheduled a therapeutic intervention to correct the problem. As you have already learned, you must read the guidelines and the code descriptions carefully.

EXAMPLE

Dr. Aspiras performed a carotid arterial angiography to check for blockage and immediately performed an intervention procedure. You would report this by using code 36227.

2. In other cases, the diagnostic angiography *should be coded separately* even though it is done at the same session as an interventional procedure. This is true if one of the following conditions has been met:

   a. A full diagnostic study is done, no prior catheter-based angiographic study is available, and the decision to intervene is determined by the diagnostic study.

   b. The patient's condition has changed since a previously done study.

   c. The patient's condition changes during the interventional procedure that requires a diagnostic procedure to look at vessels outside of the area.

   d. The prior diagnostic angiography did not show the applicable anatomy and/or pathology being treated at the session.

EXAMPLE

Denise Casson had a diagnostic angiography of her adrenal gland 1 year ago. Since then, her condition has deteriorated. Therefore, Dr. Reginald first performs a diagnostic procedure. Because this shows changes, at the same session he performs an interventional procedure.

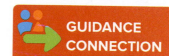

GUIDANCE CONNECTION

Additional explanation can be found in the guidelines within the **Radiology** section, subhead **Vascular Procedures,** subsection **Aorta and Arteries,** in your CPT book.

3. Diagnostic angiography is included with the code for an interventional procedure and should *not* be coded separately when that diagnostic angiography is performed for any of the following:

   a. Vessel measurement.

   b. Postangioplasty or stent angiography.

   c. Contrast injections, angiography, road mapping, and/or fluoroscopic guidance for the interventional procedure.

LET'S CODE IT! SCENARIO

Norma Washington, a 57-year-old female, has had two mild heart attacks in the past 2 years. Today, Norma is at the Fairfield Ambulatory Surgical Center for a diagnostic angiography to quantify the degree of blockage suspected in her left renal artery. Dr. Johannson performs the procedure that includes placing the catheter directly in the renal artery. Later that day, Dr. Johannson dictates a report indicating that Norma's left renal artery is 50% percent blocked.

Let's Code It!

The notes indicate that a *left renal angiography* was performed on Norma. Let's go to the Alphabetic Index and look up *angiography*. You know that Norma's renal artery was examined, and the index suggests codes 36251–36252. Let's check the complete descriptions in the numerical listings:

36251 Selective catheter placement (first-order), main renal artery and any accessory renal artery(s) for renal angiography, including arterial puncture and catheter placement(s), fluoroscopy, contrast injection(s), image postprocessing, permanent recording of images, and radiological supervision and interpretation, including pressure gradient measurements when performed, and flush aortogram when performed; unilateral

36252   bilateral

The difference between these two code descriptions is that 36251 is for a unilateral procedure and 36252 is for a bilateral procedure. Norma had only her left renal artery examined. One side is unilateral, leading us to the correct code of 36251.

Diagnostic Venography

The codes for reporting diagnostic **venography** have guidelines similar to those for diagnostic angiography.

1. Some interventional procedure codes include the diagnostic venography when done at the same time as the procedure. You must read the descriptions carefully to determine if this is the case.

2. Diagnostic venography done at the same time as an interventional procedure *should be coded separately* if one of the following conditions has been met:

    a. A full diagnostic study is done, no prior catheter-based venographic study is available, and the decision to intervene is determined by this diagnostic study.

    b. The patient's condition has changed since a previously done study.

    c. The patient's condition changes during the interventional procedure and requires a diagnostic procedure to look at vessels outside of the area.

    d. The prior diagnostic venography did not show the applicable anatomy and/or pathology being treated at the session.

3. Diagnostic venography is included with the code for an interventional procedure and should *not* be coded separately when that diagnostic venography is performed for any of the following:

    a. Vessel measurement.

    b. Postangioplasty or stent venography.

    c. Contrast injections, venography, road mapping, and/or fluoroscopic guidance for the interventional procedure.

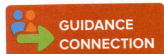

GUIDANCE CONNECTION

Additional explanation can be found in the guidelines within the **Radiology** section, directly under the subhead **Vascular Procedures,** subsection **Veins and Lymphatics,** in your CPT book.

LET'S CODE IT! SCENARIO

Natan Fawzi, a 55-year-old male, flew in yesterday from Australia, a 26-hour airplane ride. Since getting off the plane, he has been having pain in his right calf. Dr. Leventhol performed a diagnostic venography to determine if Natan has deep vein thrombosis (DVT). After completing the procedure, he wrote a report with his interpretation, which was sent to Natan's internist.

Let's Code It!

Dr. Leventhol performed a *diagnostic venography* of Natan's *right leg*. Let's go to the Alphabetic Index and find *venography*. Beneath *venography,* you see the anatomical site *leg* with the suggested code range 75820–75822. Let's look at the code descriptions in the numerical listings:

75820 Venography, extremity, unilateral, radiological supervision and interpretation

75822 Venography, extremity, bilateral, radiological supervision and interpretation

The difference between these two codes is that 75820 is a unilateral procedure and 75822 is a bilateral procedure. Natan had only his right leg examined, making it a unilateral procedure and making 75820 the correct code.

Transcatheter Procedures

Therapeutic transcatheter radiologic supervision and interpretation codes, when associated with intervention, already include

1. Vessel measurement.
2. Postangioplasty or stent venography.
3. Contrast injections, angiography/venography, road mapping, and/or fluoroscopic guidance for the interventional procedure.

Transcatheter therapeutic radiologic and interpretation services *are* separately reportable from diagnostic angiography/venography done at the same time *unless* they are specifically included in the code descriptor.

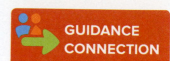

GUIDANCE CONNECTION

Additional explanation can be found in the guidelines within the **Radiology** section, directly under the subhead **Vascular Procedures**, subsection **Transcatheter Procedures**, in your CPT book.

LET'S CODE IT! SCENARIO

Dr. Jerome is in the OR today to perform a transcatheter placement of an intravascular stent, percutaneously, in Gayle Calendar's common iliac.

Let's Code It!

You are Dr. Jerome's coding specialist, so you are going to code only the radiologic supervision and interpretation of the *transcatheter* procedure, as well as the placement of the stent itself. Let's go to *transcatheter* in the Alphabetic Index. You will notice that, if you go to *placement* under *transcatheter,* you see *intravascular stents* indented below. Here, the index suggests some category III codes (the T codes, which will be reviewed in full detail in Chap. 12) along with code ranges 37215–37216, 37236–37239, and 92928–92929.

When you turn to the codes, you realize that they are in the Surgery section, not Radiology. However, they are the only codes offered by the index, so let's take a look at them all. Notice

37236 Transcatheter placement of an intravascular stent(s) (except lower extremity, cervical carotid, extracranial vertebral or intrathoracic carotid, intracranial or coronary), open or percutaneous, including radiological supervision and interpretation and including all angioplasty within the same vessel, when performed, initial artery

But we are coding for Dr. Jerome's radiologic supervision and interpretation for the procedure as well as the stent placement. Notice that the description for code 37236 includes "radiological supervision and interpretation."

Perfect!

Diagnostic Ultrasound

As the coding specialist, you must read the report and pay attention to whether the exam was "complete" or "limited" and choose the correct code. The description of an ultrasound exam as being "complete" is determined by the specific number of elements, such as organs or areas, that are surveyed during the test. However, sometimes the full list is not visualized. For example, an organ may have been previously removed surgically, or another organ may be blocking the view. The report that is submitted for the patient's record, after the exam, should note everything that was studied—as well as those elements that should have been but were not, along with why they were not.

You will find information regarding what is included in a complete exam in the guidelines shown below each of the ultrasound subheadings: Abdomen and Retroperitoneum; Pelvis—Obstetrical, Pelvis—Non-obstetrical.

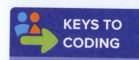

KEYS TO CODING

If the reason that an organ was not visible is documented in the patient's record, you are permitted to code this as "complete."

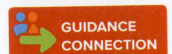
Should an ultrasound exam be performed *without* a thorough evaluation of an organ or anatomical region *and* recording of the image *and* a final, written report, you are not permitted to code the procedure separately.

EXAMPLE

ABDOMEN AND RETROPERITONEUM: A complete ultrasound examination of the abdomen (76700) consists of real-time scans of the liver, gallbladder, common bile duct, pancreas, spleen, kidney, and the upper abdominal aorta and inferior vena cava including any demonstrated abdominal abnormality.

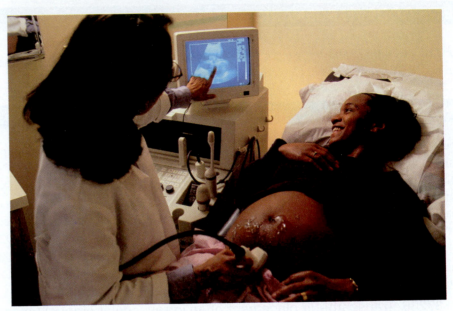

© Keith Brofsky/Getty Images

Let's say an ultrasound examination is done on Herman Smith's abdomen. The documentation includes the physician's (radiologist's) interpretation of all organs except the gallbladder. The patient had his gallbladder removed 1 year prior to this ultrasound exam. As long as this fact is also documented, code 76700 for a complete ultrasound examination of the abdomen is accurate.

You already know that an ultrasound may be called a *sonogram.* However, other definitions are important for you to know so that you can determine the best, most appropriate code. The following terms identify the type of scan:

A-mode indicates a one-dimensional ultrasonic measurement procedure.

M-mode is also a one-dimensional ultrasonic measurement procedure; however, it includes the movement of the trace so that there can be a recording of both amplitude and velocity of the moving echo-producing structures.

B-scan indicates a two-dimensional ultrasonic scanning procedure with a two-dimensional display.

Real-time scan indicates that a two-dimensional ultrasonic scanning procedure with a display was performed and included both the two-dimensional structure and motion with time.

If the report indicates that a Doppler evaluation of vascular structures, or another diagnostic vascular ultrasound study, was performed, it should be coded separately with the codes from the Noninvasive Vascular Diagnostic Studies subsection, codes 93875–93990.

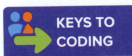

Roger Kennedy, a 63-year-old male, was sent to the Diagnostic Imaging Center by Dr. Yanksey to have an ophthalmic biometry by ultrasound echography, A-scan. After the exam, Dr. Notter, the radiologist, wrote in his report that a second test using intra-ocular lens power calculation might be necessary to further clarify the condition of the eye. Dr. Yanksey determined that Roger should wait before having the second test.

You Code It!

Go through the steps and determine the codes that should be reported for the service provided to Roger Kennedy by Dr. Notter.

Step 1: Read the case completely.

Step 2: Abstract the notes: Which key words can you identify relating to the procedures performed?

_____

Step 3: Query the provider, if necessary.

Step 4: Diagnosis: Abnormality in eye.

Step 5: Code the procedure(s).

_____

Step 6: Link the procedure codes to at least one diagnosis code.

Step 7: Back code to double-check your choices.

Answer:

Did you determine the correct code?

76516 Ophthalmic biometry by ultrasound echography, A-scan

Good job!

Mammography

Until researchers can find a way to prevent breast cancer, the best weapon in the health care arsenal is early detection—finding the malignancy when it is tiny and easier to eradicate. Mammography, low-dose radiology, is considered the best method for identifying a small, otherwise undetectable lump or microcalcification.

77055 Mammography; unilateral

77056 Mammography; bilateral

77057 Screening mammography, bilateral (2-view film study of each breast)

At times, computer-aided detection (CAD) is used in conjunction with the x-ray imaging. CAD transitions the x-ray image into a digital image, which is then scanned by a computer, searching for anything that might be abnormal. This will require another code in addition to the code for the screening or diagnostic mammogram x-ray:

+77051 Computer-aided detection (computer algorithm analysis of digital image data for lesion detection) with further

physician review for interpretation, with or without digitization of film radiographic images; diagnostic mammography

+77052 Computer-aided detection (computer algorithm analysis of digital image data for lesion detection) with further physician review for interpretation, with or without digitization of film radiographic images; screening mammography

Bone and Joint Studies

There are many reasons a physician may need information about a patient's bone structure and strength and many imaging techniques to provide the most accurate data.

- Bone age studies enable the physician to identify the degree of maturation of a child's bones.
- CT scanography has surpassed orthoroentgenogram in the last decade to determine leg length discrepancies.
- Osseous survey is a radiologic procedure used to identify fractures, tumors, and degenerative conditions of the bone.
- Bone mineral density (BMD) scanning, also called dual-energy x-ray absorptiometry (DXA or DEXA) or bone densitometry, is an enhanced form of x-ray technology that is used to measure bone loss.

LO 9.5 Radiation Oncology

radiation
The high-speed discharge and projection of energy waves or particles.

Radiation oncology is performed to treat malignant neoplasms and other carcinomas, commonly known as cancer.

The codes in this subsection already include certain services:

- Initial consultation.
- Clinical treatment planning.
- Simulation.
- Medical radiation physics.
- Dosimetry (the determination of the correct dosage).
- Treatment devices.
- Special services.
- Clinical treatment management procedures.
- Normal follow-up care during treatment and for 3 months following the completion of the treatment.

Radiation oncology services may be provided in varying degrees of intensity and are usually determined in the planning process. Therefore, the preparation for the sequence of treatments must be coded accurately. Some professionals may describe the planning as simple, intermediate, or complex. However, others may provide the detail, leaving you to match the components performed with the level of service. Here are the specifics involved in each level:

- *Simple planning* involves one treatment area with one port, or parallel opposed ports, with simple or no blocking.
- *Intermediate planning* involves two separate treatment areas, three or more converging ports, multiple blocks, or special time–dose constraints.
- *Complex planning* involves three or more separate treatment areas, highly complex blocking, custom shielding blocks, tangential ports, special wedges or compensators, rotational or special beam consideration, or a combination of therapeutic methods.

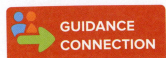

GUIDANCE CONNECTION

Additional explanation can be found in the guidelines within the **Radiology** section, directly under the subhead **Radiation Oncology**, in your CPT book.

Just to keep you on your toes, you will find the same terms (*simple, intermediate, complex*) also used to describe the simulation applied, with different definitions. The good news is that the same terms relate to the same elements involved in the process. With simulation, there is one additional descriptor:

- *Simple simulation:* a single treatment area with either a single port or parallel opposed ports. Simple or no blocking.
- *Intermediate simulation:* of three or more converging ports, two separate treatment areas, multiple blocks.
- *Complex simulation:* of tangential portals, three or more treatment areas, rotation or arc therapy, complex blocking, custom shielding blocks, brachytherapy source verification, hyperthermia probe verification, any use of contrast materials.
- *Three-dimensional computer-generated:* reconstruction of the size and mass of the tumor and the normal tissues that surround the tumor site.

If you work in a facility that provides proton beam treatments and/or clinical brachytherapy for patients, you will note that the CPT book has different definitions for the same three terms: simple, intermediate, and complex.

KEYS TO CODING

Interventional radiologic services, such as radiation oncology, are typically provided in a series over a span of time. Make certain to code dates of service accurately.

LO 9.6 Nuclear Medicine

Nuclear medicine uses tiny quantities of radioactive material, also known as tracers, in conjunction with a scintillation or gamma camera to record the emissions from the tracers to create an image of the anatomical site. Several types of nuclear medicine are tests used to identify a health concern:

nuclear medicine
Treatment that includes the injection or digestion of isotopes.

- Bone scans are used to investigate injuries (fractures, sprains, and strains) as well as tumors.
- Thyroid uptake scans are used to assess thyroid function and record the structure of the gland.
- Heart scans are used to measure heart function, evaluate the existence and extent of heart muscle damage after a heart attack, and gauge the blood flow to the heart muscle.
- Lung scans are used to determine the presence of blood clots. In addition, scans can be valuable to calculate the flow of air into and out of the lungs.
- Hepatobiliary scans can provide information to evaluate the function of the liver and the gallbladder.
- Gallium scans can be used to identify the presence of infection and some types of tumors.

In addition to the diagnostic benefits of nuclear medicine, this methodology can also be used therapeutically to treat hyperthyroidism and thyroid cancer and to help to correct blood imbalances.

One important point that you have to know as a coding specialist working with nuclear medicine procedures is that the codes presented in the CPT book do not include diagnostic or therapeutic radiopharmaceuticals (the drugs or isotopes used in the treatments). Therefore, you have to code them separately. If the insurance carrier accepts HCPCS Level II codes, you will use them. You will learn all about HCPCS Level II codes in Part 2 of this textbook.

Radiopharmaceutical therapy, the administration of nuclear drugs, whether given to the patient orally, intravenously, intracavitarily, interstitially, or intra-arterially, are reported with codes 79005–79999.

Also note that any chemical pathology or chemical analysis done in connection with the provision of nuclear medicine treatments should be coded separately from the Pathology and Laboratory section of the CPT book.

Florence Spevack, a 37-year-old female, had gained a great deal of weight recently, with no change in her diet or exercise regimen. After a thorough examination, Dr. Sundance ordered nuclear imaging of her thyroid, with uptake. Radiopharmaceuticals were administered intravenously. The report came back to Dr. Sundance with the multiple determinations of Florence's exam.

You Code It!

Go through the steps of coding and determine the radiology code or codes that should be reported for this encounter between Dr. Sundance and Florence Spevack.

Step 1: Read the case completely.

Step 2: Abstract the notes: Which key words can you identify relating to the procedures performed?

_____

Step 3: Query the provider, if necessary.

Step 4: Diagnosis: Unexplained weight gain.

Step 5: Code the procedure(s).

_____

Step 6: Link the procedure codes to at least one diagnosis code.

Step 7: Back code to double-check your choices.

Answer:

Did you determine the correct code?

78014 Thyroid imaging (including vascular flow, when performed; with single or multiple quantitative measurement(s) (including stimulation, suppression, or discharge, when performed)

Great job!

Chapter Summary

Health care technology has advanced tremendously in the area of radiology and imaging. It is important that, as a coding specialist, you understand the differences among the types of radiologic methods, as well as the components of each. Procedures with contrast and without contrast, CT scans, MRIs, sonograms, and so many more enable professionals to look inside the patient in a noninvasive manner, and it is your job to obtain the correct reimbursement for every procedure.

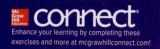

Using Terminology

Match each key term to the appropriate definition.

_____ **1.** LO 9.4 The imaging of a vein after the injection of contrast material.

_____ **2.** LO 9.1 The use of sound waves to record images of internal organs and tissues; also called an *ultrasound.*

_____ **3.** LO 9.4 The imaging of blood vessels after the injection of contrast material.

_____ **4.** LO 9.3 A piece of equipment that emits x-rays through a part of the patient's body onto a fluorescent screen, causing the image to identify various aspects of the anatomy by density.

_____ **5.** LO 9.3 A three-dimensional radiologic technique that uses nuclear technology to record pictures of internal anatomical sites.

_____ **6.** LO 9.3 A specialized computer scanner with very fine detail that records imaging of internal anatomical sites; also known as computerized axial tomography (CAT).

_____ **7.** LO 9.5 The high-speed discharge and projection of energy waves or particles.

_____ **8.** LO 9.3 The recording of a picture of an anatomical joint after the administration of contrast material into the joint capsule.

_____ **9.** LO 9.6 Treatment that includes the injection or digestion of isotopes.

_____ **10.** LO 9.3 MR imaging of an anatomical joint after the administration of contrast material into the joint capsule.

_____ **11.** LO 9.3 A CT scan using contrast materials to visualize arteries and veins all over the body.

A. Angiography

B. Arthrography

C. Computed tomography (CT)

D. Computed tomography angiography (CTA)

E. Fluoroscope

F. Magnetic resonance arthrography (MRA)

G. Magnetic resonance imaging (MRI)

H. Nuclear medicine

I. Radiation

J. Sonogram

K. Venography

Checking Your Understanding

Choose the most appropriate answer for each of the following questions.

1. LO 9.1 The professional components of radiologic services include

   a. repair of the equipment.

   b. interpretation of the imaging.

   c. supplies.

   d. training.

2. LO 9.2/9.4/9.5 Interventional radiologic services are provided with the intent of all *except*

   a. diagnosing a condition.

   b. preventing the spread of a disease.

   c. measuring the progress of a disease.

   d. testing the equipment.

3. LO 9.1 Sonograms use _____ to record images.

   a. nuclear isotopes.
   b. radiation.
   c. 3-D contrast reflection.
   d. sound waves.

4. LO 9.3 The phrase "with contrast" means that the technician or radiologist

   a. administered a substance to enhance the image.
   b. used a black background behind the patient.
   c. took the image a second time, to compare to the first.
   d. used a blue background beneath the patient.

5. LO 9.2 If the code description includes the phrase "two views" and the radiology reports show that only one view was taken, you should code the service

   a. with that code alone.
   b. with that code plus the modifier 52.
   c. with that code plus the modifier 53.
   d. with that code plus the modifier 22.

6. LO 9.4 Angiography is the imaging of

   a. bone.
   b. internal organs.
   c. blood vessels.
   d. an anatomical joint.

7. LO 9.2 RPO stands for

   a. right procedure operation.
   b. regional protocol obstetric.
   c. right posterior oblique.
   d. right preventive oblique.

8. LO 9.5 Radiation for the treatment of a malignant neoplasm is most often used for

   a. diagnostic purposes.
   b. therapeutic purposes.
   c. research purposes.
   d. prevention purposes.

9. LO 9.2/9.3 An x-ray is the same as

   a. a CTA.
   b. a CT.
   c. an MRI.
   d. none of these.

10. LO 9.3 MRI stands for

   a. magnetic radiologic image.
   b. medical reduction imaging.
   c. magnetic resonance imaging.
   d. master radiologic imagery.

Applying Your Knowledge

1. LO 9.1 Differentiate between technical components and professional components. _____
_____

2. LO 9.1 What modifier identifies the professional component? _____
_____

3. LO 9.1 What is a sonogram, and what is another term for it? _____
_____

4. LO 9.2 What is the difference between a screening image and a diagnostic image? Why is it important for the professional coder to know the difference? _____
_____

5. LO 9.2 When a screen test turns into a diagnostic test, what service(s) should be reported? _____
_____

6. LO 9.3 What does the phrase "with contrast" mean? _____
_____

7. LO 9.4 What is the difference between an angiography and a venography? _____
_____

8. LO 9.5 What is radiation oncology? What do the codes in this subsection already include? _____
_____

9. LO 9.6 What is nuclear medicine? _____
_____

10. LO 9.6 What are the types of nuclear medicine tests that are used to identify a health concern? _____
_____

Using the techniques described in this chapter, carefully read through the case studies and determine the most accurate radiology CPT code(s) and modifier(s), if appropriate, for each case study.

1. Jonelle Graybar, a 37-year-old female, is pregnant for the first time and is approximately 12 weeks' gestation. She is brought into the diagnostic center for a fetal biophysical profile with nonstress testing.

   _____

2. Max Wellington, a 15-year-old male, is brought into Dr. Eller's office with severe right leg pain. Dr. Eller takes x-rays of his right femur, AP and PA, to determine whether Max's leg is fractured.

   _____

3. Brandy Sorenna, a 75-year-old female, was brought into Dr. Appleton's office by her daughter because Brandy was complaining of a sharp pain in her chest. After a negative EKG, Dr. Appleton had a quantitative differential pulmonary function study taken, which confirmed a pulmonary embolism. Brandy was taken immediately by ambulance to the hospital. Code the quantitative differential pulmonary perfusion and ventilation study only.

   _____

4. Dr. Zeigleman saw Vernon Unger, a 31-year-old male, with a swollen right eye and loss of vision. Dr. Zeigleman ordered a CT with contrast of the right eye and area, which revealed marked proptosis of the right orbit, thrombosis, and enlargement of the right superior ophthalmic vein.

   _____

5. Xavier Pollack, a 51-year-old male, was diagnosed with intrinsic laryngeal cancer, supraglottic T1 tumor. With the tumor confined to one subsite in the supraglottis, Dr. Westerman provided radiation treatment delivery, with a single port, simple block, of 4.5 MeV.

   _____

6. Carol-Ann Springer, a 22-year-old female, came into the Diagnostic Imaging Center for her annual screening mammogram. Due to her family history of malignant neoplasms of the breast (both her mother and sister have been diagnosed), the mammogram was ordered with computer-aided detection (CAD).

   _____

7. Conrad Michaelson, a 29-year-old male, is brought into Dr. Culverwell's office with sharp pains in his lower right abdomen, shooting across to the left side. Dr. Culverwell ordered some blood work and an MRA to confirm the suspected diagnosis of acute appendicitis. Code the MRA.

_____

8. Alden Roberts, a 33-year-old male, was in training at Cape Canaveral when he hit his head in a weightlessness simulator, causing him to lose consciousness for 3 minutes. Alden was transported to the local hospital where Dr. Astrone, the ED on-call physician, took a skull x-ray, three views, and did an MRI without contrast of Alden's brain.

_____

9. Olivia Kane, a 61-year-old female, was experiencing pain in her back that radiated around her trunk. She was also suffering with spastic muscle weakness. Dr. Neumours ordered a radioisotope bone scan of Olivia's lumbar spinal area. The scan identified a metastatic invasion of L1–L3.

_____

10. Olivia Kane, newly diagnosed with metastatic lumbar spinal tumors, has been referred to Dr. Duncan for the creation of a simple radiation therapy plan.

_____

11. Jason Miolo had been diagnosed with a malignancy and came today for intravenous radiopharmaceutical therapy.

_____

12. Before beginning a series of treatments, Brianna Logan came to the Diagnostic Imaging Center for a metabolic evaluation PET scan of her brain.

_____

13. Carl Gadsden, a 13-month-old male, was brought to radiology for a real-time, limited, static ultrasound of his hips.

_____

14. Miriam Lightfoot, a 55-year-old female, arrived at the Barton Imaging Center to have a SPECT (single photon emission computed tomography) performed on her left kidney.

_____

15. Dr. Morrison performed a complete ultrasound evaluation of Eliot Shapin's pelvis. The procedure included evaluation and measurement of Eliot's urinary bladder, evaluation of his prostate and seminal vesicles, and pathology of his enlarged prostate.

_____

The following exercises provide practice in the application of abstracting the physicians' notes and learning to work with SOAP notes from our health care facility, Cipher, Victors & Associates. These case studies (SOAP notes) are modeled on real patient encounters. Using the techniques described in this chapter, carefully read through the case studies and determine the most accurate radiology CPT code(s) and modifier(s), if appropriate, for each case study. You are coding for the radiologist.

CIPHER, VICTORS & ASSOCIATES
A Complete Health Care Facility
234 MAIN STREET • ANYTOWN, FL 32711 • 407-555-1234

PATIENT:	HENLEY, VANESSA
ACCOUNT/EHR #:	HENLVA001
DATE:	09/17/18

Procedure Performed:	X-rays, front/lat, chest
	X-rays, AP, shoulder
	C-spine AP/lat
	MRI, shoulder joint

Radiologist:	Keith Robbins, MD
Referring Physician:	James I. Cipher, MD

INDICATIONS: R/O torn ligament, shoulder after MVA

IMPRESSIONS: X-rays of all areas are unremarkable
C-spine, negative for fracture or trauma
MRI indicates a torn coracohumeral ligament, right side.

Keith Robbins, MD

KR/mg   D: 09/17/18 09:50:16 T: 09/20/18 12:55:01

Determine the most accurate radiology CPT code(s) and modifier(s), if appropriate.

_____

_____

_____

CIPHER, VICTORS & ASSOCIATES
A Complete Health Care Facility
234 MAIN STREET • ANYTOWN, FL 32711 • 407-555-1234

PATIENT: PANUCCI, JOEL
ACCOUNT/EHR #:   PANUJO001
DATE: 10/01/18

Procedure Performed: X-rays, skull, two views
                                 CT, soft tissue of neck, with contrast
                                 MRI, brain stem

Radiologist: Keith Robbins, MD
Referring Physician: Valerie R. Victors, MD

INDICATIONS: Concussion, after fall from ladder

IMPRESSIONS: X-rays negative for fracture
                                 CT negative
                                 MRI indicates subdural hematoma.

Keith Robbins, MD

KR/mg   D: 10/01/18 09:50:16   T: 10/02/18 12:55:01

Determine the most accurate radiology CPT code(s) and modifier(s), if appropriate.

_____

_____

_____

CIPHER, VICTORS & ASSOCIATES
A Complete Health Care Facility
234 MAIN STREET • ANYTOWN, FL 32711 • 407-555-1234

PATIENT: WESTON, AMY
ACCOUNT/EHR #:   WESTAM001
DATE: 10/17/18

Procedure Performed: Screening mammogram, bilateral, two views each breast

Radiologist: Keith Robbins, MD
Referring Physician: Valerie R. Victors, MD

INDICATIONS: Routine annual assessment

IMPRESSIONS: Mammogram unremarkable

Keith Robbins, MD

KR/mg   D: 10/17/18 09:50:16   T: 10/20/18 12:55:01

Determine the most accurate radiology CPT code(s) and modifier(s), if appropriate.

_____

_____

_____

CIPHER, VICTORS & ASSOCIATES
A Complete Health Care Facility
234 MAIN STREET • ANYTOWN, FL 32711 • 407-555-1234

PATIENT: APPLETON, KYLE

ACCOUNT/EHR #:   APPLKY001

DATE: 11/05/18

Procedure Performed: Radiation treatment delivery

Radiologist: Keith Robbins, MD

Referring Physician: James I. Cipher, MD

INDICATIONS: Kaposi's sarcoma, extracutaneous, lungs, and GI tract (esophagus)

IMPRESSIONS: 15 MEV, two separate treatment areas

___

Keith Robbins, MD

KR/mg   D: 11/05/18 09:50:16   T: 11/07/18 12:55:01

Determine the most accurate radiology CPT code(s) and modifier(s), if appropriate.

___

___

___

CIPHER, VICTORS & ASSOCIATES
A Complete Health Care Facility
234 MAIN STREET • ANYTOWN, FL 32711 • 407-555-1234

PATIENT: HAWTHORNE, RAUL
ACCOUNT/EHR #:   HAWTRA001
DATE: 09/29/18

Procedure Performed: CT angiography of the head, without contrast and with contrast

Radiologist: Keith Robbins, MD
Referring Physician: James I. Cipher, MD

INDICATIONS: Left CVA

IMPRESSIONS:
The current study is compared with the previous one of 09-25-12.
    Compared with the previous study, there is a focal area of hypodensity present in the right posterior cerebral arterial distribution adjacent to the falx, a finding suspicious for a small acute infarction, nonhemorrhagic, most likely the parieto-occipital branch.
    No other abnormality detected. There are no intra- or extra-axial hemorrhages. There is no significant midline shift or hydrocephalus.
    Small new area as described above is suspicious for an area of acute infarction in the right posterior cerebral arterial distribution, likely the occipital branch. Please clinically correlate.

Keith Robbins, MD

KR/mg   D: 09/29/18 09:50:16   T: 09/30/18 12:55:01

Determine the most accurate radiology CPT code(s) and modifier(s), if appropriate.

_____

_____

_____

PATHOLOGY AND LABORATORY CODING

10

Learning Outcomes *After completing this chapter, the student should be able to:*

LO 10.1 Translate the guidelines for accurately coding clinical chemistry procedures.

LO 10.2 Apply the in-section guidelines regarding molecular diagnostic testing.

LO 10.3 Correctly apply guidelines for reporting hematology and coagulation tests.

LO 10.4 Discern cytopathology and cytogenetic studies.

LO 10.5 Interpret the guidelines for accurately coding surgical pathology.

LO 10.6 Determine how and when to use modifiers.

As physicians and health care professionals work to help their patients, very often they need medical science to guide them. The guidance frequently comes from tests performed by professionals working in a **laboratory,** studying the evolution of a patient's disease. Such study is called **pathology,** which includes **etiology.**

Pathology and lab testing help detect the early presence of disease, ruling out or confirming conditions that might have similar symptoms yet need to be treated differently, and predict the occurrence of disease in the future. You probably already know from your own experiences the importance of such work. Your annual physical has possibly included blood tests to measure your cholesterol. Physicians order blood work to confirm pregnancy or a urinalysis to determine if a symptom could be the result of an infection. Testing takes time and the expertise of professionals educated in interpreting the results. It also takes materials and resources.

As a coding specialist, you may work for a health care organization that has a laboratory within its facilities, a billing company that codes everything, or an independent facility that does nothing other than taking and analyzing the **specimen.** In any case, you should understand the different aspects of pathology and lab testing and procedures, as well as the guidelines involved in coding the services.

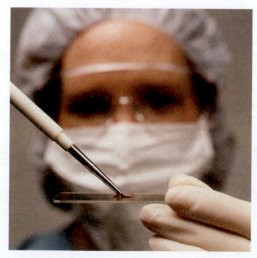

© Don Farrall/Getty Images

Key Terms

Cytology

Etiology

Gross examination

Laboratory

Microscopic examination

Pathology

Qualitative

Quantitative

Specimen

Surgical pathology

```
                              LIPID PROFILE
-----------------------------------------------------------------------------
Day                          2
Date                  05/16/05
Time                     0610                          Reference          U
-----------------------------------------------------------------------------
    CHOLESTEROL              166                        (140-200)          M
    TRIGLYCERIDE             104                        (35-160)           M
    HDL                       83                        (35-85)            M
    LDL (CALC)                63(a)                     (60-129)           M
    VLDL (CALC)               20                        (5-40)             M
    CHOL/HDL RATIO           2.0(b)                                        R


    NOTES:   (a)   LDL GOAL:
                   <100 FOR PATIENTS WITH CHD, DM OR VASCULAR DISEASE.
             (b)   LOWEST CHD RISK
```

FIGURE 10-1 Sample Lab Report

laboratory
A location with scientific equipment designed to perform experiments and tests.

pathology
The study of the nature, etiology, development, and outcomes of disease.

etiology
The study of the causes of disease.

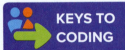

KEYS TO CODING

When you code pathology and laboratory work, you may code for the professional in charge of performing the test and interpreting the results or the facility that provided the testing.

specimen
A small part or sample of any substance obtained for analysis and diagnosis.

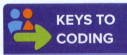

KEYS TO CODING

Remember that the codes for testing a specimen do not include collecting the specimen. Collection, such as performing a biopsy, venipuncture, or fine-needle aspiration, is coded separately by the coder for the professional who performed the collection.

The specimen sent to the lab for testing may be from any number of different sources: patients' blood, urine, or other bodily fluids; tissue; or an organ.

Panels

When you turn to the Pathology and Laboratory section of the CPT book, you will notice that many codes include a long list of elements within the code's description. These groupings of tests commonly performed at the same time are called *panels*.

EXAMPLE

80051 Electrolyte panel

This panel must include the following: Carbon dioxide (82374); Chloride (82435); Potassium (84132); and Sodium (84295)

The example shows you that, in order for code 80051 to be the most accurate code, the lab must have performed all four tests: carbon dioxide, chloride, potassium, and sodium.

If the lab performs fewer than *all* the tests listed in a panel, you must code the tests separately; you are *not* permitted to use the panel code.

You may find a report, such as the one shown in Figure 10-1, that itemizes the tests performed for the patient along with the results of each test.

Again, the CPT book will help you. Should you have to code any of the tests separately, each test code is given in parentheses right next to the name of the test listed there. From our example, next to carbon dioxide, you will notice the number 82374. Turn to code 82374, and you will see that it is the code for testing carbon dioxide alone.

Let's say, instead of fewer tests than those listed in a panel, the lab performs more. The guidelines state that you are to report those additional tests not included in the panel code separately and additionally.

LET'S CODE IT! SCENARIO

Concerned that Anna Donner, a 43-year-old female, might be suffering from hypercholesterolemia, Dr. Raider ordered some blood work, including a total cholesterol serum test, lipoprotein (direct measurement of high-density lipoprotein), and triglycerides. He also added a potassium serum test to the order.

The lab performed four tests: *total cholesterol serum test, lipoprotein (direct measurement of high-density lipoprotein), triglycerides,* and *potassium serum.* When you look up the tests individually, you are directed to codes for each. However, when it comes to pathology and laboratory coding, you must take an extra step. Turn to the numerical listings to the beginning of the Pathology and Laboratory section, where you find the standardized panels listed. Review the list of tests included in each of the panels, and match it with the list of tests Dr. Raider ordered. You see that code 80061 Lipid Panel includes three of the four tests performed. Since none of the panels includes all four tests, you use the lipid panel code and code the potassium test additionally, code 84132.

> **84132 Potassium; serum, plasma, or whole blood**

Therefore, you have two codes for the lab work's claim: 80061, 84132. Good job!

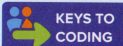

KEYS TO CODING

When all the included tests of a panel are performed, you must use the panel code. Coding the tests individually is considered unbundling. You will remember from Chap. 1 that unbundling is unethical and illegal. If fewer tests are performed, using a panel code with the modifier 52 Reduced Services is *not* permitted. You must code the tests individually.

Testing Methodology and Sources

Although no one expects you, as the coding specialist, to be completely knowledgeable about the details of laboratory and pathologic testing, you will need certain information regarding the performance of the tests in order to code them correctly. This may begin with exactly what is being tested, going beyond just the name of the test itself.

One aspect of the testing performed will be identifying if the test is **quantitative** or **qualitative.**

GUIDANCE CONNECTION

Additional explanation can be found in the guidelines within the **Pathology and Laboratory** section, directly under the subhead **Organ or Disease-Oriented Panels,** in your CPT book.

EXAMPLE

> 82355 Calculus; qualitative analysis
> 82360   quantitative analysis, chemical

quantitative
The counting or measurement of something.

qualitative
The determination of character or essential element(s).

The guidelines tell you that, if the documentation does not specify, you may assume that the examination performed was quantitative. However, remember that documentation is absolute in the health care industry. Therefore, it is recommended that you query the lab technician or pathologist and request that the paperwork include this important detail.

All the details regarding the specimen and the testing are important. There are times when the code descriptions include the type of test, the type of specimen, or both.

Let's look back at Anna Donner's cholesterol test. Go to the alphabetic index and look up *cholesterol.*

EXAMPLE

> **Cholesterol**
> Measurement   83721
> Serum   82465
> Testing   83718–83719

KEYS TO CODING

Experience and practice will help you learn the elements easily. After working at a lab or for a facility with a lab, you will recognize the lab tests that are typically performed together and possibly have a panel code grouping them. Should a test not be in a panel, the alphabetic index will direct you to the correct individual code for that test.

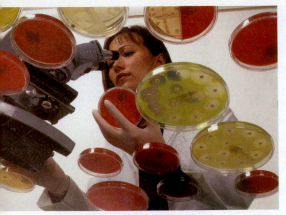

You can see that the fact that Dr. Raider ordered a total cholesterol *serum* test makes a difference in which code is best. In addition, *cholesterol, serum* (82465) is the test included in the lipid panel code we used for reporting Anna's tests. If Dr. Raider had ordered a cholesterol *measurement* test instead of the serum test, you would not be able to use the 80061 lipid panel test code. Then, you would have to code each of Anna's tests separately. Our example highlights the importance of reading the details of the testing beyond the element or category.

In addition to how the test is performed, you must also know the type of specimen involved in the testing and, sometimes, how many specimens or sources are involved. First, the type of specimen being tested may change the code. Let's look again at Anna Donner's case, specifically at her potassium test. Let's go to the alphabetic index for *potassium*.

EXAMPLE

Potassium	84132
Urine	84133

The first code in the example, listed next to the word *potassium,* is code 84132, but it does not contain any additional descriptors. However, the second code, listed under potassium, indicates that it would be the code used if the potassium were tested from Anna's urine rather than her blood (serum). When you look at the codes' complete descriptions in the numerical listing, you see the details shown.

EXAMPLE

84132	Potassium; serum, plasma, or whole blood
84133	urine

The listings clearly show that there is a difference in which code is correct based on the source of the specimen.

In certain circumstances, an analysis may be performed on multiple specimens collected at different times or from different sources. In such cases, the guidelines tell you to code each source and each specimen separately. However, be certain to always read the code descriptions carefully. Some codes already include multiple tests and/or multiple sources.

LET'S CODE IT! SCENARIO

Marlene Saunders, RN, performs a rapid influenza test using a commercial test kit in the office to determine if Jess Burns has the virus so that results can be provided while Jess is still in with Dr. Chipton. When complete, Nurse Saunders visually reads the result as positive.

Let's Code It!

For this scenario, you are going to focus only on reporting the provision of the rapid influenza test. The first place you look in the CPT alphabetic index is under the word *Test.* However, there is nothing there, so let's look up the term *Influenza.* There are several choices. Let's analyze them.

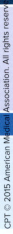

The first two choices are titled *Influenza A* and *Influenza B*. There is nothing in the notes about which this might be. Before querying the nurse or doctor, let's keep reading.

The next listing is *Influenza Vaccine*. There is nothing in the notes stating that Jess was given a vaccination, so this is not applicable to this encounter.

The last listing category is titled *Influenza Virus*. This could be possible because the notes state the test was given to "determine if Jess Burns has the virus." Two codes are suggested here:

Antibody...86710

By Immunoassay, with direct optical observation.....87804

Let's turn to the main portion of CPT, look for these two possible codes in the Pathology and Laboratory section, and read the complete code descriptions.

86710 Antibody; influenza virus

87804 Infectious agent antigen detection by immunoassay with direct optical observation; influenza

When you read the scenario and the complete code description, you can see how code 87804 matches accurately.

LO 10.1 Clinical Chemistry

The lab tests that are most commonly performed use chemical processes to distinguish qualities and quantities of elements in the specimens provided. Typically, the specimens are samples of a patient's blood or urine. Tests with which you might be familiar include the following:

- *Blood glucose* (sugar) is used to diagnose conditions such as diabetes mellitus (hyperglycemia) or hypoglycemia.
- *Electrolytes* are used to diagnose metabolic or kidney disorders.
- *Enzymes* can be released into the bloodstream by a damaged or diseased organ. The presence of creatine kinase can indicate damage after a heart attack, or amylase and lipase elevations may be a sign of cancer of the pancreas and/or pancreatitis.
- *Hormones,* such as cortisol, in quantities too high or too low might indicate the malfunction of the patient's adrenal glands.
- *Lipids* (fatty substances) can signal coronary heart disease or liver disease.
- *Metabolic substances,* such as uric acid, at incorrect levels can identify the presence of gout.
- *Proteins* identified at the wrong levels on electrophoresis can point to malnutrition or certain infections.

Many tests can be easily performed in the physician's office with a small amount of blood or urine. Companies have created kits that make measuring such elements as simple as dipping a little slip of special paper into the patient's specimen. It means that you have a much greater opportunity to code any number of tests.

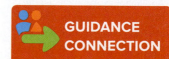

GUIDANCE CONNECTION

Additional explanation can be found in the guidelines within the **Pathology and Laboratory** section, directly under the subhead **Chemistry,** in your CPT book.

YOU CODE IT! CASE STUDY

Jeffrey Farthington, a 27-year-old male, is an up-and-coming stockbroker who does not pay much attention to a proper diet. He came to see his physician, Dr. Stanley, because he has been experiencing episodes of light-headedness. Dr. Stanley asks his assistant, Marlene Fleet, to do a quantitative blood glucose test using a reagent strip. Marlene takes a capillary stick (on Jeff's fingertip), goes to the back, and checks the specimen. The results indicate that Jeff has hypoglycemia.

You Code It!

Go through the steps and determine the pathology/lab code(s) that should be reported for this encounter.

Step 1: Read the case completely.

Step 2: Abstract the notes: Which key words can you identify relating to the procedures performed?

_____

Step 3: Query the provider, if necessary.

Step 4: Diagnosis: Hypoglycemia.

Step 5: Code the procedure(s).

_____

Step 6: Link the procedure codes to at least one diagnosis code.

Step 7: Back code to double-check your choices.

Answer:

Did you determine the correct code?

82948 Glucose; blood, reagent strip

Good work!

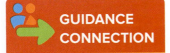

GUIDANCE CONNECTION

Additional explanation can be found in the guidelines within the **Pathology and Laboratory** section, **Molecular Pathology** in your CPT book.

LO 10.2 Molecular Diagnostics

Molecular diagnostic tests investigate infectious disease, oncology concerns (malignant neoplasms), hematology (the study of blood and its disorders), neurology, and inherited disorders (genetics).

For genetics tests, you must include the appropriate modifier from the special list of genetic testing code modifiers found in Appendix I. These modifiers are to be used with both CPT and HCPCS Level II codes, as appropriate, to specify the probe type or the condition being tested. By using special modifiers, more detailed information can be gathered for statistical and other important data without requiring the rewriting of any of the existing code descriptions. The genetic testing code modifiers consist of two characters: the first a number (0 through 9) and the second a letter (A through Z).

YOU CODE IT! CASE STUDY

Marcus Angelli, a 3-year-old male, has a cousin who was diagnosed with cystic fibrosis last year. Recently, he has been wheezing and has a dry, nonproductive cough. The fact that his cousin has cystic fibrosis means that Marcus has a 25% chance of carrying the disease. Therefore, Dr. Cauldwell ordered a molecular diagnostic test for the mutation of delta F 508 deletion in his DNA by sequencing, single segment.

Go through the steps and determine the pathology/lab code(s) that should be reported for this encounter.

Step 1:   Read the case completely.

Step 2:   Abstract the notes: Which key words can you identify relating to the procedures performed?

_____

Step 3:   Query the provider, if necessary.

Step 4:   Diagnosis: Family history of cystic fibrosis.

Step 5:   Code the procedure(s).

_____

Step 6:   Link the procedure codes to at least one diagnosis code.

Step 7:   Back code to double-check your choices.

Answer:

Did you determine the correct code?

81220 CFTR (cystic fibrosis transmembrane conductance regulator) (e.g., cystic fibrosis) gene analysis; common variants (e.g., ACMG/ACOG guidelines)

Good job!

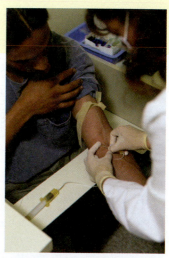

© Photodisc/Getty Images

LO 10.3   Hematology and Coagulation

The study of blood and its disorders is called *hematology*. Hematologic tests can help diagnose such conditions and diseases as anemia, hemophilia, and leukemia. Very often, these tests are referred to by their initials, so let's go over the most common tests and their acronyms:

- CBC = Complete blood count, which includes the following tests.
- WBC = White blood cell count.
- RBC = Red blood cell count.
- PLT = Platelet count, which is used to diagnose or monitor bleeding and clotting disorders.
- HCT = Hematocrit.
- HGB = Hemoglobin concentration, which is the concentration of the oxygen-carrying pigment in red blood cells.
- DIFF = Differential blood count.

In addition, one other test is used frequently:

- PT = Prothrombin time, which is used to evaluate bleeding and clotting disorders.

Abbreviations for pathology and laboratory tests are used in reports from labs all over the country. Some of the most common are shown in Table 10-1.

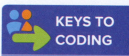

KEYS TO CODING

Remember that the CBC includes the WBC, RBC, HCT, HGB, platelet count, and differential count. Therefore, you are not to code those tests separately.

TABLE 10-1 Abbreviations and Acronyms for Most Common Diagnostic and Laboratory Tests

ABG	Arterial blood gases	DIC	Disseminated intra-vascular coagulation	NEUT	Neutrophils
ACE	Angiotensin-converting enzyme	DIFF	Differential	PAP	Prostatic acid phosphatase
ACT	Activated clotting time	EIA	Enzyme immunoassay	PH	Hydrogen ion concentration
AFP	Fetoprotein	EOS	Eosinophil count	PLT	Platelet
A/G	Albumin/globulin ratio	ESR	Erythrocyte sedimentation rate	PSA	Prostate-specific antigen
AIT	Agglutination inhibition test	FBS	Fasting blood sugar	PT	Prothrombin time
ALT	Alanine aminotransferase	GTT	Glucose tolerance test	PTT	Partial thromboplastin time
ALP	Alkaline phosphatase	HCT	Hematocrit	RBC	Red blood cells
AMA	Antimitochondrial antibody	HDL	High-density lipoprotein	RDW	Red cell distribution width
ANA	Antinuclear antibody	HGB	Hemoglobin	RF	Rheumatoid factor
APTT	Activated partial thrombo-plastin time	HPF	High-power field	RPR	Rapid plasma reagin test
		INR	International normalization ratio	SEGS	Segmented neutrophils
AST	Aspartate aminotransferase			SGOT	Serum glutamicoxaloacetic transaminase
BMC	Bone mineral content	LD	Lactic dehydrogenase	SGPT	Serum glutamicpyruvic transaminase
BMD	Bone marrow density	LDL	Low-density lipoprotein		
BASO	Basophiles	LFT	Liver function tests	SMA	Sequential multiple analyzer
BST	Blood serologic test	LPF	Low-power field		
BUN	Blood urea nitrogen	LYMPHS	Lymphocytes	SP GRAV	Specific gravity
CBC	Complete blood count	MCH	Mean corpuscular hemoglobin	STS	Serologic test for syphilis
CEA	Carcinoembryonic antigen	MCHC	Mean corpuscular hemo-globin concentration	T&C	Type and crossmatch
CK	Creatine kinase			TSH	Thyroid-stimulating hormone
CMV	Cytomegalovirus	MCV	Mean corpuscular volume	UA	Urinalysis
CO_2	Carbon dioxide	MONO	Monocyte count	WBC	White blood cell
CPK	Creatine phosphokinase	MPV	Mean platelet volume		

Immunology

Immunology is the study of the body's immune system—how it works and what can go wrong. Immunologic tests identify problems that may occur when a disease causes the body's defense system to attack itself (called an *autoimmune disease*) or when a disease causes a malfunction of the body's immune system (called an *immunodeficiency disorder*). The tests can also evaluate the compatibility of tissues and organs for transplantation.

Conditions and diseases that you may be familiar with, which fall into this category, include rheumatoid arthritis, allergies, and, of course, human immunodeficiency virus (HIV).

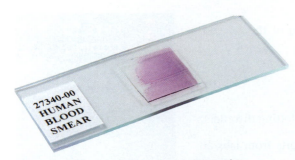

© McGraw-Hill Education/Jacques Cornell photographer

Alfred Manning, a 49-year-old male, was diagnosed with hemophilia many years ago. As a result of a blood transfusion, he contracted HIV. He has come today for lab work to check on his T-cell count, an indicator of whether the HIV is progressing.

Let's Code It!

Alfred is having a test to determine the *count* of *T cells* in his blood. Let's turn to the alphabetic index to the letter *T*. Are you surprised at the many listings with *T cell* in the heading? Read through them all carefully. Remember that Alfred does not have leukemia; he has HIV. Keep going down the list to *T cells*, under which you see *count*, with the suggested code 86359.

The complete code description in the numerical listing shows us

86359 T cells; total count

Good job!

Microbiology

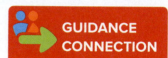

GUIDANCE CONNECTION

Additional explanation can be found in the guidelines within the **Pathology and Laboratory** section, directly under the subhead **Microbiology,** in your CPT book.

Microbiologic tests use many different methods to study bacteria, fungi, parasites, and viruses. The specimens used in the tests might be blood, urine, sputum (mucus, also called *phlegm*), feces (stool), cerebrospinal fluid (CSF), and other bodily fluids. Blood cultures are used to diagnose bacterial infections of the blood, sputum cultures can identify respiratory infections like pneumonia, and stool cultures can confirm the presence of pinworms and other parasites.

Code descriptions in this subsection may include some specific terms, such as

- *Presumptive identification.* This is the pathologic identification of colony morphology; growth on selective media (such as a culture or slide); gram stains; or other tests such as catalase, oxidase, indole, or urease.
  - Example: 87081 Culture, presumptive, pathogenic organisms, screening only.
- *Definitive identification.* This is the pathologic identification of the genus or species that requires additional testing, such as biochemical panels or slide cultures.
  - Example: 87106 Culture, fungi, definitive identification, each organism, yeast.

Veronica Adderson, a 5-year-old female, went to a picnic at the park with her playgroup and had a rare hamburger. Later that evening, her parents rushed her to the hospital because she was vomiting and had severe diarrhea. Dr. Calvinelli ordered an infectious agent antigen enzyme immunoassay for E. coli 0157. Fortunately, the test was negative, and it turned out that she just had eaten too much ice cream and milk.

Let's Code It!

Dr. Calvinelli ordered "an infectious agent antigen enzyme immunoassay" for Veronica to determine if she was suffering from *Escherichia coli (E. coli)*. Let's go to the alphabetic index to *immunoassay* and find *infectious agent* below it, with the suggested codes 86317–86318, 87449–87451. Let's go to the numerical listings and read the complete code descriptions.

> **86317** Immunoassay for infectious agent antibody, quantitative, not otherwise specified (For immunoassay techniques for antigens, see 83516, 83518, 83519, 83520, 87301–87450, 87810–87899.)

The code description states *antibody,* but the notes say *antigen.* Luckily, the CPT book is guiding you via the parenthetical notation below the code description, which directs you to a long list of codes. The descriptions for 83516, 83518, 83519, and 83520 do not come any closer to Dr. Calvinelli's notes. Let's turn to the next set of suggested codes:

> **87301** Infectious agent antigen detection by enzyme immunoassay technique, qualitative or semiquantitative, multiple step method; adenovirus enteric types 40/41

Read down the list a little farther:

> **87335** Escherichia coli 0157

When you read the complete description, you get the following:

> **87335** Infectious agent antigen detection by enzyme immunoassay technique, qualitative or semiquantitative, multiple step method; Escherichia coli 0157

Sometimes, even with the CPT book pointing at codes, it may take a lot of reading to be certain you have the best, most appropriate code.

LO 10.4 Cytopathology and Cytogenetic Studies

cytology
The investigation and identification of cells.

Cytology is the study of one cell at a time to discover abnormal cells present in tissue or bodily fluids. Cytologic testing is used to detect cancer cells and infectious organisms and to screen for fetal abnormalities.

Specimens used in cytopathologic testing are obtained by fine-needle aspirations (as in amniocentesis), scraping of tissue surfaces (as in Pap smears), and collection of bodily fluids (as with sputum or seminal fluid, or sperm).

LET'S CODE IT! SCENARIO

Barbara Rosen, a 51-year-old female, came to see Dr. Farber for her annual well-woman checkup. In addition to the examination, Dr. Farber took a Pap smear, to be examined using the Bethesda reporting system with manual screening. Barbara's examination showed she was completely healthy.

Let's Code It!

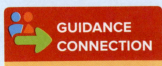

GUIDANCE CONNECTION

Additional explanation can be found in the guidelines within the **Pathology and Laboratory** section, directly above code 88141, in your CPT book.

Dr. Farber took a *smear* of tissue for a cytopathologic examination of Barbara's cervical cells using *the Bethesda system.* Let's go to the alphabetic index to *cytopathology, smears, cervical or vaginal,* with the suggested codes 88141–88167 and 88174–88175. However, in this case, you can also go to *Pap smears* and see the suggested codes 88141–88155, 88164–88167, and 88174–88175. Note that there is a difference: Codes 88160, 88161, and 88162 are not included in the listing under Pap smears. Let's go to the numerical listings and read the complete code descriptions.

Before you begin reading all the code descriptions, read the paragraph of instructions directly before code 88141. You will note that these instructions tell you to

"Use codes 88164–88167 to report Pap smears that are examined using the Bethesda System of reporting." That saves you quite a lot of time. Reading that one small paragraph directs you to the four best codes:

88164 Cytopathology, slides, cervical or vaginal (the Bethesda System); manual screening under physician supervision

88165 Cytopathology, slides, cervical or vaginal (the Bethesda System); with manual screening and rescreening and under physician supervision

88166 Cytopathology, slides, cervical or vaginal (the Bethesda System); with manual screening and computer-assisted rescreening under physician supervision

88167 Cytopathology, slides, cervical or vaginal (the Bethesda System); with manual screening and computer-assisted rescreening using cell selection and review under physician supervision

Which of these four codes most accurately describes the pathology test done for Barbara? No rescreening or computer-assisted rescreening is documented. This means the most accurate code for this test is

88164 Cytopathology, slides, cervical or vaginal (the Bethesda System); manual screening under physician supervision

Great job!

LO 10.5 Surgical Pathology

When a biopsy is taken during a surgical procedure (or is the surgical procedure itself), the specimen is sent to the lab for testing. The testing, typically performed immediately upon receipt from the OR, is called **surgical pathology.** Its purpose, much like that of other testing and studies, is to provide the information necessary to diagnose a disease or condition and to set forth a treatment plan. In such cases, all the steps (taking the specimen, testing, diagnosis, and treatment) may occur during one surgical session. The benefit of this quick and immediate process is that there is less trauma for the patient, who has to undergo anesthesia and an invasive procedure only once. In addition, it saves money for the patient, the facility, and the third-party payer.

Codes 88300–88309 represent six levels of surgical pathologic testing. The codes include accession, the testing itself, and the written report from the pathologist. The codes (with the exception of 88300) also include both **gross examination** (also known as macroscopic examination) of the specimen and **microscopic examination.**

The first level, code 88300, is applicable for any and all specimens that are examined only by visual, or gross, examination. It means that the sample has not been looked at under a microscope.

88300 Level I—Surgical pathology, gross examination only

Codes 88302–88309 recognize the various amounts of work required by the pathologist or physician doing the examination to determine the accurate condition of the specimen. Don't worry—you don't have to study pathology to decide which level to use properly to represent the work done. Each code level is determined by the anatomical site from where the specimen was taken. Under each, the sites are listed in alphabetic order. However, you have to know what happened in the OR to find the correct code because that will change the level involved.

You may find a report, such as the one shown in Figure 10-2, that shows the results of the surgical pathology along with the pathologist's interpretation.

surgical pathology
The study of tissues removed from a living patient during a surgical procedure.

gross examination
The visual study of a specimen (with the naked eye).

microscopic examination
The study of a specimen using a microscope (under magnification).

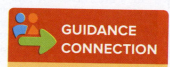
GUIDANCE CONNECTION

Additional explanation can be found in the guidelines within the **Pathology and Laboratory** section, directly under the subhead **Surgical Pathology,** in your CPT book.

HILL MCGRAW PATHOLOGY LABORATORIES INC.
Warren R. Mulford, MD,. Director
123 Learning Way • Academia, FL 12345

PATIENT INFORMATION	PHYSICIAN INFORMATION

Name: NICOLE GABRINI
Sex: Female
D.O.B: 09/07/01
Patient ID: 55899
Patient Phone: 555-456-5555

JOSE MARKETTEN, MD
456 Healing Lane
Suite 505
Academia, FL 12345
555-399-5555

SPECIMEN INFORMATION

COLLECTED: 04/29/16
Reported: 05/01/16
Received: 04/30/16

Accession # IF_16_6971
Other Accession (IC):

PATHOLOGY REPORT

CLINICAL INFORMATION

A. Right upper extremity—Scabies vs Eczema
B. Left lower extremity—Scabies vs Eczema
C. Right lower extremity—Scabies vs Eczema

Terrell Rodriguez, PA-C

SPECIMEN DATA

GROSS DESCRIPTION:
A. The specimen is a punch biopsy received in immunofluorescence transport medium that measures 0.1 × 0.4 × 0.1 cm. The specimen is flash frozen and multiple 4 micron sections are cut for manual immunofluorescence staining. The sections are probed with fluorescein labeled antihuman antibodies against IgG, IgA, IgM, C3, C5b-9, and fibrinogen.

B. Received is a 0.2 cm punch biopsy of skin, submitted complete. The specimen is received in formalin.

C. Received is a 0.2 cm punch biopsy of skin, submitted complete. The specimen is received in formalin.

MICROSCOPIC DESCRIPTION:
All positive and negative controls stained appropriately as required.

RESULTS

DIAGNOSIS:
A. DIRECT IMMUNOFLUORESCENCE, RIGHT UPPER EXTREMITY—NEGATIVE (See Note)
Note: There is no IgG, IgA, IgM, C3, C5b-9, and fibrinogen deposition seen in this specimen. There is no immunofluorescence evidence of connective tissue, vasculitis, dermatitis herpetiformis, porphyria cutanea tarda, pseudoporphyria, or autoimmune blistering disease; however, clinical histologic and, if pertinent, serologic correlation is recommended. Multiple immunoreactant dilutions and sections were performed.

B. PUNCH BIOPSY, LEFT LOWER EXTREMITY—STASIS ECZEMA, TRAUMATIZED AND IMPETIGINIZED
Note: PAS is negative for fungus. Multiple deepersections have been reviewed and no mite or mite elements identified. There is an impetiginized ulcer with bacterial colonization of the stratum corneum containing neutrophils and serum exudate. The papillary dermis contains a capillary proliferation, a few neutrophils, rare eosinophils and dermal cicatrix. These histopathologic features are consistent with traumatized and impetiginized stasis eczema. There is no evidence of scabies.

C. PUNCH BIOPSY, RIGHT LOWER EXTREMITY—STASIS ECZEMA, TRAUMATIZED AND IMPETIGINIZED Note: PAS is negative for fungus. Multiple deeper sections have been reviewed and no mite or mite elements identified. There is an impetiginized ulcer with bacterial colonization of the stratum corneum containing neutrophils and serum exudate. The papillary dermis contains a capillary proliferation, a few neutrophils, rare eosinophils and dermal cicatrix. These histopathologic features are consistent with traumatized and impetiginized stasis eczema. There is no evidence of scabies.

Noah W. Wegner, MD Dermatopathologist (electronic signature)

FINAL REPORT

Figure 10-2 Sample Pathology Report

After the listings for the six levels of surgical pathologic examinations, there are other codes and descriptions for services that may be performed in addition to the gross and microscopic examinations of the specimen. Should any of those services be performed instead of, or in addition to, the surgical pathologic examination, it should be coded separately.

YOU CODE IT! CASE STUDY

Trent Bingham, an 11-year-old male, was taken to the OR to have his tonsils removed. However, due to additional symptoms, Dr. Ellendale did a biopsy and sent a specimen of Trent's tonsil to the lab for surgical pathologic examination. The report came back from the lab that Trent had a malignant neoplasm of his tonsils. Dr. Ellendale surgically removed additional sections to be certain that the entire tumor had been removed. Trent tolerated the procedure well and was taken to the recovery room.

You Code It!

Go through the steps and determine the pathology/lab code(s) that should be reported for this encounter.

Step 1: Read the case completely.

Step 2: Abstract the notes: Which key words can you identify relating to the procedures performed?

_____

Step 3: Query the provider, if necessary.

Step 4: Diagnosis: Malignant neoplasm, tonsil.

Step 5: Code the procedure(s).

_____

Step 6: Link the procedure codes to at least one diagnosis code.

Step 7: Back code to double-check your choices.

Answer:

Did you determine the correct code?

88305 Level IV; Tonsil, Biopsy

Good work!

Pathologic Testing on Bone Marrow

Although not performed as commonly as blood tests or urinalysis (because obtaining the specimen is complex), pathologic examination of a patient's bone marrow has many possible uses, including

- As a diagnostic tool for suspected myeloma, leukemia, myelodysplastic syndromes, and myeloproliferative disorders.
- To assess a current diagnosis of thrombocytopenia, anemia, or leukopenia.
- To measure quantities of stored iron and marrow cellularity.
- To determine neoplasm, infection, fibrosis, or other infiltrative bone disease.
- To enable staging of lymphoma and/or other malignant neoplasms.

A patient may have abnormal blood counts for which an explanation has yet to be identified, or the patient may have other abnormal cells evidenced in circulating blood. These, as well as a current diagnosis of a bone marrow–related disease (such as lymphoma) or indications that a malignancy has metastasized into the marrow, are standard-of-care justifications to obtain and study a bone marrow specimen.

Typically, the specimen is taken from the posterior superior iliac spine of the pelvis to acquire a sampling of the blood-forming cells in the marrow space. Evaluation of a specimen taken by biopsy is considered to be more accurate than one obtained by aspiration because the quantity of material gathered is greater and therefore more likely to provide a representative sampling of a wider scope.

When coding for bone marrow biopsy, the first procedure to be reported is for obtaining the specimen, using either 38220 Bone marrow; aspiration only or 38221 Bone marrow, biopsy, needle or trocar.

Note that the abstraction of bone marrow from a patient is not performed solely for the lab. Therefore, it is very important to identify, from the documentation, not only how the bone marrow was taken but also for what purpose. For example, bone marrow aspiration for platelet rich stem cell injections are not reported with 38220 but with code 0232T Injection(s), platelet-rich plasma, any site, including image guidance, harvesting and preparation when performed. Harvesting bone marrow for transplantation is reported with either 38230 Bone marrow harvesting for transplantation; allogeneic or 38232 Bone marrow harvesting for transplantation; Autologous.

When both a bone marrow biopsy and a bone marrow aspiration are performed on a Medicare beneficiary during the same encounter, do not report code 38220. Instead, use code G0364 Bone marrow aspiration performed with bone marrow biopsy through the same incision on the same date of service.

Pathologic Testing Next, the specimen will be sent to the laboratory for analysis. A bone marrow specimen, obtained by either biopsy or aspiration, can enable a hematologist/pathologist to investigate the patient's hematopoiesis (the process of forming blood cells), as well as the shape, size, and quantity of red and white blood cells and megakaryocytes (very large bone marrow cells that produce blood platelets). Blood cell formation is primarily the responsibility of the red bone marrow, specifically in the sternum, ribs, and iliac bones (pelvis).

Code 88305 Level IV Surgical pathology, gross and microscopic examination reports both evaluation of the bone marrow biopsy specimen by the naked eye (gross examination) and visualization of the specimen using a microscope. When the documentation states that the specimen was obtained by aspiration, instead of 88305, the analysis is reported with 85097 Bone marrow; smear interpretation.

It is not uncommon for a decalcification procedure and/or iron staining to be performed at the same time as the surgical pathologic examination. When documentation confirms this, report these procedures separately using +88311 Decalcification procedure (list separately in addition to code for surgical pathology examination) and/or 88313 Special stain including interpretation and report; Group II, all other (e.g., iron, trichrome) except stain for microorganisms, stains for enzyme constituents, or immunocytochemistry and immunohistochemistry.

Per CPT parenthetical instruction, you should report one unit of 88313 for each special stain on each surgical pathologic block, cytologic specimen, or hematologic smear. Check documentation or query the pathologist performing the testing to ensure that the notes are clear as to how many blocks, specimens, or smears are tested so that you can report the accurate number of codes.

Immunophenotyping by flow cytometery provides the identification of cell-specific antibodies, enabling a more accurate determination of cell percentages as well as identification of abnormal cell patterns. Report this test using 88184 Flow cytometry, cell surface, cytoplasmic, or nuclear marker, technical component only; first marker and +88185 each additional marker, as appropriate.

Because 88184 and 88185 are specifically limited to the technical component only, you will need a code to report the interpretation service separately. Note that no modifiers (TC nor 26) are necessary because these details are already included in the code descriptors, as follows:

> 88187 Flow cytometery, interpretation; 2 to 8 markers
>
> 88188 Flow cytometery, interpretation; 9 to 15 markers
>
> 88189 Flow cytometery, interpretation; 16 or more markers

Fluorescent in situ hybridization (FISH) analysis (88365 In situ hybridization [e.g., FISH], each probe) is usually performed after the analysis of the bone marrow, the results of which will direct the specific DNA probes to be conducted. FISH analysis is better than an overall karyotype test because it can find smaller pieces of chromosomes that may be missing or may have extra copies.

YOU CODE IT! CASE STUDY

Heloise Abelardo, a 43-year-old female, has a history of chronic myeloid leukemia (CML) and came to our facility today for a bone marrow aspiration, right side posterior iliac crest. Dr. Nicholas used a 15-gauge needle to obtain the aspirate including an aspirate clot. The patient tolerated the procedure well.

You Code It!

Part 1: Go through the steps of coding, and determine the code or codes that should be reported for this encounter between Dr. Nicholas and Heloise Abelardo.

Step 1: Read the case completely.

Step 2: Abstract the notes: Which key words can you identify relating to what procedure Dr. Nicholas performed on Heloise?

_____

Step 3: Query the provider, if necessary.

Step 4: Code the diagnosis or diagnoses: History of CML.

Step 5: Code the procedure(s).

_____

Step 6: Link the procedure codes to at least one diagnosis code to confirm medical necessity.

Step 7: Back code to double-check your choices.

Answer:

Did you determine the correct code for obtaining the bone marrow specimen to be

38220 Bone marrow; aspiration only

Part 2: Dr. Alfredo, a certified pathologist, wrote this report after testing the bone marrow:

PATHOLOGY REPORT:

The following specimens were reviewed: peripheral smear of bone marrow aspirate and clot section; iron stain.

Did you determine the correct code for the pathology testing to be:

85097 Bone marrow; smear interpretation

88313 Special stain including interpretation and report; Group II, all other (e.g., iron, trichrome) except stain for microorganisms, stains for enzyme constituents, or immunocytochemistry and immunohistochemistry

LO 10.6 Modifiers for Laboratory Coding

If your health care facility uses an outside laboratory that bills your office, you include the charges for the lab work on the claim form that you file. In such instances, you must append the CPT code for the lab test with modifier 90. If the outside lab bills the patient's insurance directly, you will not include the test code or modifier on the claim form you submit.

90 **Reference (Outside) Laboratory:** When laboratory procedures are performed by a party other than the treating or reporting physician, the procedure may be identified by adding modifier 90 to the usual procedure number.

Also on occasion, you may find that a lab test has to be repeated, on the same day for the same patient, in order to get several readings of a level or measurement.

91 **Repeat Clinical Diagnostic Laboratory Test:** In the course of treatment of the patient, it may be necessary to repeat the same laboratory test on the same day to obtain subsequent (multiple) test results. Under these circumstances, the laboratory test performed can be identified by its usual procedure number and the addition of modifier 91. (Note: This modifier may not be used when tests are rerun to confirm initial results; due to testing problems with specimens or equipment; or for any other reason when a normal, one-time, reportable results is all that is required. This modifier may not be used when other code[s] describe a series of test results [e.g., glucose tolerance tests, evocative/suppression testing]. This modifier may only be used for laboratory test[s] performed more than once on the same day on the same patient.)

The use of testing kits is increasing in health care facilities because they make it easier to obtain fast, accurate results. When a testing kit is being used, append modifier 92.

92 **Alternative Laboratory Platform Testing:** When laboratory testing is being performed using a kit or transportable instrument that wholly or in part consists of a single use, disposable analytical chamber, the service may be identified by adding modifier 92 to the usual laboratory procedure code.

Chapter Summary

Pathology and laboratory tests provide health care professionals with definitive evidence as to the condition that may be interfering with a patient's good health. That proof will help direct the physician toward a more accurate diagnosis and a beneficial treatment plan. Lab tests are an invaluable part of the health care toolbox and must be coded accurately.

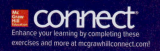

Using Terminology

Match each key term to the appropriate definition.

_____ **1.** LO 10.4 The investigation and identification of cells.

_____ **2.** LO 10.1 The counting or measurement of something.

_____ **3.** LO 10.5 The study of tissues removed from a living patient during a surgical procedure.

_____ **4.** LO 10.5 The study of a specimen using a microscope (under magnification).

_____ **5.** LO 10.1 A location with scientific equipment designed to perform experiments and tests.

_____ **6.** LO 10.1 The study of the nature, etiology, development, and outcomes of disease.

_____ **7.** LO 10.5 The visual study of a specimen (with the naked eye).

_____ **8.** LO 10.1 The study of the causes of disease.

_____ **9.** LO 10.1 A small part or sample of any substance obtained for analysis and diagnosis.

_____ **10.** LO 10.1 The determination of character or essential element(s).

A. Cytology

B. Etiology

C. Gross examination

D. Laboratory

E. Microscopic examination

F. Pathology

G. Qualitative

H. Quantitative

I. Specimen

J. Surgical pathology

Checking Your Understanding

Choose the most appropriate answer for each of the following questions.

1. LO 10.1 Laboratory tests can be performed

   a. in a free-standing lab.

   b. in a hospital.

   c. at a physician's office.

   d. all of these.

2. LO 10.1 Most often, the coding specialist responsible for reporting the lab work is employed by

   a. the physician who ordered the tests.

   b. the facility that performed the tests.

   c. the hospital.

   d. the third-party payer.

3. LO 10.1 A specimen can be

   a. blood.

   b. urine.

   c. sputum.

   d. all of these.

4. LO 10.1 When not all of the tests listed in a panel are performed, you should

   a. code the panel with modifier 52.

   b. code the panel alone.

   c. code the tests individually.

   d. code the panel with modifier 53.

5. LO 10.1 When more tests are performed, including all those listed in a panel, you should

    a. code the panel with modifier 22.
    b. code the panel alone.
    c. code the panel, plus the additional tests performed.
    d. code all the tests individually.

6. LO 10.2 Genetic testing code modifiers are used when reporting

    a. clinical chemistry.
    b. molecular diagnostics.
    c. hematology.
    d. immunology.

7. LO 10.3 CBC stands for

    a. comprehensive blood cytology.
    b. concentration blood count.
    c. cellular blind concentration.
    d. complete blood count.

8. LO 10.3 CBC includes

    a. WBC.
    b. RBC.
    c. HCT.
    d. all of these.

9. LO 10.5 Surgical pathology may include

    a. gross examination.
    b. microbiology.
    c. genetic testing.
    d. nuclear medicine.

10. LO 10.1 Quantitative testing is

    a. the determination of essential elements.
    b. the listing of all components.
    c. the measurement of an element.
    d. the total assessment.

Applying Your Knowledge

1. LO 10.1 Differentiate between pathology and etiology. _____

_____

2. LO 10.1 What is the difference between *quantitative* and *qualitative?* _____

_____

3. LO 10.1 List six familiar clinical chemistry tests. _____

_____

4. LO 10.2 Explain molecular diagnostics. Why do they need special modifiers? What do those modifiers identify? In what appendix are the modifiers found? _____

_____

5. LO 10.3 What is hematology, and what can hematologic tests help diagnose? _____

_____

6. LO 10.3 What does the acronym CBC stand for, and what tests does it include? _____

_____

7. LO 10.4 What is cytopathology? What is cytologic testing used for, and how are specimens obtained? _____

_____

8. LO 10.5 What are the purpose and benefit of surgical pathology? _____

_____

9. LO 10.5 Explain the difference between gross examination and microscopic examination. _____

_____

10. LO 10.6 If your health care facility uses an outside laboratory that bills your office, and you include the charges for the lab work on the claim form, what modifier must you append? _____

_____

YOU CODE IT! Practice
Chapter 10: Pathology and Laboratory Coding

Using the techniques described in this chapter, carefully read through the case studies and determine the most accurate pathology and laboratory CPT code(s) and modifier(s), if appropriate, for each case study.

1. Leroy Matheson, a 39-year-old male, was feeling rundown and tired all the time. So Dr. Lowe, thinking that Leroy might have anemia, ordered a complete CBC, automated with an automated differential WBC count.

   _____

2. Tiffany Deloach, an 18-year-old female, has been living on the street and in shelters and comes to the free clinic for a checkup because she is 5 months' pregnant. Dr. Jacobs orders a complete CBC; automated and appropriate manual differential WBC count; hepatitis B surface antigen, rubella antibody, qualitative syphilis test, RBC antibody screening, blood typing ABO, and Rh factor.

   _____

3. Caitlyn Calhoun, a 2-year-old female, is at the office of her pediatrician, Dr. Childers, for her regular checkup. Dr. Childers notices that Caitlyn is very small for her age and orders a growth hormone stimulation panel to be done.

   _____

4. Sean McCully, a 27-year-old male, went to the shore with his friends and feasted on raw oysters and beer. About 5 hours later, after getting home, he began to cough and vomit, and he found blood in his stool. He went to the walk-in clinic, where Dr. Ferguson ran a smear test for ova and parasites, particularly *Anisakis*.

   _____

5. Chad Tanger, a 33-year-old male, was diagnosed with prostate cancer last week. Before beginning radiation treatments, which will make him unable to have children, he comes today to submit his sperm for cryopreservation.

   _____

6. Rulon Porter, a 67-year-old male, has a history of gastrointestinal problems, including intestinal polyps. After taking a special kit home, he submits fecal specimens for an occult blood test by immunoassay.

   _____

7. Margaret Kahlil, a 29-year-old female, just got a new job with the space industry. As a condition of her employment, she came to the lab today for drug screening of alcohol, amphetamines, and barbiturates. The test was confirmed to be negative for all drugs by immunoassay.

   _____

8. Reyna Cutler, a 23-year-old female, was found unconscious by her roommate and brought into the emergency department by ambulance. The roommate stated that Reyna was very depressed, and she feared that Reyna might have taken an overdose of her medication. Dr. Farmer ordered a therapeutic drug assay for phenobarbital.

_____

9. Edward Stuart, a 15-year-old male, is overweight, bordering on obese, and Dr. Swenson is concerned that he may be developing diabetes, so he orders an insulin tolerance panel for adrenocorticotropic hormone (ACTH) insufficiency.

_____

10. Georgia Olin, a 44-year-old female, goes to her physician, Dr. Rodriguez, for her annual checkup, which includes a non-automated urinalysis with microscopy for glucose, ketones, and leukocytes. Dr. Rodriguez's assistant, Tracy, performs the test, by dipstick, in the office. The results are normal.

_____

11. Jolene Abernathy, a 19-year-old female, got drunk at a party and had unprotected sex. She came into the clinic today for an HIV-1 and HIV-2 single assay test.

_____

12. At the doctor's suggestion, Jolene was also tested for syphilis, qualitative (VDRL).

_____

13. Vivian Zeeman, a 41-year-old female, is pregnant for the first time. Dr. Lanahan performed an amniocentesis to do a chromosome analysis, count 15 cells, 1 karyotype, with banding. The results showed that the baby is fine.

_____

14. Jay Winegarten, a 53-year-old male, was in the operating room for Dr. Ashley to perform a subtotal resection of his pancreas. Surgical pathology showed no malignancy.

_____

15. Walter Praxis, a 15-day-old male, was born at 33 weeks' gestation, and there is concern that he may have hyperbilirubinemia. Therefore, Dr. Stevenson performed a total transcutaneous bilirubin.

_____

The following exercises provide practice in the application of abstracting the physicians' notes and learning to work with SOAP notes from our health care facility, Cipher, Victors & Associates. These case studies (SOAP notes) are modeled on real patient encounters. Using the techniques described in this chapter, carefully read through the case studies and determine the most accurate pathology and laboratory CPT code(s) and modifier(s), if appropriate, for each case study. You are coding for the pathologist.

CIPHER, VICTORS & ASSOCIATES
A Complete Health Care Facility
234 MAIN STREET • ANYTOWN, FL 32711 • 407-555-1234

PATIENT: FRANKLIN, FRANCES
ACCOUNT/EHR #:   FRANFR001
DATE: 10/17/18

Procedure Performed: Comprehensive metabolic panel

Pathologist: Caryn Simonson, MD

Referring Physician: Valerie R. Victors, MD

INDICATIONS: Routine physical exam

IMPRESSIONS:

Albumin	3.9
Bilirubin	Small*
Calcium	8.9
Carbon dioxide (CO_2)	28
Chloride	96 L C
Creatinine	1.2
Glucose	102
Phosphatase, alkaline	90
Potassium	3.9
Protein, total	30*
Sodium	138
Transferase, alanine amino (ALT)(SGPT)	30
Transferase, aspartate amino (AST)(SGOT)	29
Urea nitrogen (BUN)	18

* = Abnormal, L = Low, H = High

Caryn Simonson, MD

CS/mg   D: 10/17/18 09:50:16   T: 10/20/18 12:55:01

Determine the most accurate pathology and laboratory CPT code(s) and modifiers, if appropriate.

_____

_____

_____

CIPHER, VICTORS & ASSOCIATES
A Complete Health Care Facility
234 MAIN STREET • ANYTOWN, FL 32711 • 407-555-1234

PATIENT: TRANSIL, BRENT
ACCOUNT/EHR #:   TRANBR001
DATE: 09/29/18

Procedure Performed: Tissue, skin, head, mutation identification

Pathologist: Caryn Simonson, MD

Referring Physician: James I. Cipher, MD

INDICATIONS: Suspected melanoma

IMPRESSIONS: Abnormal cells present
Molecular diagnostics; mutation identification by sequencing, single segment

Caryn Simonson, MD

CS/mg   D: 09/29/18 09:50:16   T: 09/30/18 12:55:01

Determine the most accurate pathology and laboratory CPT code(s) and modifiers, if appropriate.

_____

_____

_____

CIPHER, VICTORS & ASSOCIATES
A Complete Health Care Facility
234 MAIN STREET • ANYTOWN, FL 32711 • 407-555-1234

PATIENT: HAVERSTROM, OLIVIA
ACCOUNT/EHR #: HAVEOL001
DATE: 11/15/18

Procedure Performed: Surgical pathology, gallbladder, gross and microscopic examination

Pathologist: Caryn Simonson, MD

Referring Physician: Valerie R. Victors, MD

INDICATIONS: R/O malignancy

IMPRESSIONS: All tissues unremarkable
Surgical pathology, gross and microscopic examination of gallbladder

_____

Caryn Simonson, MD

CS/mg   D: 11/15/18 09:50:16   T: 11/20/18 12:55:01

Determine the most accurate pathology and laboratory CPT code(s) and modifiers, if appropriate.

_____

_____

_____

CIPHER, VICTORS & ASSOCIATES
A Complete Health Care Facility
234 MAIN STREET • ANYTOWN, FL 32711 • 407-555-1234

PATIENT: FRIEDMAN, DORIS
ACCOUNT/EHR #:   FRIEDO001
DATE: 19/23/18

Procedure Performed: Rectal biopsies, gross and microscopic examination

Pathologist: Caryn Simonson, MD

Referring Physician: Matthew Appellet, MD

INDICATIONS: Inflammatory bowel disease

IMPRESSIONS: All tissues normal
                            Surgical pathology, gross and microscopic examination, colon biopsy

---

Caryn Simonson, MD

CS/mg   D: 09/23/18 09:50:16   T: 09/25/18 12:55:01

Determine the most accurate pathology and laboratory CPT code(s) and modifiers, if appropriate.

_____

_____

_____

CIPHER, VICTORS & ASSOCIATES
A Complete Health Care Facility
234 MAIN STREET • ANYTOWN, FL 32711 • 407-555-1234

PATIENT: FRANKS, ELMER
ACCOUNT/EHR #:   FRANEL001
DATE: 06/17/18

Procedure Performed: Mass (fat tissue), upper eyelid gross and microscopic
examination

Pathologist: Caryn Simonson, MD

Referring Physician: Mark C. Welby, MD

INDICATIONS: Herniated orbital fat pad, OD

IMPRESSIONS: Carcinoma in situ
Surgical pathology, gross and microscopic examination,
soft tissue tumor, extensive resection

Caryn Simonson, MD

CS/mg   D: 06/17/18 09:50:16   T: 06/20/18 12:55:01

Determine the most accurate pathology and laboratory CPT code(s) and modifiers, if appropriate.

_____

_____

_____

11

MEDICINE CODING

Learning Outcomes *After completing this chapter, the student should be able to:*

LO 11.1 Interpret the guidelines for coding the administration of immunizations.

LO 11.2 Apply the guidelines to accurately report injections and infusions.

LO 11.3 Determine the correct coding parameters for reporting psychiatric services.

LO 11.4 Abstract physicians' notes to accurately report dialysis services.

LO 11.5 Identify specifics to correctly report ophthalmology services.

LO 11.6 Determine how to accurately report cardiovascular services.

Key Terms

Ablation

Catheter

Duplex scan

Immunization

Infusion

Injection

Ophthalmologist

Optometrist

Otorhinolaryngology

Push

The Medicine section of the CPT book has codes for services that are supplied by health care professionals but not represented in any other sections. Services reported using codes from the Medicine section include

- Flu shots.
- Vaccinations for the kids to go back to school.
- Allergy shots.
- Chiropractic services.
- Psychotherapy.
- Dialysis.
- Hearing evaluations.
- Vision checks.
- Chemotherapy.
- Acupuncture.

Wherever you work as a coding specialist, there is an excellent chance you will be using this section. Let's go through it together.

LO 11.1 Immunizations

Immunization of a patient has two parts to the process: the medication itself and the administration of the medication. Each part is coded separately.

The medication may be an immune globulin, an antitoxin, a vaccine, or a toxoid. Codes 90281–90399 and 90476–90749 are available for you to identify the specific drug.

Medications can be given, or administered, to the patient in several different ways: percutaneous, intradermal, subcutaneous (SC), or intramuscular (IM) injections; intranasal (INH) or oral (ORAL); intra-arterial (IA) or intravenous (IV). The method of administration will help you find the correct administration codes 90460–90461 and 90471–90474.

When more than one vaccine is provided on the same date, use the add-on codes for the administration of the additional injections. You will find that most of the codes are offered in sets: the first injection, administration, or hour and then the add-on code for each additional injection, administration, or hour.

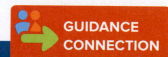

LET'S CODE IT! SCENARIO

Carlton Travella, a 5-year-old male, came to Dr. Quon for his MMR vaccine so that Carlton could start kindergarten next month. Dr. Quon administered an injection subcutaneously. Dr. Quon met face-to-face with Carlton's mother and discussed the importance of the vaccine, as well as indications of a reaction that she should watch for. Carlton chose a red balloon as his prize for being a good patient.

Let's Code It!

Dr. Quon gave Carlton *one subcutaneous injection* of the *MMR vaccine.* Do you know what *MMR* stands for? Even if you don't know that it is an acronym for *measles, mumps, and rubella,* you can look it up in the alphabetic index under *MMR shots.* The suggested code is 90707. The numerical listing confirms

90707 Measles, mumps, and rubella virus vaccine (MMR), live, for subcutaneous use.

The description matches Dr. Quon's notes exactly. However, the code will reimburse Dr. Quon's office only for the drug itself, not Dr. Quon's time and expertise in administering the injection and counseling the family. You could go back to the alphabetic index, or you could read the instructional paragraph at the beginning of the Vaccines, Toxoids subsection (where you found the code 90707). You will see that this paragraph tells you that you must use these codes "in addition to an immunization administration code(s) 90460–90474." Let's turn to the first code, 90465, and read the description:

90460 Immunization administration through 18 years of age via any route of administration, with counseling by physician or other qualified health care professional; first or only component of each vaccine or toxoid administered

Now, you have the codes to reimburse Dr. Quon for the drug, as well as his time and expertise in administering the injection and talking with Carlton's mother.

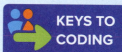

LO 11.2 Injections and Infusions

The administration of fluids (such as saline solution to hydrate a patient suffering from dehydration), pharmaceuticals (such as medications for treatment or preventive purposes), or dyes (such as those used for diagnostic testing) is coded from the Injections and Infusions subsection, which includes codes 96360–96379.

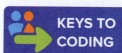

infusion
The introduction of a fluid into a blood vessel.

injection
Compelling a fluid into tissue or cavity.

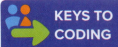

KEYS TO CODING

The administration of chemotherapy drugs is not coded from the Injections and Infusions subsection, but from the Chemotherapy Administration subsection, codes 96401–96549.

push
The delivery of an additional drug via an intravenous line over a short period of time.

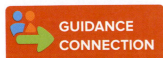

GUIDANCE CONNECTION

Additional explanation can be found in the guidelines within the **Medicine** section, directly under the subhead **Hydration, Therapeutic, Prophylactic, Diagnostic Injections and Infusions, and Chemotherapy and Other Highly Complex Drug or Highly Complex Biologic Agent Administration,** in your CPT book.

The **infusion** and **injection** codes include certain standard parts involved in administering liquids. Services included and therefore not reported separately are

- The administration of a local anesthetic.
- The initiation of the IV.
- Accessing an indwelling IV, subcutaneous catheter, or port.
- Flushing the line at the completion of the infusion.
- The appropriate supplies: tubing, syringes, and so on.

The guidelines for coding injections and infusions provide further direction when coding these services:

- When more than one infusion is provided into one IV site, report only the first service.
- Should more than one IV site be used, report the appropriate services for each site.
- Report different drugs or materials and that service separately.
- Report infusion time as the actual time the fluid is provided.

An IV or intra-arterial **push** is described by the CPT guidelines as

- An injection administered to the patient and then observed continuously by the health care professional who administered the drug.

  or

- An infusion that lasts 15 minutes or less.

Multiple Administrations

When more than one injection or infusion is provided to a patient at the same encounter, there is a specific order in which you need to report the codes. The sequencing guidelines are different for those reporting physician services than for those reporting for the facility.

When you are reporting for the physician's, or other health care professional's, services, you must read the notes carefully to determine the main diagnosis or reason for the treatment. The primary reason for the injection or infusion should be reported first, as the "initial" service, no matter in what order the injections were administered.

EXAMPLE

Mary comes to see her physician because she has been vomiting a lot over the last several days. Dr. Palmer identifies that she has become dehydrated, due to this excessive vomiting. Dr. Palmer gives Mary an intramuscular (IM) injection of an antiemetic (a drug to stop vomiting) and then gives her an IV infusion, 45 minutes, of normal saline for hydration. The primary reason for the encounter is Mary's excessive vomiting; therefore, the injection of the antiemetic is the "initial" service, followed by the hydration infusion service.

> 96372 Therapeutic, prophylactic, or diagnostic injection; subcutaneous or intramuscular
> 96360 Intravenous infusion, hydration; initial, 31 minutes to 1 hour

When you are reporting services on behalf of a facility rather than the providing professional, the order is determined by the type of service provided as well as the reason for that service:

1. Chemotherapy service.
2. Therapeutic, prophylactic, and diagnostic services
3. Hydration services.

Then, the specific service hierarchy is

1. Infusions
2. Pushes
3. Injections

LET'S CODE IT! SCENARIO

Allison Bradley, a 45-year-old female, postmastectomy for malignant neoplasm of the breast, has been having chemotherapy treatments. She was seen today for nausea and vomiting as a result of this therapy. Dr. Eider ordered an antiemetic 10 mg IV push and another antiemetic IV infusion over 30 minutes.

Let's Code It!

Allison received two medications via two different routes of administration: *IV push* and *IV infusion*. Therefore, you need two codes.

The notes report that an intravenous push, which is an injection given intravenously, was given. Let's turn to the alphabetic index and look up *injection, intravenous.*

Injection

Intravenous   96379

Keep reading below that and you will see

Injection

Intravenous push   96374–96376

That looks perfect. Turn to the numerical listing, and read the complete descriptions. You see that 96374 matches the notes:

96374 Therapeutic, prophylactic or diagnostic injection (specify substance or drug); intravenous push, single or initial substance/drug

You also know that Allison was given an *infusion, intravenously,* and that it was for *therapeutic* reasons—to eliminate her nausea and vomiting. Let's go to the alphabetic index and look up *infusion, intravenous, therapeutic.*

Infusion

Intravenous

Therapeutic   96365–96368, 96379

When you turn to the numerical listing to check the code descriptions, you see that codes 96360–96361 are for hydration only. Look through the complete descriptions for the next grouping, 96365–96368, and you see that the best, most accurate code is

96367 Intravenous infusion, for therapy, prophylaxis, or diagnosis (specify substance or drug); additional sequential infusion of a new drug/substance, up to one hour

The notes indicate that Allison was given the infusion after the first (sequentially) for 30 minutes. Excellent!

Therefore, the claim form for this encounter with Allison will show 96374, 96367. Great job!

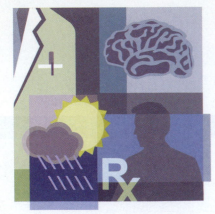

LO 11.3 Psychiatry, Psychotherapy, and Biofeedback

Sometimes we become so focused on physical health care issues that we forget the health care professionals who treat mental health concerns. This area is a great opportunity for coding specialists because more and more health care plans cover psychotherapy and psychiatric services. Codes 90785–90911 provide details on such services.

When coding psychotherapy services, the best, most appropriate code is determined first by the location [where the therapeutic services were provided, which is similar to when you code evaluation and management (E/M) services]:

- Office or other outpatient facility.
- Inpatient hospital or residential care facility.

Next, review the documentation to determine the type of therapy provided:

- Insight-oriented/behavior modification/supportive.
- Interactive using play equipment, physical devices, language interpreter, or other mechanisms of nonverbal communication.

Once the type of therapy is determined, the next factor to consider is how much time the provider spent face-to-face with the patient.

Last, you must find out from the documentation whether the physician or therapist provided medical E/M services in addition to the therapy session at the same time or on the same day. If such services were provided but not at the same time or on the same day, then a code from the Evaluation and Management section of the CPT book may be appropriate.

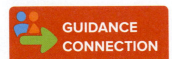

GUIDANCE CONNECTION

Additional explanation can be found in the guidelines within the **Medicine** section, directly under the subhead **Psychiatry,** in your CPT book.

LET'S CODE IT! SCENARIO

Rick Springer, a 29-year-old male, was sent to Dr. Wheeler for psychotherapy to deal with anger management issues. Dr. Wheeler spent 45 minutes with Rick in her office.

Let's Code It!

Rick saw Dr. Wheeler in *her office* for psychotherapy for *45 minutes.* Let's look in the alphabetic index under *psychotherapy,* beneath which you see *family* or *group* as choices. The notes indicate that Rick had an individual psychotherapy session. The Alphabetic Index suggests codes 90832–90834 and 90836–90838. Let's look at the numerical listing and see which of these matches Dr. Wheeler's notes.

> **90834** Psychotherapy, 45 minutes with patient and/or family member
>
> **+90836** Psychotherapy, 45 minutes with patient and /or family member when performed with an evaluation and management service (List separately in addition to the code for primary procedure)

The next issue to consider is whether Dr. Wheeler provided medical E/M services at the same time. According to her notes, she did not. This means that code 90834 is the code to report.

Great job!

LO 11.4 Dialysis

Dialysis is an artificial process used to clean the blood by removing excess water and waste products when the individual's body cannot do this. In addition to hospitals providing this service, independent centers and home health agencies help patients receive treatment. The correct code for reporting dialysis service is determined by the patient's age, where the services are provided, and the level of physician services during the encounters.

Physician services provided during a dialysis month included in these codes are

- Determination of the dialysis cycle.
- Outpatient E/M of the dialysis visits.
- Telephone calls.
- Patient management.
- Face-to-face visit with the patient.

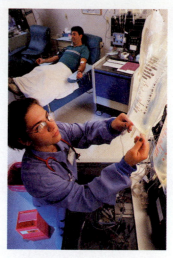

You should code the treatment of patients who receive dialysis but are not diagnosed with end-stage renal disease (ESRD) with 90935, 90937, 90945, or 90947, whether the services are provided on an outpatient or inpatient basis.

Due to the regularity of dialysis for those with ESRD, codes 90951–90966 represent a full month of dialysis services and, therefore, are reported only once a month. If a facility does not provide a full month of services to a patient, for whatever reason, then the coder should use codes 90967–90970, accordingly, multiplied by each day of service.

For ESRD patients who receive dialysis as an inpatient, code 90935 or 90937 for hemodialysis or 90945 or 90947 for dialysis other than hemodialysis during the hospitalization.

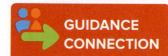

GUIDANCE CONNECTION

Additional explanation can be found in the guidelines within the **Medicine** section, directly under the subhead **Dialysis,** subsections **Hemodialysis, Miscellaneous Dialysis Procedures,** and **End-Stage Renal Disease Services,** in your CPT book.

LET'S CODE IT! SCENARIO

Verna Abernathy, a 63-year-old female, was diagnosed with ESRD 6 months ago. She has just moved to Mayfield to be closer to her daughter and began her daily dialysis on June 20 at the Mayfield Dialysis Center. Prepare the claim for dialysis services for June.

Let's Code It!

Verna has *ESRD* and has received *dialysis* as an *outpatient* from Mayfield Dialysis Center. Let's look up *dialysis* in the alphabetic index. You can see the listing for *end-stage renal disease,* with the suggested code range of 90951–90970. When you turn to the numerical listing, you read that codes 90951–90966 are only for a full month of treatment. Verna received *11 days* of treatment from the facility (June 20 through June 30 is 11 days). So you have to find the code to report each day of service to Verna. Codes 90967–90970 are chosen by the patient's age. Verna is *63 years old,* bringing us to the following code:

90970 End-stage renal disease (ESRD) related services (less than full month), per day; for patients twenty years of age and over

Great! So the code will read 90970 × 11.

Gastroenterology

A limited number of tests and services for the gastroenterological system—from the patient's mouth down the esophagus to the stomach through the intestinal tract to the rectum—are included in the Medicine section of the CPT book. The alphabetic index will guide you to the best, most appropriate code in the best section, depending upon the service provided.

Sabrina Gentry, a 42-year-old female, has been battling with indigestion for over a year. After trying virtually every over-the-counter medication possibility, she came to see Dr. Michaels, who decided to administer an esophageal acid reflux test. The test was administered in the office using a nasal catheter intraluminal impedance electrode. The 45-minute test was recorded and analyzed and interpreted by Dr. Michaels.

You Code It!

Go through the steps and determine the procedure code(s) that should be reported for the test provided by Dr. Michaels to Sabrina Gentry.

Step 1:   Read the case completely.

Step 2:   Abstract the notes: Which key words can you identify relating to the procedures performed?

_____

Step 3:   Query the provider, if necessary.

Step 4:   Diagnosis: Possibly esophageal acid reflux.

Step 5:   Code the procedure(s).

_____

Step 6:   Link the procedure codes to at least one diagnosis code.

Step 7:   Back code to double-check your choices.

Answer:

Did you determine the correct code?

91037   Esophageal function test, gastroesophageal reflux test with nasal catheter intraluminal impedance electrode(s) placement, recording, analysis and interpretation

LO 11.5 Ophthalmology

ophthalmologist
A physician qualified to diagnose and treat eye disease and conditions with drugs, surgery, and corrective measures.

optometrist
A professional qualified to carry out eye examinations and to prescribe and supply eyeglasses and contact lenses.

Ophthalmologists are commonly called *eye doctors* or *vision specialists*. However, be careful not to confuse them with **optometrists,** who are eyeglass specialists.

The Ophthalmology subsection of the CPT book reports services provided by an ophthalmologist. General services, codes 92002–92014, are divided in two ways:

1. *The relationship between the patient and the physician: new patient or established patient.* Remember this from E/M coding? As a reminder, a new patient is one who has not received any services or treatments from the ophthalmologist (or any other physician with the same specialty in the same group practice) within the last 3 years.

2. *The level of service: intermediate or comprehensive.* An intermediate service is similar to a problem-focused evaluation. That is, the patient has a new or existing specific condition to be addressed by the physician. The comprehensive service is more of a general evaluation of the patient's entire visual system.

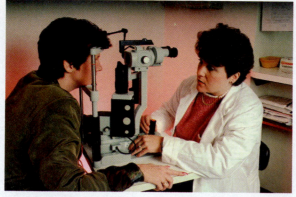
© Larry Mulvehill/Corbis

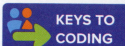
It is important to remember that these general services include both technical examinations and medical decision-making services. Therefore, it is not appropriate to code any of those services separately.

However, special services may be coded separately if provided at the same time as general services or E/M services. The documentation must be specific in its identification of the additional services. (Of course, special services can be provided alone and coded as such.) Codes 92015–92499 are used to report other ophthalmologic services.

LET'S CODE IT! SCENARIO

Raymond Nailer, a 55-year-old male, has been having a problem with blurred vision and pain in his eyes. His father has glaucoma, which makes Raymond at high risk for the disease. Therefore, Dr. Roberts is going to perform a bilateral visual field examination and a serial tonometry with multiple measurements. None of these services is done as a part of a general ophthalmologic service provided to Raymond.

Let's Code It!

Dr. Roberts is giving Raymond a "bilateral visual field examination and a serial tonometry" today. Let's go to the alphabetic index and look at *visual field exam.* The index suggests codes 92081–92083. Let's take a look at the numerical listing's code description:

92081 Visual field examination, unilateral or bilateral, with interpretation and report; limited examination (e.g., tangent screen, Autoplot, arc perimeter, or single stimulus level automated test, such as Octopus 3 or 7 equivalent)

It matches the notes. Now, you need to code the second test, the tonometry. You see that the alphabetic index shows *tonometry, serial* and suggests code 92100. Let's take a look at the complete code description:

92100 Serial tonometry (separate procedure) with multiple measurements of intraocular pressure over an extended time period with interpretation and report, same day (e.g., diurnal curve or medical treatment of acute elevation of intraocular pressure)

That's great! You are ready to create the claim form for Raymond's tests: codes 92081, 92100. Good job!

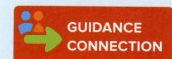

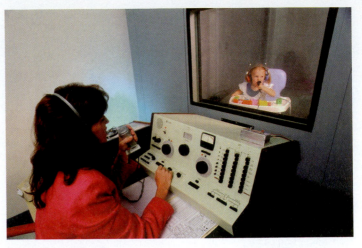
© Larry Mulvehill/Corbis

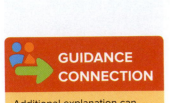

GUIDANCE CONNECTION

Additional explanation can be found in the guidelines within **Medicine** section, directly under the subhead **Special Otorhinolaryngologic Services,** in your CPT book.

otorhinolaryngology
The study of the human ears, nose, and throat (ENT) systems.

Otorhinolaryngologic Services

In the otorhinolaryngologic services portion of the Medicine section are codes for special services that are not usually included in an office visit or evaluation encounter in the field of **otorhinolaryngology.**

Throughout the listings for codes 92502–92700, you will see all types of tests and services that can help health care professionals diagnose and treat conditions relating to a patient's ears, nose, and throat and their functions.

YOU CODE IT! CASE STUDY

Kim Whirlon came with her husband, Arlen, to see Dr. Dean because of the problems Arlen has been having sleeping. Kim noticed that Arlen snores terribly during the night and has, at times, abruptly stopped. She is concerned that he may actually stop breathing during one of his episodes. Dr. Dean performed a nasopharyngoscopy with an endoscope to check Arlen's adenoids and lingual tonsils. The results of the exam indicated that Arlen is suffering from sleep apnea.

You Code It!

Go through the steps and determine the code(s) that should be reported for this test provided by Dr. Dean to Arlen Whirlon.

Step 1: Read the case completely.

Step 2: Abstract the notes: Which key words can you identify relating to the procedures performed?

_____

Step 3: Query the provider, if necessary.

Step 4: Diagnosis: Sleep apnea.

Step 5: Code the procedure(s).

_____

Step 6:   Link the procedure codes to at least one diagnosis code.

Step 7:   Back code to double-check your choices.

Answer:

Did you determine the correct code?

92511   Nasopharyngoscopy with endoscope (separate procedure)

That is exactly what Dr. Dean did. In addition, he did not perform it as a part of any other service, so it was a separate procedure. Excellent!

LO 11.6 Cardiovascular Services

In cardiovascular services you will find both diagnostic and therapeutic services for conditions of the heart and its vessels. As you look through the descriptions of the codes in this section, you might think that some appear to be surgical in nature (an atherectomy), while others appear to be imaging (radiologic), such as an echocardiogram. Regardless of what you think, the CPT book is structured the way it is, and it is your job as a coding specialist to find the best, most appropriate code to represent the service or treatment provided by the physician or other health care professional for whom you are reporting. Again, this is why it is so important that you take nothing for granted, read all notations and instructions carefully, and use the alphabetic index to guide you through the numerical listings.

Cardiovascular Therapeutic Services: 92950–92998

A variety of procedures relating to the heart are included in the Cardiovascular Therapeutic Services subsection that might seem more appropriate for other places in the CPT book. For example, intravascular ultrasound or percutaneous transluminal coronary balloon angioplasty illustrates the importance of using the alphabetic index to locate the correct range of codes for the procedures performed.

YOU CODE IT! CASE STUDY

Josiah Moore was in Dr. Toller's office when Josiah went into cardiac arrest. Dr. Toller immediately performed cardiopulmonary resuscitation (CPR). The nurse called 911, and Josiah was taken to the hospital after regaining consciousness and being stabilized.

You Code It!

Go through the steps and determine the code(s) that should be reported for the service provided by Dr. Toller for Josiah Moore.

Step 1:   Read the case completely.

Step 2:   Abstract the notes: Which key words can you identify relating to the procedures performed?

_____

Step 3:   Query the provider, if necessary.

Step 4:   Diagnosis: Cardiac arrest.

Step 5:   Code the procedure(s).

_____

Step 6:   Link the procedure codes to at least one diagnosis code.

Step 7:   Back code to double-check your choices.

Answer:

Did you determine the correct code?

92950 Cardiopulmonary resuscitation (e.g., in cardiac arrest)

It matches the notes perfectly. Good work!

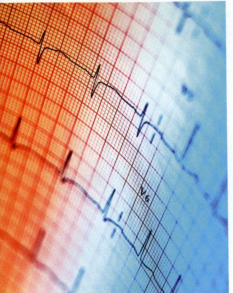

Cardiography: 93000–93278

The electronic measurement of heart rhythms very often uses an electrocardiograph (ECG, also called an EKG, machine). Services involving an electrocardiogram are coded from the Cardiography subsection.

> ### EXAMPLE
>
> Mary Alice Fallon experienced a rapid heartbeat and mild pain in her chest. Dr. Jacobson took a 12-lead routine ECG to rule out a heart attack. He interpreted the tracing and wrote a report for the file. The code is
>
> 93000 Electrocardiogram, routine ECG with at least 12 leads; with interpretation and report

Implantable and Wearable Cardiac Device Evaluations: 93279–93299

Technology has provided physicians with the ability to monitor a person's heart function under various circumstances. The incredible measuring devices that do this must be programmed, and then data must be gathered by using in-person and/or remote transmission and interpreted by the physician. The codes in this subsection report these services.

Echocardiography: 93303–93355

Echocardiography is different from electrocardiography. As the name indicates, an echocardiogram uses ultrasound (sound waves to produce an echo), rather than a measurement by electronic impulses, as with the ECG.

When coding echocardiography, the codes already include:

- The exam (the recording of the images of the organ or anatomical areas being studied).
- The interpretation and report of the findings.

You are not permitted to use these codes for echocardiograms that have been taken when no interpretation or report has been done.

Cardiac Catheterization: 93451–93462 + 93530–93533

The codes available for reporting cardiac catheterization include the following:

- The introduction of the **catheter**(s).
- The positioning and repositioning of the catheter(s).

KEYS TO CODING

The provision of a cardiac catheterization may require as many as five codes. It will depend upon for whom you are coding (which professional or facility) that will determine how many of these codes you are responsible for reporting:

1. The professional service for the catheterization . . . procedure code + modifier 26.
2. The administration of the dye . . . procedure code + modifier 51.
3. The radiologist's supervision and interpretation for the guidance for the injection of the dye . . . procedure code + modifier 26.
4. The procedure itself, such as coronary artery angiography.
5. The radiologist's supervision and interpretation of the images.

- Recording of the intracardiac and intravascular pressure.
- Obtaining blood samples for the measurement of blood gases, dilution curves, and/or cardiac output with or without electrode catheter placement.
- Final evaluation and report of the procedure.

catheter
A thin, flexible tube, inserted into a body part, used to inject fluid, to extract fluid, or to keep a passage open.

LET'S CODE IT! SCENARIO

Vladimir Susnow, a 5-month-old male, was experiencing cyanotic episodes, known as "blue" spells. Dr. Isaacson, his pediatrician, performed a transthoracic echocardiogram, which identified a ventricular septal defect and hypertrophied walls of the right ventricle. He then performed a right cardiac catheterization that confirmed a diagnosis of a tetralogy of Fallot.

Let's Code It!

Dr. Isaacson performed two tests on little Vladimir: first, a *transthoracic echocardiogram* and, second, a *right cardiac catheterization*. Let's go to the alphabetic index and look for the echocardiogram. Beneath it, you see *transthoracic* with a series of suggested codes. But before you go on, take a look at the indented listing below *transthoracic* for *congenital anomalies*. Vladimir is only 5 months old, and his heart problems are congenital; therefore, those are likely the more accurate codes. Let's take a look at the complete descriptions in the numerical listing for the suggested codes 93303–93304.

> **93303** Transthoracic echocardiography for congenital cardiac anomalies; complete

This matches the notes. Now, we must code the catheterization. In the alphabetic index, under *catheterization*, you find *cardiac*, and indented below that you find *right heart*. And look what is indented below that: *congenital cardiac anomalies*. Let's take a look at the complete description:

> **93530** Right heart catheterization, for congenital cardiac anomalies

Excellent. Now, you can see how terms you learned from coding the first procedure—congenital cardiac anomalies—make coding the second procedure easier. It is a small example of how practice and experience will make the entire coding process go more smoothly for you.

Electrophysiological Procedures: 93600–93662

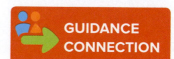
GUIDANCE CONNECTION

Intracardiac electrophysiologic studies (EPS) codes include

- The insertion of the electrode catheters (usually performed with two or more catheters).
- The repositioning of the catheters.
- Recording of electrograms both before and during the pacing or programmed stimulation of multiple locations of the heart.
- Analysis of the recorded electrograms.
- Report of the procedure and the findings.

There are cases when a diagnostic EPS is followed by treatment (**ablation**) of the problem at the same encounter. When ablation is done at the same time as an EPS, you must code it separately.

Additional explanation can be found in the guidelines within the **Medicine** section, directly under the subhead **Intracardiac Electrophysiological Procedures/Studies,** in your CPT book.

ablation
The destruction or eradication of tissue.

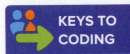
duplex scan
An ultrasonic scanning procedure to determine blood flow and pattern.

Noninvasive Vascular Studies

Codes 93880–93998 are provided for reporting noninvasive vascular studies of the arteries and veins of a patient and include the following:

- Preparation of the patient for the testing.
- Supervision of the performance of the tests.
- Recording of the study.
- Interpretation and report of the findings.

Codes are chosen by the type of study done: noninvasive physiologic, transcranial Doppler (TCD), or **duplex scan.**

YOU CODE IT! CASE STUDY

Dr. Unger was giving Itzel Malaga her annual physical examination. She had a low-grade fever and swelling and cyanosis was evident on her lower right leg. Concerned that she might have deep-vein thrombophlebitis, he performed a duplex Doppler ultrasonogram to study the arteries in her leg.

You Code It!

Go through the steps and determine the code(s) that should be reported for this test performed on Itzel Malaga.

Step 1: Read the case completely.

Step 2: Abstract the notes: Which key words can you identify relating to the procedures performed?

_____

Step 3: Query the provider, if necessary.

Step 4: Diagnosis: Cyanosis of lower limb, swelling of lower limb, fever.

Step 5: Code the procedure(s).

_____

Step 6: Link the procedure codes to at least one diagnosis code.

Step 7: Back code to double-check your choices.

Answer:

Did you determine the correct code?

93926 Duplex scan of lower extremity arteries or arterial bypass grafts; unilateral or limited study

Good job!

Pulmonary

Codes 94002–94799 in the Pulmonary subsection identify procedures and tests on the pulmonary system and include

- The exam and/or laboratory procedure.
- Interpretation of the findings.

Cahlil Cabel, a 2-day-old male, was born at 35 weeks' gestation, with a birthweight of 1,450 g. After exhibiting hypotension, peripheral edema, and oliguria, Cahlil was diagnosed by Dr. Redmon with respiratory distress syndrome. Dr. Redmon performed the initiation of continuous positive airway pressure ventilation (CPAP).

You Code It!

Go through the steps and determine the code(s) that should be reported for this treatment provided to Cahlil Cabel.

Step 1: Read the case completely.

Step 2: Abstract the notes: Which key words can you identify relating to the procedures performed?

_____

Step 3: Query the provider, if necessary.

Step 4: Diagnosis: Respiratory distress syndrome.

Step 5: Code the procedure(s).

_____

Step 6: Link the procedure codes to at least one diagnosis code.

Step 7: Back code to double-check your choices.

Answer:

Did you determine the correct code?

94660 Continuous positive airway pressure ventilation (CPAP) initiation and management

Excellent!

Allergy and Clinical Immunology

Codes 95004–95199 cover allergy and clinical immunology procedures. Allergies can be responsible for many different reactions in the human body. Beyond the typical sneezing and watery eyes, outcomes can cause anything from hives and rashes to behavioral problems, sleeplessness, and even death.

Often, when there is concern or suspicion that a patient may be suffering from an allergic reaction, the physician will begin with allergy sensitivity tests. In these cases, small yet potent samples of the suspected allergen are given to the patient in one of a number of methods: percutaneously (scratch, puncture, or prick), intracutaneously (intradermal), inhalation, or ingestion. Then the patient is watched, and the body's reaction to the allergen is documented. The results of the tests tell the physician to which elements the patient is considered allergic.

Once an allergy is identified, immunotherapy may be provided. The therapy is a way of retraining the patient's immune system, or desensitizing it, so that the body no longer views the particles as a threat.

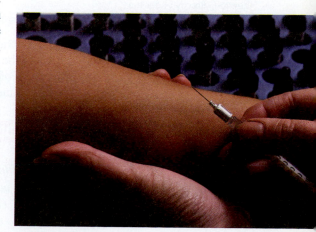

© PhotoLink/Getty Images

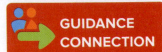
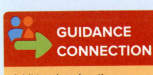
Neurology and Neuromuscular Procedures

As with so many other headings in this section, the neurology and neuromuscular procedure codes (95803–96020) include the recording of the test as well as the physician's interpretation and report of the findings.

Acronyms often seen in this arena of health care services include

EEG Electroencephalogram

EMG Electromyogram

EOG Electrooculogram

MEG Magnetoencephalography

LET'S CODE IT! SCENARIO

Alberto Hernandez, a 37-year-old male, was having a hard time staying awake during the day and asleep during the night. Dr. Hartford sent him down the hall to have a polysomnography, with three additional parameters, to rule out sleep apnea.

Let's Code It!

Dr. Hartford performed a *polysomnography* on Alberto to see if he has *sleep apnea.* Let's turn to the alphabetic index and find

Polysomnography   95808–95811

As you read through the complete code descriptions in the numerical listing, you will see that, because Dr. Hartford ordered *three additional parameters,* the best code is

95808 Polysomnography; sleep staging with 1–3 additional parameters of sleep, attended by a technologist

Excellent!

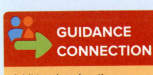
Central Nervous System Assessments

When a patient exhibits problems with cognitive processes, testing may evaluate the extent of the condition so that a treatment plan can be established. It is expected that the results of the tests in the Central Nervous System subsection (codes 96101–96127) will be formulated into a report to be used in the creation of a treatment plan.

YOU CODE IT! CASE STUDY

Chase Baltich, a 3-year-old male, does not appear to be meeting certain milestones. Dr. Reese performed a developmental test known as an Early Language Milestone Screening. Once the test was interpreted, he sent his report and contacted a speech therapist to consult on a treatment plan.

Go through the steps and determine the code(s) that should be reported for this screening test performed on Chase Baltich.

> Step 1:   Read the case completely.
>
> Step 2:   Abstract the notes: Which key words can you identify relating to the procedures performed?
>
> _____
>
> Step 3:   Query the provider, if necessary.
>
> Step 4:   Diagnosis: Delayed development of speech.
>
> Step 5:   Code the procedure(s).
>
> _____
>
> Step 6:   Link the procedure codes to at least one diagnosis code.
>
> Step 7:   Back code to double-check your choices.

Answer:

Did you determine the correct code?

96111 Developmental testing, (includes assessment of motor, language, social, adaptive, and/or cognitive functioning by standardized developmental instruments) with interpretation and report

Good work!

Chemotherapy Administration

Codes 96401–96549 cover the different methods of chemotherapy dispensation that may be used with one patient. Each method (such as steroidal agents and biologic agents) and/or each technique (such as infusion or IV push) should be coded separately. The codes include the following services:

- The administration of a local anesthetic.
- The initiation of the IV.
- Accessing an indwelling IV, subcutaneous catheter, or port.
- Flushing the line at the completion of the infusion.
- The appropriate supplies: tubing, syringes, and so on.
- The preparation of the chemotherapy agent(s).

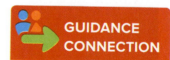

GUIDANCE CONNECTION

Additional explanation can be found in the guidelines within the **Medicine** section, directly under the subhead **Chemotherapy and Other Highly Complex Drug or Highly Complex Biologic Agent Administration** in your CPT book.

Gary Whitworth is admitted today for his chemotherapy, which consists of an antineoplastic drug, 500 mg IV infusion over 3 hours. Dr. Thatcher is in attendance during Gary's treatment.

Go through the steps and determine the code(s) that should be reported for this encounter between Dr. Thatcher and Gary Whitworth.

Step 1: Read the case completely.

Step 2: Abstract the notes: Which key words can you identify relating to the procedures performed?

_____

Step 3: Query the provider, if necessary.

Step 4: Diagnosis: Chemotherapy.

Step 5: Code the procedure(s).

_____

Step 6: Link the procedure codes to at least one diagnosis code.

Step 7: Back code to double-check your choices.

Answer:

Did you determine the correct codes?

96413 Chemotherapy administration, intravenous infusion technique; up to 1 hour, single or initial substance/drug

+96415 each additional hour, 1 to 8 hours (for second hour)

+96415 each additional hour, 1 to 8 hours (for third hour)

Physical Medicine and Rehabilitation

Throughout the Physical Medicine and Rehabilitation heading and its subheadings, read codes 97001–97799 carefully because some groups of codes require the provider to have direct (face-to-face) contact with the patient during the course of the treatment and others do not.

> ### EXAMPLE
>
> Codes 97010–97028, "Application of a modality to one or more areas," *do not* require provider-patient contact during the treatment; however, codes 97597–97610 *do* require a personal encounter.

Acupuncture

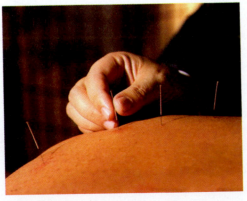
© Guy Cali/Corbis

The health care industry is always evolving and incorporating new techniques into its accepted methods for helping patients. The techniques of acupuncture (codes 97810–97814) are thousands of years old but are newly accepted by western medicine and health insurance payers.

Acupuncture services are measured in 15-minute increments of direct provider-patient contact. While the needles may be in place for a longer period of time, you are permitted to report only the time actually spent with the patient.

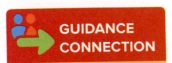

GUIDANCE CONNECTION

Additional explanation can be found in the guidelines within the **Medicine** section, directly under the subhead **Acupuncture,** in your CPT book.

Charlene Brown, a 55-year-old female, was having a problem with menopause. Because of the reported concerns about hormone replacement therapy (HRT), she decided to try acupuncture. After discussing her symptoms and a treatment plan, Dr. Kini inserted several needles. The needles were removed 20 minutes later. Dr. Kini reviewed the follow-up plan and made an appointment for Charlene's next visit. Dr. Kini spent 30 minutes in total face-to-face with Charlene, who reported marked improvement.

Let's Code It!

Dr. Kini's treatment of Charlene included *30 minutes face-to-face time* and *several needles* during the *acupuncture* treatment. Let's turn to the alphabetic index and look up *acupuncture.*

> **Acupuncture**
>
> **With Electrical Stimulation**   97813–97814
>
> **Without Electrical Stimulation** 97810–97811

There is no mention of electrical stimulation being used in Charlene's treatment, so turn to the codes recommended for *without electrical stimulation.*

97810 Acupuncture, 1 or more needles; without electrical stimulation, initial 15 minutes of personal one-on-one contact with the patient

+97811 without electrical stimulation, each additional 15 minutes of personal one-on-one contact with the patient, with reinsertion of needles(s) (List separately in addition to code for primary procedure.)

The first code, 97810, reports Dr. Kini's services, but only for the first 15 minutes. You have to add the second code, 97811, to report the remainder of the time so that the doctor can be reimbursed for the total 30 minutes for the session.

Osteopathic Manipulative Treatments

Codes 98925–98929, to report osteopathic manipulative treatments (OMT), are defined by the number of body regions involved in the encounter. Ten regions are identified with the codes:

- Head
- Cervical
- Thoracic
- Rib cage
- Upper extremities
- Lumbar
- Sacral
- Abdominal/visceral
- Pelvic
- Lower extremities

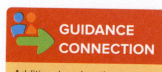

GUIDANCE CONNECTION

Additional explanation can be found in the guidelines within the **Medicine** section, directly under the subhead **Osteopathic Manipulative Treatment,** in your CPT book.

Chiropractic Manipulative Treatment

Similar to the osteopathic treatment codes, chiropractic manipulative treatment (CMT) codes 98940–98943 are determined by the number of regions treated during an encounter. The codes use spinal or extraspinal descriptions and are identified as follows:

SPINAL REGIONS

- Cervical, including atlanto-occipital joint.
- Thoracic, including costovertebral and costotransverse joints.
- Lumbar.
- Sacral.
- Pelvic, including the sacroiliac joint.

EXTRASPINAL REGIONS

- Head, including temporomandibular joint (but not the atlanto-occipital).
- Upper extremities.
- Rib cage, excluding costotransverse and costovertebral joints.
- Abdomen.
- Lower extremities.

GUIDANCE CONNECTION

Additional explanation can be found in the guidelines within the **Medicine** section, directly under the subhead **Chiropractic Manipulative Treatment,** in your CPT book.

YOU CODE IT! CASE STUDY

Ivan Lampkin, a 23-year-old male who is 6 ft 6 in. tall, has pain in his neck and spine. Dr. Turner, a chiropractor, provides CMT to his cervical, thoracic, lumbar, sacral, and pelvic regions to alleviate Ivan's pain.

You Code It!

Go through the steps and determine the code(s) that should be reported for this CMT encounter between Dr. Turner and Ivan Lampkin.

Step 1: Read the case completely.

Step 2: Abstract the notes: Which key words can you identify relating to the procedures performed?

_____

Step 3: Query the provider, if necessary.

Step 4: Diagnosis: Pain, neck, and spine.

Step 5: Code the procedure(s).

_____

Step 6: Link the procedure codes to at least one diagnosis code.

Step 7: Back code to double-check your choices.

Answer:

Did you determine the correct code?

98942 Chiropractic manipulative treatment (CMT); spinal, five regions

Good job!

Education and Training for Patient Self-Management

Technological and other health care treatment and pharmaceutical advancements have made it easier for the average patient to care for him- or herself or for a caregiver to administer treatments formerly provided exclusively by a physician. Of course, this is not something that should be done without guidance, so it is important that the patient or caregiver is taught how to administer treatment properly. Education and training for patient self-management is reported by using codes 98960–98962.

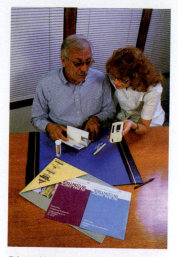

© Larry Mulvehill/Corbis

EXAMPLE

- Teaching a diabetic patient how to self-administer insulin injections.
- Teaching a caregiver how to change a dressing.

Non–Face-to-Face Nonphysician Services

Nurses and allied health care professionals extend the ability of a physician to communicate with patients. When a qualified nonphysician member of the health care team provides an assessment and management service to an established patient via telephone or on-line electronic contact, this service is reported with a code from 98966–98969.

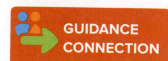

GUIDANCE CONNECTION

Additional explanation can be found in the guidelines within the **Medicine** section, directly under the subhead **Non–Face-to-Face Nonphysician Services,** in your CPT book.

Special Services, Procedures, and Reports

There are times when a health care professional is required to provide a service or write a report that is outside the normal realm of his or her responsibilities or outside of the scope of other codes in the CPT book. In those cases, match the circumstance to one of the descriptions in the Special Services, Procedures, and Reports subsection (codes 99000–99091). Each code identifies a different special situation.

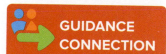

GUIDANCE CONNECTION

Additional explanation can be found in the guidelines within the **Medicine** section, directly under the subhead **Special Services, Procedures and Reports,** in your CPT book.

EXAMPLE

Dr. Jocamona comes into the office to meet Drew Larson on Thanksgiving because Drew was bitten by his nephew's pet snake and Dr. Jocamona has the only antidote for that species. You would use the following code:

99050 Services provided in the office at times other than regularly scheduled office hours, or days when the office is normally closed (e.g., holidays, Saturday or Sunday), in addition to basic service

Qualifying Circumstances for Anesthesia

You should remember the qualifying circumstances codes from Chap. 6, "Anesthesia Coding." The codes are not only shown in the guidelines pages directly in front of the Anesthesia section of the CPT book but also repeated in the Qualifying Circumstances for Anesthesia subsection of the Medicine section, in their numerical order, for your reference. The codes are added to the claim form when an anesthesiologist provides services to a patient with any of four complications:

+ 99100 Extreme age (younger than one year or older than 70).

+ 99116 Utilization of total body hypothermia.

+ 99135 Utilization of controlled hypotension.

+ 99140 Emergency conditions.

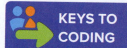

KEYS TO CODING

These qualifying circumstances codes, along with their descriptions, are also repeated in the guidelines pages directly before the **Anesthesia** section of CPT.

Moderate (Conscious) Sedation

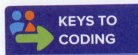
In Chap. 6, "Anesthesia Coding," Chap. 7, "Surgery Coding, Part 1," and Chap. 8, "Surgery Coding, Part 2," you learned the details of moderate (conscious) sedation (codes 99143–99150), used when a patient is given medication to reduce anxiety and possibly cause sleepiness but not unconsciousness. The correct code is determined by the age of the patient, the length of time, and the professional providing the sedation.

These codes may only be used when conscious sedation is not already included in the procedure code. (Remember, when conscious sedation is included in the procedure code, this is indicated with a bull's-eye [⊙] symbol shown to the left of that procedure code.)

Home Health Procedures/Services

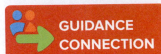
In Chap. 5, "Evaluation and Management Codes, Part 2," we studied codes 99341–99350 for services provided by a physician at the patient's home. However, occasionally a health care professional in your facility *other than the physician* provides services to a patient at his or her home. The person may be a nurse or therapist, for example. For nonphysician clinical professionals, you must use the codes 99500–99602 from the home health procedures/services in the Medicine section.

EXAMPLE

Margaret Sanders, RN, stopped by Terrell Anderson's home to give him an injection of morphine sulfate, 10 mg, IM for pain management. Report Nurse Sanders's visit with 99506 Home visit for intramuscular injections.

Medication Therapy Management Services

When a patient is prescribed multiple medications, especially when ordered by multiple providers, a pharmacist may step in to assess the list and intervene as necessary. The pharmacist can provide insights into potential drug interactions and duplications caused by secondary ingredients.

Medication Therapy Management Services (MTMS) codes can be reported when the following has been documented:

- Review of the pertinent patient history.
- Review of medication profile for prescription, non-prescription, and herbal.
- Specific recommendations for improving patient health outcomes.
- Recommendations to support the patient's treatment compliance.

The codes available to report these services are

99605   Medication therapy management service(s) provided by a pharmacist, individual, face-to-face with patient, with assessment and intervention, if provided; initial 15 minutes, new patient

99606   Medication therapy management service(s) provided by a pharmacist, individual, face-to-face with patient, with assessment and intervention, if provided; initial 15 minutes, established patient

+99607   each additional 15 minutes (List separately in addition to code for primary service)

As stated in the CPT guidelines, these codes should not be used to report the provision of product-specific information at the time the product is provided to the patient or any other routine dispensing-related activities.

Modifiers

There are many codes in the Medicine section of the CPT book that include interpretation and the report along with the particular service or exam, such as neurologic and nonvascular studies. You may remember the details of modifier 26 from Chap. 9, "Radiology Coding," but a little reminding never hurt anyone. Therefore, when you are using any of the codes from the Medicine section and your health care professional is interpreting the findings and writing the report but did not perform the test or procedure, you must append the procedure code with modifier 26.

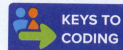

KEYS TO CODING

For physician interpretation and report only, append modifier 26 Professional Component to the correct procedure code from the **Neurology and Neuromuscular** subsection.

> **26 Professional Component:** Certain procedures are a combination of a physician component and a technical component. When the physician component is reported separately, the service may be identified by adding modifier 26 to the usual procedure number.

Chapter Summary

Many services provided by physicians, therapists, chiropractors, and other trained health care professionals deserve to receive reimbursement. The Medicine section contains information about these services. The variety of services included in the Medicine section emphasizes the fact that finding the correct code begins in the alphabetic index and culminates in the numerical listings.

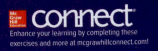

Using Terminology

Match each key term to the appropriate definition.

_____ **1.** LO 11.2 The introduction of a fluid into a blood vessel.

_____ **2.** LO 11.6 The destruction or eradication of tissue.

_____ **3.** LO 11.2 The delivery of an additional drug via an intravenous line over a short period of time.

_____ **4.** LO 11.6 A thin, flexible tube, inserted into a body part, used to inject fluid, to extract fluid, or to keep a passage open.

_____ **5.** LO 11.5 A professional qualified to carry out eye examinations and to prescribe and supply eyeglasses and contact lenses.

_____ **6.** LO 11.2 Compelling a fluid into tissue or cavity.

_____ **7.** LO 11.5 A physician qualified to diagnose and treat eye disease and conditions with drugs, surgery, and corrective measures.

_____ **8.** LO 11.6 An ultrasonic scanning procedure to determine blood flow and pattern.

_____ **9.** LO 11.5 The study of the human ears, nose, and throat (ENT) systems.

_____ **10.** LO 11.1 To make someone resistant to a particular disease by vaccination.

A. Ablation

B. Catheter

C. Duplex scan

D. Immunization

E. Infusion

F. Injection

G. Ophthalmologist

H. Optometrist

I. Otorhinolaryngology

J. Push

Checking Your Understanding

Choose the most appropriate answer for each of the following questions.

1. LO 11.1 When an immunization is given, you will need

   a. one code for administering the immunization.

   b. two codes: one for the administration and one for the drug.

   c. one code for the medication or drug.

   d. one HCPCS Level II code.

2. LO 11.1 Vaccinations and immunizations can be administered

   a. percutaneously.

   b. intradermally.

   c. subcutaneously.

   d. all of these.

3. LO 11.2 When a patient receives infusion therapy via more than one site, code

   a. only the first site.

   b. all appropriate sites.

   c. infusion time instead of number of sites.

   d. only when chemotherapy is infused.

4. LO 11.3 Psychotherapy services are coded first by

   a. location.
   b. relationship of the patient.
   c. type of therapy.
   d. qualifications of the treating health care professional.

5. LO 11.4 Dialysis codes are reported by

   a. the patient's age.
   b. the number of days treated.
   c. the location of treatment (inpatient or outpatient).
   d. all of these.

6. LO 11.5 An optometrist is qualified to

   a. diagnose and treat eye diseases.
   b. supply glasses and contact lenses.
   c. write prescriptions for the treatment of eye diseases.
   d. perform surgery.

7. LO 11.5 An otorhinolaryngologist treats all *except*

   a. ear.
   b. nose.
   c. throat.
   d. stomach.

8. LO 11.6 Duplex scans are

   a. ultrasonic.
   b. noninvasive.
   c. records of blood patterns and flow.
   d. all of these.

9. LO 11.6 Acupuncture codes are determined by

   a. the age of the patient.
   b. the time spent face-to-face with the patient.
   c. whether electrical stimulation was used.
   d. both the time spent face-to-face with the patient and whether electrical stimulation was used.

10. LO 11.6 Chiropractic treatment codes are chosen by

   a. the time spent face-to-face with the patient.
   b. the total number of treatments in a month.
   c. the number of regions treated.
   d. the age of the patient.

Applying Your Knowledge

1. LO 11.1 List eight services reported using codes from the Medicine section. _____
   _____

2. LO 11.1 What are the parts of the process when a patient receives an immunization? _____
   _____

3. LO 11.1 List five ways medication can be administered to the patient. _____
   _____

4. LO 11.2 What are the standard parts included in infusion and injection codes? _____
   _____

5. LO 11.2 How do the CPT guidelines describe an IV or intra-arterial push? _____
   _____

6. LO 11.3 When coding psychotherapy services, what is the first thing a coder must determine in order to assign the
   most appropriate code? _____
   _____

7. LO 11.3 What are the types of psychotherapy? _____
   _____

8. LO 11.4 What determines the correct code for reporting dialysis service? _____
   _____

9. LO 11.4 What physician services are included in the codes during a dialysis month? _____
   _____

10. LO 11.5 What is the difference between an ophthalmologist and an optometrist? _____
    _____

11. LO 11.5 How is the Ophthalmology subsection of CPT divided? _____
    _____

12. LO 11.6 What do the available codes for reporting a cardiac catheterization include? _____
    _____

YOU CODE IT! Practice
Chapter 11: Medicine Coding

Using the techniques described in this chapter, carefully read through the case studies and determine the most accurate Medicine section CPT code(s) and modifier (s), if appropriate, for each case study.

1. Roberta Crushey, a 71-year-old female, has been suffering from bronchitis off and on for 2 years. Dr. Martin has ordered a pulmonary stress test for her. Dr. Martin notes that he wants her CO_2 and O_2 uptake measured during the test as well as an electrocardiogram to be recorded.

   _____

2. David Pinchot, a 61-year-old male, has uncontrolled diabetes and comes into the emergency department complaining of signs of hyperglycemia. Dr. Tennison gives him insulin subcutaneous and IV push to bring his blood sugar down.

   _____

3. After finding relief nowhere else, Felicia Heath, a 39-year-old female, goes to Dr. Kini, an acupuncturist, for treatment of her osteoarthritic knee. Dr. Kini spends 15 minutes with the patient, reviewing history and symptoms and palpating and locating the points to treat, and he inserts the needles and applies electrical stimulation. Felicia is asked to rest. Dr. Kini comes back in about 10 minutes and spends 5 minutes monitoring the patient and restimulating the needles. Ten minutes later, Dr. Kini sees that the pain and swelling in Felicia's knee have reduced, removes the needles, and instructs Felicia on home care measures. Dr. Kini spent a total of 30 minutes in direct contact with Felicia.

   _____

4. Alice Gardener, a 6-year-old female, is brought to Dr. Kaplan by her mother after a referral from the school counselor and her pediatrician. Alice is having difficulties with class work. Mrs. Gardener also tells Dr. Kaplan that Alice has a problem understanding speech in noisy environments. Alice may have a hearing deficiency that has not shown up in hearing tests before, and it may account for her declining work in class. Dr. Kaplan performs a central auditory function evaluation, which takes 1 hour with report.

   _____

5. Jalel Covington, a 15-year-old male, suffered from a severe asthma attack while at the playground. He was rushed to the clinic, where he was given a nebulizer treatment (nonpressurized inhalation).

   _____

6. Rubina Kalish, a 35-year-old female, broke out in a rash, which would not go away. After trying multiple over-the-counter treatments, she went to Dr. Brown, who did a series of 11 allergenic extract scratch tests to see if he could identify an allergen. The tests pointed to an allergy to her new kitten.

   _____

7. Rubina (from the previous scenario) didn't want to give away her new kitten, so Dr. Brown prepared the allergenic extract and began immunotherapy injections. She received the first injection today.

_____

8. Elijah Gersten, a 44-year-old male, is beginning chemotherapy today with the administration of methotrexate, via IV push.

_____

9. Paul Cantrel, a 21-year-old male, is a lifeguard at the beach and came into the emergency clinic with uncontrolled nausea and vomiting. Paul told Dr. Guerva that he was on the beach for 12 hours straight with no breaks because his replacement didn't show up. Dr. Guerva diagnosed him with severe dehydration and ordered 20 minutes of Zofran, IV infusion, and then saline for 4 hours.

_____

10. Zena Eggerton, a 27-year-old female, comes to Patricia Tallman, a licensed massage therapist, as prescribed by Dr. Ulverton. Zena is pregnant and has been suffering from acute lower back pain for over a month. Patricia performs therapeutic massage with effleurage on the left side and kneading on the iliac band, nerve stroking, and light compression on the gluteus.

_____

11. Kenya Kensington, a 7-day-old male, was born prematurely, and Dr. Valentine is concerned about Kenya's heart. He performs a combined right heart catheterization and transseptal left heart catheterization through the intact septum, in order to measure the blood gases and record Kenya's intracardiac pressure. Dr. Valentine provides conscious sedation to Kenya before beginning the procedure.

_____

12. Darlene Conner, a 6-year-old female, comes to see Dr. Beech for an evaluation of her cochlear implant. Dr. Beech reprograms the implant to improve Darlene's reception.

_____

13. Rasheem Overton, a 66-year-old male, came to see Dr. Macinaw, his ophthalmologist, for an annual checkup of his eyes. Dr. Macinaw does a general evaluation of Rasheem's complete visual system.

_____

14. Grant Johnston, a 55-year-old male, came to see Dr. Hawkins because he was having chest pain. Dr. Hawkins performed a routine ECG with 15 leads. After talking with Grant and reviewing the ECG results, Dr. Hawkins determined that Grant was having a bout of indigestion.

_____

15. Marlene Smith, a 20-year-old female, is a professional gymnast who pulled a muscle in her shoulder. Today, Dr. Tunner measured her range of motion in the shoulder to confirm that the area has healed completely. Dr. Tunner then wrote and signed the report.

_____

YOU CODE IT! Application
Chapter 11: Medicine Coding

The following exercises provide practice in the application of abstracting the physicians' notes and learning to work with SOAP notes from our health care facility, Cipher, Victors & Associates. These case studies (SOAP notes) are modeled on real patient encounters. Using the techniques described in this chapter, carefully read through the case studies and determine the most accurate Medicine section CPT code(s) and modifier(s), if appropriate, for each case study.

CIPHER, VICTORS & ASSOCIATES
A Complete Health Care Facility
234 MAIN STREET • ANYTOWN, FL 32711 • 407-555-1234

PATIENT: NETTLES, DUANE
ACCOUNT/EHR #:   NETTDU001
DATE: 10/13/18

Attending Physician: James I. Cipher, MD

S: This new Pt is a 35-year-old male who works in a mattress factory. He states that he has had a piercing ringing sound in his left ear that began 6 months ago. He noticed the ringing sound in his ear upon awakening one morning, and it remains a considerable annoyance all day long, interfering with his ability to enjoy television, movies, and even conversation. Pt states he has trouble sleeping, as well.

O: Pt taken to testing suite for a bilateral tinnitus assessment: pitch (frequency) matching; loudness matching; and masking procedures are included. Findings of the testing indicate a positive determination of tinnitus. Patient is informed of the outcome, along with the recommendations for remediation therapy.

A: Acute tinnitus

P: Follow-up with masking therapy treatment plan

James I. Cipher, MD

JIC/mg   D: 10/13/18 09:50:16   T: 10/15/18 12:55:01

Determine the most accurate Medicine section CPT code(s) and modifier(s), if appropriate.

_____

_____

_____

CIPHER, VICTORS & ASSOCIATES
A Complete Health Care Facility
234 MAIN STREET • ANYTOWN, FL 32711 • 407-555-1234

PATIENT: MCDANIEL, CICI
ACCOUNT/EHR #:   MCDACI001
DATE: 10/21/18

Attending Physician: Sigmund Freund, MD

Pt is a 16-year-old female who was recently released from a residential drug rehabilitation program and has moved back into the family home. Her therapy plan calls for a combination of individual counseling and family psychotherapy to help all members of the household understand the circumstances of her addiction and how to help her maintain a healthy, drug-free lifestyle.

   Today is the first family psychotherapy session. Present are Helen McDaniel, the patient's mother; Raul Esponoza, the patient's stepbrother; Jake Esponoza, the patient's stepfather; and Lucy McDaniel, the patient's paternal grandmother. The patient, Cici McDaniel, is also present.

   The group talks openly and shows genuine concern for the patient. The session lasts 50 minutes.

P: 1. Individual session: scheduled next Monday
   2. Next family session: 2 weeks

_____

Sigmund Freund, MD

SF/mg   D: 10/21/18 09:50:16   T: 10/25/18 12:55:01

Determine the most accurate Medicine section CPT code(s) and modifier(s), if appropriate.

_____

_____

_____

CIPHER, VICTORS & ASSOCIATES
A Complete Health Care Facility
234 MAIN STREET • ANYTOWN, FL 32711 • 407-555-1234

PATIENT: ROSSEN, EDWARD
ACCOUNT/EHR #:   ROSSED001
DATE: 09/30/18

Attending Physician: Laverne Aspiras, MD

This new Pt is a 9-year-old male with ESRD, here for dialysis, monitoring, assessment, and counseling with parents.

PROCEDURE: Dialysis services for month of September—30 days

_____

Laverne Aspiras, MD

LA/mg   D: 09/30/18 09:50:16   T: 09/30/18 12:55:01

Determine the most accurate Medicine section CPT code(s) and modifier(s), if appropriate.

_____

_____

_____

CIPHER, VICTORS & ASSOCIATES
A Complete Health Care Facility
234 MAIN STREET • ANYTOWN, FL 32711 • 407-555-1234

PATIENT: LUELLEN, JOYCE
ACCOUNT/EHR #:   LUELJO001
DATE: 10/07/18

Attending Physician: Walter P. Henricks, DC
Referring Physician: Valerie Victors, MD

This new Pt is a 36-year-old female who was in a car accident 1 month ago. She is diagnosed with whiplash.

    She presents today for chiropractic manipulative treatment of her cervical spine.

    Treatment plan calls for one treatment a week for 2 months, at which point her status will be reevaluated.

_____

Walter P. Henricks, DC

WPH/mg   D: 10/07/18 09:50:16   T: 10/09/18 12:55:01

Determine the most accurate Medicine section CPT code(s) and modifier(s), if appropriate.

_____

_____

_____

CIPHER, VICTORS & ASSOCIATES
A Complete Health Care Facility
234 MAIN STREET • ANYTOWN, FL 32711 • 407-555-1234

PATIENT: SLATON, AMBER
ACCOUNT/EHR #:   SLATAM001
DATE: 10/15/18

Attending Physician: Rhonda E. Beardall, MD
Referring Physician: James I. Cipher, MD

Pt is a 75-year-old female who recently had a stroke. She is here on referral from Dr. Cipher for an assessment of her aphasia.
   Assessment of expressive and receptive speech and language function: language comprehension, speech production ability, reading, spelling, writing, using Boston Diagnostic Aphasia Examination.

Interpretation and report to follow.

Total time: 60 minutes

_____

Rhonda E. Beardall, MD

REB/mg   D: 10/15/18 09:50:16   T: 10/17/18 12:55:01

Determine the most accurate Medicine section CPT code(s) and modifier(s), if appropriate.

_____

_____

_____

12

CATEGORY II AND CATEGORY III CODING

Learning Outcomes *After completing this chapter, the student should be able to:*

LO 12.1 Interpret the guidelines for using Category II codes.

LO 12.2 Obtain the most current information about Category II codes.

LO 12.3 Correctly use Category II code modifiers.

LO 12.4 Utilize the details on quality reporting for physician bonus payments.

LO 12.5 Identify the guidelines for using Category III codes.

LO 12.6 Correctly follow notational instructions with Category III codes.

Key Terms

Category I codes

Category II codes

Category III codes

Customary clinical documentation

Experimental

Intervention

Medical exclusion criteria

Patient population

Performance measure

Unlisted codes

Category II codes are used for statistical purposes and to track and measure performance and the quality of care in a health care facility. They are not used as part of the reimbursement process and may not be used in substitution for a **Category I codes** (codes from the main text of the CPT book). Category II codes are optional, so you may never use them. However, they are important to the growth of the health information management industry.

The Physician Quality Reporting System (PQRS), signed into law on December 20, 2006, by the president as a part of the Tax Relief and Health Care Act of 2006 (TRHCA), instructs eligible professionals to report on designated sets of quality measures using CPT Category II codes.

Category III codes offer the opportunity to collect detailed information on the use of new technological advancements, services, and procedures at their entry point into health care practices throughout the United States. Each code identifies an innovative procedure that is at the forefront of the health care industry but not yet widely used or accepted as a standard of care. It is why the codes in this section of the CPT book are considered temporary.

LO 12.1 Category II Codes

Category II codes are listed directly after the Medicine section of the CPT book. The listing is used in conjunction with the web-based "Alphabetic Index of Performance Measure by Clinical Condition or Topic" available from the American Medical Association (AMA) website (www.ama-assn .org/go/cpt).

While the number of Category II codes is small, the codes identify services and test results that physicians should provide to their patients, that is, specific services that have been proved to be connected to quality patient care.

Each code's description explains clinical fundamentals (such as vital signs), lab test results, patient education, or other facets that might be provided within a typical office visit. However, individually, these component services do not have any billable value and, therefore, are not assigned a code from Category I CPT codes. Assigning Category II codes simply is a way for the industry and the government to specifically calculate how often these services are being provided.

The Centers for Medicare and Medicaid Services (CMS), in response to the TRHCA's mandate for a physician quality reporting system, created the PQRS. This program provides for a bonus payment to those eligible professionals who meet the criteria for successful reporting.

Category II codes have five characters: four numbers followed by the letter *F*.

> ## EXAMPLE
>
> 0001F Heart failure assessed
> 3006F Chest x-ray results documented and reviewed

They are compiled into categories:

- Composite measures.
- Patient management.
- Patient history.
- Patient examination.
- Diagnostic/screening processes or results.
- Therapeutic, preventive, or other interventions.
- Follow-up or other outcomes.
- Patient safety.
- Structural measures.

These categories were determined by content from **customary clinical documentation** formatting.

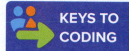

LO 12.2 Alphabetic Measure Index of Performance Measures

As a coding specialist, you must refer to the additional data included in the chart in the web-based document "Alphabetic Measure Index of **Performance Measures** by Clinical Type." The chart shows specific details regarding the following:

- Complete explanation of what is being measured within the component.
- Characteristics of patients that would make them eligible for this report.
- Factors that would automatically include or exclude a particular patient.

Let's look at one example, shown in Figure 12-1.

Right after the phrase "Avoidance of (Inappropriate) Antibiotic Treatment in Adults with Acute Bronchitis[2]," you will notice a superscript number 2. It directs you to footnote 2, which references the National Committee on Quality Assurance (NCQA), Health Employer Data Information Set (HEDIS), www.ncqa.org.

Other items in the index show additional references:

Superscript number 1 refers to the Physician Consortium for Performance Improvement (PCPI), www.physicianconsortium.org.

Superscript number 3 refers to the Joint Commission, ORYX Initiative Performance Measures, www.jointcommission.org/PerformanceMeasurement.

Superscript number 4 refers to National Diabetes Quality Improvement Alliance (NDQIA) performance measures, www.nationaldiabetesalliance.org. Superscript numbers 5 and 6 have been added to identify measures from the Physician Consortium and NCQA, as well as the Society of Thoracic Surgeons and the National Quality Forum.

customary clinical documentation
The usual contents of the notes or reports written by the provider after a health care encounter.

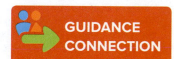

performance measure
Criteria for gathering specific data about actions to study.

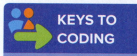

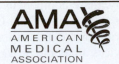

Acute Bronchitis (A-BRONCH)		
Brief Description of Performance Measure and Source and Reporting Instructions	**CPT Category II Code(s)**	**Code Descriptor(s)**
Avoidance of (Inappropriate) Antibiotic Treatment in Adults with Acute Bronchitis[2] To assess the percentage of adults 18–64 years of age with a diagnosis of acute bronchitis who were not dispensed an antibiotic prescription on or within 3 days after the date of service. **Numerator:** Patients who were dispensed an antibiotic prescription on or three days after the episode date. **Denominator:** All patients aged 18 – 64 years of age with a diagnosis of acute bronchitis. **Exclusion(s):** Documentation of medical reasons for prescribing or dispensing an antibiotic **Percentage** of adults 18–64 years of age with a diagnosis of acute bronchitis who were not dispensed an antibiotic prescription on or 3 days after the episode date. **Reporting Instructions:** Report one of these codes for a patient identified in the eligible population. For patient with appropriate medical exclusion criteria report 4120F with modifier 1P. There are no exclusions for 4124F.	4120F 4124F	Antibiotic prescribed or dispensed Antibiotic neither prescribed nor dispensed

Footnotes
[1] Physician Consortium for Performance Improvement, www.physicianconsortium.org
[2] National Committee on Quality Assurance (NCQA), Health Employer Data Information Set (HEDIS®), www.ncqa.org
[3] Joint Commission on Accreditation of Healthcare Organizations (JCAHO), ORYX Initiative Performance Measures, www.jcaho.org/pms
[4] National Diabetes Quality Improvement Alliance (NDQIA), www.nationaldiabetesalliance.org
[5] Joint measure from The Physician Consortium for Performance Improvement, www.physicianconsortium.org and National Committee on Quality Assurance (NCQA), www.ncqa.org
[6] The Society of Thoracic Surgeons, http://www.sts.org, National Quality Forum, http://www.qualityforum.org
[7] Ingenix, www.ingenix.com
[8] American Academy of Neurology, www.aan.com/go/practice/quality/measurements or quality@aan.com

FIGURE 12-1 Performance Measure: Acute Bronchitis

patient population
A group with common traits among patients using the same health care facility or health care provider.

intervention
Action taken to change or prevent something that is happening, most often to stop or prevent something undesirable.

Superscript number 5 refers to a joint measure of the PCPI and the NCQA.

Superscript number 6 references a study by the Society of Thoracic Surgeons and the National Quality Forum.

Superscript number 7 references Ingenix.

Superscript number 8 refers to the American Academy of Neurology.

Many clinical measurement sets focus on specific **patient populations,** such as those 18 years of age or older or patients diagnosed with coronary artery disease (CAD). The reason for this is the large amount of scientific evidence that exists to indicate that a particular **intervention** is important to the health or continued health of that type of patient.

EXAMPLE

- The Tobacco Use measurement set covers patients aged 18 years and older.

- The Adult Influenza Immunization measurement set focuses on patients 50 years and older.

Dr. Pinnati's practice is located near a large university. Most of his patients are in their twenties. Statistically, 75% of his established patients (his patient population) are between the ages of 18 and 34.

Dr. Seng's practice is located in a neighborhood where most of the residents have been living for 20 years or more. About 70% of Dr. Seng's patient population is aged 50 and older.

Therefore, in terms of Category II coding, it would make sense for Dr. Pinnati's coding specialist to include data related to the tobacco use performance measurement and for Dr. Seng's coding specialist to include data about patient flu shots. The guidelines recommend that health care facilities do this—pick the individual measurement set(s) that make sense for their circumstances. No one wants anyone wasting time. That is not productive.

The health care professional will be reimbursed for the evaluation and discussion with the patient, most often by reporting an evaluation and management (E/M) code. However, an E/M code does not provide the specific details in a manner that will enable statistical research. This is the reason for Category II codes—to enable calculation and evaluation of individual health care services.

LO 12.3 Category II Modifiers

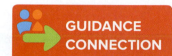

GUIDANCE CONNECTION

Additional explanation can be found in the guidelines in the **Category II Codes** section, subheading **Modifiers,** in your CPT book.

Performance measurement modifiers are used *only* with Category II codes and explain that the specific service indicated by the code was *not* actually provided. You might look at this as coding a service that was not performed, and you would be correct. In such cases, the research wants to quantify how often the physician recommends a service, even if the patient does not accept the recommendation. When you think about it, how else can researchers learn these facts? They may know if a patient agrees to smoking-cessation therapy, for example, by tracking the prescription for the medication. However, if the patient refuses the physician's urging to quit, without these codes the information is restricted to the patient's chart.

The fact that the physician made the recommendation, along with the reasons the service might not be performed, must be documented. The reasons may be medical circumstances or personal issues vocalized by the patient and will be reported by you using one of the modifiers in this section.

Category II code modifiers include the following:

- **1P.** Performance measure exclusion modifier due to medical reasons.
  Includes
  - Not indicated (absences of organ/limb, already received/preformed, other).
  - Contraindicated (patient allergic history, potential adverse drug interaction, other).
  - Other medical reasons.

- **2P.** Performance measure exclusion modifier due to patient reasons.
  Includes
  - Patient declined.
  - Economic, social, or religious reasons.
  - Other patient reasons.

- **3P.** Performance measure exclusion modifier due to system reasons.

  Includes
  - Resources to perform the services not available.
  - Insurance coverage/payor-related limitations.
  - Other reasons attributable to health care delivery system.

- **8P.** Performance measure reporting modifier—action not performed, reason not otherwise specified.

Certain Category II codes are exempt from these modifiers. In such cases, a notation is included below the code description.

Take a look at the following code:

4015F Persistent asthma, preferred long term control medication or an acceptable alternative treatment, prescribed (Asthma)[1]

(Note: There are no medical exclusion criteria.)

(Do not report modifier 1P with 4015F.)

(To report patient reasons for not prescribing, use modifier 2P.)

> **medical exclusion criteria**
> Medical reasons a patient's data should *not* be reported with a certain code.

You can see that the CPT book, once again, reminds you of the guidelines, as they relate to the use of these modifiers.

LET'S CODE IT! SCENARIO

Candace Sheridan, a 69-year-old female, comes to see Dr. Devin for her annual checkup. After the examination, Dr. Devin discusses smoking. He offers Candace, a smoker for over 20 years, a prescription for a nicotine patch to help her quit. She thanks him but says no.

Let's Code It!

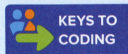

KEYS TO CODING

The superscript number 1 shown after the word (*Asthma*) in the description of code 4015F refers to the footnote showing the sponsoring organization of the study.

Of course, you know that you will use an E/M code for the encounter, along with any specific tests or exams that Dr. Devin ordered as a part of Candace's annual physical to make certain Dr. Devin is properly reimbursed for his work. If Candace had accepted his offer for the prescription, a diagnosis code for long-term tobacco use could support the writing of the prescription. However, there is no place in the standard reporting codes of the CPT book to document that Dr. Devin counseled her about her smoking and offered pharmacologic therapy to a patient who is a known tobacco user, because she turned him down. This is an excellent example of the benefits of Category II codes. Turn to the Category II code section.

Under the heading *Patient History,* find the code that identifies this patient as a current tobacco user (smoker). You will see code

1034F Current tobacco smoker (CAD, CAP, COPD, PV)[1] (DM)[4]

(Note: PV stands for Preventive.)

You know from the notes that Dr. Devin talked with her about her smoking and offered Candace a prescription, so that would lead us to

4000F Tobacco use cessation intervention, counseling (COPD, CAP, CAD)[1](DM)[4](PV)[2]

4001F Tobacco use cessation intervention, pharmacologic therapy (COPD, CAD, CAP, PV)[1] (DM)[4](PV)[2]

Next, you must reference the Performance Measure Index and look through the qualifiers for these codes. Look at this specific measure, shown in Figure 12-2.

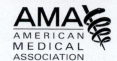

Preventive Care & Screening (PV) <u>Back to Top</u>		
Brief Description of Performance Measure & Source and Reporting Instructions	**CPT Category II Code(s)**	**Code Descriptor(s)**
or more times **Numerator:** Patients who were queried about tobacco use one or more times **Denominator:** All patients aged > 18 years at the beginning of the two-year measurement period **Percentage** of patients queried about tobacco use one or more times during the two-year measurement period **Reporting Instructions:** When reporting 1000F, it is required to report 1034F, and/or 1035F, or 1036F. There are no performance exclusions for this measure; modifiers 1P, 2P and 3P may not be used.	1035F 1036F	Current smokeless tobacco user (*eg*, chew, snuff) Current tobacco non-user
Tobacco Use Intervention[1] Whether or not patient identified as a tobacco user received cessation intervention **Numerator:** Patients identified as tobacco users who received cessation intervention **Denominator:** All patients > 18 years at the beginning of the two-year measurement period identified as tobacco users **Percentage** of patients identified as tobacco users who received cessation intervention during the two year measurement period **Reporting Instructions:** Report 1034F, 1035F or 1036F for each patient. If patient is a tobacco user (1034F or 1035F) and received cessation intervention, report 4000F or 4001F or both. There are no performance exclusions for this measure; modifiers 1P, 2P and 3P may not be used.	4000F 4001F **Denominator Codes:** 1034F 1035F 1036F	Tobacco use cessation intervention, counseling Tobacco use cessation intervention, pharmacologic therapy Current tobacco smoker Current smokeless tobacco user (*eg*, chew, snuff) Current tobacco non-user
Advising Smokers to Quit[2] To assess the percentage of patients who have received advice to quit smoking from a doctor or other health provider	1034F	Current tobacco smoker

Footnotes
[1] Physician Consortium for Performance Improvement, <u>www.physicianconsortium.org</u>
[2] National Committee on Quality Assurance (NCQA), Health Employer Data Information Set (HEDIS®), <u>www.ncqa.org</u>
[3] Joint Commission on Accreditation of Healthcare Organizations (JCAHO), ORYX Initiative Performance Measures, <u>www.jcaho.org/pms</u>
[4] National Diabetes Quality Improvement Alliance (NDQIA), <u>www.nationaldiabetesalliance.org</u>
[5] Joint measure from The Physician Consortium for Performance Improvement, www.physicianconsortium.org and National Committee on Quality Assurance (NCQA), <u>www.ncqa.org</u>
[6] The Society of Thoracic Surgeons, <u>http://www.sts.org</u>, National Quality Forum, <u>http://www.qualityforum.org</u>
[7] Ingenix, <u>www.ingenix.com</u>
[8] American Academy of Neurology, <u>www.aan.com/go/practice/quality/measurements</u> or <u>quality@aan.com</u>

CPT is a registered trademark of the American Medical Association
Copyright 2009 American Medical Association All rights reserved
Last Updated July 2, 2010

FIGURE 12-2 Preventive Care and Screening: Tobacco Use Intervention

You will see that the chart shows

Tobacco Use Intervention[1]—whether or not patient identified as a tobacco user received cessation intervention

Numerator: Patients identified as tobacco users who received cessation intervention

Denominator: All patients >18 years at the beginning of the two-year measurement period identified as tobacco users

Percentage of patients identified as tobacco users who received cessation intervention during the two-year measurement period

Reporting Instructions: Report 1034F, 1035F, or 1036F for each patient. If patient is a tobacco user (1034F or 1035F) and received cessation intervention, report 4000F or 4001F or both.

There are no exclusions for this measure; modifiers 1P, 2P, and 3P may not be used.

This is in direct agreement with the physician's notes, and there is nothing in the patient's chart that would exclude her from the measurement set. There is just one more step.

You'll remember that Category II codes require a modifier if the service was not, in fact, provided. The notes indicate that the patient *says no* to the pharmacologic therapy (the prescription). Let's go to the list in the beginning of the Category II section and review the definitions of the modifiers. You see that the modifier 2P matches perfectly.

2P Performance measure exclusion modifier due to patient reasons; including patient declined

But wait a minute; look back at the performance measure details (in Figure 12-2). It clearly states that modifiers may not be used. This means that you cannot report 4001F because the pharmacologic therapy was not provided (she said no) and 4001F-2P is not permitted. Therefore, the accurate way to report this is with 4000F. The physician did provide counseling.

So your report for this encounter includes the Category II codes 1034F and 4000F.

LO 12.4 Physician Quality Reporting System (PQRS)

A health care provider who participates in the PQRS program may receive bonus monies when meeting all of the criteria. CMS has outlined four steps to properly report quality measurement data:

1. Eligible clinicians must identify Medicare-covered patients who are qualified for one or more reportable quality measures.
2. The provider must document the fulfillment of the measure or measures in the notes for the encounter.
3. Assign the appropriate Category II codes to accurately report the documented service, in addition to the proper CPT Category I codes for the visit. If appropriate Category II codes are not available, HCPCS Level II G codes may be used. (More about G codes appears in Chap. 13 of this textbook.)
4. Submit the claim form with the appropriate diagnosis and procedure codes for normal billing plus the performance measurement codes with a charge of $0.00 (no more than $1.00).

The bonus payments are based on the "successful reporting" of designated quality data. CMS defines the term "successful reporting" as the submission of correctly presented data for at least 80% of the eligible cases for at least three quality measures.

This percentage is evaluated for each provider, based on the national provider identifier (NPI) shown on each submitted Medicare Part B claim.

Eligible individual providers who successfully submit PQRS quality measures data will qualify to earn an incentive payment equal to 0.5% of their total estimated Medicare Part B Physician Fee Schedule (PFS) allowed charges for professional services furnished during that same reporting period. While 0.5% may seem like a small amount, 0.5% of $1 million means the physician is getting a bonus of $5,000.

Each year, the PQRS quality measures must

- Be adopted by a consensus organization such as the National Quality Forum (NQF).
- Include measures that have been submitted by a physician specialty.
- Be identified by CMS as having used a consensus-based process for development.
- Include structural measures, such as the use of electronic health records and electronic prescribing technology.

Proposed quality measures for the following year are published in the *Federal Register* in August, with the final set published by November of the previous year.

Category II codes are updated twice each year with new codes, deletions, and other changes on January 1 and June 1. The most current listing, along with guidelines, can be found at www.ama-assn.org/go/cpt.

LO 12.5 Category III Codes

Newspapers and television are always mentioning new drugs, cures, and procedures that allow a longer, better quality of life than ever before. Whether a new use for a laser or the latest surgical method, it must go through continued evaluation in the health care industry before becoming an accepted component of the standard of care.

Category III codes are the internship for potential Category I codes (the codes in the main text of the CPT book). New procedures and services are assigned a Category III code so that actual usage can be accurately measured. They are placed in this section of the CPT book and given a code that has five characters: four numbers followed by the letter *T* (for *temporary*) in the fifth position.

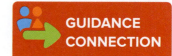

GUIDANCE CONNECTION

Additional explanation can be found in the guidelines directly under the section heading **Category III Codes** in your CPT book.

EXAMPLE

0085T Breath test for heart transplant rejection
0198T Measurement of ocular blood flow by repetitive intraocular pressure sampling, with interpretation and report

The use of Category III codes is mandatory, as appropriate, according to the physician's notes. If there aren't any accurate Category I codes in the CPT book to report the physician's services, you must check the Category III section for an appropriate code *before* you are permitted to use a Category I **unlisted code.** The good news is that the CPT book will continue to help you. Category III codes are included in the alphabetic index. In addition, there are notations throughout the main text (numerical) listings that will direct you to a Category III code, if applicable.

unlisted codes
Codes shown at the end of each subsection of the CPT used as a catch-all for any procedure not represented by an existing code.

EXAMPLE

In the Medicine section of the CPT book, beneath code 95930, you will see a notation:

(For screening of visual acuity using automated visual evoked potential devices, use 0333T)

Allen Jamison, a 58-year-old male, came into the office so that Dr. Goodman could evaluate how well his cardioverter-defibrillator device was working and program this single lead implanted device to ensure optimal values. Dr. Goodman analyzed the system while asking Allen questions about how he was feeling.

Let's Code It!

The notes document that Dr. Goodman evaluated the functioning of the system while Allen was in his office and programmed it to ensure optimal function. Turn to the alphabetic index and find

Evaluation

Implantable Cardiovascular-Defibrillator Device

    Interrogation. 0327T, 93289

    Programming. 0328T, 93282-93284

Let's compare the complete code descriptions to find which accurately reports what Dr. Goodman did for Allen.

0328T   Programming device evaluation (in person) with iterative adjustment of the implantable device to test the function of the device and select optimal permanent programmed values with analysis, implantable subcutaneous lead defibrillator system

93282   Programming device evaluation (in person) with iterative adjustment of the implantable device to test the function of the device and select optimal permanent programmed values with analysis, review and report by a physician or other qualified health care professional; single lead implantable cardioverter-defibrillator system

93283   Programming device evaluation (in person) with iterative adjustment of the implantable device to test the function of the device and select optimal permanent programmed values with analysis, review and report by a physician or other qualified health care professional; dual lead implantable cardioverter-defibrillator system

93284   Programming device evaluation (in person) with iterative adjustment of the implantable device to test the function of the device and select optimal permanent programmed values with analysis, review and report by a physician or other qualified health care professional; multiple lead implantable cardioverter-defibrillator system

You are just learning, so the differences between these code descriptions have been highlighted. All of the other words are the same. Which description matches Dr. Goodman's notes most accurately? This should lead you to report code 93282. Good job!

LO 12.6 Category III Notations

Once a procedure or service has been accepted by health care professionals and is found to be effective, safe, and beneficial in clinical practice, the code will be "promoted" to a Category I code. At that time, the T code is deleted, and the procedure is given a five-digit code and placed in the appropriate section of the main text of the CPT book. A notation is placed in the Category III section that states the T code has been deleted and refers you to the new five-digit code.

> ### EXAMPLE
>
> (0162T has been deleted. To report, see 95980-95982)

As a new coder, this will not affect you very much. Such notations will be helpful once you have been coding for a while in a particular health care facility that might use such codes frequently. If a code used in your office changes, you need the notation to direct you to the new code. Remember, your claim form may be rejected or denied if it includes a deleted code.

Similar to notations in the main text of CPT, you may see the direction to use a specific Category III code along with a CPT code. This will help you properly report the addition of new technology being used along with a standard procedure.

> ### EXAMPLE
>
> +0164T Removal of total disc arthroplasty, anterior approach, lumbar, each additional interspace
> (Use 0164T in conjunction with 22865.)

Notations in this section will also highlight mutually exclusive codes—those codes that cannot be reported on the same claim form as another.

> ### EXAMPLE
>
> 0230T Injection(s), anesthetic agent and/or steroid, transforaminal epidural, with ultrasound guidance, lumbar or sacral; single level
> (Do not report 0228T–0231T in conjunction with 76942, 76998, 76999)

Sometimes, the notation explains that, if an alternative to the code description is performed, another code is correct.

> ### EXAMPLE
>
> 0201T Percutaneous sacral augmentation (sacroplasty), bilateral injections, including the use of a balloon or mechanical device, when used, 2 or more needles
> (If bone biopsy is performed, see 20220, 20225)

You will also find that extensive guidelines are included within the section, just as you saw in CPT. These paragraphs, such as the guidelines provided under the subheading *Remote Real-Time Interactive Videoconferenced Critical Care Services* guideline paragraph above code 0188T will help you to report these codes correctly.

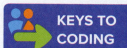

KEYS TO CODING

Use a Category III code when both the following conditions are true:

1. A regular CPT code *is not* appropriate.
2. A Category III code *is* appropriate.

Use an unlisted code when both of these conditions are true:

1. A regular CPT code *is not* appropriate.
2. A Category III code *is not* appropriate.

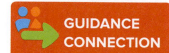

GUIDANCE CONNECTION

Additional explanation can be found in the guidelines directly under the section heading **Category III Codes** in your CPT book.

It is important that you are aware of the fact that Category III codes represent up-and-coming technology. Because of this, the third-party payers from whom you seek reimbursement may consider some services **experimental.** When you work in a health care facility that uses any procedures or services identified by a Category III code, it is critical that you determine the carrier's rules and coverage with regard to the treatment or test. Should the carrier exclude it and refuse to pay, the patient and your office are better off knowing it as soon as possible. You may be able to petition the payer, convince them of the medical necessity and the cost efficiency of the new technology, and receive an approval after all. Waiting for the denial notice is not the efficient way to handle the situation. That is also not respectful to the patient.

A particular Category III code, once assigned, is reserved for 5 years, whether the code is upgraded to a Category I code or deleted altogether. It allows for the fact that certain technologies or procedures may take time to find acceptance and it prevents confusion.

YOU CODE IT! CASE STUDY

Henry Battsmann, a 47-year-old male, had a heart transplant 2 months ago. He has been unwell, so Dr. Rufani performs a breath test for heart transplant rejection. This test is experimental, but it is noninvasive.

You Code It!

Go through the steps of coding and determine the code(s) that should be reported for this test provided by Dr. Rufani to Henry Battsmann.

Step 1: Read the case completely.

Step 2: Abstract the notes: Which key words can you identify relating to the procedures performed?

_____

Step 3: Query the provider, if necessary.

Step 4: Diagnosis: Heart transplant follow-up.

Step 5: Code the procedure(s).

_____

Step 6: Link the procedure codes to at least one diagnosis code.

Step 7: Back code to double-check your choices.

Answer:

Did you determine the correct code?

0085T Breath test for heart transplant rejection

Good work!

Chapter Summary

Category III codes, like Category II codes, are updated twice a year. The latest adjustments are released on January 1 and June 1. So if you are working as a coding specialist for a health care facility that uses any Category III codes, you will be responsible for staying on top of the changes. The most current listing, along with guidelines, can be found at www.ama-assn.org/go/cpt.

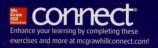
Enhance your learning by completing these exercises and more at mcgrawhillconnect.com!

Using Terminology

Match each key term to the appropriate definition.

_____ 1. LO 12.1/12.2/12.3 Codes for performance measurement and tracking.

_____ 2. LO 12.3 Medical reasons a patient's data should *not* be reported with a certain code.

_____ 3. LO 12.5 Codes shown at the end of each subsection of the CPT used as a catch-all for any procedure not represented by an existing code.

_____ 4. LO 12.2 Action taken to change or prevent something that is happening; most often to stop or prevent something undesirable.

_____ 5. LO 12.1 The usual contents of the notes or reports written by the provider after a health care encounter.

_____ 6. LO 12.2 Criteria for gathering specific data about actions to study.

_____ 7. LO 12.1 The codes listed in the main text of the CPT book, also known as CPT codes.

_____ 8. LO 12.1/12.5/12.6 Codes for emerging technology.

_____ 9. LO 12.6 A procedure or treatment that has not yet been accepted by the health care industry as the standard of care.

_____ 10. LO 12.2 A group with common traits among patients using the same health care facility or health care provider.

A. Category I codes
B. Category II codes
C. Category III codes
D. Customary clinical documentation
E. Experimental
F. Intervention
G. Medical exclusion criteria
H. Patient population
I. Performance measure
J. Unlisted codes

Checking Your Understanding

Choose the most appropriate answer for each of the following questions.

1. LO 12.1/12.5 Category I codes are also known as

   a. temporary codes.
   b. experimental codes.
   c. CPT codes.
   d. modifiers.

2. LO 12.1 Category II codes are used for reporting

   a. emerging technology.
   b. experimental procedures.
   c. performance measurement.
   d. neurologic procedures.

3. LO 12.1/12.2 When coding Category II codes, you have to also reference

   a. performance measures.
   b. *Merck Manual.*
   c. *Physicians' Desk Reference.*
   d. CMS conditions of participation.

4. LO 12.3 The modifiers 1P and 2P are used with

   a. CPT codes.

   b. Category II codes.

   c. Category III codes.

   d. all of these.

5. LO 12.1 An example of a Category II code is

   a. 11111.

   b. 1111T.

   c. 1111F.

   d. H1111.

6. LO 12.5 Category III codes should be used

   a. only if no unlisted codes are appropriate.

   b. only if no Category I codes are appropriate.

   c. first.

   d. only if no Category II codes are appropriate.

7. LO 12.5 An unlisted code should only be used when

   a. an accurate Category I code is not available.

   b. an accurate Category III code is not available.

   c. an accurate Category I code is not available *and* an accurate Category III code is not available.

   d. an accurate Category I code is not available *or* an accurate Category III code is not available.

8. LO 12.5/12.6 Category III codes are updated

   a. once a year.

   b. twice a year.

   c. once every 2 years.

   d. quarterly.

9. LO 12.1 The use of Category II codes is

   a. optional.

   b. mandatory for reimbursement.

   c. determined by each individual third-party payer.

   d. none of these.

10. LO 12.1/12.5 Coding for reimbursement properly may include all *except*

   a. CPT codes.

   b. Category II codes.

   c. Category III codes.

   d. HCPCS Level II codes.

Applying Your Knowledge

1. LO 12.1/12.2/12.5 Differentiate between Category I codes, Category II codes, and Category III codes. _____

   _____

2. LO 12.1/12.2 Explain what a Category II code is. Where are they located in the CPT book, and what does each Category II code's description explain? _____

   _____

3. LO 12.2 Why is the Alphabetic Measure Index of Performance Measures important? _____

   _____

4. LO 12.6 How often are the Category II codes updated, and when are the adjustments released? _____

   _____

5. LO 12.1 What letter denotes a Category II code? _____

   _____

6. LO 12.3 List the Category II modifiers, and include what each modifier identifies. _____

   _____

7. LO 12.4 What does PQRS stand for? What are the steps to properly report quality measurement data? _____

   _____

8. LO 12.5 What are Category III codes, and are they required? _____

   _____

9. LO 12.6 What is a Category III notation? _____

   _____

10. LO 12.5/12.6 Where can you find the most current listing, along with the guidelines, for Category III codes? _____

    _____

Using the techniques described in this chapter, carefully read through the case studies and determine the most accurate Category II or Category III code(s) and modifier(s), if appropriate, for each case study.

1. Renya Ryan, a 68-year-old female, has a history of back pain. Renya comes to see Dr. Mendelsohn today for a back pain and function assessment.

   _____

2. Arlene Register, a 25-year-old female, came for her first prenatal care visit. She enrolled in a managed care organization just 10 days before she conceived. She is now 2 months pregnant.

   _____

3. Ellis Fenton, a 16-year-old male, has a history of wheezing and respiratory infections, so Dr. Zelna performs an asthma risk assessment.

   _____

4. Ann Hovenarian, a 69-year-old female, has been diagnosed with Parkinson disease, stage 3. Dr. Smyth counseled Ann's caregiver about various safety issues dealing with this stage of the disease.

   _____

5. Bernard Hodges, a 61-year-old male, had an artificial heart implanted 3 months ago. Today, Dr. Yamagucci replaced the thoracic unit of Bernard's heart.

   _____

6. Shirley Kiley, a 73-year-old female, was diagnosed with coronary artery disease (CAD) last year. During her regular checkup with Dr. Pauli, her blood pressure was measured.

   _____

7. Dr. Spevack completed a 67-lead electrocardiogram on Marilyn Porter, with graphic presentation, analysis, interpretation, and a report to the attending physician.

   _____

8. Fonda Gold, a 27-year-old female, is having an intrastromal corneal ring segment implanted by Dr. Berntini.

   _____

9. Dr. Forrest performs a physiologic recording of the frequency and amplitude of Jason Kinnear's tremors using an accelerometer. His interpretation was included in his report to the attending physician. Determine the most accurate Category I code.

_____

10. Dr. Francetti inserted an anterior segment aqueous drainage device, using an internal approach, on Patria Maladrova's left eye. There was no extraocular reservoir included.

_____

11. Ava Vitasek, a 66-year-old female, had a myocardial infarction (MI) last year and has since been diagnosed with coronary artery disease (CAD). Dr. Loreneta prescribed beta-blocker therapy for her at this visit.

_____

12. Frank Milotti, a 43-year-old male, had a heart transplant 5 months ago. He is beginning to show signs that he may be rejecting the heart, so Dr. Yuan gives him a breath test.

_____

13. Kelly Scotcia, a 58-year-old female, was diagnosed with ventricular tachyarrhythmias and a subcutaneous implantable defibrillator (S-ICD) system was implanted 6 months ago. Today, Dr. Neumann is removing the S-ICD and the electrodes. Determine the most accurate Category I code.

_____

14. Edward Rotan, a 79-year-old male, has been having back pain for about 4 months. Today, Dr. Lipsitz is following up with him on the instruction he has been getting on therapeutic exercise.

_____

15. Maria Vasquez, a 71-year-old female, has type I diabetes and was diagnosed with coronary artery disease (CAD). Dr. Willimina prescribed an angiotensin-converting enzyme (ACE) inhibitor for her.

_____

The following exercises provide practice in the application of abstracting the physicians' notes and learning to work with SOAP notes from our health care facility, Cipher, Victors & Associates. These case studies (SOAP notes) are modeled on real patient encounters. Using the techniques described in this chapter, carefully read through the case studies and determine the most accurate Category III code(s) for each case study. Code for the attending physician's services.

CIPHER, VICTORS & ASSOCIATES
A Complete Health Care Facility
234 MAIN STREET • ANYTOWN, FL 32711 • 407-555-1234

PATIENT: GEICCOR, MORRIS
ACCOUNT/EHR #:   GEICMO001
DATE: 11/13/18

Diagnosis: Osteoporotic compression fracture, S1-2

Procedure: Sacroplasty, percutaneous, LT

Physician: Marion M. March, MD

Anesthesia: Local

PROCEDURE: Patient is a 39-year-old male, with chronic back pain. The patient was positioned on the table, prepped, and draped in a sterile fashion. Anesthetic was injected, and fluoroscopy was used to localize the area. A spinal needle was placed adjacent to the S1-2 disc, the depth was measured, and local anesthetic was injected. An introducer needle was placed into the disc and advanced obliquely into the anterolateral quadrant of the disc space. This position was confirmed by fluoroscopy. The balloon was advanced through the introducer needle and navigated into the area of disc pathology. Final positioning was again confirmed by fluoroscopy.

Bone cement was injected into the disc. The catheter and needle were removed. Dressings were applied. Patient tolerated the procedure well and was taken to the recovery room.

Marion M. March, MD

MMM/mg   D: 11/13/18 09:50:16   T: 11/13/18 12:55:01

Determine the most accurate Category III code(s).

_____

_____

_____

CIPHER, VICTORS & ASSOCIATES
A Complete Health Care Facility
234 MAIN STREET • ANYTOWN, FL 32711 • 407-555-1234

PATIENT: SAMPORO, ELIJAH
ACCOUNT/EHR #:   SAMPEL001
DATE: 10/20/18

Attending Physician: James I. Cipher, MD

S: Pt is a 72-year-old male, with a history of hypercholesterolemia, diabetes, and hypertension. The patient is experiencing chest pain and tightness. Dr. Cipher discussed the possibility of doing a coronary artery obstruction severity assessment, which the patient agreed to undergo.

O: Pt taken to the test suite, where a coronary artery obstruction severity assessment, 64 ECG lead, was performed. Patient tolerated the procedure well.

A: Coronary artery disease

P: Follow-up in 1 week

_____

James I. Cipher, MD

JIC/mg   D: 10/20/18 09:50:16   T: 10/23/18 12:55:01

Determine the most accurate Category III code(s).

_____

_____

_____

CIPHER, VICTORS & ASSOCIATES
A Complete Health Care Facility
234 MAIN STREET • ANYTOWN, FL 32711 • 407-555-1234

PATIENT: CHEN, REBECCA
ACCOUNT/EHR #:   CHENRE001
DATE: 11/15/18

Diagnosis: Malignant neoplasm, urinary bladder

Procedure: Compensator-based beam modulation treatment

Physician: Marion M. March, MD

Anesthesia: Local

PROCEDURE: Patient is a 47-year-old female, brought in to undergo external beam radiation to the bladder with dose escalation to 32 Gy. A fluence map was generated for a 5-field compensator-based beam modulation technique to treat this patient while meeting the required constraints. Once this was approved, the final plan was generated using a single compensator for each beam of varying thickness throughout its area to generate the required fluence map. The compensator was milled according to specifications. The treatment was delivered to a film phantom using these compensators and images overlaid well with the dose distributions. The treatments were delivered as prescribed: daily for 5 days.

Marion M. March, MD

MMM/mg   D: 11/15/18 09:50:16   T: 11/21/18 12:55:01

Determine the most accurate Category I or Category III code(s).

_____

_____

_____

CIPHER, VICTORS & ASSOCIATES
A Complete Health Care Facility
234 MAIN STREET • ANYTOWN, FL 32711 • 407-555-1234

PATIENT: WYNDHAM, MAXWELL
ACCOUNT/EHR #:   WYNDMA001
DATE: 11/15/18

Procedure Performed: Cerebral perfusion analysis, CT scan

Radiologist: Keith Robbins, MD

Referring Physician: James I. Cipher, MD

INDICATIONS: R/o vascular obstruction

IMPRESSIONS: With contrast administration. Postprocessing of parametric maps with determination of cerebral blood flow, cerebral blood volume, and mean transit time.

_____

Keith Robbins, MD

KR/mg   D: 11/15/18 09:50:16   T: 11/17/18 12:55:01

Determine the most accurate Category III code(s).

_____

_____

_____

CIPHER, VICTORS & ASSOCIATES
A Complete Health Care Facility
234 MAIN STREET • ANYTOWN, FL 32711 • 407-555-1234

PATIENT:	COLLIER, ANITA
ACCOUNT/EHR #:	COLLAN001
DATE:	11/11/18

Diagnosis: Uterine leiomyomata

Procedure: Ultrasound ablation of uterine leiomyomata

Physician: Marion M. March, MD

Anesthesia: General

PROCEDURE: Patient is a 51-year-old female, brought into the OR and placed on the table in the lithotomy position. The patient is draped in a sterile fashion. Using magnetic resonance-guided focused ultrasound, the beams are focused on the fibroids, temperature within the tissue reached 75°, destroying the diseased tissue; total leiomyomata volume is 135 cc.

Marion M. March, MD

MMM/mg   D: 11/11/18 09:50:16   T: 11/12/18 12:55:01

Determine the most accurate Category III code(s).

_____

_____

_____

PART II

HCPCS LEVEL II

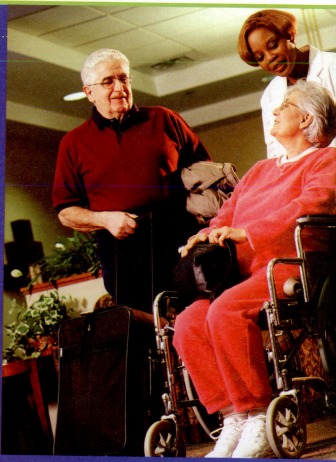

© Dynamic Graphics/JupiterImages

13

HCPCS LEVEL II CODING: INTRODUCTION AND GUIDELINES

Learning Outcomes *After completing this chapter, the student should be able to:*

LO 13.1 Identify the scope of categories reported with HCPCS Level II codes.

LO 13.2 Correctly use the alphabetic index within HCPCS Level II codes.

LO 13.3 Confirm codes suggested by the index in the alphanumeric listing.

LO 13.4 Interpret the meanings of the notations and symbols.

LO 13.5 Apply the additional information provided by the appendixes.

Key Terms

Chelation therapy

Durable medical equipment (DME)

Durable medical equipment regional carrier (DMERC)

Enteral

Not otherwise specified (NOS)

Orthotic

Parenteral

Prosthetic

There is another portion to the procedure coding system that professional coding specialists use to report services and treatments. HCPCS (pronounced "hick-picks") is the acronym for Health care Common Procedure Coding System. You may remember the following from Chap. 2 in this textbook:

- HCPCS Level I codes are commonly known as CPT codes.
- HCPCS Level II codes are referred to as HCPCS codes.

LO 13.1 HCPCS Level II Categories

HCPCS Level II codes and modifiers are listed in their own book and are used to report a service, a procedure, and supplies that are not properly described in the CPT book. There are almost 5,000 HCPCS codes, each represented by five characters: one letter followed by four numbers.

EXAMPLE

C1715   Brachytherapy needle
M0075   Cellular therapy

HCPCS Level II codes cover specific aspects of health care services, including

- Durable medical equipment (such as a wheelchair or a humidifier).
- Pharmaceuticals administered by a health care provider (such as a saline solution or a chemotherapy drug).
- Medical supplies provided for the patient's own use (such as an eye patch or gradient compression stockings).

- Dental services (such as all services provided by a dental professional).
- Transportation services (such as ambulance services).
- Vision and hearing services (such as trifocal spectacles or a hearing screening).
- **Orthotic** and **prosthetic** procedures (such as scoliosis braces or postsurgical fitting).

Not all insurance carriers accept HCPCS Level II codes, but Medicare and Medicaid want you to use them. It is your responsibility as a coding specialist to find out whether each third-party payer with which your facility works accepts HCPCS Level II codes. If not, you have to ask for the payer's policies on reporting the services and supplies covered by HCPCS Level II.

EXAMPLE

Medicare accepts HCPCS Level II codes and therefore requires you to code an injection of tetracycline, 200 mg, with two codes (for administration of the shot and the drug inside the syringe).

96372 Therapeutic, prophylactic or diagnostic injection (specify substance or drug injected); subcutaneous or intramuscular

J0120 Injection, tetracycline, up to 250 mg

Barton Health Insurance does not accept HCPCS Level II codes. This payer includes reimbursement for the drug in the CPT code for the actual injection. Therefore, you would report only the one code to get paid for both the service (the giving of the shot) and the material (the drug inside the syringe).

96372 Therapeutic, prophylactic or diagnostic injection (specify substance or drug injected); subcutaneous or intramuscular

The process for using HCPCS Level II codes is the same as you have learned throughout this book for coding from the CPT book. You abstract the key words from the physician's notes regarding the services and procedures, look those key words up in the alphabetic index of the appropriate book (CPT or HCPCS), confirm the code in the numerical listing, and report the service using that code. You know how to do this already! However, there are specific elements unique to HCPCS Level II coding that you need to know. You will learn them here, in Chap. 14, and Appendix B.

Understanding how to use HCPCS codes accurately will open new employment opportunities for you. In addition to hospitals, physicians' offices, and outpatient clinics, nursing homes, home health care agencies, health care equipment and supply companies, and other facilities use these codes quite extensively.

LO 13.2 The Alphabetic Index

Like the other coding books, the HCPCS Level II book has an alphabetic index as well as an alphanumeric listing.

The alphabetic index lists the Level II code descriptions in alphabetic order from *A* to *Z*. After abstracting the key words from the provider's notes, you can look up the key words in the index by using the following:

- Brand name of the drug.
- Generic name of the drug.
- Medical supply item.
- Orthotic.
- Prosthetic.
- Service.
- Surgical supply.

The index will suggest a code or a range of codes, similarly to CPT's alphabetic index. Then, as you have done before, you look the suggestions up in the alphanumeric listing, read the complete description(s), and determine the best, most accurate code. (*Note:* The alphabetic index in the HCPCS Level II book does not list all the codes included in the alphanumeric listing. So if you can't find what you are looking for in the index, you might want to find something closely related to get you to the appropriate section of the book and then look around.)

This index includes many alternate terms identified by notations in the alphanumeric listings.

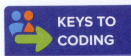

EXAMPLE

In the alphabetic index, you will see

    Abciximab, J0130

    ReoPro, TRH, J0130

In the alphanumeric listing, you will see

    J0130 Injection, abciximab, 10 mg

        Use this code for ReoPro.

Deleted code descriptions are not included in the alphabetic index. However, the new code(s) that are to be used instead of the deleted codes are listed.

EXAMPLE

In the alphabetic index, you will see

    Wheelchair,

        Cushion

            Seat E2610, E2622-E2625

            General, E2601, E2602

In the alphanumeric listing, you will see

    E2601 General use wheelchair seat cushion, width less than 22 in. any depth

    E2602 General use wheelchair seat cushion, width 22 in. or greater, any depth

    E2610 Wheelchair seat cushion, powered

When the alphanumeric listing shows a notation to use one code with another code, the alphabetic index often provides you with the same direction.

EXAMPLE

In the alphabetic index, you will see

    Prefabricated post and core, dental, D2954, D6972

    Each additional (same tooth), D2957, D6977

In the alphanumeric listing, you will see

    D6977 Each additional prefabricated post—same tooth

        Report this code in addition to code D6972.

HCPCS Level II codes are listed in sections, grouped by the type of service, the type of supply item, or the type of equipment they represent. However, you should not assume that a particular item or service is located in a specific section. Use the alphabetic index to direct you to the correct category in the alphanumeric listing of the book. One type of service or procedure might be located under several different categories depending upon the details.

EXAMPLE

Transportation services may be identified by A, Q, R, S, T, or V codes.
Transportation
Ambulance, A0021–A0999
Corneal tissue, V2785
EKG (portable), R0076
Waiting time, T2007

LO 13.3 The Alphanumeric Listing Overview

The alphanumeric listing presents the codes in alphabetic order by the first letter and then numerical order beginning with the first number of that code.

Let's go through all the sections together so that you can get a general idea of the procedures, services, and supplies that are reported using these codes. Chap. 14 will provide more in-depth discussion of several of these areas.

A0000–A0999 Transportation Services Including Ambulance

Details about reporting transportation services are in Chap. 14, page 391.

GUIDANCE CONNECTION

Additional explanation can be found in the guidelines within the **A** section, directly under the subhead **Transportation Services Including Ambulance A0000–A0999** in your HCPCS Level II book.

EXAMPLE

A0021 Ambulance service, outside state per mile, transport
A0420 Ambulance waiting time (ALS or BLS), one-half hour increments

A4000–A8999 Medical Supplies

These codes cover medical supplies, surgical supplies, and some services related to **durable medical equipment (DME)** (see Chap. 14, page 394).

EXAMPLE

A4245 Alcohol wipes, per box
A4452 Tape, waterproof, per 18 sq in.
A4490 Surgical stocking above knee length, each
A4637 Replacement, tip, cane, crutch, walker, each

durable medical equipment (DME)
Apparatus and tools that help individuals accommodate physical frailties, provide pharmaceuticals, and provide other assistance that will last for a long time and/or be used to assist multiple patients over time.

A9000–A9999 Administrative, Miscellaneous, and Investigational

You will find codes in the Administrative, Miscellaneous, and Investigational section for:

- Nonprescription drugs (also known as over-the-counter drugs).
- Exercise equipment.

- Radiopharmaceutical diagnostic imaging agents.
- Non-covered items and services.

(Note: An item or service may be non-covered with regard to national standards but covered by your state or other third-party carrier. Never take anything for granted. Always ask!)

EXAMPLE

A9280 Alert or alarm device, not otherwise classified
A9505 Thallium T1-201, thallous chloride diagnostic, per millicurie

LET'S CODE IT! SCENARIO

Anabelle Simpson, a 67-year-old female, has been diagnosed with malignant neoplasm of the liver. She has lost all her hair because of the chemotherapy and radiation treatments. Dr. Tippin prescribed a wig to help lift her spirits and self-esteem.

Let's Code It!

You have to submit a claim to Medicare for the wig. Let's go to the alphabetic index of the HCPCS Level II book and find the *W* section. Beneath this, find

Wig, A9282

Go to the alphanumeric listing to confirm it is the best code:

A9282 Wig, any type, each

enteral
Within, or by way of, the gastrointestinal tract.

parenteral
By way of anything other than the gastrointestinal tract, such as intravenous, intramuscular, intramedullary, or subcutaneous.

B4000–B9999 Enteral-Parenteral Therapy

The B codes cover supplies, formulas, nutritional solutions, and infusion pumps for **enteral-parenteral** therapy.

EXAMPLE

B4083 Stomach tube—Levine type
B9006 Parenteral nutrition, infusion pump, stationary

C1000–C9999 Outpatient PPS

Codes from the *outpatient PPS* category are used to report drugs, biologicals, devices for transitional pass-through payments for hospitals, and items classified in new-technology ambulatory payment classifications.

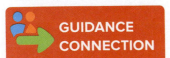

GUIDANCE CONNECTION

Additional explanation can be found in the guidelines within the **C** section, directly under the subhead **Outpatient PPS C1300–C9899,** in your HCPCS Level II book.

EXAMPLE

C1724 Catheter, transluminal atherectomy, rotational
C2636 Brachytherapy linear source, nonstranded, palladium 103, per 1 mm
C9364 Porcine implant (Permacol), per square cm

D0000–D9999 Dental Procedures

The *dental procedures* category is the Current Dental Terminology (CDT) code set, copyrighted by the American Dental Association. The codes are used to report dental services.

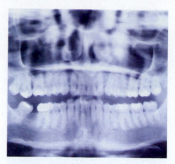

> ### EXAMPLE
>
> D0240 Intraoral—occlusal film
> D1110 Prophylaxis—adult
> D3310 Endodontic therapy, anterior tooth (excluding final restoration)

Prophylaxis is also known as a dental cleaning, and *anterior (excluding final restoration)* is one of the codes that can be used to report root canal therapy.

LET'S CODE IT! SCENARIO

Daniel Roseman, a 73-year-old male, came to Dr. Franks for a complete maxillary denture. His old one was broken beyond repair, so Daniel needed something immediately.

Let's Code It!

Dr. Franks provided Daniel with a *complete maxillary denture*. Let's go to the HCPCS Level II alphabetic index:

> Dentures (removable)
>> Adjustments, D5410–D5422
>> Complete, D5110–D5140

As you read the full list, you see that the reference matches Dr. Franks's notes. Next, turn to the alphanumeric listing to see which code is the most accurate.

> D5110 Complete denture—maxillary
> D5120 Complete denture—mandibular
> D5130 Immediate denture—maxillary
> D5140 Immediate denture—mandibular

Is there additional information in the notes that will help you determine the best code? They state that Daniel needed the denture *immediately*. It leads you directly to

> D5130 Immediate denture—maxillary

Excellent!

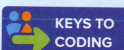

KEYS TO CODING

The CDT code set is published as an individual book but includes the same codes given here.

E0100–E9999 Durable Medical Equipment

The E codes are used to identify certain pieces of durable medical equipment (DME) provided to a patient.

> ### EXAMPLE
>
> E0105 Cane, quad, or 3-prong, includes canes of all materials, adjustable or fixed, with tips
> E0156 Seat attachment, walker
> E0242 Bathtub rail, floor base

KEYS TO CODING

Be careful not to confuse the E codes with ICD-9-CM E codes, which report how and where an injury occurred.

E0980 Safety vest, wheelchair:

Letter followed by four numbers (from HCPCS).

E980.0 Poisoning, unknown, analgesics:

Letter followed by three numbers, a period, and possibly additional numbers (from ICD-9-CM).

More information about durable medical equipment (DME) codes is in Chap. 14, page 394.

G0000–G9999 Procedures/Professional Services (Temporary)

Codes from this section are used to report services and procedures that do not have an accurate code description in the main portion of the CPT book.

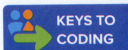
> ### EXAMPLE
>
> G0102 Prostate cancer screening; digital rectal examination
> G0151 Services of physical therapist in home health or hospice setting, each 15 minutes
> G0268 Removal of impacted cerumen (one or both ears) by physician on same date of service as audiologic function testing

H0001–H2037 Alcohol and Drug Abuse Treatment Services

When alcohol and drug treatment, as well as some other mental health services, are provided, some state Medicaid agencies will have you use codes from the *alcohol and drug abuse treatment services* category.

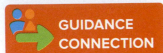
> ### EXAMPLE
>
> H0005 Alcohol and/or drug services; group counseling by a clinician
> H0038 Self-help/peer services, per 15 minutes
> H2020 Therapeutic behavioral services, per diem

J0000–J9999 Drugs Administered Other Than Oral Method

As the title so clearly states, the *drugs administered other than oral method* category provides you with codes to identify drugs that are given to the patient by a health care professional in any way other than by mouth. This includes chemotherapy drugs, immunosuppressive drugs, inhalation solutions, and other miscellaneous drugs and solutions.

> ### EXAMPLE
>
> J0207 Injection, amifostine, 500 mg
> J7100 Infusion, dextran 40, 500 mL
> J7610 Albuterol, inhalation solution, compounded product, administered through DME, concentrated form, 1 mg

You will find that drugs identified in the code descriptions are most often the chemical, or generic, name of the pharmaceutical. At times the brand, or trade, name is listed in the alphabetic index and/or in the Table of Drugs in Appendix 1 of your HCPCS Level II book. If your provider notes refer to a name that you cannot find in this book, you might need to look in the *Physician's Desk Reference* (PDR) to find an alternate name for the drug. Chap. 15, page 419 of this text will go into more detail.

Take these two prescription drugs: Zenapax, generic name daclizumab, and CellCept, generic name mycophenolate mofetil.

- Zenapax is listed in the alphabetic index of HCPCS.
- CellCept is not listed by trade name, only by its generic name, in the alphabetic index. However, it is listed by trade name in the Table of Drugs in Appendix 1.

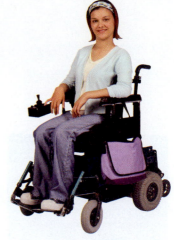

© Amos Morgan/Getty Images

K0000–K9999 Temporary Codes

The K codes were developed for **durable medical equipment regional carriers (DMERCs)** to report services that are not currently identified by other codes.

EXAMPLE

K0001 Standard wheelchair
K0462 Temporary replacement for patient owned equipment being repaired, any type

durable medical equipment regional carrier (DMERC)
A company designated by the state or region to act as the fiscal intermediary for all DME claims.

L0000–L4999 Orthotic Procedures and L5000–L9999 Prosthetic Procedures

The codes included in the *orthotic procedures and prosthetic procedures* categories identify orthotic devices, orthopedic shoes, prosthetic devices, prosthetic implants, and scoliosis equipment.

EXAMPLE

L0170 Cervical, collar, molded to patient model
L0984 Protective body sock, each
L5050 Ankle, Symes, molded socket, SACH foot

M0000–M0301 Medical Services

The codes in the *medical services* category cover cellular therapy, prolotherapy, intragastric hypothermia, intravenous **chelation therapy,** and fabric wrapping of an abdominal aneurysm (MNP).

EXAMPLE

M0075 Cellular therapy
M0301 Fabric wrapping of abdominal aneurysm

chelation therapy
The use of a chemical compound that binds with metal in the body so that the metal will lose its toxic effect. It might be done when a metal disc or prosthetic is implanted in a patient, eliminating adverse reactions to the metal itself as a foreign body.

P0000–P9999 Pathology and Laboratory

HCPCS Level II codes in the *pathology and laboratory* category include codes for services not listed in the CPT book, including chemistry, toxicology, microbiology, screening Papanicolaou (Pap) procedures, and numerous blood products.

P2031 Hair analysis (excluding arsenic)
P7001 Culture, bacterial, urine; quantitative, sensitivity study
P9051 White blood or red blood cells, leukocytes reduced, CMV-negative, each unit

Q0035–Q9968 Q Codes (Temporary)

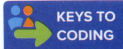

The Q codes replace the less specific codes that you may find elsewhere in the coding process for casting and splinting supplies when a health care professional cares for a patient with a fracture. The section also includes codes for certain drugs and services having nothing to do with the management of a fracture.

EXAMPLE

Q0113 Pinworm examination
Q2017 Injection, teniposide, 50 mg
Q4049 Finger splint, static

R0000–R5999 Diagnostic Radiology Services

The codes in the *diagnostic radiology services* category are used to report the hauling of portable radiologic equipment.

EXAMPLE

R0070 Transportation of portable x-ray equipment and personnel to home or nursing home, per trip to facility or location, one patient seen
R0076 Transportation of portable EKG to facility or location, per patient

S0000–S9999 Temporary National Codes (Non-Medicare)

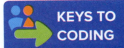

The *temporary national codes* category was developed by the Health Insurance Association of America (HIAA) and the Blue Cross Blue Shield Association (BCBSA) for use by the Medicaid program and other third-party payers. The codes cover supplies, services, and drugs for which there are no other codes.

EXAMPLE

S0081 Injection, piperacillin sodium, 500 mg
S0317 Disease management program; per diem
S2060 Lobar lung transplantation
S9015 Automated EEG monitoring

T1000–T9999 National T Codes Established for State Medicaid Agencies

Planned for use by state agencies that administer Medicaid programs, the T codes are used to report services not otherwise described by any other code. Services represented in this category include nursing facility and home health–related services, substance abuse treatment, and training-related procedures.

EXAMPLE

    T1013 Sign language or oral interpretive services, per 15 minutes
    T2022 Case management, per month
    T2045 Hospice general inpatient care; per diem

V0000–V2999 Vision Services

If not represented by any other codes, ophthalmic and optometric services and sup-plies may be coded from this V code category, including contact lenses, intraocular lenses, miscellaneous lenses, prostheses, spectacles, and other vision-related supplies.

EXAMPLE

    V2118 Aniseikonic lens, single vision
    V2321 Lenticular lens, per lens, trifocal
    V2530 Contact lens, scleral, gas impermeable, per lens

V5000–V5999 Hearing Services

Services related to hearing and speech-language pathology are included in this V code category. It covers hearing tests, repair of augmentative communicative systems, speech-language pathology screenings, and other hearing test–related supplies and equipment.

EXAMPLE

    V5008 Hearing screening
    V5100 Hearing aid, bilateral, body worn
    V5364 Dysphagia screening

YOU CODE IT! CASE STUDY

Eric Ziambi, a 17-year-old male, lost his eye in a skiing accident and has come to see Dr. Voltain to receive his prosthetic eye. It is a custom-made, plastic prosthesis. Code for the prosthesis only.

You Code It!

Go through the steps of coding and determine the code(s) that should be reported for the prostheic provided by Dr. Voltain to Eric Ziambi.

Step 1: Read the case completely.

Step 2: Abstract the notes: Which key words can you identify relating to the item provided?

_____

Step 3: Query the provider, if necessary.

Step 4: Diagnosis: Acquired absence of eye.

Step 5:   Code the item(s).

_____

Step 6:   Link the item code(s) to at least one diagnosis code.

Step 7:   Back code to double-check your choices.

Answer:

Did you determine the correct code?

V2623 Prosthetic eye, plastic, custom

Good job!

LO 13.4 Symbols And Notations

Throughout many versions of a HCPCS Level II codebook, you may see notations that will help you use the codes correctly and determine the best, most appropriate code available.

Symbols

● A large bullet, or solid circle, shown next to a code indicates that it is the first year that the code is included in this code set.

▲ A solid triangle shown next to a code lets you know that the code's description has been changed or adjusted since last year or that a rule or guideline regarding the code has changed.

○ An open circle next to a code identifies that the code had been deleted but now has been restored (reinstated).

⊘ A circle with a slash through it, in the HCPCS Level II book, identifies a code that is not covered under the skilled nursing facility prospective payment system (SNFPPS).

☑ A check mark inside a square box marks a code description that identifies a specific quantity of material or supply. It is a reminder for you to check the detail in the notes and report the code not only for the item it represents but for the amount as well.

> ## EXAMPLE
>
> J0894 Injection, decitabine, 1 mg
> K0073 Caster pin lock, each

♂ The male symbol is placed next to codes that identify procedures, services, and equipment that can *only* be performed or used on a male patient.

> ## EXAMPLE
>
> L3219 Orthopedic footwear, man's shoes, Oxford, each ♂
> L8330 Truss, addition to standard pad, scrotal pad ♂

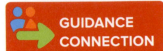

GUIDANCE CONNECTION

Additional explanation and guidelines can be found in the **Introduction** section in your HCPCS Level II book.

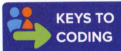

KEYS TO CODING

In CPT, the symbol ⊘ means that the code may not be used with modifier 51. In HCPCS Level II, this symbol means not covered under SNFPPS.

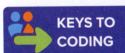

KEYS TO CODING

Should the provider administer less than the indicated amount in the code descriptor, you are permitted to simply report the code as shown. For example, if the provider administered 0.5 mg of decitabine, you would report J0894.

When more than the quantity shown in the code description is indicated in the provider's notes, report the appropriate code in the proper number. For example, if the provider gave the patient 2 mg of decitabine, you would report J0894 ×2 to indicate two units.

♀ The female symbol identifies codes used to report procedures, services, and equipment that can *only* be performed or used on a female patient.

> ## EXAMPLE
>
> A4286 Locking ring for breast pump, replacement ♀
>
> L8600 Implantable breast prosthesis, silicone or equal ♀

A The "A" symbol highlights the fact that a code is used only for procedures, services, and equipment that are performed or used on a patient of a certain age group. Read the code description carefully to ensure that the age limitation of the code matches the patient.

M The "M" symbol is used to remind you that the code describes maternity procedures, services, and equipment that are performed or used on a pregnant female 12–55 years of age.

~~**Z1111**~~ A line through the center of a code and its description means that the code has been deleted and may no longer be used.

Notations

Just as in the CPT book, you will find notations (below code descriptions in the alphanumeric listing) that guide you on the proper use of HCPCS Level II codes.

Always Report Concurrent to the *xxx* Procedure This notation directs you to always report this code with a code for another specific procedure. The notation is similar to the "code also" instruction found in CPT or ICD-10-CM.

> ## EXAMPLE
>
> A4263 Permanent, long-term, non-dissolvable lacrimal duct implant, each
>
> Always report concurrent to the implant procedure.

In the example, the "A" code is for the implant itself, and the note reminds you that you have to code the physician's services for putting the implant into the patient.

See Also Code Z1111 The *see also code* notation cross-references this code with another code that may be similar in description. The notation serves as a reminder for you to double-check that you are using the most accurate code.

> ## EXAMPLE
>
> A4450 Tape, non-waterproof, per 18 sq in.
>
> See also code A4452
>
> A4452 Tape, waterproof, per 18 sq in.
>
> See also code A4450

Clarifications of Coverage *Clarifications of coverage* notations are worded differently from code to code but indicate when to use or *not* use the code. However, always check with the specific payer to whom you will be sending the claim.

> **EXAMPLE**
>
> A4565 Slings
>
> Dressings applied by a physician are included as part of the professional service. Surgical dressings obtained by the patient to perform homecare as prescribed by the physician are covered.

Report in Addition to Code Z1111 When one code is to be reported with other codes, a notation *Report in addition to* (a particular *code*) will identify those circumstances. It not only tells you the circumstances but also tells you which code to use. You may notice that it is similar to an add-on code in CPT.

> **EXAMPLE**
>
> D2953 Each additional indirectly fabricated post—same tooth
>
> Report in addition to code D2952

See Code Z1111 When a code has been deleted, you may find a notation that directs you to another HCPCS Level II code that can be used instead.

> **EXAMPLE**
>
> J0560 Injection, penicillin G benzathine, up to 600,000 units
>
>   To report, see J0561

See Code(s): 00000 The notation *See* (a particular *code*) refers you to a CPT code for a description that is *potentially* better and may be more specific for reporting what was actually done or given to the patient.

> **EXAMPLE**
>
> E1130 Standard wheelchair, fixed full-length arms, fixed, or swing-away
>   detachable footrests
>
> See code(s): K0001
>
> K0001 Standard wheelchair

Determine If an Alternative HCPCS Level II or a CPT Code Better Describes . . . You will see the notation *Determine if an alternative HCPCS Level II or a CPT code better describes* beneath each miscellaneous, unlisted, unclassified, not otherwise classified (NOC), not otherwise listed, or **not otherwise specified (NOS)** code. The notation serves as a warning to you to make certain that there is no better or more specific code either in the CPT or elsewhere in this HCPCS Level II book that correctly reports the services or procedures performed.

not otherwise specified (NOS)
An indication that more detailed information is not available from the physician's notes.

> **EXAMPLE**
>
> L0999 Addition to spinal orthosis, not otherwise specified
>
> Determine if an alternative HCPCS Level II or a CPT code better describes the service being reported. This code should be used only if a more specific code is unavailable.

Use This Code For . . . The notation *Use this code for* provides you with alternative names, brand names, and other terms that are also represented by the code's description.

> ### EXAMPLE
>
> B4150 Enteral formula, nutritionally complete with intact nutrients, includes proteins, fats, carbohydrates, vitamins and minerals, may include fiber, administered through an enteral feeding tube, 100 calories = 1 unit
>
> Use this code for Enrich, Ensure, Ensure HN, Ensure Powder, Isocal, Lonalac Powder, Meritene, Meritene Powder, Osmolite, Osmolite HN, Portagen Powder, Sustacal, Renu, Sustagen Powder, Travasorb.

Pertinent Documentation to Evaluate Medical Appropriateness Should Be . . .

Some procedures are not automatically accepted as being medically necessary. The notation *Pertinent documentation to evaluate medical appropriateness should be* warns you up front that you should include the proper documentation along with the claim *the first time* you submit it, rather than wait to be asked by the third-party payer, which would delay payment.

> ### EXAMPLE
>
> D2980 Crown repair, by report
>
> Pertinent documentation to evaluate medical appropriateness should be included when this code is reported.

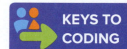

KEYS TO CODING

When you determine from the documentation that a different code may be more accurate than one indicated by the physician, you should query the physician to have him or her document agreement with your decision.

Do Not Use This Code to Report . . .

The notation *Do not use this code to report* warns you of circumstances when you are not permitted to use a code.

> ### EXAMPLE
>
> D3220 Therapeutic pulpotomy (excluding final restoration)—removal of pulp coronal to the dentinocemental junction and application of medicament
>
> Do not use this code to report the first stage of root canal therapy.

Medicare Covers . . .

Throughout the HCPCS Level II book, you will see notations giving you information about coverage, particularly Medicare and Medicaid coverage. You should note that the book covers the entire nation and that both programs are state-administered. This means that you should still confirm the terms and policies of what is covered with your own state's fiscal intermediary (FI)—the agency or organization that is in charge of reimbursement for your state's program. Also check with other third-party payers to see if they will cover this item or service.

> ### EXAMPLE
>
> E0607 Home blood glucose monitor
>
> Medicare covers home blood-testing devices for diabetic patients when the devices are prescribed by the patient's physicians. Many commercial payers provide this coverage to non–insulin dependent diabetics as well.

Code with Caution When you see the notation *Code with caution* beneath a code, you need to go back and double-check the provider's notes carefully. If this is what was actually done, then be certain to attach documentation explaining why that method was used instead of the newer technique because it is surely going to be questioned.

YOU CODE IT! CASE STUDY

Dr. Yawia modified Arthur Wassau's left orthopedic shoe by inserting a between-sole metatarsal bar wedge to accommodate Arthur's shrinking Achilles tendon. Dr. Yawia checked off the code L3649 on the superbill. In your judgment as the professional coding specialist, is this the best code available?

You Code It!

Go through the steps of coding and determine the code(s) that should be reported for this product provided by Dr. Yawia.

Step 1: Read the case completely.

Step 2: Abstract the notes: Which key words can you identify relating to the service performed?

_____

Step 3: Query the provider, if necessary.

Step 4: Diagnosis: Contracture of Achilles tendon (acquired).

Step 5: Code the procedure(s).

_____

Step 6: Link the procedure codes to at least one diagnosis code.

Step 7: Back code to double-check your choices.

Answer:

Did you determine the correct codes?

L3410 Metatarsal bar wedge, between sole

That's a much more specific code. Good job!

LET'S CODE IT! SCENARIO

Kim Whirlon came with her husband, Arlen, to see Dr. Dean because of the problems Arlen was having sleeping. You may remember their case from Chap. 11 in the text when you coded the nasopharyngoscopy with an endoscope that Dr. Dean performed to confirm that Arlen had sleep apnea. Dr. Dean supplied Arlen and Kim with an apnea monitor, complete with a recording feature, so that Arlen's sleep could be monitored and Dr. Dean could further evaluate his condition.

In Chap. 11, you found the CPT code for the *nasopharyngoscopy with an endoscope*—code 92511. Now, you see that Dr. Dean supplied Arlen with an *apnea monitor with a recording feature*. This machine is considered durable medical equipment (DME). Arlen's insurance carrier accepts HCPCS Level II codes. Therefore, you have to add another code to the claim form for the encounter so that Dr. Dean can be reimbursed for the machine. Let's go to the alphabetic index and look up the word *monitor* because that is the key word that best describes this item. Beneath the word *monitor*, indented slightly, you see the word *apnea* and the suggestion for the code E0618. This seems to be exactly what Dr. Dean described in his notes, so let's turn to the alphanumeric listing to read the complete description of the code.

E0618 Apnea monitor, without recording feature

This matches the notes with one big exception. The code description specifically states *without* recording feature. Dr. Dean documented giving Arlen a monitor *with* a recording feature. Keep reading, and you will find

E0619 Apnea monitor, with recording feature

Excellent! It matches perfectly.

LET'S CODE IT! SCENARIO

Dr. Porter provided Janine Matlock, a 73-year-old female, with a quad cane, after putting on a new handgrip. Code for the supply only.

Let's Code It!

When you pull out the key words that describe the items for which Dr. Porter should be reimbursed, you see that Janine was provided with a *quad cane* and *new handgrip*.

It wouldn't be out of line to think that the codes are automatically going to be listed in the Durable Medical Equipment section, codes E0100–E9999. If you turned to that section directly, you would find the code for the quad cane rather quickly. It's right in the front. However, you could examine and search through the entire listing of 9,899 possible codes in the section and never find the correct code for the replacement handgrip. When you look these key words up in the alphabetic index first, you see very quickly, and more efficiently, that the codes you need are

E0105 Cane, quad or 3-prong, includes canes of all materials, adjustable or fixed, with tips

A4636 Replacement, handgrip, cane, crutch, or walker, each

It's great when the process works, isn't it? You bet!

LO 13.5 Appendixes

The HCPCS Level II book provides you with additional information in the back of the book to help you code more accurately. (Note: The content of appendixes may vary depending upon the publisher of the HCPCS Level II book used.)

Appendix 1: Table of Drugs. Appendix 1 is an alphabetic listing of drug names, along with the standard unit of administration, a particular method of administration, and a reference to its HCPCS Level II code.

Appendix 2: Modifiers. This is an alphabetic list of all HCPCS Level II modifiers. You will learn more about these modifiers in Chapter 14 of this text.

Appendix 3: Abbreviations and Acronyms. Abbreviations and acronyms are used throughout the health care industry. Appendix 3 lists those used in HCPCS Level II descriptions to help you better understand the meaning of the codes.

Appendix 4: PUB100 References. Certain components of the coding system change from time to time. Up-to-date manuals and information can be found on-line in the Centers for Medicare and Medicaid Services (CMS) manual system found at www.cms.hhs.gov/manuals. Included in each annual edition of some printed HCPCS Level II books are references to national coverage determinations made just prior to publication. As a student, this may be outside the scope of your studies. As you mature in your career, this reference will be very handy.

Appendix 5: New, Changed, Deleted, and Reinstated HCPCS Codes. This appendix lists all HCPCS Level II codes that have experienced a change since the previous year's printed book. As a student, this will have little relevance for you. But when the new book comes out, it serves as an excellent reference for someone who may use the same code or codes over and over again.

Appendix 6: Place of Service and Type of Service Codes. Appendix 6 offers you a thorough explanation of each place of service (POS) and type of service (TOS) code required for boxes 24B and 24C of the CMS 1500 claim form.

Chapter Summary

HCPCS Level II codes are updated quarterly and are officially effective January 1 of each year, with no grace period. Most printed versions of the book are published with those codes posted by the Centers for Medicare and Medicaid Services (CMS) as of November 1. Read the following notation in the introduction of the HCPCS Level II book:

> *Because of the unstable nature of HCPCS Level II codes, everything has been done to include the latest information available at print time. Unfortunately, HCPCS Level II codes, their descriptions, and other related information change throughout the year. Consult the patient's payer and the CMS website to confirm the status of any HCPCS Level II code. The existence of a code does not imply coverage under any given payment plan.*

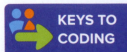

KEYS TO CODING

The list in Appendix 3 is not inclusive of all abbreviations and acronyms used in the health care industry. It is a good idea to keep a medical dictionary close by to reference those abbreviations not included in this appendix.

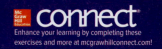

Using Terminology

Match each key term to the appropriate definition.

_____ 1. LO 13.3 A company designated by the state or region to act as the Medicare Administrative Contractor (fiscal intermediary) for all DME claims.

_____ 2. LO 13.3 By way of anything other than the gastrointestinal tract, such as intravenous, intramuscular, intramedullary, or subcutaneous.

_____ 3. LO 13.4 An indication that more detailed information is not available from the physician's notes.

_____ 4. LO 13.1 A device used to correct or improve an orthopedic concern.

_____ 5. LO 13.3 Apparatus and tools that help individuals accommodate physical frailties, provide pharmaceuticals, and provide other assistance that will last for a long time and/or be used to assist multiple patients over time.

_____ 6. LO 13.3 Within, or by way of, the gastrointestinal tract.

_____ 7. LO 13.1 Fabricated artificial replacement for a damaged or missing part of the body.

_____ 8. LO 13.3 The use of a chemical compound that binds with metal in the body so that the metal will lose its toxic effect. It might be done when a metal disc or prosthetic is implanted in a patient, eliminating adverse reactions to the metal itself as a foreign body.

A. Chelation therapy

B. Durable medical equipment (DME)

C. Durable medical equipment regional carrier (DMERC)

D. Enteral

E. Not otherwise specified (NOS)

F. Orthotic

G. Parenteral

H. Prosthetic

Checking Your Understanding

Choose the most appropriate answer for each of the following questions.

1. LO 13.4 The symbol of a circle with a line through it ⊘ means

   a. a new code.
   b. a revised code.
   c. a code exempt from a particular modifier.
   d. a service not covered under the skilled nursing facility payment system.

2. LO 13.4 The little box with a check mark in it ☑ indicates a code description that

   a. includes a quantity measurement.
   b. is always covered by Medicare.
   c. is approved for reimbursement at a higher rate.
   d. includes refills.

3. LO 13.3 The J codes are used to bill insurance carriers for

   a. prescription drugs patients get at the drugstore.
   b. drugs administered by a health care professional.
   c. nothing; they are deleted codes.
   d. items not accepted by Medicaid in any state for any reason.

4. LO 13.1 HCPCS Level II codes are used, most often, to report all *except*

   a. drugs used for treatment of a patient.
   b. equipment provided to a patient.
   c. anesthesia administered by an anesthesiologist.
   d. dental services.

5. LO 13.3 The acronym DME stands for

   a. determination of medical effectiveness.
   b. durable medical equipment.
   c. donated medical equipment.
   d. diluted medicine equivalent.

6. LO 13.1 HCPCS Level II codes are presented as

   a. five numbers.
   b. one letter followed by four numbers.
   c. four numbers followed by one letter.
   d. five letters.

7. LO 13.1 HCPCS is an acronym that stands for

   a. Health care Professional Classification Systems.
   b. Health and Caretaker Providers Coding Series.
   c. Home Care Providers Coding System.
   d. Health care Common Procedure Coding System.

8. LO 13.3 The code D1110 is an example of a

   a. HCPCS Level I code, also known as a CPT code.
   b. HCPCS Level II code.
   c. HCPCS Level III code.
   d. HCPCS Level IV code.

9. LO 13.3 The D0000–D9999 codes are created and maintained by the

   a. American Medical Association.
   b. American Dental Association.
   c. Centers for Medicare and Medicaid Services.
   d. Department of Health and Human Services.

10. LO 13.5 HCPCS Level II Appendix 5 provides additional information on

    a. New, Changed, Deleted, and Reinstated HCPCS Codes.
    b. Abbreviations and Acronyms.
    c. Modifiers.
    d. Place of Service and Type of Service codes.

11. LO 13.3 The E codes shown in the HCPCS Level II book are

    a. an expansion of the E codes in the ICD-9-CM book.
    b. used to identify DME provided to a patient.
    c. not accepted by Medicaid.
    d. always listed first on a claim form.

12. LO 13.3 An example of DME is

    a. an injection of Demerol.
    b. a prosthetic ankle.
    c. a three-prong cane.
    d. home infusion therapy.

13. LO 13.4 A line through the center of a code and its description means

    a. the procedure is obsolete.
    b. the service is no longer reimbursable.
    c. the code is reinstated.
    d. the code had been deleted and may no longer be used.

14. LO 13.3 Alcohol intervention treatment might be coded from

    a. H0001–H2037.
    b. H5000–H9999.
    c. F1000–F9999.
    d. G0000–G9999.

15. LO 13.4 A code with an *A* next to it means that

    a. a drug was administered intravenously.
    b. the machine can only be used for infusion therapy.
    c. the service is limited to a specific age group.
    d. the equipment is illegal in some states.

Applying Your Knowledge

1. LO 13.1 List four specific aspects for health care services covered by HCPCS Level II codes. _____

_____

2. LO 13.1 Do all insurance carriers accept HCPCS Level II codes? What is the responsibility of the coding specialist in regard to billing third-party payers? _____

_____

3. LO 13.2 What does the alphabetic index list? _____

_____

4. LO 13.2 List five ways to look up the key words after abstracting them from the provider's notes. _____

_____

5. LO 13.3 What HCPCS Level II code range represents medical supplies? _____

_____

6. LO 13.3 B4000–B9999 represent what HCPCS Level II procedures, services, and/or supplies? _____

_____

7. LO 13.3 What HCPCS Level II codes represent procedures/professional services (temporary)? _____

_____

8. LO 13.3 Explain what chelation is. _____

_____

9. LO 13.4 What does the "M" symbol represent? _____

_____

10. LO 13.4 What do 'notations' help the coding specialist with? _____

_____

11. LO 13.4 What does the notation *Use this code for* . . . indicate? _____

_____

12. LO 13.5 List the six appendixes in HCPCS Level II, including what each appendix contains or identifies. _____

_____

Using the techniques described in this chapter, carefully read through the case studies and determine the most accurate HCPCS Level II code(s) and modifier(s), if appropriate, for each case study.

Note: All insurance carriers and third-party payers for the patients accept HCPCS Level II codes and modifiers.

1. Oona Garrity, a 13-year-old female, has severe asthma. Dr. Summers ordered a nebulizer, with compressor, for her to use at home. Code for the home health agency that supplied the equipment.

   _____

2. Leo Pennuzo, a 45-year-old male with end-stage renal disease (ESRD), was fitted for a reciprocating peritoneal dialysis system. Code the supply of the equipment.

   _____

3. Due to his condition, Leo Pennuzo (previous case study) had an unscheduled dialysis treatment at the nearest hospital outpatient department. This hospital is not certified as an ESRD facility.

   _____

4. Melissa Hallmark, a 19-year-old female with a history of bipolar disorder, was given an injection IM of Thorazine, 45 mg. Code for the drug.

   _____

5. Thomas Roberts, a 37-year-old male, was being prepared for his kidney transplant. The nurse administered 100 mg of Zenapax, IV, parenteral. Code the drug.

   _____

6. After Thomas Roberts (previous case study) received his kidney transplant, the nurse gave him an oral dose of 250 mg of CellCept (mycophenolate mofetil) in the hospital. Code the drug.

   _____

7. Latonya Terranzano, a 93-year-old female, was having trouble eating for such a long period of time that she was exhibiting signs of malnutrition. Therefore, Dr. Pollack ordered enteral formula (Ensure) to be administered through a feeding tube at 500 calories per day. Code for the nutritional supplement only.

   _____

8. Marion Caulder, a 23-year-old male, came to see Dr. Kinder, his dentist, for an implant-supported porcelain crown on his back tooth. Code the implant supported porcelain crown.

_____

9. Felicia Simon, a 13-year-old female, lost her retainer at camp. She is at Dr. York's office to get a replacement. Code the replaced retainer.

_____

10. Andrew Reynolds, a 10-year-old male, sat in poison ivy while camping in the woods. Dr. Storm prescribed a portable sitz bath for him to use at home. Code the portable sitz bath.

_____

11. Gina Campbell, a 49-year-old female, was recuperating from surgery to repair a complex fracture of her tibia and a compound fracture of her ankle. To help her be more comfortable, Dr. Matson ordered a fixed-height hospital bed, without side rails and with a mattress, for her to use at home. Code for the DME only.

_____

12. Lawrence Tieborn, a 77-year-old male, was on complete bed rest while recuperating from surgery. Because his skin was very sensitive, he was particularly prone to decubitus ulcers. Dr. Ellington prescribed a lamb's wool sheepskin pad to help prevent any ulcers from forming. Code the sheepskin pad.

_____

13. Dr. Rossini provided a complete set of dentures, maxillary and mandibular, for Allison Porter. Code the dentures.

_____

14. Fred Plantman, a 55-year-old male, had surgery on his left foot. To enable him to take a shower safely, Dr. Porteous gave him a tub stool to sit on. Code the stool.

_____

15. Roger Madison came home from serving in the Marines a double amputee, having had both legs damaged badly in a suicide bomber's attack. Dr. Leventhol supplied him with an amputee wheelchair, desk height, with detachable arms and no footrests or leg rests. Code the wheelchair.

_____

The following exercises provide practice in the application of abstracting the physicians' notes and learning to work with SOAP notes from our health care facility, Cipher, Victors & Associates. These case studies (SOAP notes) are modeled on real patient encounters. Using the techniques described in this chapter, carefully read through the case studies and determine the most accurate CPT and/or HCPCS Level II code(s) and modifier(s), if appropriate, for each case study.

Note: All insurance carriers and third-party payers for the patients accept HCPCS Level II codes and modifiers.

CIPHER, VICTORS & ASSOCIATES
A Complete Health Care Facility
234 MAIN STREET • ANYTOWN, FL 32711 • 407-555-1234

PATIENT: KELLER, ANDRIENNE
ACCOUNT/EHR #:   KELLAN001
DATE: 12/21/18

Attending Physician: James I. Cipher, MD

S: This Pt is a 35-year-old female who was here 6 months ago for her annual physical. Today, she presents with a cut in the palm of her right hand. Pt states that she was hanging ornaments on her tree and a glass ball broke in her hand. She is otherwise healthy and has no other stated health concerns.

O: Pt lies back on the examination table and her right hand is draped in a sterile fashion. A topical antiseptic is applied and the superficial laceration, measuring 2.0 cm in length, is checked for residual glass shards. None are found and the wound is cleansed, and a simple repair is accomplished with a tissue adhesive.

A: Superficial laceration of the right hand, 2.0 cm

P: Follow-up in 10 days

James I. Cipher, MD

JIC/mg   D: 12/21/18 09:50:16   T: 12/22/18 12:55:01

Determine the most accurate CPT and/or HCPCS Level II code(s) and modifier(s), if appropriate.

_____

_____

_____

CIPHER, VICTORS & ASSOCIATES
A Complete Health Care Facility
234 MAIN STREET • ANYTOWN, FL 32711 • 407-555-1234

PATIENT: GRANT, AMOS
ACCOUNT/EHR #:   GRANAM001
DATE: 11/05/18

Attending Physician: Valerie R. Victors, MD

S: This Pt is a 15-year-old male. I have not seen this patient since last July when he came in for a certificate to play sports in school. Today he is brought in by his father after being tackled during football practice and hurting his left wrist. He is complaining of pain upon flexing and is having difficulty moving his fingers.

O: Tenderness and swelling of the wrist is observed. Pt can move his fingers slightly, indicating no fracture; however, AP/lat x-rays are taken to confirm. X-ray does confirm the wrist is sprained. A conforming, nonelastic (nonsterile) bandage, 2″ × 35″, is applied.

A: Sprain, radiocarpal ligament, wrist

P: Follow-up in 1 week

_____

Valerie R. Victors, MD

VRV/mg   D: 11/05/18 09:50:16   T: 11/08/18 12:55:01

Determine the most accurate CPT and/or HCPCS Level II code(s) and modifier(s), if appropriate.

_____

_____

_____

CIPHER, VICTORS & ASSOCIATES
A Complete Health Care Facility
234 MAIN STREET • ANYTOWN, FL 32711 • 407-555-1234

PATIENT: WEINGARTEN, LEONORA
ACCOUNT/EHR #:   WEINLE001
DATE: 10/26/18

Attending Physician: Valerie R. Victors, MD

S: Pt is a 71-year-old female whom I diagnosed with type II diabetes mellitus 2 years ago. She comes in complaining of cramps and aching in her calves. Pt states that most times she can relieve the symptoms, but lately the pain has not subsided during rest.

O: Ht. 5′ 2″, Wt 165 lb, comprehensive metabolic panel blood test taken. Each extremity is examined with special attention to lower leg, ankle, and feet. Lab results indicate that glucose levels are abnormal. Gradient compression stockings are applied to each leg, below knee, 18–30 mmHg. Patient is given instructions for proper use of these stockings.

A: Suspected peripheral arterial disease (PAD), uncontrolled diabetes mellitus type II

P: 1. Order for computed tomographic scans of both legs, with contrast
   2. Follow-up after results of CT scans

_____

Valerie R. Victors, MD

VRV/mg   D: 10/26/18 09:50:16   T: 10/27/18 12:55:01

Determine the most accurate CPT and/or HCPCS Level II code(s) and modifier(s), if appropriate.

_____

_____

_____

CIPHER, VICTORS & ASSOCIATES
A Complete Health Care Facility
234 MAIN STREET • ANYTOWN, FL 32711 • 407-555-1234

PATIENT: ABERNATHY, CARTER
ACCOUNT/EHR #:   ABERCA001
DATE: 10/15/18

Attending Physician: Valerie R. Victors, MD

S: Pt is a 45-year-old male diagnosed with carcinoma of the inner cheek 3 months ago. He has chewed tobacco for the last 20 years. Pt states he quit chewing 6 weeks ago. He presents today for his daily therapeutic injection.

O: Pt is brought into the examining room and given an injection of Interferon Alfa-2a, 3 million units, IM.

A: Malignant carcinoma, cheek, internal

P: Series of injections to continue on daily basis

_____

Valerie R. Victors, MD

VRV/mg   D: 10/15/18 09:50:16   T: 10/17/18 12:55:01

Determine the most accurate CPT and/or HCPCS Level II code(s) and modifier(s), if appropriate.

_____

_____

_____

CIPHER, VICTORS & ASSOCIATES
A Complete Health Care Facility
234 MAIN STREET • ANYTOWN, FL 32711 • 407-555-1234

PATIENT: FISCHER, ELVIRA
ACCOUNT/EHR #:   FISCEL001
DATE: 12/09/18

Attending Therapist: Stephen L. Brooks, MPT

Pt is a 37-year-old female hurt during a waterskiing accident. She was performing in a ski show at Water World Adventure Park when she came off the ski jump ramp at the wrong angle and hit the water unevenly, twisting her knee. Her physician, Dr. Cipher, ordered her to use a wheelchair for the next 6 weeks.

    I delivered a standard wheelchair with fixed full-length arms and swing-away, detachable footrests to the patient's home. I spent 15 minutes instructing the patient on the proper way to use the chair, transfer from the chair to standard furniture and back, and transfer to other function furniture including the toilet and the bed. She was instructed on how to stop and start the chair with the least amount of strain on her upper extremities and how to apply the brakes. Patient stated she clearly understood all instructions.

DX: Torn meniscus, lateral, knee

P: Patient given instruction booklet and technical support number

_____
Stephen L. Brooks, MPT

SLB/mg   D: 12/09/18 09:50:16   T: 12/11/18 12:55:01

Determine the most accurate CPT and/or HCPCS Level II code(s) and modifier(s), if appropriate.

_____

_____

_____

14 HCPCS LEVEL II MODIFIERS

Learning Outcomes *After completing this chapter, the student should be able to:*

LO 14.1 Apply the guidelines to correctly use HCPCS Level II modifiers.

LO 14.2 Append multiple modifiers in the proper sequence.

LO 14.3 Determine when to appropriately use HCPCS Level II modifiers.

LO 14.4 Distinguish among the various functions of HCPCS Level II modifiers.

LO 14.5 Utilize HCPCS Level II modifiers for statistical analysis of services.

Key Terms

Class A finding

Class B finding

Class C finding

Clinical Laboratory Improvement Amendment (CLIA)

Early and Periodic Screening, Diagnostic, and Treatment (EPSDT)

End-stage renal disease (ESRD)

Locum tenens physician

Liters per minute (LPM)

Parenteral enteral nutrition (PEN)

Urea reduction ratio (URR)

Chapter 3 of this textbook introduced you to CPT modifiers. This chapter introduces you to HCPCS Level II modifiers. The modifiers can be used with both CPT (HCPCS Level I) codes and HCPCS Level II codes. However, you can append them only when submitting data to a third-party payer or an organization that accepts Level II codes.

HCPCS Level II modifiers are two-character codes that are appended to the main code, as necessary, to provide additional information about a particular health care encounter. The modifiers have either two letters (alpha) or one letter and one number (alphanumeric). You will find the complete, and very long, list of the modifiers in Appendix 2 of the HCPCS Level II code book.

EXAMPLE

Q3 Live kidney donor surgery and related services

ST Related to trauma or injury

LO 14.1 Level II Modifier Guidelines

Just as with CPT modifiers, HCPCS modifiers are used to add detail or information to the description of the code. It is your responsibility to read the code's description carefully to make certain the information is not already there. As a coding specialist, you must determine whether or not a modifier is required.

EXAMPLE

> 96154 Health and behavior intervention, each 15 minutes, face-to-face; family (with the patient present)
>
> When you carefully read this code's description, you can see that appending the modifier that follows would be duplicating information.
>
> Modifier HR Family/couple with client present repeats information already in the 96154 code description

KEYS TO CODING

HCPCS Level II modifiers can be appended to either CPT codes or HCPCS Level II codes.

In other cases, adding a modifier can provide important additional information to help care for the patient more effectively, now and in the future. Modifiers can be used to help avoid what might appear to the insurance carrier as a duplicate billing.

EXAMPLE

> 28008 Fasciotomy, foot and/or toe
>
> Adding a modifier such as T7 would include very important information to the claim, especially if the patient had a preexisting condition involving a different toe.
>
> T7 Right foot, third digit

YOU CODE IT! CASE STUDY

On January 5, a respiratory suction pump was provided to Annabelle Anderson, who was diagnosed with emphysema. On January 6, another suction pump was delivered to Annabelle. The first unit had to be replaced because of a defective piece.

You Code It!

Go through the steps and determine the HCPCS Level II code(s) that should be reported for this service for Annabelle Anderson.

Step 1: Read the case completely.

Step 2: Abstract the notes: Which key words can you identify relating to the procedures performed?

_____

Step 3: Query the provider, if necessary.

Step 4: Diagnosis: Emphysema.

Step 5: Code the provision of the original pump and the replacement pump.

_____

Step 6: Link the procedure codes to at least one diagnosis code.

Step 7: Back code to double-check your choices.

Answer:

Did you determine the correct codes?

January 5: E0600 Respiratory suction pump, home model, portable or stationary, electric

January 6: E0600-RA Respiratory suction pump, home model, portable or stationary, electric; replacement of DME

Without the RA modifier to add the information that this code was to replace or repair the first pump, the insurance carrier would be certain to believe that the January 6 claim was a case of double billing.

LO 14.2 Multiple Modifiers

When you need more than one modifier with a procedure or service code, you must place the modifiers in order of specificity, with the most important, most precise modifier closest to the main code.

YOU CODE IT! CASE STUDY

Dr. Curtis drained an abscess on Barry McClintock's left great toe and another on his second toe. Both were simple procedures.

You Code It!

Go through the steps of coding and determine the codes that should be reported for this encounter between Dr. Curtis and Barry McClintock.

Step 1: Read the case completely.

Step 2: Abstract the notes: Which key words can you identify relating to the procedures performed?

_____

Step 3: Query the provider, if necessary.

Step 4: Diagnosis: Abscess, great toe; abscess, second toe.

Step 5: Code the procedure(s).

_____

Step 6: Link the procedure codes to at least one diagnosis code.

Step 7: Back code to double-check your choices.

Answer:

Did you determine the correct codes?

10060-TA Incision and drainage of abscess, simple or single; left foot, great toe

10060-T1-59 Incision and drainage of abscess, simple or single; left foot, second digit; separate procedure

Without the modifiers *TA* for left foot, great toe; *T1* for left foot, second digit; and *59* for distinct procedural service, the claim form could not clearly communicate that Dr. Curtis did work on two different toes.

LO 14.3 The Modifiers

The modifiers are listed in alphabetic order in a separate section of the HCPCS Level II code book. They are not grouped with regard to what each modifier represents anywhere in the HCPCS Level II book. In this chapter, the modifiers have been reorganized and grouped by content to help you better understand when to use each one.

LO 14.4 Providers

The modifiers shown in this section specifically identify the qualifications of the health care professional who provided the service reported by the code to which this modifier is being attached. You will note that some of the modifier descriptions also include a location as a part of its meaning.

EXAMPLE

GF Non-physician services in a critical access hospital

AQ Physician providing a service in an unlisted health professional shortage area (HPSA)

Other modifiers identify the special training that the provider has.

EXAMPLE

SD Services provided by registered nurse with specialized, highly technical home infusion training

Provider Modifiers

AE	Registered dietician
AF	Specialty physician
AG	Primary physician
AH	Clinical psychologist
AI	Principal physician of record
AJ	Clinical social worker
AK	Nonparticipating physician
AM	Physician, team member service
AQ	Physician providing service in unlisted HPSA
AR	Physician provider services in a physician scarcity area
AS	Physician assistant, nurse practitioner, or clinical nurse specialist services for assistant at surgery
DA	Oral health assessment by professional other than a dentist
GC	Service performed in part by a resident under the direction of a teaching physician
GE	Service performed by a resident without the presence of a teaching physician under the primary care exception
GF	Nonphysician services in a critical access hospital

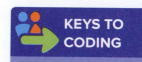

KEYS TO CODING

A nonphysician can be a nurse practitioner, certified registered nurse anesthetist, certified registered nurse, clinical nurse specialist, or physician assistant.

GJ	"Opt out" physician or practitioner emergency or urgent service
GV	Attending physician not employed or paid under arrangement by the patient's hospice provider
HL	Intern
HM	Less than bachelor degree level
HN	Bachelors degree level
HO	Masters degree level
HP	Doctoral level
HT	Multidisciplinary team
Q4	Service for ordering/referring physician that qualifies as a service exemption
Q5	Service furnished by a substitute physician under a reciprocal billing arrangement
Q6	Service furnished by a **locum tenens physician**
SA	Nurse practitioner rendering service in collaboration with a physician
SB	Nurse midwife
SD	Services provided by registered nurse with specialized, highly technical home infusion training
SW	Services provided by a certified diabetic educator
TD	Registered nurse (RN)
TE	Licensed practical nurse (LPN) or LVN

locum tenens physician
A physician that fills in, temporarily, for another physician.

Wound Care

Typically, a dressing change is required for a wound many times throughout the healing process. In addition, it is not unusual that a patient might have more than one wound that needs care at the same time. Therefore, to make the coding process easier and more efficient, one modifier can explain the extent of such care so that listing the same code multiple times is not necessary. The following list contains the modifiers for multiple wounds:

A1	Dressing for one wound
A2	Dressing for two wounds
A3	Dressing for three wounds
A4	Dressing for four wounds
A5	Dressing for five wounds
A6	Dressing for six wounds
A7	Dressing for seven wounds
A8	Dressing for eight wounds
A9	Dressing for nine or more wounds

LET'S CODE IT! SCENARIO

Victor Hirsch, a 29-year-old male, is a firefighter who sustained partial-thickness burns the entire length of his right arm when something exploded. He comes in to see Dr. Malvern to have the dressings changed on four wounds.

Victor comes in to have his *dressings changed* on *four* burn wounds. First, you must find the CPT code for the procedure; second, you can address the modifier. Let's go to the alphabetic index and look up *dressings*. You find

Dressings

Burns   16020–16030

Change

   Anesthesia   15852

You know that Dr. Malvern is changing Victor's dressings; however, there is nothing in the notes that states anesthesia was involved. In addition, Victor's wounds are burns, so let's turn to the numerical listing and carefully read the descriptions for the codes shown next to *burns*. Do you agree that the best code is

16025 Dressings and/or debridement of partial-thickness burns, initial or subsequent; medium (e.g., whole face or whole extremity, or 5% to 10% total body surface area)

The notes indicate that Dr. Malvern changed the dressings for *four wounds*. So rather than just list this code four times, we can use a modifier to communicate this fact: 16025-A4 tells the whole story clearly.

Good work!

Anesthesia Services

You should remember anesthesia modifiers from Chap. 3, "Introduction to CPT Modifiers," and Chap. 6, "Anesthesia Coding," of this textbook. The following modifiers, used only with anesthesia codes, are actually HCPCS Level II modifiers:

AA   Anesthesia services that are performed personally by anesthesiologist
AD   Medical supervision by a physician: more than four concurrent anesthesia procedures
G8   Monitored anesthesia care (MAC) for deep complex, complicated, or markedly invasive surgical procedure
G9   Monitored anesthesia care for patient who has history of severe cardiopulmonary condition
QK   Medical direction of two, three, or four concurrent anesthesia procedures involving qualified individuals
QS   Monitored anesthesia care (MAC) service
QX   CRNA service: with medical direction by a physician
QY   Medical direction of one certified registered nurse anesthetist (CRNA) by an anesthesiologist
QZ   CRNA service without medical direction by a physician

Ophthalmology/Optometry

Sometimes, when ophthalmic or optometric services are provided, more detail is necessary to ensure proper reimbursement. Following are the HCPCS Level II modifiers used with these services:

AP   Determination of refractive state was not performed in the course of diagnostic ophthalmologic examination
LS   FDA-monitored intraocular lens implant
PL   Progressive addition lenses
VP   Aphakic patient

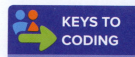

KEYS TO CODING

Chap. 6, "Anesthesia Coding," reviews the use of anesthesia modifiers thoroughly, including the P1–P6 physical status modifiers.

ESRD/Dialysis

Dialysis and other services for a patient with renal conditions, including those with **end-state renal disease** (**ESRD**), may involve extenuating circumstances requiring further explanation. The following dialysis modifiers provide that information.

CB   Service ordered by a renal dialysis facility (RDF) physician as part of the beneficiary's benefit is not part of the composite rate and is separately reimbursable

CD   AMCC test has been ordered by an ESRD facility or MCP physician that is part of the composite rate and is not separately billable

CE   AMCC test has been ordered by an ESRD facility or MCP physician that is a composite rate test but is beyond the normal frequency covered under the rate and is separately reimbursable based on medical necessity

CF   AMCC test has been ordered by an ESRD facility or MCP physician that is not part of the composite rate and is separately billable

EM   Emergency reserve supply (for ESRD benefit only)

G1   Most recent **urea reduction ratio (URR)** reading of less than 60

G2   Most recent URR reading of 60 to 64.9

G3   Most recent URR reading of 65 to 69.9

G4   Most recent URR reading of 70 to 74.9

G5   Most recent URR reading of 75 or greater

G6   ESRD patient for whom less than six dialysis sessions have been provided in a month

---

end-stage renal disease (ESRD)
Chronic, irreversible kidney disease requiring regular treatments.

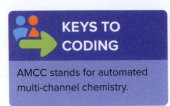

KEYS TO CODING

AMCC stands for automated multi-channel chemistry.

urea reduction ratio (URR)
A formula to determine the effectiveness of hemodialysis treatment.

LET'S CODE IT! SCENARIO

Naomi Bridges, a 41-year-old female, was diagnosed with ESRD. Dr. Nashman prescribed her treatments to begin on May 29 at the Hammerlin Dialysis Center (HDC). Code for the services provided at HDC for the month of May.

Let's Code It!

As you remember from Chap. 11, "Medicine Coding," ESRD services are billed on a monthly basis. However, Naomi only received 3 days of services during the month of May (May 29, May 30, and May 31) from Hammerlin Dialysis Center. In the alphabetic index, you will find no listings for ESRD or end-stage renal disease. That is the patient's diagnosis. You need to turn to the listing for the procedure that was done:

Dialysis

End-stage renal disease   **90951–90970**

After reading the complete code descriptions in the suggested range, you find the best procedure code to be:

90970   End-stage renal disease (ESRD) related services (less than full month), per day; for patients twenty years of age and over

This means you will have to list the code three times because the code description says per day. The modifier that will complete this report is G6 because she has had fewer than six sessions in 1 month: 90970-G6; 90970-G6; 90970-G6 or 90970-G6 ×3. Good job!

Pharmaceuticals

Pharmaceuticals, the industry term for drugs, are items that must be monitored very carefully: the purchase, the storage, and the dispensing. The following modifiers provide important information that must be tracked.

Modifier RD indicates that a particular pharmaceutical was given to the patient but not administered. In other words, the provider may have given the patient the drugs in a bottle or other container but did not inject or use any other means to deliver the drug into the patient's biologic system.

Modifier SV might be used by a mail-order pharmaceutical service to show that the medications were delivered to the patient's house but have nothing to do with how, when, or if the patient uses those drugs.

EXAMPLE

RD Drug provided to beneficiary, but not administered "incident to"

SV Pharmaceuticals delivered to patient's home but not utilized

Pharmaceutical Modifiers

JW	Drug amount discarded/not administered to any patient
KD	Drug or biological infused through DME
KO	Single drug unit dose formulation
KP	First drug of a multiple drug unit dose formulation
KQ	Second or subsequent drug of a multiple drug unit dose formulation
QE	Prescribed amount of oxygen is less than 1 **liter per minute (LPM)**
QF	Prescribed amount of oxygen exceeds 4 LPM and portable oxygen is prescribed
QG	Prescribed amount of oxygen is greater than 4 LPM
QH	Oxygen-conserving device is being used with an oxygen delivery system
RD	Drug provided to beneficiary but not administered "incident to"
SL	State-supplied vaccine
SV	Pharmaceuticals delivered to patient's home but not utilized

liters per minute (LPM)
The measurement of how many liters of a drug or chemical are provided to the patient in 60 seconds.

Items/Services

The following modifiers cover a variety of circumstances relating to the provision of an item or a service.

AU	Item furnished in conjunction with a urologic, ostomy, or tracheostomy supply
AV	Item furnished in conjunction with a prosthetic device, prosthetic or orthotic
BA	Item furnished in conjunction with **parenteral enteral nutrition (PEN)** services
BL	Special acquisition of blood and blood products
BO	Orally administered nutrition, not by feeding tube
EY	No physician or other licensed health care provider order for this item or service
GK	Reasonable and necessary item/item associated with GA or GZ modifier
GL	Medically unnecessary upgrade provided instead of standard item, no charge, no advance beneficiary notice (ABN)
GY	Item or service statutorily excluded or does not meet the definition of any Medicare benefit, not a contract benefit

parenteral enteral nutrition (PEN)
Nourishment delivered using a combination of means other than the gastrointestinal tract (such as IV) in addition to via the gastrointestinal tract.

GZ	Item or service expected to be denied as not reasonable and necessary
KS	Glucose monitor supply for diabetic beneficiary not treated with insulin
KZ	New coverage not implemented by managed care
Q1	Routine clinical service provided in a clinical research study in a an approved clinical research study
QW	**Clinical Laboratory Improvement Amendment (CLIA)** waived test
SC	Medically necessary service or supply
SF	Second opinion ordered by a professional review organization (PRO)
SM	Second surgical opinion
SN	Third surgical opinion
SQ	Item ordered by home health

Purchase/Rental Items

Often, when durable medical equipment (DME) is supplied, the patient has a choice to rent the equipment or purchase it outright. This will depend upon the patient's personal situation.

BP	The beneficiary has been informed of the purchase and rental options and has elected to purchase the item
BR	The beneficiary has been informed of the purchase and rental options and has elected to rent the item
BU	The beneficiary has been informed of the purchase and rental options and after 30 days has not informed the supplier of his/her decision
KH	DMEPOS item, initial claim, purchase or first month rental
KI	DMEPOS item, second or third month rental
KJ	DMEPOS item, parenteral enteral nutrition (PEN) pump or capped rental, months four to fifteen
KR	Rental item, billing for partial month
LL	Lease/rental (use when DME rental payments are to be applied against the purchase price)
MS	Six-month maintenance and servicing fee for reasonable and necessary parts and labor not covered under any manufacturer or supplier warranty
NR	New when rented
RR	Rental DME

YOU CODE IT! CASE STUDY

Nickolas Sawyer, a 67-year-old male, fell and broke his hip last winter. Even though it healed, Nickolas experienced difficulty in walking long distances. Dr. Estevez prescribed a power wheelchair for him. Nickolas decided to purchase a lightweight, portable, motorized/power wheelchair from Wentworth Medical Supply Systems.

You Code It!

Go through the steps of coding and determine the codes that should be reported for the supply of Nickolas Sawyer's new equipment.

Step 1: Read the case completely.

Step 2: Abstract the notes: Which key words can you identify relating to the procedures performed?

_____

Step 3: Query the provider, if necessary.

Step 4: Diagnosis: Osteoarthrosis, pelvic region and thigh.

Step 5: Code the provision of the wheelchair.

Step 6: Link the procedure codes to at least one diagnosis code.

Step 7: Back code to double-check your choices.

Answer:

Did you determine the correct code to be

K0012-KH Lightweight portable motorized/power wheelchair;
DMEPOS item, initial claim, purchase or first month rental

Good work!

Deceased Patient

Should a patient expire (die) while services are in the process of being rendered, certainly the situation changes and there must be some indication of the death. The following modifiers are used in such circumstances:

CA   Procedure payable only in the inpatient setting when performed emergently on an outpatient who expires prior to admission

QL   Patient pronounced dead after ambulance called

LO 14.5 Claims and Documentation

The following modifiers directly provide additional information relating to the claims and documentation involved in certain health care encounters:

CC   Procedure code change (used to indicate that a procedure code previously submitted was changed either for an administrative reason or because an incorrect code was filed)

GA   Waiver of liability statement issued, individual case

GB   Claim being resubmitted for payment because it is no longer covered under a global payment

KB   Beneficiary requested upgrade for ABN, more than four modifiers identified on claim

KX   Requirements specified in the medical policy have been met

QP   Documentation is on file showing that the laboratory test(s) was ordered individually or ordered as a CPT-recognized panel other than automated profile codes 80002–80019, G0058, G0059, and G0060

Anatomical Sites

In Chap. 3, some of the HCPCS Level II modifiers were reviewed that identify a very specific anatomical site upon which a procedure was performed. The following list contains all these modifiers:

E1   Upper left eyelid

E2   Lower left eyelid

E3   Upper right eyelid

E4   Lower right eyelid

FA   Left hand, thumb

F1   Left hand, second digit

F2	Left hand, third digit
F3	Left hand, fourth digit
F4	Left hand, fifth digit
F5	Right hand, thumb
F6	Right hand, second digit
F7	Right hand, third digit
F8	Right hand, fourth digit
F9	Right hand, fifth digit
LC	Left circumflex coronary artery
LD	Left anterior descending coronary artery
LT	Left side (i.e., left side of the body)
RC	Right coronary artery
RT	Right side (i.e., right side of the body)
TA	Left foot, great toe
T1	Left foot, second digit
T2	Left foot, third digit
T3	Left foot, fourth digit
T4	Left foot, fifth digit
T5	Right foot, great toe
T6	Right foot, second digit
T7	Right foot, third digit
T8	Right foot, fourth digit
T9	Right foot, fifth digit

YOU CODE IT! CASE STUDY

Gregory Kendall, a 51-year-old male, had a mass on his left upper eyelid. Dr. Denning performed a biopsy on the eyelid. The pathology report determined it was a benign neoplasm.

Let's Code It!

Go through the steps of coding and determine the codes that should be reported for this encounter between Dr. Denning and Gregory Kendall.

Step 1: Read the case completely.

Step 2: Abstract the notes: Which key words can you identify relating to the procedures performed?

_____

Step 3: Query the provider, if necessary.

Step 4: Diagnosis: Neoplasm, benign, eyelid.

Step 5: Code the procedure(s).

_____

Family Services

Services provided under Medicaid's **Early and Periodic Screening, Diagnostic, and Treatment (EPSDT)** program must be identified with the EP modifier. In addition, other family services may benefit from further explanation by the use of one of the modifiers found in this list:

Early and Periodic Screening, Diagnostic, and Treatment (EPSDT)
A medicaid preventive health program for children under 21.

EP Service provided as part of Medicaid early periodic screening diagnosis and treatment (EPSDT) program

FP Service provided as part of family planning program

G7 Pregnancy resulted from rape or incest or pregnancy certified by physician as life threatening

TL Early intervention/individualized family service plan (IFSP)

TM Individualized education plan (IEP)

TR School-based individualized education program (IEP) services provided outside the public school district responsible for the student

Treatments/Screenings

The modifiers shown in the following list are directly related to the provision of mammography and infusion therapeutic services:

GG Performance and payment of a screening mammogram and diagnostic mammogram on the same patient, same day

GH Diagnostic mammogram converted from screening mammogram on same day

SH Second concurrently administered infusion therapy

SJ Third, or more, concurrently administered infusion therapy

Transportation

The following list has the modifiers that provide additional details with relation to transportation services provided to patients:

GM Multiple patients on one ambulance trip

LR Laboratory round trip

QM Ambulance service provided under arrangement by a provider of services

QN Ambulance service furnished directly by a provider of services

TK Extra patient or passenger, non-ambulance

TP Medical transport, unloaded vehicle

TQ Basic life support transport by a volunteer ambulance provider

Funded Programs

When a service or treatment is provided under the terms or conditions of a formalized program or plan, the services must be identified so that statistical tracking can be accomplished accurately and reimbursement is not received from two sources. The modifiers in the following list enable such tracking:

GN   Services delivered under an outpatient speech language pathology plan of care

GO   Services delivered under an outpatient occupational therapy plan of care

GP   Services delivered under an outpatient physical therapy plan of care

H9   Court-ordered

HA   Child/adolescent program

HB   Adult program, nongeriatric

HC   Adult program, geriatric

HE   Mental health program

HF   Substance abuse program

HG   Opioid addiction treatment program

HH   Integrated mental health/substance abuse program

HI   Integrated mental health and mental retardation/developmental disabilities program

HJ   Employee assistance program

HK   Specialized mental health programs for high-risk populations

HU   Funded by child welfare agency

HV   Funded by state addictions agency

HW   Funded by state mental health agency

HX   Funded by county/local agency

HY   Funded by juvenile justice agency

HZ   Funded by criminal justice agency

SE   State and/or federally funded programs/services

Individual/Group

Most often, modifiers for individuals or groups are going to be used in conjunction with psychiatric and psychotherapeutic codes to clarify how many patients were involved in the session. These modifiers relate to the number, and sometimes the type, of patient(s) being helped at one time:

HQ   Group setting

HR   Family/couple with client present

HS   Family/couple without client present

TJ   Program group, child and/or adolescent

TT   Individualized service provided to more than one patient in same setting

UN   Two patients served

UP   Three patients served

UQ   Four patients served

UR   Five patients served

US   Six or more patients served

Prosthetics

When services are provided relating to the supply or adjustment of a prosthetic device, you might have to include additional information by using one of the following modifiers:

K0   Lower extremity prosthesis functional level 0—does not have the ability or potential to ambulate or transfer safely with or without assistance and prosthesis does not enhance his or her quality of life or mobility

K1   Lower extremity prosthesis functional level 1—has the ability or potential to use a prosthesis for transfers or ambulation on level surfaces at fixed cadence, typical of the limited and unlimited household ambulatory

K2   Lower extremity prosthesis functional level 2—has the ability or potential for ambulation with the ability to traverse low-level environmental barriers such as curbs, stairs, uneven surfaces, typical of limited community ambulatory

K3   Lower extremity prosthesis functional level 3—has the ability or potential for ambulation with variable cadence. Typical of the community ambulatory who has the ability to traverse most environmental barriers and may have vocational, therapeutic, or exercise activity that demands prosthetic utilization beyond simple locomotion

K4   Lower extremity prosthesis functional level 4—has the ability or potential for prosthetic ambulation that exceeds the basic ambulation skills, exhibiting high impact, stress, or energy levels, typical of the prosthetic demands of the child, active adult, or athlete

KM   Replacement of facial prosthesis including new impression/ moulage

KN   Replacement of facial prosthesis using previous master model

LET'S CODE IT! SCENARIO

Rafael Longbranch, a 23-year-old male, returned home after being in a rehabilitation center for 3 months. He had a below knee amputation (BKA) after he was hurt in a rescue mission following a major hurricane. Carol Ann Burkett fitted him for an initial, below-knee patellar tendon bearing (PTB) type socket prosthesis because he has the ability to walk on and even maneuver over such low obstacles as sidewalk curbs and stairs.

Let's Code It!

Carol Ann Burkett ordered and supplied an *initial, below-knee PTB type socket prosthesis*. In the HCPCS Level II alphabetic index, you find

Prosthesis

Fitting, L5400–L5460, L6380–L6388

The notes did say that Carol Ann fitted him, so this should provide a good lead. When you get to this section, beginning with L5400, you find a code whose description matches the notes very well:

L5500   **Initial, below knee PTB type socket, non-alignable system, pylon, no cover, SACH foot, plaster socket, direct formed.**

(Note: SACH stands for solid ankle, cushioned heel.)

You also have to support the service with a modifier to explain Rafael's abilities:

K2 Lower extremity prosthesis functional level 2—has the ability or potential for ambulation with the ability to traverse low-level environmental barriers such as curbs, stairs, or uneven surfaces. Typical of the limited community ambulator

Durable Medical Equipment

When the services relate to the provision of or adjustments to a piece of durable medical equipment (DME), a modifier from the following list may be needed to clarify a certain condition or circumstance:

KA	Add on option/accessory for wheelchair
KC	Replacement of special power wheelchair interface
KF	Item designated by FDA as Class III device
NB	Nebulizer system, any type, FDA-cleared for use with specific drug
NR	New when rented
NU	New equipment
TW	Backup equipment
UE	Used durable medical equipment (DME)

Location

The following modifiers describe situations when you will need to clarify the location at which services were provided:

SG	Ambulatory surgical center (ASC) facility service
SU	Procedure performed in physician's office (i.e., to denote use of facility and equipment)
TN	Rural/outside providers' customary service area

Podiatric Care

There are times when particular services are recategorized, determined by certain signs and/or symptoms that the patient may be exhibiting. The following list identifies modifiers used to indicate some of these circumstances when a podiatrist provides treatment to a patient:

Q7	One **class A finding**
Q8	Two **class B findings**
Q9	One class B and two **class C findings**

Recording

The following modifiers indicate the use of recording equipment as a part of the service, treatment, or procedure provided to the patient:

QC	Single-channel monitoring
QD	Recording and storage in solid-state memory by a digital recorder
QT	Recording and storage on tape by an analog tape recorder

Other Services

The following modifiers do not seem to fit into any of the other categories we have established. Review all the modifiers in the list, and see if you can come up with examples of how and when they would be used.

---

class A finding
Nontraumatic amputation of a foot or an integral skeletal portion.

class B finding
Absence of a posterior tibial pulse; absence or decrease of hair growth; thickening of the nail, discoloration of the skin, and/or thinning of the skin texture; and/or absence of a posterior pedal pulse.

class C finding
Edema, burning sensation, temperature change (cold feet), abnormal spontaneous sensations in the feet, and/or limping.

AT	Acute treatment (to be used only with 98940, 98941, 98942)
EJ	Subsequent claims for a defined course of therapy
ET	Emergency services
GQ	Via asynchronous telecommunications system
GT	Via interactive audio and video telecommunication systems
GW	Service not related to the hospice patient's terminal condition
QJ	Services/items provided to a prisoner or patient in state or local custody, however, the state or local government, as applicable, meets the requirements in 42CFR411.4(B)
Q2	HCFA/ORD demonstration project procedure/service
Q3	Live kidney donor surgery and related services
SK	Member of high-risk population (use only with immunization codes)
ST	Related to trauma or injury
SY	Persons who are in close contact with member of high-risk population (use with immunization codes only)
TC	Technical component
TG	Complex/high-tech level of care
TH	Obstetrical treatment/services, prenatal or postpartum
TS	Follow-up service
UF	Services provided in the morning
UG	Services provided in the afternoon
UH	Services provided in the evening
UJ	Services provided at night
UK	Services provided on behalf of the client to someone other than the client (collateral relationship)

Medicaid Services

Each state administers its own version of the federal Medicaid program and determines its own specific descriptions of the different levels of care. To maintain consistency, HCPCS Level II has the following modifiers that can be used nationwide—even though the description of each modifier will change, as defined by each state.

U1	Medicaid level of care 1, as defined by each state
U2	Medicaid level of care 2, as defined by each state
U3	Medicaid level of care 3, as defined by each state
U4	Medicaid level of care 4, as defined by each state
U5	Medicaid level of care 5, as defined by each state
U6	Medicaid level of care 6, as defined by each state
U7	Medicaid level of care 7, as defined by each state
U8	Medicaid level of care 8, as defined by each state
U9	Medicaid level of care 9, as defined by each state
UA	Medicaid level of care 10, as defined by each state
UB	Medicaid level of care 11, as defined by each state
UC	Medicaid level of care 12, as defined by each state
UD	Medicaid level of care 13, as defined by each state

Special Rates

The following two modifiers are used to indicate that a service or procedure was provided to a patient during an unusual time frame, that is, not during regular working hours:

TU   Special payment rate, overtime

TV   Special payment rates, holidays/weekends

LET'S CODE IT! SCENARIO

Betsy Conchran, a 43-year-old female, came into the hospital for a screening mammogram with computer-aided detection, due to a lump that Dr. Erlich had found in her left breast during her annual checkup. Betsy has a prior history of breast cancer. Later that day, after the films were analyzed, Dr. Erlich made the decision to perform a simple, complete mastectomy. Betsy agreed, and she was immediately taken to the OR for the surgery.

Let's Code It!

Betsy came in for a screening mammogram with computer-aided detection on her left breast. Let's go to the alphabetic index of the CPT book and find the best, most appropriate procedure code or codes:

77057 Screening mammography, bilateral (two view film study of each breast)

77052 Computer-aided detection (computer algorithm analysis of digital image data for lesion detection) with further physician review for interpretation, with or without digitization of film radiographic images; screening mammography (List separately in addition to code for primary procedure.)

There are two points you must address with regard to the preceding codes. First, Betsy had only one breast examined, but code 77057 describes a bilateral exam. Therefore, you must use a modifier to identify what was actually done.

77057-52 Screening mammography, bilateral (two view film study of each breast), reduced services

The addition of modifier 52 explains that the services were for only one side (unilateral), not two sides (bilateral).

Second, once the results of the mammogram became the basis for a decision to have surgery, the screening mammogram became a diagnostic mammogram. Betsy's insurance carrier accepts HCPCS Level II codes and modifiers, so you must adapt the definition of the mammogram from screening to diagnostic by appending a modifier: 77057-52-GH. The GH modifier means that a diagnostic mammogram was converted from a screening mammogram on the same day. This is also why you use 77052 for the computer-aided detection.

Dr. Erlich then performed a "simple, complete mastectomy" on Betsy's *left breast*. The alphabetic index directs you to 19303. The numerical listing shows the complete description:

19303 Mastectomy, simple, complete

You know that Betsy's insurer accepts HCPCS Level II codes and modifiers, so you need to complete the description of the procedure Dr. Erlich performed.

19303-LT Mastectomy, simple, complete, left side

Great job!

Chapter Summary

The general concept of using modifiers is the same for both HCPCS Level II and CPT modifiers, as you learned here and in Chap. 3 of this text. The two-character HCPCS Level II codes help identify specific situations or conditions that are out of the ordinary and enable your facility to receive additional compensation. At the very least, you know that modifiers help offer additional information that may avoid a delay in payment from the insurance carrier or third-party payer.

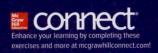

Using Terminology

Match each key term to the appropriate definition.

_____ 1. LO 14.5 Nontraumatic amputation of a foot or an integral skeletal portion.

_____ 2. LO 14.5 A Medicaid preventive health program for children under 21.

_____ 3. LO 14.4 Nourishment delivered using a combination of means other than the gastrointestinal tract (such as IV) in addition to via the gastrointestinal tract.

_____ 4. LO 14.5 Edema, burning sensation, temperature change (cold feet), abnormal spontaneous sensations in the feet, and/or limping.

_____ 5. LO 14.4 Chronic, irreversible kidney disease requiring regular treatments.

_____ 6. LO 14.5 Absence of a posterior tibial pulse; absence or decrease of hair growth; thickening of the nail, discoloration of the skin, and/or thinning of the skin texture; and/or absence of a posterior pedal pulse.

_____ 7. LO 14.4 The measurement of how many liters of a drug or chemical are provided to the patient in 60 seconds.

_____ 8. LO 14.4 A physician that fills in, temporarily, for another physician.

_____ 9. LO 14.4 Federal legislation created for the monitoring and regulation of clinical laboratory procedures.

_____ 10. LO 14.4 A formula to determine the effectiveness of hemodialysis treatment.

A. Class A finding

B. Class B finding

C. Class C finding

D. Clinical Laboratory Improvement Amendment (CLIA)

E. Early and Periodic Screening, Diagnostic, and Treatment (EPSDT)

F. End-stage renal disease (ESRD)

G. Locum tenens physician

H. Liters per minute (LPM)

I. Parenteral enteral nutrition (PEN)

J. Urea reduction ratio (URR)

Checking Your Understanding

Choose the most appropriate answer for each of the following questions.

1. LO 14.1 HCPCS Level II Modifiers can be appended to

   a. Level II codes only.
   b. CPT codes only.
   c. Category III codes only.
   d. Level II codes or CPT codes.

2. LO 14.1/14.2/14.3/14.5 HCPCS Level II modifiers can identify

   a. an anatomical part.
   b. a replacement part.
   c. a professional's qualifications.
   d. all of these.

3. LO 14.4 LPM stands for

   a. local procedure modality.
   b. liters per minute.
   c. licensed practical medicine.
   d. local patient median.

4. LO 14.2 When both a CPT modifier and a HCPCS Level II modifier are needed, place them in the following order:
   a. CPT and then HCPCS Level II.
   b. HCPCS Level II and then CPT.
   c. They cannot be reported together.
   d. The most important modifier should be placed closest to the code.

5. LO 14.5 An example of a DME is
   a. aspirin.
   b. the administration of a vaccination.
   c. a wheelchair.
   d. the removal of a cyst.

6. LO 14.4 CLIA stands for
   a. Clinical Laboratory Internal Assessment.
   b. Clinical Laboratory Improvement Amendment.
   c. Catastrophic Laboratory Inventory Allotment.
   d. Clinical Lateral Improvement Amendment.

7. LO 14.5 Early and Periodic Screening, Diagnosis, and Treatment is a program of
   a. Medicare.
   b. Medicaid.
   c. BlueCross BlueShield Association.
   d. The American Medical Association.

8. LO 14.5 A prosthetic is
   a. a treatment plan.
   b. a type of diagnostic exam.
   c. an artificial body part.
   d. a specially trained health care professional.

9. LO 14.5 A podiatric Class C finding includes all *except*
   a. edema.
   b. bleeding.
   c. a burning sensation.
   d. temperature change.

10. LO 14.5 Medicaid provides modifiers at _____ levels for use by each state.
    a. 10.
    b. 5.
    c. 13.
    d. 12.

Applying Your Knowledge

1. **LO 14.1** What are HCPCS Level II modifiers used for, and where can you append a HCPCS Level II modifier? ____

   _____

2. **LO 14.2** Explain how to sequence multiple modifiers. _____

   _____

3. **LO 14.3** How are HCPCS Level II modifiers listed in the HCPCS Level II code book? How are they reorganized in this chapter, and why? _____

   _____

4. **LO 14.4** List six functions of HCPCS Level II modifiers. _____

   _____

5. **LO 14.5** What claims and documentation modifier represents a waiver of liability statement issued by individual case? _____

   _____

6. **LO 14.5** What is the anatomical site modifier that represents the right hand, fifth digit? _____

   _____

7. **LO 14.5** What does transportation modifier TQ represent? _____

   _____

8. **LO 14.5** Explain the difference between a Class A finding, a Class B finding, and a Class C finding. _____

   _____

YOU CODE IT! Practice
Chapter 14: HCPCS Level II Modifiers

Using the techniques described in this chapter, carefully read through the case studies and determine the most accurate HCPCS Level II modifier(s) for each case study. *Note:* All insurance carriers and third-party payers for the patients accept HCPCS Level II codes and modifiers.

1. Dr. Mathers performed a blepharotomy on Georgie Anne McAfee, draining the abscess on her upper left eyelid.

   _____

2. Wilma Certifano, a nurse midwife, helped Cloris Dana deliver her first baby, a girl.

   _____

3. Jasper Jons, a 71-year-old male diagnosed with terminal bone cancer, has been in the hospice facility for 3 weeks and is showing signs of an ear infection. Dr. Lieber was called in to attend Jasper's ear problem.

   _____

4. Frank Ferguson, an EMT, answered a call, with his partner, to Barton Nursing Home. There was a small fire in the laundry room, and two patients were overcome by smoke enough to require hospitalization. Frank transported both patients at the same time in his ambulance and made one trip to the hospital.

   _____

5. Allen Ashcroft, a licensed psychotherapist, began the first of a series of court-ordered therapy sessions with Neil Scranton.

   _____

6. Dr. Horvath was called in to provide monitored anesthesia care for a procedure that will be performed on Sophia Applot. Sophia has a history of acute cardiopulmonary problems.

   _____

7. Juan Gonzalez, a registered nurse, works at the Barton Nursing Facility. He changed the dressing on three wounds that Miriam Warner had on her leg.

   _____

8. Elaine Everidge is the coding specialist for Barton Dialysis Center. She is preparing the claim for services provided to Grace Boxer, a patient with ESRD, who moved to the area just last week. Barton Dialysis provided four dialysis treatments for Grace during the month.

_____

9. Linda Meyers, one of the coding specialists at Barton Hospital, discovered that a claim had been submitted with an incorrect code. She has corrected the procedure code and is resubmitting the claim.

_____

10. Nadine Stuart works at Barton Medical Equipment Inc. She meets with Arthur Lynch, who was recently prescribed an electric wheelchair by Dr. Bryan. Nadine explains the options of purchasing and renting the chair, and Arthur decides to purchase the wheelchair.

_____

11. Dr. Quimby excised a lesion from Gary McDonald's right thumb.

_____

12. Glenda Javlin gave Blanche Hansel, a 77-year-old female, a flu shot.

_____

13. Dr. Helen Messina saw Virginia Cromwell and provided service defined as level 3 by Medicaid in her state.

_____

14. Ashley Polk is a certified diabetic educator. She met with Amos Brahma to provide services.

_____

15. The peer review organization (PRO) ordered Dr. Filippelli to provide a second opinion on the surgical options for Marcel Daquan.

_____

The following exercises provide practice in the application of abstracting the physicians' notes and learning to work with SOAP notes from our health care facility, Cipher, Victors & Associates. These case studies (SOAP notes) are modeled on real patient encounters. Using the techniques described in this chapter, carefully read through the case studies and determine the most accurate CPT and/or HCPCS Level II code(s) and *necessary* modifier(s) for each case study. *Note:* All insurance carriers and third-party payers for the patients accept HCPCS Level II codes and modifiers.

CIPHER, VICTORS & ASSOCIATES
A Complete Health Care Facility
234 MAIN STREET • ANYTOWN, FL 32711 • 407-555-1234

PATIENT: LEE, CHARLENE
ACCOUNT/EHR #:   LEECHA001
DATE: 11/23/18

Attending Physician: James I. Cipher, MD

S: New Pt is a 67-year-old female who works at a car dealership and spends a lot of time on her feet. She has been suffering from a cyst on the fourth toe of her left foot that is filled with fluid. She presents today to have the cyst drained.

O: Pt lies back on the examination table, and her left foot is elevated and draped in a sterile fashion. A topical antiseptic is applied, and I incised the cyst located below the fascia and drained it. The tendon sheath is not involved. The incision area is bandaged. The patient tolerated the procedure well.

A: Cyst of bursa

P: Follow-up in 2 weeks

James I. Cipher, MD

JIC/mg   D: 11/23/18 09:50:16   T: 11/25/18 12:55:01

Determine the most accurate CPT and/or HCPCS Level II code(s) and necessary modifier(s).

_____

_____

_____

CIPHER, VICTORS & ASSOCIATES
A Complete Health Care Facility
234 MAIN STREET • ANYTOWN, FL 32711 • 407-555-1234

PATIENT: GENTRY, BRIAN
ACCOUNT/EHR #:   GENTBR001
DATE: 11/10/18

Attending Physician: James I. Cipher, MD

S: Pt is a 36-year-old male who has not been seen in the office in just over a year. He recently began working for a landscaping company and presents today with a rash covering both hands and arms up to the elbow. Pt states that the rash itches and is uncomfortable. Scabs have formed over spots where he scratched and bled. Patient has no history of allergies or other dermatologic reactions. However, he also states that he has not previously worked with pesticides, particularly the new brand being used at his job.

O: HEENT is unremarkable with the exception of some redness in the back of the throat. Upper extremities show pustular eruptions anteriorly and posteriorly. Herve Sanchez, a nurse practitioner, in collaboration with me, gave the patient an injection subcutaneously of Benadryl, 40 mg.

A: Exanthem

P: 1. Rx Benadryl ointment prn
   2. Follow-up in 2 weeks

_____

James I. Cipher, MD

JIC/mg   D: 11/10/18 09:50:16   T: 11/12/18 12:55:01

Determine the most accurate CPT and/or HCPCS Level II code(s) and necessary modifier(s).

_____

_____

_____

CIPHER, VICTORS & ASSOCIATES
A Complete Health Care Facility
234 MAIN STREET • ANYTOWN, FL 32711 • 407-555-1234

PATIENT: BRINKLEY, ALISSA
ACCOUNT/EHR #:   BRINAL001
DATE: 11/21/18

Attending Physician: Rodney Southern, MD
Referring Physician: Valerie R. Victors, MD

S: Pt is a 41-year-old female who was injured in a car accident. She presents today, at the recommendation of Dr. Victors, for a fitting for a prosthetic spectacle.

O: HEENT is unremarkable. Monofocal measurements are taken, and data for the creation of an appropriate prosthesis are recorded.

A: Aphakia, left eye

P: Return in 2 weeks for final fitting

_____

Rodney Southern, MD

RS/mg   D: 11/21/18 09:50:16   T: 11/23/18 12:55:01

Determine the most accurate CPT and/or HCPCS Level II code(s) and necessary modifier(s).

_____

_____

_____

CIPHER, VICTORS & ASSOCIATES
A Complete Health Care Facility
234 MAIN STREET • ANYTOWN, FL 32711 • 407-555-1234

PATIENT: DAHL, WILLIAM
ACCOUNT/EHR #:   DAHLWI001
DATE: 12/10/18

Attending Physician: Kristen Tremaine, MD
Referring Physician: James I. Cipher, MD

Upon orders from Dr. Cipher, I transported a portable x-ray machine to the Barton Nursing Facility to take a chest x-ray, one view—frontal, of each of three patients with suspicion of tuberculosis.

Patients served:
- Joselyn Gano, a 73-year-old female
- Barbara Ann Forrester, an 83-year-old female
- Martin Bloomington, a 79-year-old male

All three patients show nodular lesions and patchy infiltrates in the upper lobes.

_____

Kristen Tremaine, MD

KT/mg   D: 12/10/18 09:50:16   T: 12/12/18 12:55:01

Determine the most accurate CPT and/or HCPCS Level II code(s) and necessary modifier(s).

_____

_____

_____

CIPHER, VICTORS & ASSOCIATES
A Complete Health Care Facility
234 MAIN STREET • ANYTOWN, FL 32711 • 407-555-1234

PATIENT: TRUMBLE, HORACE
ACCOUNT/EHR #:   TRUMHO001
DATE: 09/07/18

Locum Tenens Physician: Roxan J. Platt, MD
Attending Physician: James I. Cipher, MD

S: Pt is a 17-year-old male who has been a patient of Dr. Cipher for many years. He presents today with a sore throat. I explained to the patient that I am filling in for Dr. Cipher while he is on vacation.

O: HEENT is relatively unremarkable with the exception of white spots in the back of the throat. Patient still has his tonsils. His throat is swabbed for a culture (immunoassay with direct optical observation to detect Streptococcus group B).

A: Streptococcal sore throat

P: 1. Rx antibiotic
    2. Follow-up in 10 days

_____

Roxan J. Platt, MD

RJP/mg   D: 09/07/18 09:50:16   T: 09/09/18 12:55:01

Determine the most accurate CPT and/or HCPCS Level II code(s) and necessary modifier(s).

_____

_____

_____

15

CODING MEDICAL SUPPLIES, DURABLE MEDICAL EQUIPMENT, PHARMACEUTICAL, AND AMBULANCE AND OTHER TRANSPORTATION SERVICES

Learning Outcomes *After completing this chapter, the student should be able to:*

LO 15.1 Interpret correctly the rules and guidelines for coding medical supplies.

LO 15.2 Apply the instructions for properly coding durable medical equipment.

LO 15.3 Report the accurate codes for pharmaceutical services.

LO 15.4 Distinguish between the generic and brand names of drugs.

LO 15.5 Utilize the guidelines for coding transportation services.

LO 15.6 Calculate correct waiting time for transportation services.

Key Terms

Advanced life support (ALS)

Basic life support (BLS)

Cannula

Decubitus ulcer

DMEPOS

Incontinence

Ostomy

Self-administer

Specialty care transport (SCT)

Transcutaneous electrical nerve stimulators (TENS)

The most common items and services that are coded from the HCPCS Level II code set include medical supplies, durable medical equipment (DME), pharmaceuticals administered by a health care professional, and transportation services. This chapter will review what you should know when coding these.

LO 15.1 Coding Medical Supplies

In almost every health care encounter, materials and supplies are used. The paper used to cover the examination table and the disposable cover on the digital thermometer are good examples. Such medical supplies are used by the health care facility itself. However, they are *not* the types of medical and surgical supplies to which the HCPCS Level II book refers. The codes in the HCPCS Level II book are for reporting supplies given to a patient to **self-administer** health care at home.

A Codes and B Codes

Let's begin by reviewing the subheadings throughout the A code and B code sections to get a good idea of which items are covered.

Miscellaneous Supplies A4206–A4290 The supplies used by a physician in the course of treatment (syringes, alcohol wipes, urine test strips, and so on) are included in the amount reimbursed for the provision of that treatment or service. The codes in miscellaneous supplies (HCPCS Level II) are used to report, and be reimbursed for, supplies provided to patients for their own use at home. For example, if a diabetic patient requires a daily insulin shot at home, he or she would need to have syringes available.

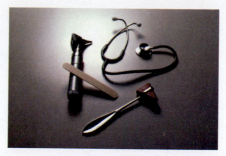

EXAMPLE

A4252 Blood ketone test or reagent strip, each
A4250 Urine test or reagent strips or tablets (100 tablets or strips)

self-administer
To give medication to oneself, such as a diabetic giving herself an insulin injection.

Vascular Catheters A4300–A4306 In the subheading for vascular catheters, you will find codes to report the use of a disposable drug delivery system (DDS) as well as implantable access catheters. The codes are not for reporting the physician's work to implant the catheter but for the facility to be reimbursed for the cost of the catheter itself.

EXAMPLE

A4300 Implantable access catheter, external access
A4306 Disposable drug delivery system, flow rate of 5 mL or less than 50 ml per hour

Incontinence Appliances and Care Supplies A4310–A4355
External Urinary Supplies A4356–A4360 The sections Incontinence Appliances and Care Supplies and External Urinary Supplies cover urinary supplies that a patient uses when he or she has been diagnosed with permanent, or chronic, **incontinence.**

incontinence
The inability to control urination or fecal expulsion.

EXAMPLE

A4330 Perianal fecal collection pouch with adhesive, each
A4349 Male external catheter, with or without adhesive, disposable, each

Ostomy Supplies A4361–A4434 Patients who have had surgery to create an **ostomy** need supplies every day to make their medical situation easier to deal with and to enable them to live their lives more normally.

ostomy
An artificial opening made in the body surgically.

EXAMPLE

A4404 Ostomy ring, each
A4416 Ostomy pouch, closed, with barrier attached, with filter (one piece), each

Additional Miscellaneous Supplies A4450–A4608 *Additional miscellaneous supplies represent a grouping of codes for other necessary items.*

EXAMPLE

A4458 Enema bag with tubing, reusable
A4510 Surgical stocking full-length, each

YOU CODE IT! CASE STUDY

Carmella Sanfilippo, a 65-year-old female, was diagnosed with acute varicose veins in her legs. Dr. Bennett gave her a prescription for a pair of thigh-length surgical stockings. She received two pairs from Thompson Health care Supplies and Service.

You Code It!

Go through the steps of coding and determine the code(s) that should be reported for the stockings provided to Carmella Sanfilippo.

Step 1: Read the case completely.

Step 2: Abstract the notes: Which key words can you identify relating to the procedures performed?

_____

Step 3: Query the provider, if necessary.

Step 4: Diagnosis: Acute varicose veins.

Step 5: Code for the provision of the stockings.

_____

Step 6: Link the procedure codes to at least one diagnosis code.

Step 7: Back code to double-check your choices.

Answer:

Did you determine the correct code ?

A4495 × 4 Surgical stocking thigh length, each, four stockings

Good job!

Supplies for Oxygen and Related Respiratory Equipment A4611–A4629

Supplies for Other Durable Medical Equipment A4630–A4640

Here, and in other portions of the subsections for coding respiratory supplies and other DME, you will find the ancillary supplies and items used in conjunction with DME, such as a **cannula** or a cleaning brush.

cannula
A tube that is inserted into the body to either deliver or extract fluid, such as a nasogastric tube.

EXAMPLE

A4615 Cannula, nasal
A4626 Tracheostomy cleaning brush, each
A4637 Replacement, tip, cane, crutch, walker, each

Benjamin Stiles, a 77-year-old male, diagnosed with acute emphysema, used a ventilator purchased by him last year. Walter Synder, from Miller Medical Supplies, brought a new, heavy-duty replacement battery for the ventilator and installed it.

You Code It!

Go through the steps of coding and determine the code(s) that should be reported for the replacement battery provided to Benjamin Stiles.

Step 1: Read the case completely.

Step 2: Abstract the notes: Which key words can you identify relating to the procedures performed?

_____

Step 3: Query the provider, if necessary.

Step 4: Diagnosis: Acute emphysema.

Step 5: Code the replacement battery.

_____

Step 6: Link the procedure codes to at least one diagnosis code.

Step 7: Back code to double-check your choices.

Answer:

Did you determine the correct code?

A4611 Battery, heavy duty; replacement for patient-owned ventilator

Excellent!

Supplies for Radiologic Procedures A4641–A4932 Similar to other cases in this book, the codes for radiologic procedure supplies represent the ancillary items needed during and/or after some procedures—not the actual procedure itself.

> ## EXAMPLE
>
> A4648 Tissue marker, implantable, any type, each
> A4770 Blood collection tube, vacuum, for dialysis, per 50
> A4931 Oral thermometer, reusable, any type, each

Additional Ostomy Supplies A5051–A5093
Additional Incontinence Appliances/Supplies A5102–A5114
Supplies for Either Incontinence or Ostomy Appliances A5120–A5200 These subsections—Additional Ostomy Supplies, Additional Incontinence Appliances/Supplies, and Supplies for Either Incontinence or Ostomy Appliances—are additional codes for items needed by patients with medical problems.

EXAMPLE

A5055 Stoma cap

A5093 Ostomy accessory; convex insert

A5120 Skin barrier, wipes or swabs, each

Diabetic Shoes, Fitting, and Modifications A5500–A5511 One thing you are certain to notice is that every one of the codes under Diabetic Shoes, Fitting, and Modifications begins with the same three words, "for diabetics only." Another detail you should notice is that each code specifies coverage of only one shoe. Therefore, if the patient gets a pair of shoes, you must report the appropriate code twice.

EXAMPLE

A5508 For diabetics only, deluxe feature of off-the-shelf depth-inlay shoe or custom-molded shoe, per shoe

YOU CODE IT! CASE STUDY

Jerry Gaynor, a 71-year-old male, has type 1 diabetes mellitus with peripheral neuropathy with evidence of callus formation, particularly on his left foot. He came today so that Marilyn Requin could do a fitting for a pair of custom-molded shoes.

You Code It!

Go through the steps and determine the code(s) that should be reported for the fitting of shoes for Jerry Gaynor.

Step 1: Read the case completely.

Step 2: Abstract the notes: Which key words can you identify relating to the procedures performed?

_____

Step 3: Query the provider, if necessary.

Step 4: Diagnosis: Diabetic, peripheral neuropathy.

Step 5: Code for the shoes.

_____

Step 6: Link the procedure codes to at least one diagnosis code.

Step 7: Back code to double-check your choices.

Answer:

Did you determine the correct code?

A5501 × 2 For diabetics only, fitting (including follow-up) custom preparation and supply of shoe molded from cast(s) of patient's foot (custom-molded shoe), per shoe, two shoes

Great!

Dressings A6000–A8004 Wound care requires a lot of supplies, such as bandages that need to be changed frequently to ensure a clean and sterile environment for healing. Different wounds involve different types of dressings.

EXAMPLE

A6154 Wound pouch, each

A6215 Foam dressing, wound filler, per gram

A6410 Eye pad, sterile, each

YOU CODE IT! CASE STUDY

Beverly Schuck, a 19-year-old female, was riding with her boyfriend on his motorcycle and burned her right calf on the tailpipe. Her friend told her to put butter on the burn, and Beverly's calf became badly infected. After debriding the wound, Dr. Errol applied an alginate dressing, 15 sq in., because the wound was oozing fluid. Dr. Errol provided Beverly with one additional dressing so that she could change the wound cover in 1 week.

You Code It!

Go through the steps and determine the code(s) that should be reported for the wound cover provided to Beverly Schuck.

Step 1:   Read the case completely.

Step 2:   Abstract the notes: Which key words can you identify relating to the procedures performed?

_____

Step 3:   Query the provider, if necessary.

Step 4:   Diagnosis: Infected burn, lower leg, right.

Step 5:   Code for the alginate dressing.

_____

Step 6:   Link the procedure codes to at least one diagnosis code.

Step 7:   Back code to double-check your choices.

Answer:

Did you determine the correct code?

A6196 Alginate or other fiber gelling dressing, wound cover, sterile, pad size 16 sq in. or less, each dressing

You got it!

Administrative, Miscellaneous, and Investigational A9000–A9999

Administrative, Miscellaneous, and Investigational provides a catch-all for items such as nonprescription medications, exercise equipment, and other supplies that may be provided for home care.

EXAMPLE

A9280 Alert or alarm device, not otherwise classified

A9504 Technetium Tc 99m apcitide, diagnostic, per study dose, up to 20 millicuries

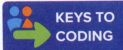

Enteral Formulae and Enteral Medical Supplies B4034–B4162
Parenteral Nutrition Solutions and Supplies B4164–B5200
Enteral and Parenteral Pumps B9000–B9999 The codes in the Enteral Formulae and Enteral Medical Supplies, Parenteral Nutrition Solutions and Supplies, and Enteral and Parenteral Pumps sections report the supply of items related to providing nutrition to a patient by alternate means—other than by mouth and/or the digestive tract.

EXAMPLE

B4081 Nasogastric tubing with stylet

B4178 Parenteral nutrition solution; amino acid, greater than 8.5% (500 mL = 1 unit), home mix

B9004 Parenteral nutrition infusion pump, portable

LET'S CODE IT! SCENARIO

Jan Bagwell, a 71-year-old female, was diagnosed with a malignant neoplasm of the rectum. As a result, last month Dr. Garwood performed a colostomy on her. She is fitted with a drainable, rubber colostomy pouch with faceplate and drain along with a protective solid skin barrier, four by four.

Let's Code It!

The notes tell us that Dr. Garwood gave Jan a "drainable, rubber colostomy pouch with faceplate and drain," as well as a "protective solid skin barrier." Let's begin coding the pouch by going to the alphabetic index and looking up *pouch.* As you review the indented terms beneath, you notice immediately that there is no listing for *colostomy;* however, there are a few choices you can follow:

Pouch, drainable, A4388–A4389, A5061

Pouch, ostomy, A4375–A4378, A4387–A4391, A5051–A5054, A50061-A5063, A4416-A4420, A4423-A4434

Go to the alphanumeric listing, and read the complete description of each of the suggested codes. Did you find the one that matches the notes most accurately?

A4376 Ostomy pouch, drainable, with faceplate attached, rubber, each

Next, you want to code the skin barrier. Let's go back to the alphabetic index and look under *skin.* You find the suggested codes:

Skin, barrier, Ostomy, A4362, A4369, A4385

Check the complete code descriptions in the alphanumeric listing. While there is great similarity between A4362 and A4385, you notice that Dr. Garwood's notes say nothing about its being an extended wear barrier. Therefore, A4362 is most accurate. Your claim form for the supplies Dr. Garwood provided to Jan shows

A4376 Ostomy pouch, drainable, with faceplate attached, rubber, each

A4362 Skin barrier, solid, 4 × 4 or equivalent; each

Excellent! This matches perfectly.

LO 15.2 Coding Durable Medical Equipment (DME)

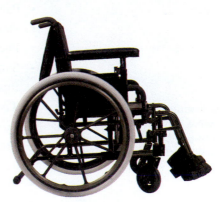

© Ingram Publishing/Alamy

Science and technology have provided our society with great innovations that make life easier and more functional. Canes, walkers, and wheelchairs, among other items, help individuals move from one place to another without further assistance. Portable oxygen, humidifiers, vaporizers, and other equipment assist breathing, and pacemakers and electrical nerve stimulators help keep a heart beating. Some items are so commonplace that we take them for granted, yet only 10 years ago, patients would be forced to stay home all day every day. Other products, such as wheelchairs, have evolved into more convenient and accommodating pieces of equipment.

Each item and every accessory costs money to build. Therefore, the health care facility or company should be reimbursed for giving, renting/leasing, or selling equipment. HCPCS Level II codes for DME are used in the reimbursement process.

Durable Medical Equipment

Durable medical equipment (DME) includes such items as canes, wheelchairs, and ventilators. However, to be accurate, Medicare has four qualifiers to determine whether an item can be classified as DME. These qualifiers are

1. The item can withstand repeated use.
2. The item is primarily used for medical purposes.
3. The item is used in the patient's home (rather than only in a health care facility).
4. The item would not be used if the individual were not ill or injured.

Most often, **DMEPOS** dealers supply DME to the patient. Such companies submit their claims not to Medicare or the state's Medicare fiscal intermediary (FI) but to their assigned durable medical equipment regional carrier (DMERC), which is contracted by Centers for Medicare and Medicaid Services (CMS).

DMEPOS
Durable medical equipment, prosthetic, and orthotic supplies.

HCPCS E Code Subheadings

The DME E code section, codes E0100–E9999, is divided into subheadings. It is not the only section in the HCPCS Level II book having codes related to DME services and supplies; however, it is the section dedicated to them. Take a minute to look through its subheadings, and you should gain a clearer understanding of the items and services included here.

- Canes
- Crutches
- Walkers

- Attachments (i.e., accessories for walkers)
- Commodes (i.e., portable toilets)
- Decubitus care equipment (i.e., care for **decubitus ulcers** and related issues)
- Heat/cold application
- Bath and toilet aids
- Hospital beds and accessories
- Oxygen and related respiratory equipment
- Intermittent positive-pressure breathing (IPPB) machines
- Humidifiers/compressors/nebulizers for use with oxygen IPPB equipment
- Suction pump/room vaporizers
- Monitoring equipment (i.e., home blood glucose monitor)
- Pacemaker monitor
- Patient Lifts (i.e., to lift a patient out of, or into, a bed, a bathtub, or other circumstance)
- Pneumatic compressor and appliances
- Safety equipment
- Restraints
- **Transcutaneous** and/or neuromuscular **electrical nerve stimulators (TENS)**
- Infusion supplies
- Traction—all types
- Traction—cervical
- Traction—overdoor
- Traction—extremity
- Traction—pelvic
- Trapeze equipment, fracture frame, and other orthopedic devices
- Rollabout chair
- Wheelchairs—fully reclining
- Wheelchair—semireclining
- Wheelchair—standard
- Wheelchair—amputee
- Wheelchair—power
- Wheelchair—special size
- Wheelchair—lightweight
- Wheelchair—heavy-duty
- Whirlpool—equipment
- Repairs and replacement supplies
- Additional oxygen-related equipment
- Artificial kidney machines and accessories
- Jaw motion rehabilitation system and accessories
- Other orthopedic devices

LET'S CODE IT! SCENARIO

Isadore McPherson, an 82-year-old male, had a stroke and is coming to live with Grace, his granddaughter. In order to properly accommodate his needs, Chuck Michaels, a representative of Peterson's Medical Equipment, has come to Grace's home to deliver and set up a hospital bed. The bed has a variable height function to make caring for Isadore easier, and it has detachable side rails. The mattress is a firm one and is supplied with the bed.

Let's Code It!

You are the coding specialist working for Peterson's Medical Equipment and must send a claim to Medicare for the bed. The bed is described as a *hospital bed, variable height,* with detachable *side rails,* and a *mattress.* Let's go to the alphabetic index in the HCPCS Level II book.

Find the term *bed,* and you see *hospital* indented below. Beneath this, indented, are more descriptors, such as full electric, manual, or safety enclosure frame. You do not have any of those terms in your notes, so let's go to the suggested codes shown next to Bed, hospital, E0250–E0270.

E0250 Hospital bed, fixed height, with any type side rails, with mattress

E0251 Hospital bed, fixed height, with any type side rails, without mattress

Neither code is accurate because they describe beds with a *fixed* height, not *variable* height, as your notes describe. Let's keep reading.

E0255 Hospital bed, variable height, hi-lo, with any type side rails, with mattress

The code description matches your notes. Great job!

LET'S CODE IT! SCENARIO

Dean Bernard, a 12-year-old male, was born with spina bifida. His power wheelchair's motor has malfunctioned, and Wayne Dolan, a repair technician for Haverty's Medical Supplies and Repairs, has come to Dean's house to install a replacement drive wheel motor.

Let's Code It!

You are the coding specialist working for Haverty's Medical Supplies and Repairs and must send a claim to Dean's insurance carrier for the *replacement motor* for the *power wheelchair.* You have checked and know that the third-party payer accepts HCPCS Level II codes.

Let's go to the alphabetic listing and find *wheelchair.* As you go down the list indented beneath the key term, you find *power.* Keep reading, and indented below *power,* you see *motor.* Hmm. This looks perfect. Let's check out Wheelchair, power, motor, E2368.

E2368 Power wheelchair component, drive wheel motor, replacement only

Cool. It couldn't be a better description if you had written it yourself!

LO 15.3 Coding Pharmaceutical Services

In Chap. 11, "Medicine Coding," you learned about coding for the administration of pharmaceuticals (drugs). Those codes are used for reporting the services—the labor—of the health care professional who gives the patient the drug. You may remember that the different methods of administering drugs include:

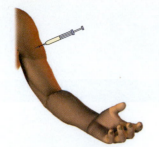

Intramuscular

IA	Intra-arterial administration
IV	Intravenous administration (e.g., gravity infusion, injections, and timed pushes)
IM	Intramuscular administration
IT	Intrathecal
SC	Subcutaneous administration
INH	Inhaled solutions
VAR	Various routes for drugs that are commonly administered into joints, cavities, tissues, or topical applications, as well as other parenteral administrations
ORAL	Administered orally
OTH	Other routes of administration, such as suppositories or catheter injections

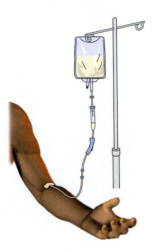

Intravenous

EXAMPLE

The CPT book has the following codes:

96372 Therapeutic, prophylactic or diagnostic injection (specify substance or drug); subcutaneous or intramuscular

96373 intra-arterial

96374 intravenous push, single or initial substance/drug

The codes in HCPCS Level II enable you to report and gain reimbursement for the actual drug or medication, as well as the syringe or IV bag used. The codes cover the pharmaceutical materials only—*not* the administration of the drug.

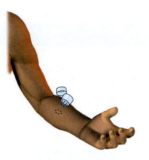

Intradermal

EXAMPLE

J0760 Injection, colchicine, per 1 mg

J7613 Albuterol, inhalation solution, FDA-approved final product, noncompounded, administered through DME, unit dose, 1 mg

S0012 Butorphanol tartrate, nasal spray, 25 mg

S5001 Prescription drug, brand name

In some cases, you may find DME has been supplied to the patient to provide medication, or drugs. When the equipment is made available to an individual, it may need to be reported separately from the drug itself.

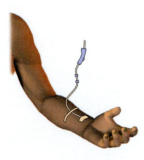

Intra-arterial

EXAMPLE

> S5560 Insulin delivery device, reusable pen; 1.5 mL size
>
> J1817 Insulin for administration through DME (i.e., insulin pump) per 50 units

Note that S5560 covers only the DME, whereas J1817 covers only the medication.

LO 15.4 Generic Names and Brand Names

As you look through the HCPCS Level II book, you will notice that the drugs are listed by their chemical, or generic, name. When the notes describe a medication or a drug by its brand name, or trade name, you may have to look for the drug in one of the following resources:

1. Alphabetic index of the HCPCS Level II book. Some—but not all—drugs are shown in the alphabetic index by both the generic name and a brand, or trade, name.
2. Appendix 1, Table of Drugs, of the HCPCS Level II book.
3. *Physicians' Desk Reference* (PDR).

The PDR has the correct generic name for any drug, along with other important data, such as indications (when the patient should be given this drug), contraindications (when a patient should *not* be given this drug), and possible side effects. Once you have the generic name for the drug supplied to the patient, you will be able to look it up in the HCPCS Level II book.

EXAMPLE

> Proventil (brand name) is listed in the Table of Drugs but not in the alphabetic index.
>
> Albuterol (generic name) is listed in both the alphabetic index and the Table of Drugs.

Appendix 1—Table of Drugs

In addition to the alphabetic index, you also have the Table of Drugs, located in Appendix 1 in the back of the HCPCS Level II book. The table lists drugs, by their generic and/or brand names, alphabetically.

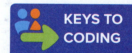

KEYS TO CODING

The Table of Drugs is no different from the primary alphabetic index. You should never code from the table. Always confirm the code by its complete description in the alphanumeric listing.

DRUG NAME	UNIT	ROUTE	CODE
Alimta	10 mg	IV	J9305
Cipro	200 mg	IV	J0744

In the first column of the table, the name of the drug is listed in alphabetic order, from *A* to *Z*.

The second column identifies the most often used unit of measurement or dose for that drug.

The third column indicates the method of administration (the route), such as intravenous (IV) or inhalation (INH).

The last column has the suggested code. You should still double-check the code's complete description in the alphanumeric listings contained in the body of the book.

You might find the table easier to use than the alphabetic index. Choose whichever helps you find the best, most accurate code for the services delivered.

Russell Bromwell, a 23-year-old male, was brought to the emergency department with severe abdominal cramps, vomiting, and nausea. Test results and examination led Dr. Camponetta to the diagnosis of an intraabdominal infection caused by exposure to Escherichia coli. *He prescribed ampicillin sodium and sulbactam sodium IV injection 1.5 g q6h. Code for the first 12 hours.*

Let's Code It!

Dr. Camponetta prescribed *ampicillin sodium and sulbactam sodium,* for *IV injection.* Let's go to the HCPCS Level II book's alphabetic index and look up the name of the drug: ampicillin sodium. You will see

Ampicillin sodium, J0290

> **sodium/sulbactam sodium, J0295**

It appears that you may need only one code for both drugs. Let's go to the alphanumeric listing to check the complete description for J0295.

J0295 Injection, ampicillin sodium/sulbactam sodium, per 1.5 g

That matches Dr. Camponetta's orders (and the nurses' notes indicate that Russell actually did receive the medication). Next, we must look at the quantity, or measurement, included in the code description and compare it with the dosage that Russell received. Russell was given a dosage of *1.5 grams* (g) and that matches the code description. Excellent! However, the case gives you the instruction to code for the first 12 hours of Russell's treatment. He was given the medication *every 6 hours* (q6h). Therefore, your claim form for Russell's first 12 hours of pharmaceutical, therapeutic treatment will show J0295 × 2. Great job!

Notations

Notations below some code descriptions include additional names, usually brand names, also represented by that code to confirm a generic drug and a brand name drug reported with the same code.

EXAMPLE

☑ J2940 Injection, somatrem, 1 mg
Use this code for Protropin

(*Note:* Protropin is listed in the table of drugs but not the alphabetic index.)

Quantity Specifications

Many codes also include the measurement of a typical dose in the code's description. You may recognize the check mark in the box symbol ☑ next to almost every code in this section. You learned earlier that the symbol means the code description includes a quantity or an amount.

EXAMPLE

☑ J9100 Injection, cytarabine, 100 mg
☑ S5011 5% dextrose in lactated ringer's, 1000 mL

TABLE 15-1 Conversions and Equivalents

Measure	Equivalent
1 L (liter)	1,000 mL (milliliter)
1 L	1,000 cc (cubic centimeter)
1 mL (milliliter)	1 cc
1 oz (fluid ounce)	8 dr (fluid drams)
1 oz	30 cc
1 g (gram)	1,000 mg
1 g	15 gr (grain)
1 mg (milligram)	1,000 mcg (microgram)
1 kg (kilogram)	1,000 g
1 kg	2.2 lb (pounds)
1 in. (inch)	2.54 cm (centimeters)
1 T (tablespoon)	3 teaspoons

In our example, J9100's amount is 100 mg. Therefore, if the procedure notes state that 200 milligrams of cytarabine were given to the patient, the correct way to report this would be written J9100, J9100 (or J9100 $\times$ 2). If only 50 mg of cytarabine were given, code J9100 would be reported once because the amount in the code means "less than or equal to."

Measurement Equivalents

As you can see, many code descriptors for medications and pharmaceuticals include dosage measurements. Of course, if the notes you are coding from are written in a different type of measurement, you have to do the math. To make it easier, Table 15-1 has conversion rates.

J Codes

The J codes (J0000–J9999) in the HCPCS Level II book are used for reporting drugs that are administered by a health care professional and *cannot,* under usual circumstances, be self-administered.

EXAMPLE

Some drugs that cannot be self-administered include chemotherapy drugs, immunosuppressive drugs, and inhalation solutions.

LO 15.5 Coding Ambulance and Other Transportation Services

If a severely ill or injured individual must be moved, whether from home or an accident scene, to a health care facility or from one health care facility to another, transportation arrangements are made. The patient may need to be lying down or receiving continuous IV. The health care professional may have to monitor the patient's vital signs and other issues constantly. The room for additional personnel, the ability to keep special equipment secure and functional, and the configuration

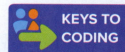

KEYS TO CODING

In order for transportation charges to be reimbursable from the third-party payer, the claim form must include diagnosis code(s) to identify the medical necessity for the special equipment.

of the seating so that everyone involved can be kept safe during the ride are all concerns that demand more than the average vehicle.

HCPCS Level II codes A0000–A0999 report the following transportation services:

- Ground ambulances.
- Air ambulances (often a helicopter but not exclusively).
- Nonemergency transportation, such as a special van, a taxi cab, a car, or even a bus.
- Additional or secondary related costs and fees.

Coding Components

The transportation section codes are determined by

1. What type of vehicle was used to transport the patient?
   a. Ground (ambulance, taxi, bus, minibus, van, etc.)
   b. Air—fixed wing (such as an airplane)
   c. Air—rotary wing (such as a helicopter)

2. What type of services did the patient need?
   a. Emergency
   b. Nonemergency
   c. **Advanced life support (ALS)**
   d. **Basic life support (BLS)**
   e. **Specialty care transport (SCT)**

3. Did the ambulance have to wait? (See Table 15-2, page 425, "Waiting Times.")
4. How many miles did the ambulance have to travel from origin to destination?
5. Were extra personnel required?

Answering the preceding questions will direct you to the best, most appropriate code or codes needed to properly report transportation services for a patient.

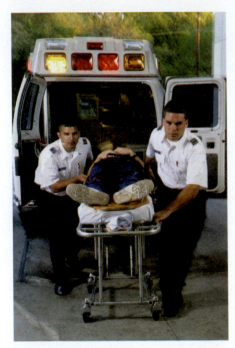
© Don Tremain/Getty Images

advanced life support (ALS)
Life-sustaining, emergency care provided, such as airway management, defibrillation, and/or the administration of drugs.

basic life support (BLS)
The provision of emergency CPR, stabilization of the patient, first aid, control of bleeding, and/or treatment of shock.

specialty care transport (SCT)
Continuous care provided by one or more health professionals in an appropriate specialty area, such as respiratory care or cardiovascular care, or by a paramedic with additional training.

EXAMPLE

Hilda Camacho, an 87-year-old female, was taken by ambulance to the ED at Barton Hospital after having a seizure and falling into a coma. The EMTs provided advanced life support (ALS) services during transport. Use code A0427 Ambulance service, ALS, emergency transport, level 1 (ALS 1).

LET'S CODE IT! SCENARIO

Abby Lennox, an emergency medical technician (EMT), was called in as an extra ambulance attendant for the ALS ground transportation of Ruby Premin, a 15-year-old autistic female.

Let's Code It!

Abby was called in as an *extra ambulance attendant*. When you look in the alphabetic index of the HCPCS Level II book, notice that this does not match any of the listings under *Ambulance* or *Attendant*. So let's turn to the range shown next to the term *Ambulance* in the index: A0021– A0999.

Although reading down the listing will take time, sometimes it is the best way to find the code you need. Fortunately, you won't have to read too far to reach

A0424 Extra ambulance attendant, ground (ALS or BLS) or air (fixed or rotary winged); (requires medical review)

Transportation Codes in Other Sections

A few transportation codes in the HCPCS Level II book are in sections other than the A codes. This, of course, is an excellent example of why you should use the alphabetic index to find the best code in the alphanumeric listing—because there may be a better, more appropriate code in a section you might not otherwise examine. In all cases of temporary codes, you must confirm the acceptance of the temporary code by the third-party payer to whom you are billing.

The S series (S0000–S9999) consists of temporary codes and is not accepted by Medicare, according to the HCPCS Level II book. Medicaid programs and some private insurers, such as Blue Cross and Blue Shield Association, do accept S codes. You must check with the organization or association in your state to confirm the acceptance of S codes. The S codes that relate to transportation are

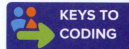

S0215 Nonemergency transportation; mileage, per mile

S9992 Transportation costs to and from trial location and local transportation costs (e.g., fares for taxicab or bus) for clinical trial participant and one caregiver/companion

The T codes (T1000–T9999) are used by Medicaid state agencies to report services, procedures, and other items for which there are no permanent national codes. You must communicate with the third-party payer to whom you are sending the claim to ensure that it accepts T codes. Transportation services that may be reported using T codes are

T2001 Non-emergency transportation; patient attendant/escort

T2002 Non-emergency transportation; per diem

T2003 Non-emergency transportation; encounter/trip

T2004 Non-emergency transport; commercial carrier, multi-pass

T2005 Non-emergency transportation; stretcher van

T2007 Transportation waiting time, air ambulance and non-emergency vehicle, one-half (½) hour increments

T2049 Non-emergency transportation; stretcher van, mileage; per mile

EXAMPLE

Chad Nevins, a 91-year-old male, is being transferred to a nursing home closer to his daughter. His health problems require him to be transported on a stretcher. Code T2005 Nonemergency transportation; stretcher van.

LET'S CODE IT! SCENARIO

Ronald Stockman, an 81-year-old male, had a stroke 3 weeks ago. He has now recovered sufficiently to be discharged from the hospital. However, he is not completely well. Ronald is being transferred to a short-term rehabilitation facility to help him

regain use of his legs and right arm. Terrell Peterson, from Link-Up Ambulance Services, drove the wheelchair van to take Ronald from Barton Hospital to Sunstate Nursing and Rehabilitation Center, a 12-mile ride.

Let's Code It!

Terrell, the driver, will submit the documentation to you. He noted that he drove a *wheelchair van* to transport Ronald from the hospital to the nursing facility. The notes also indicate that Ronald is being discharged from the hospital and there is no indication that this is an emergency. In addition, the wheelchair van does not contain emergency equipment, so we know that this is a *non-emergency* trip. Let's go to the alphabetic index and turn to *wheelchair*. Go down the list to the indented term *Van, non-emergency . . .* A0130, S0209. Turn to the alphanumeric listing to check out the complete description of the first code:

> **A0130 Non-emergency transportation: wheelchair van**

This matches Terrell's documentation, doesn't it? Yes. In addition, it is the only code shown for that portion of the service. However, you might also look in the alphabetic listing under *Transportation, non-emergency,* A0080–A0210, Q3020, T2001–T2005, T2049. Once you review the complete descriptions of the suggested codes, you will see rather quickly that A0130 is the most specific and accurate.

Now, you must include a code for the mileage traveled by the van. Under *Wheelchair, van, non-emergency* you get the suggestion for code S0209, and while under *Transportation, non-emergency, mileage,* you see S0215. Let's examine both codes.:

> **S0209 Wheelchair van, mileage, per mile**
>
> **S0215 Non-emergency transportation; mileage, per mile**

You also might notice

> **A0380 BLS mileage (per mile)**
>
> **A0390 ALS mileage (per mile)**
>
> **A0425 Ground mileage, per statute mile**

Five different codes appear applicable to report the mileage component of the service. Look at S0209 versus S0215 versus A0380, A0390, and A0425. You can see that the descriptions of A0380 and A0390 do not match your notes and would be considered upcoding! S0209 is more accurate and more specific in its description of the type of vehicle involved in the transportation. Therefore, as long as the insurance carrier accepts S codes, the claim form should show

> **A0130 Non-emergency transportation: wheelchair van**
>
> **S0209 Wheelchair van, mileage, per mile;**
>
> **Number of miles: twelve**

Great job!

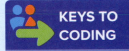

KEYS TO CODING

When you send a claim to Medicare for transportation services, you will most probably use CMS 1500. Billers need to enter the five-digit zip code of the point of pick-up (origin of service) in box 32 of the CMS 1500 form.

Ambulance Origin/Destination

When reporting transportation services to insurance carriers, you have to identify the *origin of service* and the *destination of service.*

The most common modifiers for the origin and the destination of service are one-letter codes that categorize locations. Box 15-1 shows a list of the modifiers.

BOX 15-1 Transportation Location Modifiers

D Diagnostic or therapeutic site other than "P" or "H"

E Residential domiciliary custodial facility (i.e., nursing home, but *not* a skilled nursing facility)

G Hospital-based dialysis facility (hospital or hospital-related)

H Hospital

I Site of transfer (e.g., airport or helicopter pad) between types of ambulance

J Nonhospital-based dialysis facility

N Skilled nursing facility (SNF)

P Physician's office (e.g., HMO, nonhospital facility, clinic, etc.)

R Residence

S Scene of accident or acute event

X Intermediate stop at physician's office en route to the hospital (e.g., HMO nonhospital facility, clinic, etc.)
   Note: Modifier X may be used only to identify a destination.

Source: Ambulance Claim Modifiers, HCPCS Code. Copyright © 2013 by Ambulance Claim Modifiers. All rights reserved. Used with permission.

LO 15.6 Transportation Waiting Time

The HCPCS Level II book has a table of waiting times in the A code section so that you can easily report time lapsed.

Waiting time is measured in units of 30 minutes or less but is not reported until the transportation vehicle has been waiting for 31 minutes or more. Table 15-2 shows you the waiting time data. The number of units indicated in the table tells you how many times to report either of the following codes:

A0420 Ambulance waiting time (ALS or BLS), one-half (½) hour increments

T2007 Transportation waiting time, air ambulance and non-emergency vehicle, one-half (½) hour increments

Ambulance Billing Indicators

An *ambulance billing indicator* is a two-character alphanumeric modifier consisting of one number and one letter. The modifiers can be used to supply important information regarding the patient's condition, reason for the transport, and the level of services provided during the transportation. Box 15-2 lists billing indicators.

TABLE 15-2 Waiting Times

Units	Time, in Hours
1	½ to 1
2	1 to 1½
3	1½ to 2
4	2 to 2½
5	2½ to 3
6	3 to 3½
7	3½ to 4
8	4 to 4½
9	4½ to 5
10	5 to 5½

BOX 15-2 Ambulance Billing Indicators

1A Bedridden

2A Accidental injury home/nursing home

3A Accidental injury car

4A Patient in shock

5A Oxygen used and/or heart monitor used

6A Transported by stretcher

7A Fracture to hip, leg, knee, and/or trunk (same day as ambulance trip)

8A Hospital lacks facility (patient admitted to second hospital)

9A Rectal bleeding

1B Myocardial infarction

2B Possible cerebral vascular accident (CVA)

3B Black out/passed out

4B Laceration of head

5B Dead on arrival (DOA) at hospital

6B Died en route to hospital

7B Unresponsive or coma

8B Quadriplegia

9B Stroke (same-day ambulance service)

1C Paralysis

2C Mentally retarded

Vernon Salisbury, a 31-year-old male, drove his car into an electrical pole. After the ambulance arrived at the scene, the EMTs waited 75 minutes for the electric company to turn off the power. Then the EMTs got Vernon out of the car and into the ambulance, and they drove him to the hospital. Code the waiting time.

You Code It!

Go through the steps and determine the code(s) that should be reported for this ambulance's waiting time.

Step 1: Read the case completely.

Step 2: Abstract the notes: Which key words can you identify relating to the procedures performed?

_____

Step 3: Query the provider, if necessary.

Step 4: Diagnosis: MVA.

Step 5: Code the waiting time.

_____

Step 6: Link the procedure codes to at least one diagnosis code.

Step 7: Back code to double-check your choices.

Answer:

Did you determine the correct code?

A0420× 2 Ambulance waiting time (ALS or BLS), one-half (½) hour increments; one to one and one-half hour total

Terrific!

Chapter Summary

Learning the techniques and guidelines for accurately reporting HCPCS Level II codes is mandatory for coders submitting claims for patients covered by Medicare, as well by as many other third-party payers. In addition, understanding the complexities of Level II codes opens many opportunities for employment, from skilled nursing facilities to durable medical equipment suppliers.

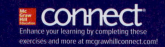

Using Terminology

Match each key term to the appropriate definition.

_____ **1.** LO 15.1 An artificial opening made in the body surgically.

_____ **2.** LO 15.2 A bedsore, or wound created by lying in the same position, on the same irritant without relief.

_____ **3.** LO 15.5 Continuous care provided by one or more health professionals in an appropriate specialty area, such as respiratory care or cardiovascular care, or by a paramedic with additional training.

_____ **4.** LO 15.5 Life-sustaining, emergency care provided, such as airway management, defibrillation, and/or the administration of drugs.

_____ **5.** LO 15.2 Durable medical equipment, prosthetic, and orthotic supplies.

_____ **6.** LO 15.5 The provision of emergency CPR, stabilization of the patient, first aid, control of bleeding, and/or treatment of shock.

_____ **7.** LO 15.2 The use of electricity to agitate the skin to relieve pain.

_____ **8.** LO 15.1 A tube that is inserted into the body to either deliver or extract fluid, such as a nasogastric tube.

_____ **9.** LO 15.1 To give medication to oneself, such as a diabetic giving herself an insulin injection.

_____ **10.** LO 15.1 The inability to control urination or fecal expulsion.

A. Advanced life support (ALS)

B. Basic life support (BLS)

C. Cannula

D. Decubitus ulcer

E. DMEPOS

F. Incontinence

G. Ostomy

H. Self-administer

I. Specialty care transport (SCT)

J. Transcutaneous electrical nerve stimulators (TENS)

Checking Your Understanding

Choose the most appropriate answer for each of the following questions.

1. LO 15.1 An example of a medical supply reported by HCPCS Level II codes is

   a. bandages for use in the office.
   b. paper liner for examination tables.
   c. paper for the office ECG machine.
   d. vascular catheter.

2. LO 15.1 Incontinence supplies, reported with HCPCS Level II codes, are used

   a. in the hospital.
   b. in the physician's office.
   c. by the patient for personal at-home use.
   d. none of these.

3. LO 15.2 DME stands for

   a. durable medical equipment.
   b. diagnostic medical equipment.
   c. diagnostic medical evaluators.
   d. durable modern escalators.

4. LO 15.2 Medicare uses all *except* one of the following qualifiers to determine an item as DME.

   a. The item can withstand repeated use.
   b. The item is used in the patient's home.
   c. The item has been paid for by the patient.
   d. The item is primarily used for medical purposes.

5. LO 15.2 An example of DME is

   a. a plaster cast.
   b. an ostomy pouch.
   c. an albuterol inhaler.
   d. a pacemaker monitor.

6. LO 15.3 A method of administering drugs in which the medication is inserted into the patient's muscle is represented by the abbreviation

   a. IA.
   b. IV.
   c. IM.
   d. IT.

7. LO 15.4 HCPCS Level II codes identify certain pharmaceuticals by brand name and/or generic name in

   a. the alphabetic index.
   b. notations beneath code descriptions.
   c. Appendix 3.
   d. the Table of Drugs.

8. LO 15.4 The J codes report drugs administered by

   a. the patient him- or herself.
   b. a family member.
   c. a health care professional.
   d. all of these.

9. LO 15.5 Coding transportation services includes specifics about all *except*

   a. the type of vehicle used.
   b. the type of insurance that covers the service.
   c. the type of service provided.
   d. whether extra personnel were required.

10. LO 15.5 The codes used for reporting transportation of a patient may be used only

   a. in cases of extreme emergency.
   b. when the patient is taken more than 10 miles.
   c. when the patient cannot afford a taxi.
   d. whenever medically necessary.

Applying Your Knowledge

1. LO 15.1 What do the medical supply codes in the HCPCS Level II book report? _____

   _____

2. LO 15.1 What do the codes in the Miscellaneous Supplies section (A4206–A4290) report? _____

   _____

3. LO 15.1 What code group represents ostomy supplies? _____

   _____

4. LO 15.1 Code group A6000–A8004 represents what type of supplies? _____

   _____

5. LO 15.2 List the four Medicare qualifiers that determine whether an item can be classified as DME. _____

   _____

6. LO 15.3 List eight methods of administering drugs to a patient. _____

   _____

7. LO 15.4 Explain the difference between a generic name and a brand name. _____

   _____

8. LO 15.4 What information can you find in the PDR, and why is it important to a coding specialist? _____

   _____

9. LO 15.5 What are the coding components that help determine the correct transportation service code? _____

   _____

10. LO 15.6 If ambulance waiting time for code A0420 were 2½ hours, what would be the correct number of waiting
    time units? _____

    _____

Using the techniques described in this chapter, carefully read through the case studies and determine the most accurate HCPCS Level II code(s) and modifier(s), if appropriate, for each case study.

Note: All insurance carriers and third-party payers for the patients accept HCPCS Level II codes and modifiers.

1. Maria Feshan, a 43-year-old female, was diagnosed with diabetes and must test her blood sugar (glucose) regularly. Grunion Medical Supplies sent her a bottle of 50 blood glucose reagent strips for use with her home glucose monitor.

   _____

2. Craig Owens, a 9-year-old male, was diagnosed with acute asthma. Johannsen Health care delivered 3000 mL of distilled water for use with his nebulizer.

   _____

3. Samantha Woods, a 5-year-old female, was diagnosed with an immature bladder. Until her bladder grows and becomes more functional, she is using a youth-sized incontinence brief. Her mother ordered two briefs.

   _____

4. Dean Mulvanney, a 50-year-old male, suffers from chronic renal failure, and Dr. Fahud has him on hemodialysis. Today, Dean receives new arterial blood tubing.

   _____

5. Ned Houston was born today with indications of spina bifida. Dr. Kensington, his pediatrician, wants to transfer him to Barton Medical Center because it has the only Level III neonatal unit in the area. The ambulance that transports Ned is equipped with a special isolette to keep Ned safe.

   _____

6. Gina Loffelin, a 77-year-old female, had a heart attack at home. During the ambulance ride to the hospital, Raul Fresca, the EMT, administered oxygen along with other advanced life support (ALS) services.

   _____

7. Jared Morrison, an 81-year-old male, was discharged from the hospital with a stress fracture of his left hip. A stretcher van was provided to take him from the hospital to the Barton Rehabilitation Center across town.

   _____

8. Paula Warren, a 23-year-old female, fell on the ski slopes. After her broken leg was stabilized by the ski patrol, she was airlifted by helicopter to the nearest hospital in Barton City.

_____

9. After a wonderful trip to South America and tours of the wilderness there, Gerard Stewart, a 41-year-old male, has signs of acute malaria. Dr. Sequoia gives him a 200-mg injection IM of chloroquine hydrochloride.

_____

10. Francine Cadwaller, a 47-year-old female, was in a great deal of pain and nothing seemed to help. Dr. Tershwell gave her an injection SC of 50 mg of codeine phosphate.

_____

11. Ryan Sparks, a 57-year-old male, was diagnosed with convulsive status epilepticus. Dr. Longwell ordered Cerebyx, with an initial dose of 100 mg.

_____

12. Karyn Monmouth, an 83-year-old female, was diagnosed with heparin-induced thrombocytopenia (HIT). Dr. Taman gave her a 25-mg injection of lepirudin.

_____

13. Roseanne Carter of Master's Medical brought a seat attachment for Joseph Starke's walker.

_____

14. Suzanne Headley's heel is irritated from the special brace ordered by her physician to assist the healing of her fractured ankle. She receives one heel protector from Jackson Medical Supplies.

_____

15. Larry Rodriguez has frequent bouts of respiratory distress, and his physician prescribed a portable negative pressure ventilator. Jason Braun delivered the equipment and taught Larry how to use it.

_____

The following exercises provide practice in the application of abstracting the physicians' notes and learning to work with SOAP notes from our health care facility, Cipher, Victors & Associates. These case studies (SOAP notes) are modeled on real patient encounters. Using the techniques described in this chapter, carefully read through the case studies and determine the most accurate HCPCS Level II code(s) and modifier(s), if appropriate, for each case study. *Note:* All insurance carriers and third-party payers for the patients accept HCPCS Level II codes and modifiers.

CIPHER, VICTORS & ASSOCIATES
A Complete Health Care Facility
234 MAIN STREET • ANYTOWN, FL 32711 • 407-555-1234

PATIENT: WEBBER, ROSE ANNE
ACCOUNT/EHR #:   WEBBRO001
DATE: 10/21/18
Representative: Elizabeth Alexander

Attending Physician: James I. Cipher, MD

The Pt is a 27-year-old female who recently returned from working in Africa. She was diagnosed with variola and has been on a gastric feeding tube to increase her fluids, electrolytes, and calories because the pharyngeal lesions make swallowing difficult. Nasogastric tubing without a stylet was supplied for this patient.

DX: Variola

P: Service number given to caregiver

Elizabeth Alexander

EA/mg   D: 10/21/18 09:50:16   T: 10/22/18 12:55:01

Determine the most accurate HCPCS Level II code(s) and modifier(s), if appropriate.

_____

_____

_____

CIPHER, VICTORS & ASSOCIATES
A Complete Health Care Facility
234 MAIN STREET • ANYTOWN, FL 32711 • 407-555-1234

PATIENT: POWELL, FARRAH
ACCOUNT/EHR #:   POWEFA001
DATE: 09/18/18
Representative Technician: LuAnn Hallmark

Attending Physician: James I. Cipher, MD

The Pt is a 69-year-old female diagnosed with adult kyphosis caused by poor posture. Dr. Cipher prescribed bed rest on a firm mattress with pelvic traction attached to the footboard. At 5:00 p.m. on this date, I delivered a bed board and the traction frame to Ms. Powell's home. I placed the bed board underneath the existing mattress in order to create a firm surface upon which the patient could sleep. I then attached the traction frame to the footboard of the existing bed. I spent 45 minutes instructing the patient, her family, and her caretaker on the proper use of the equipment, how to properly get into and out of the traction, and the expected sensations.

DX: Adult kyphosis

P: Follow-up in 2 weeks to see if patient has any questions or concerns

_____

LuAnn Hallmark

LH/mg   D: 09/18/18 09:50:16   T: 09/20/18 12:55:01

Determine the most accurate HCPCS Level II code(s) and modifier(s), if appropriate.

_____

_____

_____

CIPHER, VICTORS & ASSOCIATES
A Complete Health Care Facility
234 MAIN STREET • ANYTOWN, FL 32711 • 407-555-1234

PATIENT: YAMIN, ANTON
ACCOUNT/EHR #:   YAMIAN001
DATE: 11/12/18

Attending Physician: Jacqueline Bennett, MD

Pt is a 61-year-old male with metastatic testicular tumors. He comes in today for the administration of cisplatin solution, IV, 20 mg. It is the first of five treatments he will receive this week.
    IV infusion given over 7 hours.
    Patient reports mild nausea. Refuses any pharmaceutical treatment for that side effect of this treatment. Patient discharged at 4:15 p.m.

Jacqueline Bennett, MD

JB/mg   D: 11/12/18 09:50:16   T: 11/15/18 12:55:01

Determine the most accurate HCPCS Level II code(s) and modifier(s), if appropriate.

_____

_____

_____

CIPHER, VICTORS & ASSOCIATES
A Complete Health Care Facility
234 MAIN STREET • ANYTOWN, FL 32711 • 407-555-1234

PATIENT: STRAUSS, EMILY
ACCOUNT/EHR #:   STRAEM001
DATE: 10/04/18

Attending Physician: Jacqueline Bennett, MD

Pt is a 21-year-old female in labor. Upon examination, her cervix is dilated, and the presentation of the fetus has occurred. She is in the third stage of labor, and her uterine contractions are not strong enough to complete delivery.

    10:12 a.m. IV is started with 1.0 mU/min of oxytocin.

    10:27 a.m. increase to 2.0 mU/min

    Contractions increase to proper level and delivery is completed at 10:59 a.m. Baby girl Strauss is handed over to the pediatrics team.

    Patient is taken to the recovery room in stable condition.

Jacqueline Bennett, MD

JB/mg   D: 10/04/18 09:50:16   T: 10/05/18 12:55:01

Determine the most accurate HCPCS Level II code(s) and modifier(s), if appropriate.

_____

_____

_____

CIPHER, VICTORS & ASSOCIATES
A Complete Health Care Facility
234 MAIN STREET • ANYTOWN, FL 32711 • 407-555-1234

PATIENT: DELGATO, DESIREE
ACCOUNT/EHR #:   DELGDE001
DATE: 09/27/18

Attending Physician: James I. Cipher, MD
EMT/Attendant: Lance H. Reynoso, EMT

Pt is a 73-year-old female who appears to have suffered a myocardial infarction in her nursing home's day room. Pt complained of numbness and tingling in the left arm and sharp pains in her chest. EKG showed abnormal activity. Pulse and respiration were abnormal.

    While preparing the patient for transport, she went into arrest. Defibrillator restored heartbeat. ALS services were administered, and patient was transported immediately to Barton Hospital.

    Routine disposable supplies were used.

    Total Mileage: 4.5

Lance H. Reynoso, EMT

LHR/mg   D: 09/27/18 09:50:16   T: 09/27/18 12:55:01

Determine the most accurate HCPCS Level II code(s) and modifier(s), if appropriate.

_____

_____

_____

INPATIENT PROCEDURE CODING

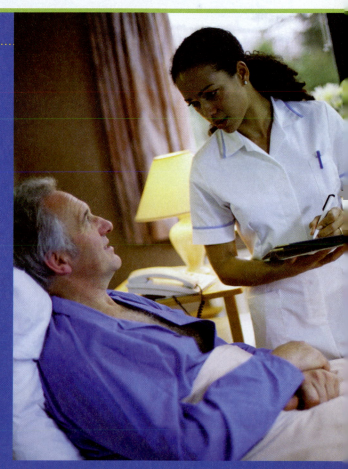

© Mark Thornton/Getty Images

437

16 INTRODUCTION TO ICD-10-PCS

Learning Outcomes *After completing this chapter, the student should be able to:*

LO 16.1 Define the objectives that guided the development of ICD-10-PCS.

LO 16.2 Properly interpret ICD-10-PCS code descriptions.

LO 16.3 Identify the structure of ICD-10-PCS codes.

LO 16.4 Recognize the proper ways to use the alphabetic index and the tables section of ICD-10-PCS.

LO 16.5 Discern the general conventions for using ICD-10-PCS.

LO 16.6 Determine the principal ICD-10-PCS code and proper sequencing for multiple procedure codes.

LO 16.7 Employ GEMS to support transitioning from ICD-9-CM Volume 3 to ICD-10-PCS.

Key Terms

Approach

Body part

Body system

Completeness

Device

Expandability

Multiaxial

Qualifier

Root operation term

Standardized terminology

Structural integrity

Unique definitions

ICD-10-PCS (*International Classification of Diseases, 10th revision, Procedure Coding System*) officially replaces ICD-9-CM Volume 3 procedure codes beginning October 1, 2015. At the same time, ICD-9-CM Volumes 1 and 2 (diagnosis codes) are replaced by ICD-10-CM—a more precise and efficient diagnostic coding system.

ICD-10-PCS provides more specificity for various procedures, as well as making it easier to incorporate new procedures as they are developed and accepted by health care professionals. To give you an idea of how much more information can be provided by this new code set, in the 2010 ICD-9-CM Volume 3, there were 3,841 ICD-9-CM procedure codes. Compare that with the 2010 ICD-10-PCS with 71,957 codes. Thank goodness you don't have to memorize them!

This chapter identifies the distinct benefits of ICD-10-PCS. Then, step by step, the chapter differentiates the way the codes look and are constructed. The notations and explanations, exclusive to ICD-10-PCS, are all reviewed. Examples are provided to illustrate the concepts and elements throughout the chapter.

LO 16.1 The Objectives for ICD-10-PCS

One of the first tasks for the development of ICD-10-PCS was to establish its specific objectives. The six objectives were identified as:

1. **Completeness:** Unique codes for each procedure and for any possible procedures have been created.
2. **Expandability:** ICD-10-PCS has been developed so that it can easily accept new procedures and incorporate them logically into the existing

list. It acknowledges the incredible speed with which technology and science are working to develop new treatments and services.

3. **Multiaxial:** The characters used in creating the codes are used consistently within each section and, whenever possible, from section to section.

4. **Standardized terminology:** ICD-10-PCS uses only one meaning for each term, even if multiple meanings are accepted in the industry. In addition, ICD-10-PCS gives you the specific definition as it is intended for each term.

5. **Unique definitions:** With the way the ICD-10-PCS codes are configured, each code can maintain its unique definition without affecting the incorporation of new methodology.

6. **Structural integrity:** The structure of the codes individually, and the system in total, can be maintained while still expanding the set to include new technology.

The successful accomplishment of these objectives will help ensure that ICD-10-PCS will make coding procedures more accurate, more efficient, and easier to assign.

LO 16.2 ICD-10-PCS Code Descriptions

ICD-10-PCS has changed the way codes are described, as compared with ICD-9-CM Volume 3.

1. *Procedure descriptions will no longer include diagnostic information.* Previously, some of the procedure codes included diagnostic statements or categories in the description of the procedure code.

EXAMPLE

ICD-9-CM Volume 3

The repair of a *rupture* of an eyeball (16.82)
Correction of *cleft palate* (27.62)

The terms *rupture* and *cleft palate* are diagnoses, meaning this code can only be used for that specific type of repair or correction.

In ICD-10-PCS, the description of each procedure code is limited to the details of the procedure itself. This will leave ICD-10-CM diagnostic codes to explain the disease or condition.

EXAMPLE: ICD-10-PCS

Percutaneous needle core biopsy of right kidney, diagnostic, 0TB03ZX
Open excision of tail of pancreas 0FBF0ZZ

2. *Not otherwise specified (NOS) options are omitted.* ICD-10-PCS requires you to have, at the very least, a minimum amount of detail regarding each portion of the procedure. In those cases in which the documentation has no additional specifics available and you cannot query the physician, ICD-10-PCS provides coding rules to guide you to the best, most appropriate code.

EXAMPLE

In ICD-9-CM Volume 3
    36.10 Aortocoronary bypass for heart revascularization, not otherwise specified
In ICD-10-PCS
No equivalent. ICD-10-PCS codes all contain a minimum level of information.

completeness
Structure that allows all procedures, services, and treatments to be represented by a code.

expandability
Structure that includes room for growth.

multiaxial
The consistent use of characters and elements throughout the book.

standardized terminology
One established meaning for each term used in code descriptions.

unique definitions
ICD-10-PCS codes are constructed of individual values that stay consistent throughout the code set.

structural integrity
The structure of the codes individually, and the system in total, can be maintained while still expanding the set to include new technology.

3. *Not elsewhere classified (NEC) options are reduced.* Due to the added levels of specificity throughout the ICD-10-PCS, the need for the NEC option is reduced. You will find the most common inclusion of NEC in procedure descriptions located in the sections on new devices and nuclear medicine because such areas are more quickly affected by new technology and science.

LO 16.3 The Structure of ICD-10-PCS Codes

Of course, the main purpose of creating ICD-10-PCS is to give you, the professional coder, an easier way to find the best, most accurate, and most specific code. That purpose has led to a new structure for the codes.

You may remember that ICD-9-CM Volume 3 procedure codes use a two-digit number to the left of a dot and up to two digits to the right of the dot for a maximum of four digits (all numbers).

EXAMPLE

18.09 Other incision of external ear (drainage, ear, external)

ICD-10-PCS codes have seven characters and are alphanumeric (both letters and numbers). Each of the seven positions in the code represents a specific piece of information relating to the procedure, service, or treatment provided.

CHARACTER POSITION—RELATED PIECE OF INFORMATION

1. *Section* of the ICD-10-PCS code set.
2. *Body system* upon which the procedure or service was performed.
3. *Root operation* explains the category or type of procedure.
4. *Body part* identifies the specific anatomical site involved in the procedure.
5. *Approach* reports which method was used to perform the service or treatment.
6. *Device* reports, when applicable, what type of device was involved in the service or procedure.
7. *Qualifier* adds any additional detail.

EXAMPLE

0990XZX Drainage, external ear, right, external approach, diagnostic

Let's go through all these elements one by one.

Sections (First Character)

The first character in the seven-character sequence identifies the section in which the procedure is listed. Box 16-1 lists the 16 section titles.

EXAMPLE

An ankle x-ray is an imaging procedure—Section B.
A breech extraction is an obstetrics procedure—Section 1.
An amputation is a surgical procedure—Section 0.

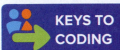

KEYS TO CODING

ICD-10-PCS codes may include any letter of the alphabet except the letters *O* and *I*. This is done to avoid any confusion between the letter *O* and the number 0, as well as any mix-up between the letter *I* and the number 1.

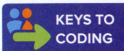

KEYS TO CODING

In ICD-10-PCS, the word *operation* has nothing to do with surgery.

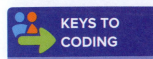

KEYS TO CODING

To help illustrate these data points, we are going to use a code as an ongoing example:

051A47Y

The following is going to show you how to take apart this code and figure out what procedure it is reporting. This should help you understand how to build a code on your own.

KEYS TO CODING

Using our example code . . .
051A47Y
First character = 0.

0 Medical and Surgical
You now know that this code is listed in the Medical and Surgical section of ICD-10-PCS.

BOX 16-1   The 16 Sections of ICD-10-PCS

0 Medical and Surgical
1 Obstetrics
2 Placement
3 Administration
4 Measurement and Monitoring
5 Extracorporeal Assistance and Performance
6 Extracorporeal Therapies
7 Osteopathic

8 Other Procedures
9 Chiropractic
B Imaging
C Nuclear Medicine
D Radiation Oncology
F Physical Rehabilitation and Diagnostic Audiology
G Mental Health
H Substance Abuse Treatment

Body Systems (Second Character)

The second character of the code reports the body system upon which the procedure, service, or treatment was performed. Box 16-2 lists the 31 body systems used for clarification and identification in the second character of codes reporting a medical or surgical procedure or service.

The Medical and Surgical section of ICD-10-PCS has the largest number of body systems to be reported, as shown in Box 16-2. Box 16-3 shows the body systems used in the other sections.

Root Operations (Third Character)

The third character in the ICD-10-PCS code reports the **root operation term**—the central aspect of the procedure or service being provided. Just as you learned when reporting procedures using CPT, you are essentially looking for the term that describes WHAT the physician did for the patient. You can see that these terms are, for the most part, familiar to you. Notice that once again the Medical and Surgical section has 31 different root operations (Box 16-4). The other sections may use some of the same terms as the Medical and Surgical section in addition to some terms specific to their

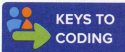

KEYS TO CODING

Using our example code . . .
0**5**1A47Y
First character   = 0
Second character = 5
0   Medical and Surgical
    5   Upper veins
You now know that this code is reporting a procedure that was performed on the patient's upper veins and is listed in the Medical and Surgical section of ICD-10-PCS.

root operation term
The category or classification of a particular procedure, service, or treatment.

BOX 16-2   Medical and Surgical Section Body Systems

0 Central nervous system
1 Peripheral nervous system
2 Heart and great vessels
3 Upper arteries
4 Lower arteries
5 Upper veins
6 Lower veins
7 Lymphatic and hemic systems
8 Eye
9 Ear, nose, sinus
B Respiratory system
C Mouth and throat
D Gastrointestinal system
F Hepatobiliary system and pancreas
G Endocrine system
H Skin and breast

J Subcutaneous tissue and fascia
K Muscles
L Tendons
M Bursae and ligaments
N Head and facial bones
P Upper bones
Q Lower bones
R Upper joints
S Lower joints
T Urinary system
U Female reproductive system
V Male reproductive system
W Anatomical regions, general
X Anatomical regions, upper extremities
Y Anatomical regions, lower extremities

BOX 16-3   Body Systems in Various Sections of ICD-10-PCS

SECTION	BODY SYSTEM(S)
Obstetrics	0 Pregnancy
Placement	W Anatomical Regions
	Y Anatomical Orifices
Administration	C Indwelling Device
	E Physiological Systems & Anatomical Regions
	0 Circulatory
Measurement and Monitoring	A Physiological Systems
	B Physiological Devices
Extracorporeal Assistance	A Physiological Systems
Extracorporeal Therapies	A Physiological Systems
Osteopathic	W Anatomical Regions
Other Procedures	A Physiological Systems
	W Anatomical Regions

SECTION	BODY SYSTEM(S)
Chiropractic	W Anatomical Regions
Imaging	[See Medical and Surgical body systems]
Nuclear Medicine	[See Medical and Surgical body systems]
Radiation Oncology	[See Medical and Surgical body systems]
Physical Rehabilitation	0 Rehabilitation* (for the second character)
Mental Health	Z None
Substance Abuse	Z None

*The Physical Rehabilitation and Diagnostic Audiology identifies the body system with the fourth character rather than the second as with other sections. The same 31 body systems used for the Medical and Surgical section apply here, as well.

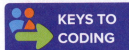

KEYS TO CODING

Using our example code . . .
051**A**47Y

First character = 0
Second character = 5
Third character = 1
Fourth character = A
  0   Medical and Surgical
     5   Upper veins
        1   Bypass
           A   Brachial vein, left

You now know that this code is reporting a bypass procedure that was performed on the patient's left (upper) brachial veins and is listed in the Medical and Surgical section of ICD-10-PCS.

---

area (Box 16-5). Try not to get overwhelmed by all these terms. You have time to learn about these procedures, look them up in a medical dictionary, and become familiar with them.

Body Part (Fourth Character)

The fourth character of the ICD-10-PCS code provides information regarding the specific body part, anatomical site, or body region upon which the procedure, service, or treatment was performed.

BOX 16-4   Root Operations—Medical and Surgical Section

0 Alteration
1 Bypass
2 Change
3 Control
4 Creation
5 Destruction
6 Detachment
7 Dilation
8 Division
9 Drainage
B Excision
C Extirpation
D Extraction
F Fragmentation
G Fusion
H Insertion

J Inspection
K Map
L Occlusion
M Reattachment
N Release
P Removal
Q Repair
R Replacement
S Reposition
T Resection
U Supplement
V Restriction
W Revision
X Transfer
Y Transplantation

BOX 16-5   Additional Root Operations—Other Sections

SECTION	ROOT OPERATION		SECTION	ROOT OPERATION
Obstetrics	A Abortion			5 Nonimaging Nuclear Medicine Probe
	E Delivery			6 Nonimaging Nuclear Medicine Assay
Placement	1 Compression			7 Systemic Nuclear Medicine Therapy
	2 Dressing		Radiation Oncology	0 Beam Radiation
	3 Immobilization			1 Brachytherapy
	4 Packing			2 Stereotactic Radiosurgery
	6 Traction			Y Other Radiation
Administration	0 Introduction		Physical Rehabilitation	0 Speech Assessment
	1 Irrigation			1 Motor and/or Nerve Function Assessment
	2 Transfusion			2 Activities of Daily Living (ADL) Assessment
Measurement and Monitoring	0 Measurement			3 Hearing Assessment
	1 Monitoring			4 Hearing Aid Assessment
Extracorporeal Assistance	0 Assistance			5 Vestibular Assessment
	1 Performance			6 Speech Treatment
	2 Restoration			7 Motor Treatment
Extracorporeal Therapies	0 Atmospheric Control			8 Activities of Daily Living (ADL) Treatment
	1 Decompression			9 Hearing Treatment
	2 Electromagnetic Therapy			B Cochlear Implant Treatment
	3 Hyperthermia			C Vestibular Treatment
	4 Hypothermia			D Device Fitting
	5 Pheresis			F Caregiver Training
	6 Phototherapy		Mental Health	1 Psychological Testing
	7 Ultrasound Therapy			2 Crisis Intervention
	8 Ultraviolet Light Therapy			3 Medication Management
	9 Shock Wave Therapy			5 Individual Psychotherapy
Osteopathic	0 Treatment			6 Counseling
Other Procedures	0 Other Procedures			7 Family Psychotherapy
Chiropractic	B Manipulation			B Electroconvulsive Therapy
Imaging	0 Plain Radiography			C Biofeedback
	1 Fluoroscopy			F Hypnosis
	2 Computerized Tomography (CT Scan)			G Narcosynthesis
	3 Magnetic Resonance Imaging (MRI)			H Group Psychotherapy
	4 Ultrasonography			J Light Therapy
Nuclear Medicine	1 Planar Nuclear Medicine Imaging			
	2 Tomographic (TOMO) Imaging			
	3 Positron Emission Tomography (PET)			
	4 Nonimaging Nuclear Medicine Uptake			

SECTION	ROOT OPERATION		SECTION	ROOT OPERATION
Substance Abuse Treatment	2 Detoxification Services			6 Family Counseling
	3 Individual Counseling			8 Medication Management
	4 Group Counseling			9 Pharmacotherapy
	5 Individual Psychotherapy			

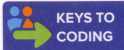

KEYS TO CODING

Using our example code . . .
051A47**Y**

First character   = 0
Second character = 5
Third character   = 1
Fourth character = A
Fifth character   = 4
Sixth character   = 7
Seventh character = Y

0   Medical and Surgical
  5   Upper veins
    1   Bypass
      A   Brachial vein, left
        4   Percutaneous
            endoscopic
          7   Autologous
              tissue
              substitute
            Y   Upper
                vein

You now know that this code is reporting a bypass procedure that was performed, using a percutaneous endoscope, with the use of autologous tissue substitute on the patient's left (upper) brachial veins and is listed in the Medical and Surgical section of ICD-10-PCS.

These characters, and what they represent, vary, determined by the section and body system. This is one of the reasons the alphabetic index will not usually reach this level of specificity.

Approach (Fifth Character)

The term *approach* as reported by the fifth character reports the technique or methodology used during the procedure, such as open or laparoscopic. However, other sections may use this character to report a different detail, such as single or multiple duration for extracorporeal therapy. The imaging section uses this position to report the use of contrast materials.

Device (Sixth Character)

Some of the sections use the sixth character to identify a device used in the procedure. To some, this term may conjure up pictures of hard, metal equipment. However, in ICD-10-PCS, the term *device* is used in a more general sense to mean any item that will remain in or with the body after the procedure is complete. So it might mean equipment, such as a pacemaker, or it may report the use of a graft.

Qualifier (Seventh Character)

The seventh character of the ICD-10-PCS code is like a wild card, reporting whatever additional information may be needed. Because the coding system is designed for future expansion, there will be cases where a specific procedure does not currently have the details to require all seven characters. In such cases, the letter *Z* is used to indicate that nothing in that position was applicable to the particular procedure.

Placeholder Characters

The letter *Z* means "not applicable" or "none." The *Z* placeholder will be used most often as the seventh character; however, it can be used in any of the seven character positions, when needed. It can also be used in multiple positions in one code.

EXAMPLE

Dr. Levinson performed a biopsy on Jerry's neck. The ICD-10-PCS code to report this would be 0WB6XZX.

0 = Medical and Surgical
W = Anatomical regions, general
B = Excision
6 = Neck
X = External
Z = No device
X = Diagnostic

There is no device, so there is nothing to report in the sixth character position. But you can't leave that part of the code out. So you put a *Z* in that spot and report that there is no device.

EXAMPLE

Dr. Odom used a percutaneous endoscope in an attempt to control post-procedural bleeding in Tina's colon, after several polyps had been removed. The ICD-10-PCS code to report this would be 0W3P4ZZ.

- 0 = Medical and Surgical
- W = Anatomical regions, general
- 3 = Control
- P = Gastrointestinal tract
- 4 = Percutaneous endoscope
- Z = No device
- Z = No qualifier

There is no device, so there is nothing to report in the sixth character position. There is no qualifier, so there is nothing to report in the seventh character position, either. By placing a *Z* in both positions, you are explaining exactly that. By the way, this is not a decision you have to make. In this subsection of ICD-10-PCS tables, Z No Device and Z No Qualifier are the only choices on the chart for those two character positions.

LO 16.4 The ICD-10-PCS Book

Just like the ICD-10-CM book and the CPT book, the ICD-10-PCS book is divided into two parts: the alphabetic index and the Tables.

The Alphabetic Index

The alphabetic index's entries are primarily sorted by root operation terms. A root operation term identifies the specific service or type of treatment that is the basis of the entire procedure.

EXAMPLE

Root operation terms include *bypass, drainage, excision,* and *insertion.*

After you find the root operation term, as stated in the physician's notes, there are subentries listed by the following:

- **Body system**

EXAMPLE

Digestive system, musculoskeletal system

body system
The physiological system, or anatomical region, upon which the procedure was performed.

- **Body part**

EXAMPLE

Arm, leg, hand, foot

body part
The anatomical site upon which the procedure was performed.

The alphabetic index also lists common terms for some procedures.

EXAMPLE

Hysterectomy is listed and then cross-referenced to *resection* (a root operation term) and *female reproductive system* (body system).

A major difference between ICD-10-PCS, ICD-9-CM Volume 3, and CPT is the fact that this alphabetic index will usually give you only the first three or four characters of the seven-character procedure code. You then must go to the tables to find the additional characters.

EXAMPLE

Fragmentation
Of the Bladder 0TF8-

You won't have to be reminded to *never code from the alphabetic index* with ICD-10-PCS in full effect. Most of the time, you won't be able to code from the alphabetic index alone anymore!

The Tables

The tables are divided by body systems, similar to ICD-9-CM Volume 3. Of course, like all the other code sets, each section is in order by the first character in the code.

Within each body system division of each section, the list continues in order by the root operation term for that procedure. Each section of the list has a grid that specifies the assigned meaning to each letter or number along with its position in the seven-character code. (See an example in Table 16-1.)

You will go through the grid and construct the correct code based on the physician's notes. As you have already learned, all ICD-10-PCS codes are seven characters. Therefore, you will build the code in this order, as directed by the grid.

First character: Section (such as Medicine, Mental Health, Imaging)

Second character: Body system

Third character: Root operation

Fourth character: Body part or region

Fifth character: **Approach**

approach
The specific technique used for the procedure.

TABLE 16-1 Sample from ICD-10-PCS Tables

0: Medical and Surgical (first character)
2: Heart and Great Vessels (second character)
7: Dilation: Expanding the orifice or the lumen of a tubular body part (third character)

Body Part Character 4	Approach Character 5	Device Character 6	Qualifier Character 7
0 Coronary Artery, One Site	0 Open	4 Drug-eluting Intraluminal Device	6 Bifurcation
1 Coronary Artery, Two Sites	3 Percutaneous	D Intraluminal Device	Z No Qualifier
2 Coronary Artery, Three Sites	4 Percutaneous Endoscopic	T Radioactive Intraluminal Device	
3 Coronary Artery, Four or More Sites		Z No Device	

Sixth character: **Device**
Seventh character: **Qualifier**

Therefore, when you review the information in Table 16-1, you can see that the correct ICD-10-PCS code for Dilation of one site of a Coronary Artery, using an open approach with an Intraluminal device is 02700DZ.

LET'S CODE IT! SCENARIO

Kenny was playing football in the park with his friends and ran to catch a pass when the ball hit him in the nose. In the emergency room, Dr. McCoy packed Kenny's nose to stop the bleeding.

Let's Code It!

What did the doctor do for Kenny? Dr. McCoy packed Kenny's nose. Sterile packing material was placed into Kenny's nose to create pressure to stop bleeding. It is always wise to begin with the actual term that the physician used in his or her notes, so let's go to the alphabetic index and look up the term *packing*.

Below the main term, *packing*, is a list of anatomical sites. What anatomical site did the packing go into? *Nose.*

Find

Packing

Nasal 2Y41X5Z

Wow! In this case, the alphabetic index suggested the entire code. Regardless, you still must go to the tables to confirm this is correct.

In the tables, turn to the Placement section: 2Y4.

2 Placement

Y Anatomical Orifices

4 Packing

Body Region Character 4	Approach Character 5	Device Character 6	Qualifier Character 7
0 Mouth and Pharynx	X External	5 Packing Material	Z No Qualifier
1 Nasal			
2 Ear			
3 Anorectal			
4 Female Genital Tract			
5 Urethra			

OK, let's build a code:

The section:	2 Placement (Dr. Coy actually placed the packing materials)
The body system:	Y Anatomical Orifices (the nose is a natural opening in the body)
The root operation:	4 Packing (as per the physician's notes)

The body part:	1 Nasal (as per the physician's notes)
The approach:	X External (the packing was placed from outside the body)
The device:	5 Packing Material (this material will stay in Kenny's nose after the procedure)
The qualifier:	Z None

The ICD-10-PCS code to report the packing of Kenny's nose is 2Y41X5Z. The reason the alphabetic index was able to provide you with all seven characters of the suggested code is that, as you can see, the last three characters have only one choice each.

LET'S CODE IT! SCENARIO

Briton was in a car accident and his right knee hit against the steering column. In the emergency room, Dr. Alberts took a high osmolar x-ray of his knee.

Let's Code It!

What did Dr. Alberta do for Briton? He x-rayed his knee.

In the alphabetic list, look up *x-ray*. The index suggests:

X-ray—*see* Plain Radiography

OK, so turn to *Plain Radiography* in the alphabetic index. Beneath this main term is a long list of anatomical sites, so read down and find

Plain Radiography
Knee
Left BQ08
Right BQ07

The alphabetic index provided only four of the seven needed characters of this suggested code, so turn to the tables to complete the code and confirm its correctness. In the tables, turn to the Imaging section: BQ07.

B Imaging
Q Non-Axial Lower Bones
0 Plain Radiography

Body Part Character 4	Contrast Character 5	Qualifier Character 6	Qualifier Character 7
7 Knee, Right	0 High Osmolar	Z None	Z None
8 Knee, Left	1 Low Osmolar		
G Ankle, Right	Y Other Contrast		
H Ankle, Left	Z None		

OK, let's build the code:

| The section: | B Imaging (you know that x-rays are a type of imaging) |

The body system:	Q Non-axial lower bones (*non-axial* means away from the central part of the body, and you know that the knee is a lower bone)
The root operation:	0 Plain Radiography (also known as x-ray)
The body part:	7 Knee, Right (as per the physician's notes)
The contrast:	0 High Osmolar (as per the physician's notes)
The qualifier:	Z None
The qualifier:	Z None

The ICD-10-PCS code to report the x-ray of Briton's knee is BQ070ZZ.

LO 16.5 ICD-10-PCS General Conventions

The ICD-10-PCS code set has its own set of guidelines, of course. The following list contains the general conventions of how the codes are constructed and how to use the tables.

Read through these 11 guidelines to get a strong start to accurately reporting inpatient procedures.

A1. ICD-10-PCS codes are composed of seven characters. Each character is an axis of classification that specifies information about the procedure performed. Within a defined code range, a character specifies the same type of information in that axis of classification.

EXAMPLE

The fifth axis of classification specifies the approach in sections 0 through 4 and 7 through 9 of the system.

A2. One of 34 possible values can be assigned to each axis of classification in the seven-character code: they are the numbers 0 through 9 and the letters of the alphabet (except I and O because they are easily confused with the numbers 1 and 0). The number of unique values used in an axis of classification differs as needed.

EXAMPLE

Where the fifth axis of classification specifies the approach, seven different approach values are currently used to specify the approach.

A3. The valid values for an axis of classification can be added to as needed.

EXAMPLE

If a significantly distinct type of device is used in a new procedure, a new device value can be added to the system.

A4. As with words in their context, the meaning of any single value is a combination of its axis of classification and any preceding values on which it may be dependent.

> ### EXAMPLE
>
> The meaning of a body part value in the Medical and Surgical section is always dependent on the body system value. The body part value 0 in the Central Nervous body system specifies Brain; the body part value 0 in the Peripheral Nervous body system specifies Cervical Plexus.

A5. As the system is expanded to become increasingly detailed, over time more values will depend on preceding values for their meaning.

> ### EXAMPLE
>
> In the Lower Joints body system, the device value 3 in the root operation Insertion specifies Infusion Device; the device value 3 in the root operation Replacement specifies Ceramic Synthetic Substitute.

A6. The purpose of the alphabetic index is to locate the appropriate table that contains all information necessary to construct a procedure code. The PCS tables should always be consulted to find the most appropriate valid code.

A7. It is not required to consult the index first before proceeding to the tables to complete the code. A valid code may be chosen directly from the tables.

A8. All seven characters must be specified to be a valid code. If the documentation is incomplete for coding purposes, the physician should be queried for the necessary information.

A9. Within a PCS table, valid codes include all combinations of choices in characters 4 through 7 contained in the same row of the table. In the example below, 0JHT3VZ is a valid code, and 0JHW3VZ is *not* a valid code.

Section: 0 Medical and Surgical

Body System: J Subcutaneous Tissue and Fascia

Operation: H Insertion: Putting in a nonbiological appliance that monitors, assists, performs, or prevents a physiological function but does not physically take the place of a body part

Body Part	Approach	Device	Qualifier
S Subcutaneous Tissue and Fascia, Head and Neck V Subcutaneous Tissue and Fascia, Upper Extremity W Subcutaneous Tissue and Fascia, Lower Extremity	0 Open 3 Percutaneous	1 Radioactive Element 3 Infusion Device	Z No Qualifier
T Subcutaneous Tissue and Fascia, Trunk	0 Open 3 Percutaneous	1 Radioactive Element 3 Infusion Device V Infusion Pump	Z No Qualifier

A10. "And," when used in a code description, means "and/or."

> ### EXAMPLE
>
> Lower Arm and Wrist Muscle means lower arm and/or wrist muscle.

A11. Many of the terms used to construct PCS codes are defined within the system. It is the coder's responsibility to determine what the documentation in the medical record equates to in the PCS definitions. The physician is not expected to use the terms used in PCS code descriptions, nor is the coder required to query the physician when the correlation between the documentation and the defined PCS terms is clear.

EXAMPLE

When the physician documents "partial resection" the coder can independently correlate "partial resection" to the root operation Excision without querying the physician for clarification.

LO 16.6 Selection of Principal Procedure

Similar to CPT and HCPCS Level II coding, ICD-10-PCS has its guidelines for determining the sequencing when reporting more than one procedure provided during an encounter. This is always going to be determined in coordination with the diagnosis codes being reported to identify the medical necessity for performing these procedures. Box 16-6 shares the official guidelines for ICD-10-PCS code sequencing.

LO 16.7 General Equivalence Mappings (GEMs)

As part of the effort to make the transition from ICD-9-CM Volume 3 to ICD-10-PCS go more smoothly, documents showing the connection between an ICD-9-CM Volume 3 code and its ICD-10-PCS code equivalent have been created. These documents are called General Equivalence Mappings, commonly known as GEMs.

Of course, the transition is not one-for-one because the new ICD-10-PCS codes are so much more specific. However, the GEMs can help you understand the conversion process of the codes and the language of procedures, services, and treatments.

BOX 16-6   Selection of Principal Procedure

The following instructions should be applied in the selection of principal procedure and clarification on the importance of the relation to the principal diagnosis when more than one procedure is performed:

1. Procedure performed for definitive treatment of both principal diagnosis and secondary diagnosis.
   a. Sequence procedure performed for definitive treatment most related to principal diagnosis as principal procedure.
2. Procedure performed for definitive treatment and diagnostic procedures performed for both principal diagnosis and secondary diagnosis.
   a. Sequence procedure performed for definitive treatment most related to principal diagnosis as principal procedure.
3. A diagnostic procedure was performed for the principal diagnosis and a procedure is performed for definitive treatment of a secondary diagnosis.

   a. Sequence diagnostic procedure as principal procedure, since the procedure most related to the principal diagnosis takes precedence.
4. No procedures performed that are related to principal diagnosis; procedures performed for definitive treatment and diagnostic procedures were performed for secondary diagnosis.
   a. Sequence procedure performed for definitive treatment of secondary diagnosis as principal procedure, since there are no procedures (definitive or nondefinitive treatment) related to principal diagnosis.

Source: ICD-10-PCS *Official Guidelines for Coding and Reporting,* 2014.

ICD-9-CM Vol. 3	Equal To (approximately)	ICD-10-PCS
65.63	≈	0UT24ZZ
Laparoscopic removal of both ovaries and tubes at same operative episode		Resection of bilateral ovaries, percutaneous endoscopic approach
		AND
		0UT74ZZ
		Resection of bilateral fallopian tubes, percutaneous endoscopic approach

You can see from this example that the one ICD-9-CM Volume 3 code is reported with two ICD-10-PCS codes because ICD-10-PCS is so much more specific in its code descriptions. Does this mean you will have to work harder to code accurately? Not at all. You will find that, when code descriptions are less ambiguous, it is easier to make the right choice.

Chapter Summary

The purpose of this chapter is to provide an overview of ICD-10-PCS, giving you an idea of what to expect, and to help you establish a comfort level so that you are not apprehensive about the new system. It's going to be great!

Additional information about ICD-10-PCS can be found at www.cms.gov/ICD10 and www.cms.gov/Medicare/Coding/ICD10/2015-ICD-10-PCS-and-GEMs.html.

CHAPTER 16 REVIEW
Introduction to ICD-10-PCS

Mc Graw Hill Education **connect**
Enhance your learning by completing these
exercises and more at mcgrawhillconnect.com!

Using Terminology

Match each key term to the appropriate definition.

_____ 1. LO 16.4 The identification of any materials or appliances that may remain in or on the body after the procedure is completed.

_____ 2. LO 16.1 One established meaning for each term used in code descriptions.

_____ 3. LO 16.1 The consistent use of characters and elements throughout the book.

_____ 4. LO 16.3 The category or classification of a particular procedure, service, or treatment.

_____ 5. LO 16.1 Structure that allows all procedures, services, and treatments to be represented by a code.

_____ 6. LO 16.4 The anatomical site upon which the procedure was performed.

_____ 7. LO 16.1 ICD-10-PCS codes are constructed of individual values that stay consistent throughout the code set.

_____ 8. LO 16.1 Structure that includes room for growth.

_____ 9. LO 16.1 The structure of the codes individually, and the system in total, can be maintained while still expanding the set to include new technology.

_____ 10. LO 16.4 Any additional feature of the procedure, if applicable.

_____ 11. LO 16.4 The physiological system, or anatomical region, upon which the procedure was performed.

_____ 12. LO 16.4 The specific technique used for the procedure.

A. Approach
B. Body part
C. Body system
D. Completeness
E. Device
F. Expandability
G. Multiaxial
H. Qualifier
I. Root operation term
J. Standardized terminology
K. Structural integrity
L. Unique definitions

Checking Your Understanding

Choose the most appropriate answer for each of the following questions.

1. LO 16.1 In ICD-10-PCS, the initials PCS stand for

   a. Popular Coding System.
   b. Procedure Coding System.
   c. Possible Coding Solutions.
   d. Proper Coding System.

2. LO 16.1 ICD-10-PCS uses only one established meaning for each term used in code descriptions, which is known as _____

   a. completeness.
   b. expandability.
   c. multiaxial.
   d. standardized terminology.

3. LO 16.2 The descriptions for procedures identified in ICD-10-PCS

  a. include diagnostic information.
  b. define the disease or condition that caused the procedure.
  c. do not include diagnostic information.
  d. match those used in the CPT book exactly.

4. LO 16.3 The structure of ICD-10-PCS codes includes

  a. three numbers.
  b. five numbers.
  c. seven characters.
  d. up to nine characters.

5. LO 16.3 ICD-10-PCS codes include

  a. only numbers.
  b. only letters.
  c. one letter followed by numbers.
  d. letters and numbers.

6. LO 16.3 An example of a root operation term is

  a. bypass.
  b. x-ray.
  c. obstetrics.
  d. hysterectomy.

7. LO 16.3 Digestive system is an example of a

  a. body part.
  b. root operation term.
  c. medical procedure.
  d. body system.

8. LO 16.3 The sections of ICD-10-PCS are identified by

  a. numbers 1–17.
  b. numbers 0–9, then letters *B–H*.
  c. letters *A–Z*.
  d. alphabetical order by the name of the section.

9. LO 16.3 Placeholders are indicated in ICD-10-PCS with

  a. the number 0.
  b. the letter *X*.
  c. the letter *Z*.
  d. the number 9.

10. LO 16.1 ICD-10-PCS is designed to replace

  a. CPT.
  b. ICD-9-CM Volume 3.
  c. ICD-10-CM.
  d. ICD-9-CM.

11. LO 16.3/16.4 An example of an approach is

    a. anterior.
    b. ileostomy.
    c. pacemaker.
    d. ventricular.

12. LO 16.3/16.4 An example of a device, for purposes of ICD-10-PCS coding, is

    a. ablation.
    b. laparoscopy.
    c. indwelling ureteral stent.
    d. allotransplantation.

13. LO 16.1 ICD-10-PCS uses characters consistently within the sections and, when possible, from section to section. This is called

    a. expandability.
    b. standardized terminology.
    c. completeness.
    d. multiaxial.

14. LO 16.3 The ICD-10-PCS code for the provision of a cesarean section would be found in

    a. Section 2 Placement.
    b. Section 1 Obstetrics.
    c. Section B Imaging.
    d. Section 6 Extracorporeal Therapies.

15. LO 16.3 Coding a chiropractic manipulative treatment would begin in

    a. Section 0 Medical and Surgical.
    b. Section 4 Measurement and Monitoring.
    c. Section 7 Osteopathic.
    d. Section 9 Chiropractic.

16. LO 16.3 What is the letter or number that represents the device in code 2W22X4Z?

    a. 2.
    b. W.
    c. 4.
    d. X.

17. LO 16.3 What is the letter or number that represents the approach in code 3E00X3Z?

    a. E.
    b. X.
    c. 0.
    d. Z.

18. LO 16.3 What is the letter or number that represents the body part in code 3E0U3HZ?

    a. 3.
    b. E.
    c. H.
    d. U.

19. LO 16.3 What is the letter or number that represents the root operation in code 3E1S38Z?

    a. 1.

    b. S.

    c. 8.

    d. E.

20. LO 16.3 What is the letter or number that represents the body system in code 5A1213Z?

    a. 5.

    b. A.

    c. 1.

    d. 3.

(Note: Until ICD-10-PCS is officially implemented, changes to the sections may still occur. This is the most recent version at the time of this publication.)

Applying Your Knowledge

1. LO 16.1 List the objectives for the development of ICD-10-PCS, including the purpose of each objective. _____

_____

2. LO 16.2 Explain the difference in code descriptions between those in ICD-9-CM Volume 3 and ICD-10-PCS. _____

_____

3. LO 16.3 How many characters does an ICD-10-PCS code have? Are the characters represented with letters, numbers, or both? _____

_____

4. LO 16.3 Which letter(s) may not be included in ICD-10-PCS codes? Why? _____

_____

5. LO 16.3 List the seven ICD-10-PCS character position related pieces of information. _____

_____

6. LO 16.3 What is the placeholder character? What does it mean? Where can it be used? _____

_____

7. LO 16.4 List the parts of the ICD-10-PCS book. _____

_____

8. LO 16.4 How are the alphabetic index's entries primarily sorted? _____

_____

9. LO 16.3/16.4 What does the root operation term identify? _____

_____

10. LO 16.4 How are the ICD-10-PCS tables divided? _____

_____

11. LO 16.5 What are the 11 ICD-10-PCS guidelines? _____

_____

12. LO 16.6 What are the instructions for selection of the principal procedure when more than one procedure is performed? _____

_____

13. LO 16.7 What does the acronym GEM stand for? What is the purpose of GEMs? _____

_____

17

ICD-10-PCS MEDICAL AND SURGICAL SECTION (0)

Learning Outcomes *After completing this chapter, the student should be able to:*

LO 17.1 Recognize the seven components of an ICD-10-PCS code.

LO 17.2 Interpret the procedure to determine the accurate root operation term.

LO 17.3 Utilize knowledge of anatomy to determine the body part treated.

LO 17.4 Identify the approach used to access the body part.

LO 17.5 Distinguish the type of device implanted, when applicable.

LO 17.6 Select the appropriate qualifier character.

Key Terms

Approach
Character
Root operation

Introduction

Medical and surgical procedures, services, and treatments are reported with codes from this first section of the tables of ICD-10-PCS (see Figure 17-1). As the codes are subdivided by anatomical site or organ system that is the focus of the procedure, you will find that building a code to report this is quite different than using the other code sets. This coding process may require you to use your knowledge in a slightly different manner.

LO 17.1 Character Definitions

As you learned earlier, every ICD-10-PCS code has seven characters, and each **character** position has a meaning. While all of these codes have the same number of characters, each section uses each character position differently. So let's review the meanings for the Medical and Surgical section characters:

Character Position	Character Meaning
1	Section of the ICD-10-PCS book
2	Body system being treated
3	Root operation term
4	Body part (specific anatomical site)
5	Approach used by physician
6	Device
7	Qualifier

Section	0	Medical and Surgical
Body System	2	Heart and Great Vessels
Operation	5	Destruction: Physical eradication of all or a portion of a body part by the direct use of energy, force, or a destructive agent

Body part	Approach	Device	Qualifier
4 Coronary Vein **5** Atrial Septum **6** Atrium, Right **8** Conduction Mechanism **9** Chordae Tendineae **D** Papillary Muscle **F** Aortic Valve **G** Mitral Valve **H** Pulmonary Valve **J** Tricuspid Valve **K** Ventricle, Right **L** Ventricle, Left **M** Ventricular Septum **N** Pericardium **P** Pulmonary Trunk **Q** Pulmonary Artery, Right **R** Pulmonary Artery, Left **S** Pulmonary Vein, Right **T** Pulmonary Vein, Left **V** Superior Vena Cava **W** Thoracic Aorta	**0** Open **3** Percutaneous **4** Percutaneous Endoscopic	**Z** No Device	**Z** No Qualifier
7 Atrium, Left	**0** Open **3** Percutaneous **4** Percutaneous Endoscopic	**Z** No Device	**K** Left Atrial Appendage **Z** No Qualifier

FIGURE 17-1 An Example from the Medical and Surgical Tables of ICD-10-PCS

Character Position 1: Medical and Surgical Section 0 (Zero)

0
Section

character
A letter or number component of an ICD-10-PCS code.

All of the codes reporting a medical or surgical procedure will begin with a zero. This is the first section of the tables, after the Alphabetic Index. When you look up a procedure in the Alphabetic Index and see that the suggested code begins with a zero, you will know immediately that you will find the rest of this code in the Medical and Surgical tables.

Character Position 2: Body System: 0–9, B–Y

0	0–9, B–Y
Section	**Body System**

In this code set, the body systems are broken down into further detail than the organ systems you learned in your anatomy and physiology course. The body systems and their corresponding characters are

0   Central Nervous System

1   Peripheral Nervous System

2   Heart and Great Vessels

3   Upper Arteries

4   Lower Arteries

5   Upper Veins

6   Lower Veins

7   Lymphatic and Hemic Systems

8   Eye

9   Ear, Nose, Sinus

B   Respiratory System

C   Mouth and Throat

D   Gastrointestinal System

F   Hepatobiliary System and Pancreas

G   Endocrine System

H   Skin and Breast

J   Subcutaneous Tissue and Fascia

K   Muscles

L   Tendons

M   Bursae and Ligaments

N   Head and Facial Bones

P   Upper Bones

Q   Lower Bones

R   Upper Joints

S   Lower Joints

T   Urinary System

U   Female Reproductive System

V   Male Reproductive System

W   Anatomical Regions, General

X   Anatomical Regions, Upper Extremities

Y   Anatomical Regions, Lower Extremities

Notice that, in this list, there is a 0 (zero) and a number 1 (one) but no letter *O* or letter *I*. The creators of this code set did this purposely to avoid confusion.

Take a look at body system 5 Upper Veins and 6 Lower Veins. As explained in the guidelines, the imaginary transverse line is at the diaphragm, dividing the body into top (upper) and bottom (lower). A procedure performed on the brachial vein, located in the arm, will be reported with body system character 5, and a procedure performed on the gastric vein, located in the stomach, is reported with body system character 6. Similarly, the same applies for characters 3 and 4 (Upper and Lower Arteries), P and Q (Upper and Lower Bones), and R and S (Upper and Lower Joints).

Now, let's look at body system characters W, X, and Y, which report anatomical regions instead of a specific body section or system. These should be used only when the documentation identifies that the procedure was performed on an anatomical cavity rather than an individual body part. You must read carefully to distinguish the details. To illustrate this, let's look at a case of a patient diagnosed with ascites (a buildup of fluid in the abdominal cavity). The physician drains this excess fluid from the abdominal cavity; therefore, it will require a character of W for the body system: Anatomical Regions, General.

You do not need to worry about remembering that the liver is part of the hepatobiliary system or that a pacemaker generator is inserted into the subcutaneous tissue and fascia and its leads are inserted into the heart. The Alphabetic Index will help you, as will the listings for body part (character position 4).

EXAMPLE

Drainage of the common bile duct...0F99

Restriction of stomach...............0DV6

LO 17.2 Character Position 3: Root Operation

0	0–9, B–Y	0–9, B–Y
Section	Body System	Root Operation

The Medical and Surgical section uses 31 **root operation** terms to describe what procedure was performed for the patient during this encounter. Don't worry—the definitions are listed in the front of the ICD-10-PCS codebook. However, you still need to learn and understand them so that you can abstract the operative report or procedure notes accurately and completely. Remember that you are required to use this definition in its entirety. Also, just as in reporting with CPT procedure codes, it is important that you understand all of the components of a specific root operation or procedure. You don't want to code inclusive components separately. Using the root operation term is the most efficient way of using the Alphabetic Index as well.

<u>Alteration</u>: Modification of a natural anatomic structure of a body part without affecting the function of the body part . . . Character: 0 (zero)

EXAMPLE

This is a procedure most often performed for cosmetic purposes, such as a face lift.

0J013ZZ Alteration of subcutaneous tissue and fascia, face, percutaneous approach

<u>Bypass</u>: Changing the route of a tubular body part's contents and how it passes through the body . . . Character: 1

Bypass procedures are coded by identifying the body part bypassed "from," identified by character 4 (Body Part), and the body part bypassed "to," identified by the character 7 (Qualifier).

EXAMPLE

As you can see from its description, a bypass can be performed only on a tubular body part, such as a vein or an artery, the esophagus, or the intestines.

02114Z8 Coronary artery bypass, one site, percutaneous endoscopic approach, rerouted to internal mammary, right side

<u>Change</u>: Taking out or off a device from a body part and putting back an identical or similar device in or on the same body part without cutting or puncturing the skin or a mucous membrane . . . Character: 2

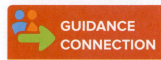

GUIDANCE CONNECTION

See ICD-10-PCS Medical and Surgical guidelines, **Body System General Guidelines; B2.1a and B2.1b,** for more details.

root operation
The term used to describe the function or purpose of the procedure.

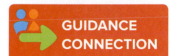

GUIDANCE CONNECTION

See ICD-10-PCS Medical and Surgical guidelines, **Root Operation; B3.1a and B3.1b,** for more details.

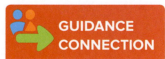

GUIDANCE CONNECTION

See ICD-10-PCS Medical and Surgical guidelines, **Bypass Procedures; B3.6a, B3.6b, and B3.6c,** for more details about reporting bypasses.

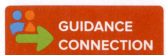
EXAMPLE

0020X0Z Changing a drainage device in the brain, external approach

Control: Stopping, or attempting to stop, postprocedural bleeding . . . Character: 3

This root operation term will lead you to the correct code when this is all that was done with regard to stopping the hemorrhage. If this attempt was unsuccessful and another procedure was performed to accomplish this task, such as excision or resection, then report the code for that root operation instead of the Control. You will not report both.

EXAMPLE

0W3B0ZZ Control post-procedural bleeding in the pleural cavity, left side, open approach

Creation: Creating a new genital structure that does not take over the function of a body part . . . Character 4

This procedure is used most often for making a new structure during sex change operations, such as creating an artificial vagina during a male-to-female procedure.

EXAMPLE

0W4N00J1 Creation of an artificial penis using synthetic substitute, open approach

0W4M00K0 Creation of an artificial vagina using nonautologous tissue substitute, open approach

Destruction: Physical eradication of all or a portion of a body part by the direct use of energy, force, or a destructive agent without replacement . . . Character 5

Several methodologies are reported as destruction, such as fulguration, the application of high-frequency electrical current when it is used to destroy tissue (typically malignant neoplasm), also known as electrofulguration. Chemical agents, such as salicylic acid, can also be used to destroy tissue.

EXAMPLE

0U5B8ZZ Fulguration of endometrium, vaginal endoscopic approach

Detachment: Cutting of all or a portion of the upper or lower extremities . . . Character 6

This is the root operation term for amputation of an arm or a leg, in whole or in part.

EXAMPLE

0Y6J0Z Amputation, below knee, left leg, open approach

Dilation: Expanding an orifice or the lumen of a tubular body part . . . Character 7

Remember, an orifice is a natural body opening (such as vagina or anus) and the lumen of a tubular body part (*lumen* = "space within the tube"). Blood vessels are tubular body parts, as are a woman's fallopian tubes.

EXAMPLE

> 037H34Z Dilation of right common carotid artery, with drug-eluting intraluminal device, percutaneous approach
> 0U7C7ZZ Dilation of the cervix, via natural opening

Division: Cutting into a body part in order to separate or transect a body part (without draining fluids and/or gases from the body part) . . . Character 8

EXAMPLE

> 0K820ZZ Division of sternocleidomastoid muscle, right side, open approach

Drainage: Taking or letting out fluids and/or gases from a body part . . . Character 9

EXAMPLE

> 0W9B30Z Drainage of excess air from left pleural cavity, percutaneous approach

Excision: Cutting out or off, without replacement a portion of a body part . . . Character B

Pay close attention to this description of excision. This term has a narrower meaning in ICD-10-PCS than it does in CPT and many physicians' notes. Excision is used in ICD-10-PCS only when a segment is cut out. This includes a biopsy, a lumpectomy, and a bone spur. However, if the entire organ or body part is removed, the root operation term used is *Resection*.

> **GUIDANCE CONNECTION**
>
> See ICD-10-PCS Medical and Surgical guidelines, **Excision vs. Resection; B3.8** and **Excision for graft; B3.9,** for more details.

EXAMPLE

> 0FB13ZX Excision, liver, right lobe, percutaneous approach, diagnostic procedure

Extirpation: Taking or cutting out solid matter from a body part . . . Character C

This reference to "solid matter" may indicate a blood clot or gallstones when surgically removed.

EXAMPLE

> 04CL0ZZ Extirpation of thrombus, femoral artery, left side, open approach

Extraction: Pulling or stripping out or off all or a portion of a body part by the use of force . . . Character D

> ## EXAMPLE
>
> 0UDB8ZZ Suction extraction of endometrium, via natural opening endoscopic approach

Fragmentation: Breaking solid matter in a body part into pieces . . . Character F

An example of fragmentation is lithotripsy—the use of shock waves to break kidney stones (renal lithiasis) into smaller pieces with the hope that the body will be able to pass them naturally.

> ## EXAMPLE
>
> 0TFCXZZ Fragmentation of stones in the bladder neck, using external approach

Fusion: Joining together portions of an articular body part rendering the articular body part immobile . . . Character G

Arthrodesis, the surgical immobilization of a joint, such as of the spine, is one type of fusion (*articular* = "joint").

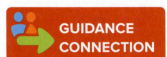

GUIDANCE CONNECTION

See ICD-10-PCS Medical and Surgical guidelines, **Fusion procedures of the spine; B3.10a, B3.10b, and B3.10c,** for more details.

> ## EXAMPLE
>
> 0RG40A0 Fusion of cervicothoracic vertebral joint, open procedure, anterior approach, anterior column, using an interbody fusion device

Insertion: Putting in nonbiological appliance that monitors, assists, performs, or prevents a physiological function but does not physically take the place of a body part . . . Character H

This is another opportunity for reading very carefully. In ICD-10-PCS, this root operation applies only to the placement into the body of a medical device, such as a pacemaker, that will remain in the body after the procedure is completed.

> ## EXAMPLE
>
> 05H933Z Insertion of catheter (infusion device) into right brachial vein, percutaneous approach

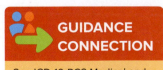

GUIDANCE CONNECTION

See ICD-10-PCS Medical and Surgical guidelines, **Inspection Procedures; B3.11a, B3.11b, and B3.11c,** for more details.

Inspection: Visually and/or manually exploring a body part . . . Character J

This root operation term is limited to the physician's looking at the body part.

> ## EXAMPLE
>
> 09JEXZZ Inspection of the left inner ear, external approach

Map: Locating the route of passage of electrical impulses and/or locating functional areas in a body part . . . Character K

Cardiac conduction mapping and brain mapping are two illustrations of this root operation. Note that this root operation term reports the examination only.

> ### EXAMPLE
>
> 00K03ZZ Mapping of brain function, percutaneous approach

Occlusion: Completing closing an orifice or lumen of a tubular body part . . . Character L

There are times when an opening, such as a fistula, or a tubular body part, such as fallopian tubes, is purposely closed off or blocked.

> ### EXAMPLE
>
> 0VLH4ZZ Occlusion of spermatic cords, bilaterally, percutaneous endoscopic approach, no device

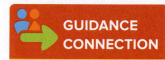

GUIDANCE CONNECTION

See ICD-10-PCS Medical and Surgical guidelines, **Occlusion vs. Restriction for vessel embolization procedures; B3.12,** for more details.

Reattachment: Putting back in or on all or a portion of a separated body part to its normal location or other suitable location . . . Character M

This word is the same as the term most often used by physicians for this procedure, such as reattaching a finger after it has been severed during an accident.

> ### EXAMPLE
>
> 0XMP0ZZ Reattachment of left index finger, open approach

Release: Freeing a body part from an abnormal physical constraint by cutting or by use of force . . . Character N

The procedure reported with this root operation term involves cutting or separation only, in order to free a body part from some type of restriction, such as tendon lengthening.

> ### EXAMPLE
>
> 0LNS0ZZ Release of right ankle tendon, open approach

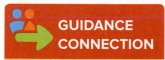

GUIDANCE CONNECTION

See ICD-10-PCS Medical and Surgical guidelines, **Release Procedures; B3.13** and **Release vs. Division, B3.14,** for more details.

Removal: Taking out or off a device from a body part . . . Character P

Read this carefully: As the description specifically states "device," this can be used only for this type of procedure, to remove a previously inserted device. As you abstract the physician's notes, be cautious of the use of this term in documentation. The removal of a mole, for example, is really an excision, not a removal.

> ### EXAMPLE
>
> 0QP304Z Removal of internal fixation device from left pelvic bone, open approach

Repair: Restoring, to the extent possible, a body part to its normal anatomic structure and function . . . Character Q

> **EXAMPLE**
>
> 0CQV8ZZ Repair of left vocal cord, via natural opening, endoscopic approach

Replacement: Putting in or on biological or synthetic material that physically takes the place and/or function of all or a portion of a body part . . . Character R

Essentially, this is the placement of a prosthetic device, such as a hip replacement or a prosthetic heart valve.

> **EXAMPLE**
>
> 02RG0JZ Replacement of mitral valve with synthetic prosthesis, open approach

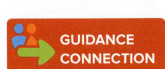

GUIDANCE CONNECTION

See ICD-10-PCS Medical and Surgical guidelines, **Reposition for fracture treatment; B3.15,** for more details.

Reposition: Moving to its normal location or other suitable location all or a portion of a body part . . . Character S

> **EXAMPLE**
>
> 0PSFXZZ Reposition humeral shaft, right side, external approach

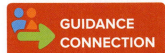

GUIDANCE CONNECTION

See ICD-10-PCS Medical and Surgical guidelines, **Excision vs. Resection; B3.8,** for more details.

Resection: Cutting out or off, without replacement, all of a body part . . . Character T

Remember how this differs from excision. When the entire body part is surgically removed, it is reported as a resection. If only a portion of the body part is removed, it is reported as an excision.

> **EXAMPLE**
>
> 0FT44ZZ Resection of gallbladder, percutaneous endoscopic approach

Restriction: Partially closing an orifice or lumen of a tubular body part . . . Character V

Compare this with the root operation term *occlusion*. Restriction is a partial closure and occlusion is a complete closure.

> **EXAMPLE**
>
> 0DV44CZ Restriction of esophagogastric junction, using extraluminal device, percutaneous endoscopic approach

Revision: Correcting, to the extent possible, a portion of a malfunctioning device or the position of a displaced device . . . Character W

Again, pay careful attention to the word *device*. This root operation term can only be used when a medical device is being fixed.

EXAMPLE

02WA0MZ Revision of cardiac lead, open approach

Supplement: Putting in or on biological or synthetic material that physically reinforces and/or augments the function of a portion of a body part . . . Character U

Note: In the tables section, *supplement* is in alphabetic order by its character *U*, not by the term *supplement*, so it falls between *resection* and *restriction*.

EXAMPLE

0TUB4JZ Supplementation of bladder, percutaneous endoscopic approach, using synthetic mesh

Transfer: Moving, without taking out, all or a portion of a body part to another location to take over the function of all or a portion of a body part . . . Character X

EXAMPLE

0JX03ZB Transfer of skin and subcutaneous tissue, scalp, percutaneous approach

Transplantation: Putting in or on all or a portion of a living body part taken from another individual or animal to physically take the place and/or function of all or a portion of a similar body part . . . Character Y

ICD-10-PCS uses this term in the same manner that physicians do. However, this includes more than just organ transplant procedures. For instance, in vitro fertilization (IVF) is included in this root operation term.

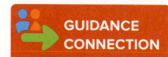

GUIDANCE CONNECTION

See ICD-10-PCS Medical and Surgical guidelines, **Transplantation vs. Administration; B3.16,** for more details.

EXAMPLE

0TY00Z0 Transplant of an allogeneic right kidney, open approach

As you abstract the physician documentation, you may need to adjust some of your interpretative processes for reporting procedures using ICD-10-PCS. The root operation term is based on the objective of the procedure. You are seeking the word describing the action, such as *excision* or *drainage*. Combination terms with which you are very familiar, such as *colonoscopy, liver biopsy,* or *appendectomy,* may describe the procedure; however, these terms do not specifically explain the action of the physician, or do they? Let's take a closer look at these terms and interpret them into the root operation terms:

Colonoscopy: *colon* = "large intestine" (anatomical site) + *-oscopy* = "to view"

In ICD-10-PCS, you would use the root operation term *Inspection: Visually and/or manually exploring a body part.*

Liver biopsy: *liver* = anatomical site + *biopsy* = "excision of tissue for diagnostic purposes"

In ICD-10-PCS, you would use the root operation term *Excision: Cutting out or off, without replacement, a portion of a body part.* In just a bit, you will learn about adding a Qualifier in the character 7 position to include the detail that this was a diagnostic excision.

Appendectomy: *append* = "appendix" (anatomical site) + *-ectomy* = "surgical removal"

In ICD-10-PCS, you would use the root operation term *Resection: Cutting out or off, without replacement, all of a body part.*

With some procedures, you will use your knowledge of the specific procedure and what it is expected to accomplish. For example, you will need to remember that lithotripsy is performed for Fragmentation: Breaking solid matter in a body part into pieces, which is done when a patient has kidney stones. Another example is thoracentesis (*thora* = "thorax [chest]" + *-centesis* = "puncture"), performed for Drainage: Taking or letting out fluids and/or gases from a body part.

YOU INTERPRET IT!

Practice interpreting from the common procedure terms used to reference the ICD-10-PCS root operation term.

Colostomy formation _____

Cautery of skin lesion _____

Transluminal angioplasty _____

Choledocholithotomy _____

Free skin graft _____

Adhesiolysis _____

Fallopian tube ligation _____

Diagnostic arthroscopy _____

Ankle arthrodesis _____

Total nephrectomy _____

Esophagogastic fundoplication _____

LO 17.3 Character Position 4: Body Part: 0–9, B–Y

0	0–9, B–Y	0–9, B–Y	0–9, B–Y
Section	Body System	Root Operation	Body Part

This character will identify the specific body part that is the focus of the procedure. The operative report or the procedure notes should be clear about these details. However, sometimes it can be a challenge to match the documentation to the choices offered in the tables. Following are some guidelines to help you determine the accurate code in ICD-10-PCS.

The notes are more specific than the code character specifics. If the physician documents that the procedure was performed on a specific anatomical site, such as the biceps femoris muscle, yet the listing of body parts under Muscles (Body System character K) does not provide this detail, you will need to code to the body part that includes this anatomical site. In this case, you would report Upper Leg Muscle.

Bilateral procedures. If the documentation identifies that a procedure was performed on both a right body part and a left body part, and a Body Part code character is available to report the bilateral procedure, that is the one code to report. However, if there is no code character available to report a bilateral procedure, then you will need to report two codes: one for each procedure.

EXAMPLE

0HRVEKZ Replacement of breasts, bilateral, percutaneous approach

0CNT8ZZ Release of right vocal cord, via natural opening endoscopic

0CNV8ZZ Release of left vocal cord, via natural opening endoscopic

Coronary arteries. While the coronary arteries are represented by one code character, there are additional characters to report when more than one site is treated in this one set of arteries.

GUIDANCE CONNECTION

See ICD-10-PCS Medical and Surgical guidelines, **B4. Body Part; General Guidelines B4.1a and B4.1b; Branches of body parts B4.2, Bilateral body part values B4.3, Coronary arteries B4.4, Tendons, ligaments, bursae, and fascia near a joint B4.5, Skin, subcutaneous tissue, and fascia overlying a joint B4.6, Fingers and toes B4.7, and Gastrointestinal Body System B4.8,** for more details.

EXAMPLE

Dr. Chrineton performed an angioplasty in the left anterior descending coronary artery in two distinct sites with two intraluminal, drug-eluting stents placed.

02713DZ Dilation of coronary artery, two sites, percutaneous approach with intraluminal device, drug-eluting

Joints and muscles. Many body systems provide individual code characters for body parts specific to a joint or a muscle. There are some cases when the Body Part characters may not be as specific as the physician's notes. The guidelines provide direction in determination of a code character to report the body part. When a procedure is performed on the skin, the subcutaneous tissue, or the fascia that is lying over a joint,

- Shoulder is reported as Upper Arm.
- Elbow is reported as Lower Arm.
- Wrist is reported as Lower Arm.
- Hip is reported as Upper Leg.
- Knee is reported as Lower Leg.
- Ankle is reported as Foot.

When a body system does not include a separate body part code character for fingers or toes:

- Finger is reported as Hand.
- Toe is reported as Foot.

Gastrointestinal body system. Certain areas within the gastrointestinal Body System tables group the individual body parts of the intestinal tract into Upper and Lower. For these cases, the Upper Intestinal Tract includes esophagus, stomach, to and including the duodenum. The Lower Intestinal Tract includes jejunum, ileus, cecum, large intestine, all the way to and including the anus.

Body Part Key Appendix in ICD-10-PCS can also help you when a specific anatomical site is documented and the Body Part components are not as specific. For instance, Stensen's duct is reported as the parotid duct, and the superior gluteal nerve is described in ICD-10-PCS as the lumbar plexus.

Practice using the *Body Part Key Appendix* and fill in the descriptions used by ICD-10-PCS for coding.

Superior olivary nucleus _____

Sigmoid vein _____

Right suprarenal vein _____

Ulnar notch _____

Ventricular fold _____

Sweat gland _____

Optic disc _____

Oropharynx _____

Nasal concha_____

Manubrium _____

Ischium _____

LO 17.4 Character Position 5: Approach

0	0–9, B–Y	0–9, B–Y	0–9, B–Y	0–9, B–Y
Section	Body System	Root Operation	Body Part	Approach

As you continue to build a code, you can see that you are telling a story. The first four characters explain what the physician did and the anatomical site upon which he or she worked. Now, with the fifth character, you are going to explain how the physician got to the anatomical site to perform the procedure. This is known as the **approach**, and seven approaches are used within the Medical and Surgical section.

approach
The path the physician took to access the body part upon which the treatment or procedure was targeted.

<u>Open</u>: Cutting through the skin or mucous membrane and any other body layers necessary to expose the site of the procedure . . . Character 0

An open procedure is the traditional approach when the physician makes an incision into the body to access an internal organ.

GUIDANCE CONNECTION

See ICD-10-PCS Medical and Surgical guidelines, **Open approach with percutaneous endoscopic assistance; B5.2,** for more details.

EXAMPLE

04H00DZ Insertion of intraluminal device into the abdominal aorta, open approach

<u>Percutaneous</u>: Entry, by puncture or minor incision, of instrumentation through the skin or mucous membrane and any other body layers necessary to reach the site of the procedure . . . Character 3

When a percutaneous approach is used, the physician cannot see inside the body. Often, a radiologist will provide imaging guidance (which would be reported separately). A needle aspiration and needle biopsy are good illustrations of a percutaneous approach.

EXAMPLE

0B9N3ZX Drainage of right pleura, percutaneous approach, diagnostic

<u>Percutaneous Endoscopic</u>: Entry, by puncture or minor incision, of instrumentation through the skin or mucous membrane and any other body layers necessary to reach and visualize the site of the procedure . . . Character 4

In this type of approach, a scope is placed through the incision or puncture. A laparoscopic procedure is a good example.

EXAMPLE

09CR4ZZ Extirpation of left maxillary sinus, percutaneous endoscopic approach

<u>Via Natural or Artificial Opening</u>: Entry of instrumentation through a natural or artificial external opening to reach the site of the procedure . . . Character 7

The natural openings to the body include the nose, mouth, ear, vagina, urethra, and anus. An artificial opening includes a stoma (an opening that has been surgically created).

EXAMPLE

08LY7DZ Occlusion of the lacrimal duct, left side, using intraluminal device, via natural or artificial opening

<u>Via Natural or Artificial Opening Endoscopic</u>: Entry of instrumentation through a natural or artificial external opening to reach and visualize the site of the procedure . . . Character 8

Note that the difference between this approach and "via natural or artificial opening" is the use of an endoscope to visualize the anatomical site upon which the procedure will be performed.

EXAMPLE

0D138Z9 Bypass from lower esophagus to duodenum, via natural or artificial opening endoscopic, no device

<u>External</u>: Procedure performed directly on the skin or mucous membrane and procedures performed indirectly by the application of external force through the skin or mucous membrane . . . Character X

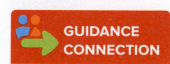

GUIDANCE CONNECTION

See ICD-10-PCS Medical and Surgical guidelines, **External approach; B5.3a and B5.3b,** for more details.

EXAMPLE

0PSJXZZ Reposition radius, left side, external approach

As you abstract the documentation and interpret the way the physician describes how the procedure was performed, you may find *Appendix F: Components of the Medical and Surgical Approach Definitions* helpful.

YOU INTERPRET IT!

Practice using Appendix F and fill in the approach used by ICD-10-PCS for coding.

Liposuction _____

Sigmoidoscopy _____

Laproscopic hysterectomy _____

Fracture manipulation (closed) _____

Traditional cholecystectomy _____

Foley catheter placement _____

Lumbar puncture _____

Breast biopsy with guidance _____

Endoscopy _____

Cesarean section _____

Blepharotomy _____

LO 17.5 Character Position 6: Device

0	0–9, B–Y	0–9, B–Y	0–9, B–Y	0–9, B–Y	0–9, B–Z
Section	Body System	Root Operation	Body Part	Approach	Device

As you can see, a character placed in the sixth position will identify a device that will remain with the patient after the procedure has been completed. ICD-10-PCS considers these generalized types of devices to qualify:

- Grafts
- Prostheses
- Implants
- Simple or mechanical appliances
- Electronic appliances

Reading through the Medical and Surgical section, with a focus on some of the options for the sixth character, you will find a limited number of descriptors. Let's take a closer look at these:

Grafts

Autologous tissue substitute . . . Character 7

    Autologous venous tissue . . . Character 9

    Autologous arterial tissue . . . Character A

This refers to a graft made with tissue from the patient's own body.

    Synthetic substitute . . . Character J

This explains that the graft material may be carbon fibers, polypropylene, or other nonhuman substance.

    Nonautologous tissue substitute . . . Character K

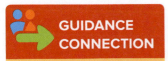

GUIDANCE CONNECTION

Guideline B6.1b. Materials such as sutures, ligatures, radiological markers and temporary post-operative wound drains are considered integral to the performance of a procedure and are not coded as devices.

This graft is made from materials other than the patient's own tissue.

>   Zooplastic tissue . . . Character 8

This identifies that the graft was made with tissue from a species other than human.

Simple or Mechanical Appliances

Drainage device . . . Character 0

Monitoring device . . . Character 2

>   Monitoring device, pressure sensor . . . Character 0

Infusion device . . . Character 3

Extraluminal device . . . Character C

Intraluminal device . . . Character D

>   Drug-eluting intraluminal device . . . Character 4

>   Bioactive intraluminal device . . . Character B

>   Radioactive intraluminal device . . . Character T

Implants and Electronic Appliances

Stimulator (cardiac) lead . . . Character M

Cardiac lead, defibrillator . . . Character K

Cardiac lead, pacemaker . . . Character J

Implantable heart assist system . . . Character Q

External heart assist system . . . Character R

Radioactive element . . . Character 1

No device . . . Character Z

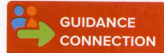

GUIDANCE CONNECTION

See ICD-10-PCS Medical and Surgical uidelines, **B6. Device: General Guidelines, B6.1a, B6.1b, and B6.1c** as well as **Drainage Device B6.2,** for more details.

In operative reports and procedure notes, when a device is placed into the patient, the notes will identify the brand name and details, rather than "synthetic substitute" or "intraluminal device." For instance, an AxiaLIF® System is an interbody fusion device used in lower joints, or Ultrapro plug is a synthetic substitute. Don't panic. You don't have to memorize these brand names. Just bookmark *Appendix D: Device Key and Aggregation Table* in your ICD-10-PCS codebook.

YOU INTERPRET IT!

Practice using Appendix D and fill in the device description used by ICD-10-PCS for coding.

>   Bovine pericardial valve _____

>   Acuity Steerable Lead_____

>   Centrimag® Blood Pump _____

>   Tissue bank graft _____

>   Pump reservoir _____

>   Lap-Band® Adjustable Gastric Banding System _____

>   Prestige cervical disc _____

>   Versa_____

>   Novacor Left Ventricular Assist Device_____

>   EndoSure® sensor _____

>   Brachytherapy seeds_____

0	0–9, B–Y	0–9, B–Y	0–9, B–Y	0–9, B–Y	0–9, B–Z	0–9, B–Z
Section	Body System	Root Operation	Body Part	Approach	Device	Qualifier

This seventh character is required. In many cases, there may be no more details to add, so you will use the placeholder Z No Qualifier—the equivalent of "not applicable."

You will find that, depending on the procedure provided, you may need to check the documentation for applicable details. For instance, when an excision is performed, you may find a Qualifier character option to explain that this was a biopsy (for diagnostic purposes . . . Character X).

Earlier in this chapter, in the section that discussed root operation terms, you learned that bypass procedures are coded by identifying the body part bypassed "from," identified by character 4 (Body Part), and the body part bypassed "to," identified by the character 7 (Qualifier). This is just a reminder that, in some cases, the Qualifier character will partner with the Body Part character to explain the whole story about the procedure.

EXAMPLE

0D164JA Gastric bypass, percutaneous endoscopic approach, rerouted from stomach to jejunum

LET'S CODE IT! SCENARIO

Faith Denarro, a 3-year-old female, was admitted to the hospital by her ophthalmologist, Dr. Kenter. Her right lacrimal duct was occluded. After sedation was administered, Dr. Kenter probed her nasolacrimal duct and inserted a transluminal balloon catheter to expand the duct. The balloon was deflated and removed. She tolerated the procedure well.

You Code It!

Let's go through the steps of coding for ICD-10-PCS and determine the code or codes that should be reported for this encounter between Dr. Kenter and Faith Denarro.

Character 1: Section: Medical and Surgical . . . Character 0
Character 2: Body System: Eye . . . Character 8
Character 3: Root Operation: Dilation . . . Character 7

Read through the scenario carefully. Dr. Kenter "expanded" the duct. The description of the term "dilation" is to expand an orifice or the lumen of a tubular body part.

Character 4: Body Part: Lacrimal Duct, Right . . . Character X

You may have been tempted to think "eye"; however, when you get to the table for Eye, Dilation . . . 087, you will see that "eye" is the Body System and not an option for Body Part.

Character 5: Approach: Via Natural or Artificial Opening . . . Character 7

Dr. Kenter inserted the catheter directly into the duct (this opening is how our tears flow from our eyes). Therefore, he used a natural opening.

Character 6: Device: No Device . . . Character Z

If Dr. Kenter inserted an intraluminal device and left it in the duct to keep it open (a stent), you would report Character D Intraluminal Device in this position.

Character 7: Qualifier: No Qualifier . . . Character Z

The ICD-10-PCS code you will report is

087X7ZZ Dilation, lacrimal duct, right, via natural or artificial opening

Good job!!

Multiple Procedures

Just because the physician performs more than one procedure does not necessarily mean you will report more than one code. The official guidelines provide four illustrations of cases when you will report multiple procedures:.

1. *The same root operation is performed on different body parts as defined by distinct values of the body part character.* Two codes are reported.
2. *The same root operation is repeated at different body sites that are included in the same body part value.* You will report the same code twice. It is recommended that a report to explain is appended.
3. *Multiple root operations with distinct objectives are performed on the same body part.* Two codes are reported, one for each root operation.
4. *The intended root operation is attempted using one approach but is converted to a different approach.* One code will report what was actually accomplished with the first approach, and a second code will report the second approach.

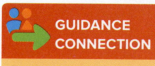

GUIDANCE CONNECTION

See ICD-10-PCS Medical and Surgical guidelines, **Multiple Procedures B3.2,** for more details.

LET'S CODE IT! SCENARIO

Justin Makelroy, a 17-year-old male, was riding his motorcycle when he skidded out. The bike fell on top of him and his left ankle was dislocated. He was admitted into the hospital and Dr. Renquist tried to manually realign the tarsal bone to its rightful position. Unfortunately, he was unable to accomplish this and had to take Justin to the OR to perform an open procedure.

Let's Code It!

Let's go through the steps of coding for ICD-10-PCS and determine the code or codes that should be reported for this encounter between Dr. Renquist and Justin Makelroy.

First code:

Character 1: Section: Medical and Surgical . . . Character 0
Character 2: Body System: Lower Bones . . . Character Q
Character 3: Root Operation: Reposition . . . Character S
Character 4: Body Part: Tarsal, left . . . Character M
Character 5: Approach: External . . . Character X
Character 6: Device: No Device . . . Character Z
Character 7: Qualifier: No Qualifier . . . Character Z

The ICD-10-PCS code you will report is

0QSMXZZ Reposition, right tarsal bone, externally

Remember the guideline about multiple procedures, part D. You will need a second code to report the second attempt to realign Justin's ankle.

Second code:

Character 1: Section: Medical and Surgical . . . Character 0

Character 2: Body System: Lower Bones . . . Character Q

Character 3: Root Operation: Reposition . . . Character S

Character 4: Body Part: Tarsal, left . . . Character M

Character 5: Approach: Open . . . Character 0

Character 6: Device: No Device . . . Character Z

Character 7: Qualifier: No Qualifier . . . Character Z

The ICD-10-PCS code you will report is

0QSM0ZZ Reposition, right tarsal bone, open approach

Finally, consider in what sequence you will report these two codes. The rule is that the most intense procedure will be reported first, so you should report the open procedure first, followed by the external approach.

0QSM0ZZ Reposition, right tarsal bone, open approach

0QSMXZZ Reposition, right tarsal bone, externally

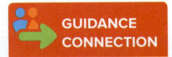

GUIDANCE CONNECTION

See ICD-10-PCS Medical and Surgical guidelines, **Discontinued Procedures B3.3,** for more details.

Discontinued Procedures

It has happened: The physician begins a procedure and for some reason must stop before accomplishing the goal originally planned. Should this occur, you are directed to report those root operations that were actually done.

EXAMPLE

The physician has planned a laparoscopic cholecystectomy. The incisions are made and the scope is inserted. The gallbladder can be visualized. However, before the organ can be surgically removed, the patient has a seizure. The physician stops the procedure and closes the incisions.

0FJ44ZZ Inspection of gallbladder, percutaneous endoscopic approach

Chapter Summary

This chapter showed you that building a code in ICD-10-PCS may require you to become familiar with a different perspective and way of interpreting the physician's notes. However, it all fits together, even though you will be using your knowledge in a slightly different way.

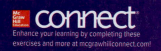

Using Terminology

Match each key term to the appropriate definition.

_____ **1.** LO 17.1 A letter or number component of an ICD-10-PCS code.

_____ **2.** LO 17.4 The path the physician took to access the body part upon which the treatment or procedure was targeted.

_____ **3.** LO 17.2 The term used to describe the function or purpose of the procedure.

A. Approach

B. Character

C. Root operation

Checking Your Understanding

Choose the most appropriate answer for each of the following questions.

1. LO 17.1 Character position 4 represents which of the following?

   a. the body system being treated.
   b. the approach used by physician.
   c. the body part (specific anatomical site).
   d. a device.

2. LO 17.1 Character position 2: Body Systems: the endocrine system is identified by what number or letter?

   a. 2.
   b. G.
   c. 7.
   d. S.

3. LO 17.1 What letters are *not* found in the list of body systems?

   a. B and H.
   b. C and W.
   c. K and Q.
   d. O and I.

4. LO 17.2 According to the official guidelines for coding and reporting B2.1a, the example "Control of postoperative hemorrhage" is coded to the _____ "Control" found in the general anatomical regions body systems.

   a. root operation.
   b. approach.
   c. device.
   d. qualifier.

5. LO 17.1 According to the official guidelines for coding and reporting B2.1b, the example "Vein body parts above the diaphragm" is found in the _____ body system.

   a. Heart and Great Vessels.
   b. Upper Veins.
   c. Anatomical Regions, Upper Extremities.
   d. Upper Arteries.

6. LO 17.2 Which character position does the root operation term represent?

   a. 1.
   b. 3.
   c. 5.
   d. 7.

7. LO 17.4 Creation of an artificial female perineum using a synthetic substitute, open approach would be coded with which of the following?

   a. 0W4M0J1.
   b. 0W4N0Z0.
   c. 0W4N0J0.
   d. 0W4N071.

8. LO 17.2 According to the official guidelines for coding and reporting B3.7, the example "Resection of spleen to stop post-procedural bleeding" is coded to

   a. resection.
   b. control.
   c. excision.
   d. incision.

9. LO 17.2 Extraction of the right cornea, external approach would be coded with which of these?

   a. 08D9XZX.
   b. 08D83ZZ.
   c. 08DKXZX.
   d. 08D8XZZ.

10. LO 17.2 The complete closing of an orifice or a lumen of a tubular body part is known as

    a. map.
    b. occlusion.
    c. fusion.
    d. detachment.

11. LO 17.2 According to the official guidelines for coding and reporting B3.14, the example "Severing a nerve root to relieve pain" is coded to the root operation term

    a. release.
    b. reposition.
    c. division.
    d. restriction.

12. LO 17.2 A diagnostic arthroscopy would be interpreted as

    a. bypass.
    b. extirpation.
    c. resection.
    d. inspection.

13. LO 17.2 An esophagogastic fundoplication would be interpreted as

    a. fusion.
    b. restriction.
    c. resection.
    d. dilation.

14. LO 17.1 The ileus is part of which body system?

    a. Upper Intestinal Tract.
    b. Upper Leg.
    c. Lower Intestinal Tract.
    d. Lower Leg.

15. LO 17.3 The appendix that helps you when a specific anatomical site is documented and the body part components are not as specific is entitled

    a. *Definition Key.*
    B. *Body Part Key.*
    C. *Device Key.*
    D. *Device Aggregation Table.*

16. LO 17.4 The approach to a procedure was entry, by puncture or minor incision, of instrumentation through the skin or mucous membrane and any other body layers necessary to reach the site of the procedure and is identified with the Character 3. What type of approach was used?

    a. open.
    b. external.
    c. percutaneous.
    d. via natural or artificial opening.

17. LO 17.4 Endoscopic repair of the urethra via natural opening would be coded with which of these?

    a. 0TQC8ZZ.
    b. 0TQD7ZZ.
    c. 0TQD4ZZ.
    d. 0TQD8ZZ.

18. LO 17.5 A cardiac lead, pacemaker implant device is represented by what sixth character?

    a. M.
    b. J.
    c. K.
    d. R.

19. LO 17.6 A diagnostic qualifier is identified by what letter?

    a. X.
    b. Z.
    c. B.
    d. F.

20. LO 17.5 Single upper tooth drainage device implant, open approach would be coded with which of the following?

    a. 0C9W000.

    b. 0C9XX02.

    c. 0C9W0Z1.

    d. 0C9W001.

Applying Your Knowledge

1. LO 17.1 List the seven character positions of an ICD-10-PCS code, including each character's meaning. _____

_____

2. LO 17.2 How many root operation terms are used in the Medical and Surgical section to describe what procedure was performed for the patient during an encounter? _____

_____

3. LO 17.2 What is the *most* efficient way of using the Alphabetic Index? _____

_____

4. LO 17.2 Explain the difference between an alteration and a bypass, including the character that represents each. _____

_____

5. LO 17.2 How are bypass procedures coded? _____

_____

6. LO 17.2 What is an extirpation, and what character represents an extirpation? Include an example. _____

_____

7. LO 17.3 What does the Character position 4 represent? _____

_____

8. LO 17.3 If the notes state a bilateral procedure was performed and there is no code character available to report a bilateral procedure, how would you report this procedure accurately? _____

_____

9. LO 17.3 What is the title of the appendix that helps you when a specific anatomical site is documented and the body part components are not as specific? _____

_____

10. LO 17.4 What character position represents the approach? _____

_____

11. LO 17.4 List the seven approaches used within the Medical and Surgical section, and explain each approach. _____

_____

12. LO 17.5 Explain what a device is and what character position represents the device. _____

_____

13. LO 17.5 List three ICD-10-PCS generalized types of devices that qualify. _____

_____

14. LO 17.6 What character position represent a qualifier? _____

_____

15. LO 17.6 The official guidelines list four cases in which you will report multiple codes. What are those four cases? _____

_____

Using the techniques described in this chapter, carefully read through the case studies and determine the most accurate ICD-10-PCS code(s) for each case study.

1. Allen Dickerson, a 9-year-old male, is experiencing obstructive sleep apnea. Dr. Harris admits Allen into the hospital and performs an adenoidectomy, open approach.

   _____

2. Charlene Bahaman, a 45-year-old female, was admitted into Barton Hospital yesterday. Dr. Jansen performs a laparoscopic cholecystectomy today.

   _____

3. Jeff Lambert, a 39-year-old male, goes to the hospital to have an endoscopic left renal artery biopsy.

   _____

4. Helene Ruboni, a 58-year-old female, has severe pain in her right foot when she walks. Upon examination, her right big toe has turned toward the second toe. Helene is admitted into the hospital, where Dr. Burton performs a bunionectomy, open approach, with a soft tissue correction.

   _____

5. Manuel Sedaka, a 19-year-old male, has had a bad cough for the last 2 months. Therefore, Dr. Fabiole admitted him into the hospital and performed a diagnostic fiberoptic bronchoscopy with hopes of determining the cause of the irritation.

   _____

6. Renee Beecher, a 39-year-old female, is a professional runner and has won three marathons. Today, she is admitted into the hospital for a total arthroplasty (replacement) of her right knee, nonautologous tissue substitute, open approach.

   _____

7. Jane Hazelrigg, a 19-year-old female, feels she has "big ears." Jane was admitted into the hospital, where her external ears were altered bilaterally, percutaneous approach.

   _____

8. Melissa Hatten, a 59-year-old female, was admitted into Barton Hospital yesterday. A middle esophagus bypass, percutaneous endoscopic approach, rerouted to stomach was performed today.

   _____

9. Frank Sox, a 14-year-old male, comes to the hospital to have his urinary bladder drainage device changed, external approach.

_____

10. Barbara Fosky, a 34-year-old female, was admitted into Barton Hospital. The patient closed the car door on her foot and severely injured her left foot. Barbara's left fifth toe is completely amputated.

_____

11. Clifton Jordan, a 63-year-old male, has had left upper quadrant pain radiating to his back. Dr. Browne admits Clifton into Barton Hospital, where he performs an endoscopic (via natural opening) inspection of the pancreatic duct.

_____

12. Roberta Richards, a 36-year-old female, gave birth to her fourth child 6 months ago. The patient presents today requesting tubal ligation. Roberta is admitted into Barton Hospital, where Dr. Gerard performs a bilateral fallopian tube ligation, percutaneous endoscopic approach.

_____

13. Anthony Kemp, a 42-year-old male, underwent an abdominal procedure this morning at Barton Hospital. After the procedure was completed, Anthony began to hemorrhage. Dr. Barnes performed a control of postoperative bleeding in the abdominal wall, open approach.

_____

14. Curt Faulks, a 72-year-old male, cannot swallow his food and has lost a substantial amount of weight. Curt is admitted into the hospital, where Dr. Kelley inserts a feeding device in Curt's stomach, percutaneous endoscopic approach.

_____

15. Shelia Hawkins, a 16-year-old female, has a history of uncontrolled motor movements and some uncontrolled eye movement. Shelia is admitted into the hospital, where Dr. Fallen performs a mapping of Shelia's basal ganglia signals, percutaneous approach.

_____

16. Robert Myson, a 43-year-old male, was admitted into Barton Hospital due to severe pain in the inguinal region. After a thorough examination, Dr. Conner diagnosed Robert with a right inguinal hernia and performed a herniorrhaphy with synthetic substitute, open approach.

_____

17. Kristen Smyth, a 66-year-old female, has a tracheostomy device and has recovered sufficiently to have the device removed. Kristen is admitted into the hospital, where Dr. Cranston removes the tracheostomy device, via natural or artificial opening endoscopic approach.

   _____

18. George Grimes, a 28-year-old male, was admitted into Barton Hospital with pain in his left arm. George was working in his yard and was hit by a falling tree limb. After a thorough examination, an external repair to his left elbow region was performed. George was discharged.

   _____

19. Sandra Hammett, a 73-year-old female, is admitted into Barton Hospital to reinforce her left acetabulum with non-autologous tissue substitute, open approach.

   _____

20. Charlie Bedser, a 48-year-old male, presents with lower back pain. After a thorough examination, Dr. James admitted Charlie into Barton Hospital, where he performed a lumbar sympathetic nerve division, percutaneous endoscopic approach.

   _____

OBSTETRICS THROUGH CHIROPRACTIC SECTIONS (0–9)

18

Learning Outcomes *After completing this chapter, the student should be able to:*

LO 18.1 Recognize the details reported in sections of ICD-10-PCS other than the Medical and Surgical section.

LO 18.2 Evaluate the details to determine the section from which to code.

LO 18.3 Determine the body system or region being treated.

LO 18.4 Interpret the procedure to determine the accurate root operation term.

LO 18.5 Utilize knowledge of anatomy to determine the body part treated.

LO 18.6 Identify the approach used to access the body part.

LO 18.7 Distinguish the type of device implanted or other qualifier, when applicable.

LO 18.8 Select the appropriate qualifier character.

Introduction

After the Medical and Surgical section (0) are additional sections with a narrower scope of details for procedures that differ from those already represented in that first section of this code set. Most of these are obvious as to their contents by their title: Obstetrics (1), Osteopathic (7), Other Procedures (8), and Chiropractics (9). Others will become clearer as you enter the sections and learn about the descriptions contained within: Placement (2), Administration (3), Measurement and Monitoring (4), Extracorporeal Assistance and Performance (5), and Extracorporeal Therapies (6).

Obstetrics Section

LO 18.1 Character Definitions

As you learned earlier, every ICD-10-PCS code has seven characters, and each character position has a meaning. While all of these codes have the same number of characters, each section uses each character position differently. So let's review the meanings for the Obstetrics section characters:

Character Position	Character Meaning
1	Section of the ICD-10-PCS book
2	Body system being treated
3	Root operation term
4	Body part (specific anatomical site)
5	Approach used by physician
6	Device, if applicable
7	Qualifier, if applicable

Key Terms

Abortifacient

Extracorporeal

Laminaria

Products of conception

Somatic

products of conception
The zygote, embryo, or fetus, as well as the amnion, umbilical cord, and placenta.

You might have noticed that these are the same meanings as for those in the Medical and Surgical section.

LO 18.2 Character Position 1: Obstetrics Section 1

1
Section

All of the codes reporting an obstetrics procedure will begin with the number one (1). You may remember that obstetrics is the care of a pregnant woman. For this reason, the only procedures reported from this section relate to the **products of conception:** zygote, embryo, or fetus, as well as the amnion, umbilical cord, and placenta. The timeline of gestation (gestational age or trimester) is not relevant to reporting procedures here.

LO 18.3 Character Position 2: Body System: 0–9, B–Y

1	0
Section	Body System

In this section there is only one body system:

0   Pregnancy

LO 18.4 Character Position 3: Root Operation

1	0	0–9, B–Y
Section	Body System	Root Operation

The Obstetrics section uses 10 root operation terms to describe what procedure was performed for the patient during this encounter. Don't worry—the definitions are listed in the front of the ICD-10-PCS codebook. However, you still need to learn and understand them so that you can abstract the operative report or procedure notes accurately and completely. Remember that you are required to use this definition in its entirety. Also, just as when reporting with CPT procedure codes, it is important that you understand all of the components of a specific root operation or procedure. You don't want to code inclusive components separately. Using the root operation term is the most efficient way of using the Alphabetic Index, as well.

Abortion: Artificially terminating a pregnancy . . . Character: A

> **EXAMPLE**
>
> 10A07ZZ Abortion of productions of conception via natural or artificial opening

Change: Taking out or off a device from a body part and putting back an identical or similar device in or on the same body part without cutting or puncturing the skin or a mucous membrane . . . Character: 2

> **EXAMPLE**
>
> 102073Z Changing a monitoring device for the products of conception via natural or artificial opening

Delivery: Assisting the passage of the products of conception from the genital canal . . . Character E

> ### EXAMPLE
>
> 10E0XZZ Delivery of a baby (products of conception), external approach

Drainage: Taking or letting out fluids and/or gases from a body part . . . Character 9

> ### EXAMPLE
>
> 10903ZU Drainage of amniotic fluid, percutaneous approach, for diagnostic purposes

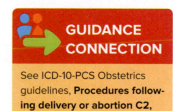

GUIDANCE CONNECTION

See ICD-10-PCS Obstetrics guidelines, **Procedures following delivery or abortion C2,** for more details.

Extraction: Pulling or stripping out or off all or a portion of a body part by the use of force . . . Character D

A great example of an extraction is a cesarean section, which is not a separate root operation because the intention is to *extract* the baby from the mother's body.

> ### EXAMPLE
>
> 10D28ZZ Extraction of ectopic products of conception via natural or artificial opening endoscopic

Insertion: Putting in nonbiological appliance that monitors, assists, performs, or prevents a physiological function but does not physically take the place of a body part . . . Character H

This is another opportunity for reading very carefully. In ICD-10-PCS, this root operation, insertion, applies only to the placement into the body of a medical device, such as a monitoring device, that will remain in the body after the procedure is completed.

> ### EXAMPLE
>
> 10H073Z Insertion of monitoring electrode via natural or artificial opening

Inspection: Visually and/or manually exploring a body part . . . Character J

This root operation term is limited to the physician's looking.

> ### EXAMPLE
>
> 10J04ZZ Inspection of productions of conception, percutaneous endoscopic approach

Removal: Taking out or off a device from a body part . . . Character P

Read this carefully: As the description specifically states "device," this can only be used for this type of procedure, to remove a previously inserted device. As you abstract the physician's notes, be cautious of the use of this term in documentation. The removal of a mole, for example, is really an excision, not a removal.

EXAMPLE

10P003Z Removal of monitoring electrode, open approach

Repair: Restoring, to the extent possible, a body part to its normal anatomic structure and function . . . Character Q

EXAMPLE

10Q03ZQ Repair of skin, percutaneous approach

Reposition: Moving to its normal location or other suitable location all or a portion of a body part . . . Character S

EXAMPLE

10S0XZZ Reposition of fetus, external approach

Resection: Cutting out or off, without replacement, all of a body part . . . Character T

Remember how this differs from excision. When the entire body part is surgically removed, it is reported as a resection. If only a portion of the body part is removed, it is reported as an excision.

EXAMPLE

10T28ZZ Resection of fallopian tube for ectopic products of conception, via natural or artificial opening endoscopic

Transplantation: Putting in or on all or a portion of a living body part taken from another individual or animal to physically take the place and/or function of all or a portion of a similar body part . . . Character Y

ICD-10-PCS uses this term in the same manner that physicians do. However, this includes more than just organ transplant procedures. For instance, in vitro fertilization (IVF) is included in this root operation term.

EXAMPLE

10Y07ZT Transplantation, via natural or artificial opening, products of conception

As you learned in previous chapters, the root operation term is based on the objective of the procedure. You are seeking the word describing the action, such as *extraction* or *transplantation*. Combination terms with which you are very familiar, such as cesarean section (c-section) or in-vitro fertilization, may describe the procedure; however, these terms do not specifically explain the action of the physician, or do they? Let's take a closer look at these terms and interpret them into the root operation terms:

> Cesarean section: What precisely is this procedure? The extraction of the baby via surgical incision. This explanation leads you to the root operation term used in ICD-10-PCS, *extraction*.

> In vitro fertilization: What precisely is this procedure? The transfer or transplantation of fertilized ova from petri dish to uterus. Again, this description directs you to the ICD-10-PCS root operation term *transplantation*.

With some procedures, you will use your knowledge of the specific procedure and what it is expected to accomplish. For example, you will need to remember that the physician supporting the natural process of a vaginal delivery is reported with the root operation term *delivery*. That one works very well in translation, doesn't it?

YOU INTERPRET IT!

Practice interpreting from the common term used to reference the ICD-10-PCS root operation term.

Amniocentesis _____

Chorionic villus sampling _____

Surgical treatment of ectopic pregnancy _____

Cerclage of cervix during pregnancy _____

Intrauterine cordocentesis (percutaneous umbilical cord blood sampling) _____

Fetal shunt placement _____

Induced abortion, by dilation and curettage _____

Uterine evacuation and curettage _____

Hysterectomy (after cesarean section) _____

Vaginal delivery _____

Hysterorrhaphy _____

LO 18.5 Character Position 4: Body Part: 0–9, B–Y

1	0	0–9, B–Y	0–2
Section	Body System	Root Operation	Body Part

The Obstetrics section focuses on three body parts, which are not specific anatomical sites with which you are familiar:

Products of conception . . . Character 0 (zero)

Products of conception, retained . . . Character 1

Products of conception, ectopic . . . Character 2

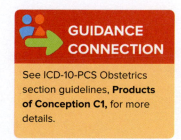

GUIDANCE CONNECTION

See ICD-10-PCS Obstetrics section guidelines, **Products of Conception C1,** for more details.

In the simplest terms, the products of conception are fertilized ova (zygote, embryo, and/or fetus) along with the components that accompany, including amnion (the inmost membrane, also known as the amniotic sac, that encloses the fetus in utero and holds the amniotic fluid), umbilical cord, and placenta. The change in the character will designate if these components are ectopic (outside of the uterus) or retained (still inside), as in an incomplete abortion.

LO 18.6 Character Position 5: Approach

1	0	0–9, B–Y	0–2	0–9, X
Section	Body System	Root Operation	Body Part	Approach

As you continue to build a code, you can see that you are telling a story. The first four characters explain what the physician did and the anatomical site upon which he or she worked. Now, with the fifth character, you are going to explain how the physician got to the anatomical site to perform the procedure. You learned in previous chapters that this is known as the approach.

<u>Open:</u> Cutting through the skin or mucous membrane and any other body layers necessary to expose the site of the procedure . . . Character 0

An open procedure is the traditional approach when the physician makes an incision into the body to access an internal organ.

EXAMPLE

10D00Z1 Cesarean section, low cervical, open incision

<u>Percutaneous:</u> Entry, by puncture or minor incision, of instrumentation through the skin or mucous membrane and any other body layers necessary to reach the site of the procedure . . . Character 3

EXAMPLE

10903Z9 Drainage of fetal blood, percutaneous approach

<u>Percutaneous Endoscopic:</u> Entry, by puncture or minor incision, of instrumentation through the skin or mucous membrane and any other body layers necessary to reach and visualize the site of the procedure . . . Character 4

EXAMPLE

10Q04ZT Repair of the female reproductive system, products of conception, via percutaneous endoscopic approach

<u>Via Natural or Artificial Opening:</u> Entry of instrumentation through a natural or artificial external opening to reach the site of the procedure . . . Character 7

EXAMPLE

10J17ZZ Inspection of retained products of conception, vaginal approach

Via Natural or Artificial Opening Endoscopic: Entry of instrumentation through a natural or artificial external opening to reach and visualize the site of the procedure . . . Character 8

EXAMPLE

10S28ZZ Reposition of products of conception from fallopian tube to uterus, via vaginal endoscopic approach

External: Procedure performed directly on the skin or mucous membrane and procedures performed indirectly by the application of external force through the skin or mucous membrane . . . Character X

EXAMPLE

10E0XZZ Delivery of neonate, vaginal delivery, no assistance

YOU INTERPRET IT!

Practice by filling in the approach used by ICD-10-PCS for coding.

Laminaria _____

Hysterorrhapy of ruptured uterus_____

Laparoscopic treatment of ectopic pregnancy _____

Episiotomy_____

Treatment of incomplete abortion, surgically _____

Cerclage of cervix, vaginal _____

Amniocentesis _____

Intrauterine cordocentesis_____

Vaginal delivery_____

Cesarean section _____

Fetal contraction stress test_____

LO 18.7 Character Position 6: Device

1	0	0–9, B–Y	0–2	0–9, X	3, Y, or Z
Section	Body System	Root Operation	Body Part	Approach	Device

As you can see, a character placed in the sixth position will identify a device that will remain with the patient after the procedure has been completed.

Fetal monitoring electrodes

Monitoring Electrode . . . Character 3

Other Device . . . Character Y

No Device . . . Character Z

Fetal monitoring can be performed either internally or externally. When done internally, the physician will place an electrode (electronic transducer) directly onto the scalp of the fetus, typically using a natural opening approach (through the vagina/cervix), with the intention of directly and continuously evaluating the fetal heart rate as well as its variability between beats, particularly in relation to the uterine contractions of labor. Another device, called an internal uterine pressure monitor (IUPM), may be used in conjunction with internal fetal heart rate monitoring. Using a catheter inserted via the vagina/cervix, an IUPM is placed inside the uterus, next to the fetus, to transmit the readings of the contraction pressure to a nearby monitor.

External fetal heart rate monitoring can be accomplished with a handheld electronic Doppler ultrasonic device, most often used at outpatient prenatal visits. Continuous electronic fetal heart monitoring, typically used during labor and delivery, consists of placing an ultrasound transducer on the mother's abdomen, where it can transfer the sounds of the fetal heart to a computer. The computer is able to show the heart pattern on a screen as well as print it out on paper similar to that used during an EKG.

LO 18.8 Character Position 7: Qualifier

1	0	0–9, B–Y	0–2	0–9, X	3, Y, or Z	0–9, B–Z
Section	Body System	Root Operation	Body Part	Approach	Device	Qualifier

The seventh character is required. In some cases, there may be no more details to add, so you will use the placeholder letter Z No Qualifier—the equivalent of "not applicable."

During a delivery, if the physician uses forceps or other assisting mechanism, this delivery becomes an *extraction,* and the additional detail will be reported with the Qualifier character:

Low forceps . . . Character 3

Mid forceps . . . Character 4

High forceps . . . Character 5

Vacuum . . . Character 6

Internal version . . . Character 7

Other . . . Character 8

Earlier you learned that a cesarean delivery is reported in ICD-10-PCS using the root operation term *extraction.* For this procedure, the Qualifier character will report:

Classical (c-section incision) . . . Character 0

Low Cervical . . . Character 1

Extraperitoneal . . . Character 2

During amniocentesis, or any other drainage procedure performed on a pregnant woman, the Qualifier character will explain exactly what was drained:

Fetal blood . . . Character 9

Fetal cerebrospinal fluid . . . Character A

Fetal fluid, other . . . Character B

Amniotic fluid, therapeutic . . . Character C

Fluid, other . . . Character D

Amniotic fluid, diagnostic . . . Character U

When the artificial termination of a pregnancy (abortion) is performed, the Qualifier character will report the methodology:

Vacuum . . . Character 6

Laminaria . . . Character W

Abortifacient . . . Character X

When an in utero procedure is performed on the fetus (root operation *repair* or *transplantation*), the Qualifier character will report the body system that was repaired or transplanted:

Nervous system . . . E	Hepatobiliary and pancreas . . . N
Cardiovascular system . . . F	Endocrine system . . . P
Lymphatics and hemic . . . G	Skin . . . Q
Eye . . . H	Musculoskeletal system . . . R
Ear, nose, and sinus . . . J	Urinary system . . . S
Respiratory system . . . K	Female reproductive system . . . T
Mouth and throat . . . L	Male reproductive system . . . V
Gastrointestinal system . . . M	Other body system . . . Y

laminaria
Thin sticks of kelp-related seaweed, used to dilate the cervix, that can induce abortive circumstance during the first 3 months of pregnancy.

abortifacient
A drug used to induce an abortion.

LET'S CODE IT! SCENARIO

Kylah Serrano, a 37-year-old female, is pregnant, G1P0, second trimester (15 weeks, 3 days) and has been admitted to have some tests, including an amniocentesis. Because she is categorized as eldergravida, Dr. Ogden is performing this test to determine the health and well-being of the fetus.

You Code It!

Let's go through the steps of coding for ICD-10-PCS and determine the code or codes that should be reported for this encounter between Dr. Ogden and Kylah Serrano.

Character 1: Section: Obstetrics . . . Character 1

Character 2: Body System: Pregnancy . . . Character 0

Character 3: Root Operation: Drainage . . . Character 9

Remember the meaning and purpose of this procedure: Amniocentesis (puncturing of the amnion) to drain amniotic fluid.

Character 4: Body Part: Products of Conception . . . Character 0

Character 5: Approach: Percutaneous . . . Character 3

Character 6: Device: No Device . . . Character Z

Character 7: Qualifier: Amniotic Fluid, Diagnostic . . . Character U

What is being drained? Amniotic fluid. Why? To test (diagnostics).

The ICD-10-PCS code you will report is

10903ZU Amniocentesis for prenatal testing

Good job!

Placement Section

LO 18.1 Character Definitions

The meanings for the Placement section characters are

Character Position	Character Meaning
1	Section of the ICD-10-PCS book
2	Anatomical region
3	Root operation term
4	Body region/orifice
5	Approach used by physician
6	Device, if applicable
7	Qualifier, if applicable

You might have noticed that these are slightly different meanings for characters 2 and 4 than those in the Medical and Surgical and Obstetrics sections.

LO 18.2 Character Position 1: Placement Section 2

2
Section

The procedures reported with codes from this section report the locating of a device either in or on a body region for protection, immobilization, stretching, compression, or packing. These procedures are some that you are familiar with, such as application of a splint to immobilize or a traction device to stretch a muscle. For the most part, the devices in this section are "off the shelf," so to speak, and not customized fabrications. (More about these devices will be discussed when we get to that character position.)

LO 18.3 Character Position 2: Body System

2	W or Y
Section	Body System

There are only two body system options:

Anatomical Regions . . . Character W
Anatomical Orifices . . . Character Y

LO 18.4 Character Position 3: Root Operation

2	W or Y	0–6
Section	Body System	Root Operation

The codes from the Placement section only report procedures that are noninvasive, meaning that the outer layer of the skin is not punctured and no incision is made.

Change: Taking out or off a device from a body part and putting back an identical or similar device in or on the same body part without cutting or puncturing the skin or a mucous membrane . . . Character: 0

Caution! This root operation term means the same as it does in the Medical and Surgical section and the Obstetrics section; however, the character used to report this in the Placement section is different.

EXAMPLE

2W05X3Z Change external back brace

Compression: Putting pressure on a body region . . . Character 1

EXAMPLE

2W1RX7Z Placement of intermittent pressure device on lower left leg

Dressing: Putting material on a body region for protection . . . Character 2

EXAMPLE

2W2EX4Z Placement of bandage on right hand

Immobilization: Limiting or preventing motion of an external body region . . . Character 3

EXAMPLE

2W3KX1Z Application of a splint to a left finger

Packing: Putting material in a body region or orifice . . . Character 4

EXAMPLE

2W48X5Z Packing to wound on right upper extremity

Removal: Taking out or off a device from a body part . . . Character 5

Read this carefully: As the description specifically states "device," this can be used only for this type of procedure, to remove a previously placed device. As you abstract the physician's notes, be cautious of the use of this term in documentation.

Caution! This root operation term means the same as it does in the Medical and Surgical section and the Obstetrics section; however, the character used to report this in the Placement section is different.

EXAMPLE

2W5TX0Z Removal of traction apparatus from left foot

Traction: Exerting a pulling force on a body region in a distal direction . . . Character 6

Notice that *Traction* is presented as a root operation term as well as traction apparatus that is offered as an option for the device used.

EXAMPLE

2W62X0Z Traction apparatus placed at neck

LO 18.5 Character Position 4: Body Region

2	W or Y	0–6	0–9, A–V
Section	Body System	Root Operation	**Body Region**

The two body systems each have a list of applicable body regions and their characters.

Anatomical Regions

Head . . . Character 0
Face . . . 1
Neck . . . 2
Abdominal Wall . . . 3
Chest Wall . . . 4
Back . . . 5
Inguinal Region, Right . . . 6
Inguinal Region, Left . . . 7
Upper Extremity, Right . . . 8
Upper Extremity, Left . . . 9
Upper Arm, Right . . . A
Upper Arm, Left . . . B
Lower Arm, Right . . . C
Lower Arm, Left . . . D
Hand, Right . . . E

Hand, Left . . . F
Thumb, Right . . . G
Thumb, Left . . . H
Finger, Right . . . J
Finger, Left . . . K
Lower Extremity, Right . . . L
Lower Extremity, Left . . . M
Upper Leg, Right . . . N
Upper Leg, Left . . . P
Lower Leg, Right . . . Q
Lower Leg, Left . . . R
Foot, Right . . . S
Foot, Left . . . T
Toe, Right . . . U
Toe, Left . . . V

Anatomical Orifices

Mouth and Pharynx . . . 0
Nasal . . . 1
Ear . . . 2
Anorectal . . . 3
Female Genital Tract . . . 4
Urethra . . . 5

LO 18.6 Character Position 5: Approach

2	W or Y	0–6	0–9, A–V	X
Section	Body System	Root Operation	Body Region	Approach

This one is easy; there is only one choice. Remember that all procedures reported from the Placement section do not involve incisions or punctures. This means all of these devices are external.

External approach . . . Character X

LO 18.7 Character Position 6: Device

2	W or Y	0–6	0–9, A–V	X	0–9, Y, Z
Section	Body System	Root Operation	Body Region	Approach	Device

It makes sense that there are several options for the character to report a device because that is really the primary activity of this section: placement of a device.

Traction apparatus . . . Character 0

Splint . . . Character 1

Cast . . . Character 2

Brace . . . Character 3

Bandage . . . Character 4

Packing Material . . . Character 5

Pressure Dressing . . . Character 6

Intermittent Pressure Device . . . Character 7

Wire . . . Character 9

Other Device . . . Character Y

No device . . . Character Z

LO 18.8 Character Position 7: Qualifier

2	W or Y	0–6	0–9, A–V	X	0–9, Y, Z	Z
Section	Body System	Root Operation	Body Region	Approach	Device	Qualifier

There are no details reported by the Qualifier position, so No Qualifier . . . character Z is the only option.

LET'S CODE IT! SCENARIO

Bruce Bruxton, a 29-year-old male, was in a fight at a bar and was punched in the face. Along with other injuries, Bruce's lower jaw was dislocated. Dr. Franklin wired the jaw to immobilize it and permit it to heal.

You Code It!

Let's go through the steps of coding for ICD-10-PCS and determine the code or codes that should be reported for this encounter between Dr. Franklin and Bruce Bruxton.

Character 1: Section: Placement . . . Character 2

Character 2: Body Region: Anatomical Regions . . . Character W

Character 3: Root Operation: Immobilization . . . Character 3

Administration Section

LO 18.1 Character Definitions

The meanings for the Administration section characters are

Character Position	Character Meaning
1	Section of the ICD-10-PCS book
2	Physiological system or anatomical region
3	Root operation term
4	Body system or region
5	Approach used by physician
6	Substance, if applicable
7	Qualifier, if applicable

For the most part, these character positions have different meanings than the other sections you have already learned about.

LO 18.2 Character Position 1: Administration Section 3

3
Section

Procedures reported from the Administration section will all begin with the number 3.

LO 18.3 Character Position 2: Physiology System

3	O, C, or E
Section	Physiology System

There are only three options for the second character:

Circulatory . . . Character 0 (This is used for transfusion procedures.)

Indwelling device . . . Character C

Physiological Systems and Anatomical Regions . . . Character E

LO 18.4 Character Position 3: Root Operation

3	O, C, or E	0–2
Section	Body System	Root Operation

There are only three root operation terms used to report procedures in this section:

<u>Introduction:</u> Putting in or on a therapeutic, diagnostic, nutritional, physiological, or prophylactic substance except blood or blood products . . . Character 0

<u>Irrigation:</u> Putting in or on a cleansing substance . . . Character 1

<u>Transfusion:</u> Putting in blood or blood products . . . Character 2

LO 18.5 Character Position 4: Body System/Region

3	O, C, or E	0–6	0–9, A–Z
Section	Body System	Root Operation	Body Region

Specifically for this section, the fourth character position will report the anatomical site into which the substance is administered. Be careful. This may be different from the site expected to benefit the ultimate effect of this substance. For example, if the substance is administered intradermally (such as an intradermal patch), the body system/region would be skin and mucous membrane, whereas an IM (intramuscular) injection would be reported as the muscle in this character position. IA (intra-arterial) or IV (intravenous) administrations would be reported to the peripheral artery or peripheral vein, respectively. However, if a catheter is used—for example, to travel to administer the substance directly to a clot—this would be reported as a central artery or central vein, per the documentation.

Oddly, there is an exception. When an irrigating substance (such as saline solution) is administered into an indwelling device (reported as body system Indwelling Device . . . C), the body system/region will be Z None.

LO 18.6 Character Position 5: Approach

3	O, C, or E	0–6	0–9, A–Z	0–8, X
Section	Body System	Root Operation	Body Region	Approach

The approaches for this section are those you have come to know: Open (0), Percutaneous (3), Via Natural or Artificial Opening (7), Via Natural or Artificial Opening Endoscopic (8), and External (X).

LO 18.7 Character Position 6: Substance

3	O, C, or E	0–6	0–9, A–Z	0–8, X	0–9, A–Y
Section	Body System	Root Operation	Body Region	Approach	Substance

In this character position, you will identify the substance being administered. Be careful! The substance and character reported for Circulatory (second character position) has different meanings for the same letter as when Physiological Systems and Anatomical Regions are reported in the second character position. This is a great example of why it is so important to read each table completely and to avoid assuming that the same letter means the same from table to table, even in the same section.

> ## EXAMPLE
>
> 30***G* = Administration, Circulatory, ***, Bone marrow *
> 3E***G* = Administration, Physiological Systems, ***, Other Therapeutic Substance *

LO 18.8 Character Position 7: Qualifier

3	O, C, or E	0–6	0–9, A–Z	0–8, X	0–9, A–Y	0–9, A–Z
Section	Body System	Root Operation	Body Region	Approach	Substance	Qualifier

This character will provide additional detail about the substance, if necessary.

> ## EXAMPLE
>
> Autologous . . . Character 0
> Nonautologous . . . 1
> Oxazolidinones . . . 8
> No Qualifier . . . Z

LET'S CODE IT! SCENARIO

Lance Franzlyn, a 37-year-old male, was admitted into McGraw Hospital. Dr. Peterson administered nonautologous pancreatic islet cells, intravenously.

You Code It!

Let's go through the steps of coding for ICD-10-PCS and determine the code or codes that should be reported for this encounter between Dr. Peterson and Lance Franzlyn.

Character 1: Section: Administration . . . Character 3

Character 2: Physiological Systems and Anatomical Regions . . . Character E

Character 3: Root Operation: Introduction . . . Character 0

Character 4: Body Region: Peripheral Vein . . . Character 3

Character 5: Approach: Percutaneous . . . Character 3

Character 6: Substance: Pancreatic Islet Cells . . . Character U

Character 7: Qualifier: Nonautologous . . . Character 1

The ICD-10-PCS code you will report is

3E033U1 Introduction of nonautologous pancreatic islet cells, percutaneous, to peripheral vein

Good job!

Measurement And Monitoring Section

LO 18.1 Character Definitions

The meanings for the Measurement and Monitoring section characters are

Character Position	Character Meaning
1	Section of the ICD-10-PCS book
2	Physiological system
3	Root operation term
4	Body system
5	Approach used by physician
6	Function/device
7	Qualifier, if applicable

For the most part, these character positions have different meanings than the other sections you have already learned about.

LO 18.2 Character Position 1: Measurement and Monitoring Section 4

4
Section

Procedures reported from the Measurement and Monitoring section will all begin with the number 4.

LO 18.3 Character Position 2: Physiology System

4	A or B
Section	Physiology System/Devices

There are only two options for the second character:

Physiological Systems . . . Character A

Physiological Devices . . . Character B

LO 18.4 Character Position 3: Root Operation

4	A or B	0 or 1
Section	Physiology System/Devices	Root Operation

There are only two root operation terms used to report procedures in this section.

<u>Measurement:</u> Determining the level of a physiological or physical function at a point in time . . . Character 0

<u>Monitoring:</u> Determining the level of a physiological or physical function repetitively over a period of time . . . Character 1

ECG reported with 4A02X4Z Measurement of cardiac electrical activity, external

Holter reported with 4A12XFZ Monitoring cardiac rhythms, externally

LO 18.5 Character Position 4: Body System/Region

4	A or B	0 or 1	0–9, A–Z
Section	Physiology System/Devices	Root Operation	**Body Region**

The specific body system being measured or monitored is identified by the character in the fourth position. Note that this section includes measurement or monitoring of a patient's metabolism, temperature, or sleep. These are reported with a body system of Z None.

> **EXAMPLE**
>
> Central Nervous system . . . Character 0
> Cardiac system . . . Character 2
> Respiratory system . . . Character 9

LO 18.6 Character Position 5: Approach

4	A or B	0 or 1	0–9, A–Z	0–8, X
Section	Physiology System/Devices	Root Operation	Body Region	Approach

The approaches for this section are those you have come to know: Open (0), Percutaneous (3), Percutaneous Endoscopic (4), Via Natural or Artificial Opening (7), Via Natural or Artificial Opening Endoscopic (8), and External (X).

LO 18.7 Character Position 6: Function/Device

4	A or B	0 or 1	0–9, A–Z	0–8, X	0–9, A–Y
Section	Physiology System/Devices	Root Operation	Body Region	Approach	Function/Device

In this character position, you will identify the specific body function being measured or monitored, such as rhythm (F) of the heart or pressure (B) of the blood within the veins. This character may also report a device, such as a pacemaker (S) or defibrillator (T).

Characters are available for measuring and/or monitoring a patient's metabolism (6), temperature (K), or sleep (Q), such as a sleep study. These three functions use a body system character of Z None.

EXAMPLE

4A0HXCZ External measurement of fetal heart rate

4A1ZXQZ 48 hour sleep study, external monitoring

LO 18.8 Character Position 7: Qualifier

4	A or B	0 or 1	0–9, A–Z	0–8, X	0–9, A–Y	0–9, A–Z
Section	Physiology System/ Devices	Root Operation	Body Region	Approach	Function/ Device	Qualifier

This character will provide additional detail about either the body part or system or the procedure performed.

EXAMPLE

4A10X4G Monitoring of central nervous system activity, intraoperatively, external

4A143J1 Monitoring of peripheral pulse, venous, external

LET'S CODE IT! SCENARIO

Winnie Carbona is a 17-year-old female with a history of asthma. Dr. Hoffman measures her respiratory volume using a spirometer.

Let's Code It!

Let's go through the steps of coding for ICD-10-PCS and determine the code or codes that should be reported for this encounter between Dr. Hoffman and Winnie Carbona.

Character 1: Section: Measurement and Monitoring . . . Character 4

Character 2: Body Region: Physiological Systems . . . Character A

Character 3: Root Operation: Measurement . . . Character 0

Character 4: Body System: Respiratory . . . Character 9

Character 5: Approach: External . . . Character X

Character 6: Function/Device: Volume . . . Character L

Character 7: Qualifier: No Qualifier . . . Character Z

The ICD-10-PCS code you will report is

4A09XLZ Measurement of respiratory volume

Good job!

Extracorporeal Assistance And Performance Section

LO 18.1 Character Definitions

The meanings for the Extracorporeal Assistance and Performance section characters are

Character Position	Character Meaning
1	Section of the ICD-10-PCS book
2	Physiological system
3	Root operation term
4	Body system
5	Duration
6	Function
7	Qualifier, if applicable

extracorporeal
Outside of the body.

For the most part, the character positions for the **Extracorporeal** Assistance and Performance section have similar meanings as the other sections about which you have already learned.

LO 18.2 Character Position 1: Extracorporeal Assistance and Performance Section 5

5
Section

Procedures reported from the Extracorporeal Assistance and Performance section will all begin with the number 5.

LO 18.3 Character Position 2: Physiology System

5	A
Section	Physiology System

There is only one option for the second character:

Physiological Systems . . . Character A

LO 18.4 Character Position 3: Root Operation

5	A	0–2
Section	Physiology System	Root Operation

There are only three root operation terms used to report procedures in this section:

<u>Assistance:</u> Taking over a portion of a physiological function by extracorporeal means . . . Character 0

<u>Performance:</u> Completely taking over a physiological function by extracorporeal means . . . Character 1

<u>Restoration:</u> Returning, or attempting to return, a physiological function to its original state by extracorporeal means . . . Character 2

EXAMPLE

5A05221 Hyperbaric oxygenation of a wound, continuous (an example of assistance because this is done to improve—or assist—the healing of the wound)

LO 18.5 Character Position 4: Body System/Region

5	A	0–2	0–9, C, D
Section	Physiology System	Root Operation	**Body System**

The specific body systems being supported by these procedures are

Cardiac system . . . Character 2
Circulatory system . . . Character 5
Respiratory system . . . Character 9
Biliary system . . . Character C
Urinary system . . . Character D

EXAMPLE

5A1D00Z Filtration of a single period of duration, urinary system (hemodialysis takes over the physiological function of the urinary system by extracorporeal means)

LO 18.6 Character Position 5: Duration

5	A	0–2	0–9, C, D	0–6
Section	Physiology System	Root Operation	Body System	Duration

The fifth character position will report the length of time, or the number of times, the patient received this treatment:

Single . . . Character 0 (one time or one session)
Intermittent . . . 1 (occasionally)
Continuous . . . 2 (nonstop ongoing)
Less than 24 consecutive hours . . . 3 (nonstop for a period of time)
24–96 consecutive hours . . . 4 (nonstop for a period of time)
Greater than 96 consecutive hours . . . 5 (nonstop for a period of time)
Multiple . . . 6 (more than one time or one session)

EXAMPLE

After the surgery, Ophelia was kept on a ventilator for 31 hours.
5A1945Z Respiratory ventilator, 25–96 consecutive hours

LO 18.7 Character Position 6: Function

5	A	0–2	0–9, C, D	0–6	0–5
Section	Physiology System	Root Operation	Body System	Duration	Function

In this character position, you will identify the specific physiological function occurring during this procedure:

Filtration . . . Character 0
Output . . . Character 1
Oxygenation . . . Character 2
Pacing . . . Character 3
Rhythm . . . Character 4
Ventilation . . . Character 5

EXAMPLE

5A2204Z Restoration of heart rhythm, single event (performing CPR)

LO 18.8 Character Position 7: Qualifier

5	A	0–2	0–9, C, D	0–6	0–5	0–9, A–Z
Section	Physiology System	Root Operation	Body System	Duration	Function	Qualifier

When a device or piece of equipment is used in the provision of the extracorporeal assistance or performance, the Qualifier will specify what was used:

Balloon pump . . . Character 0
Hyperbaric . . . Character 1
Manual . . . Character 2
Membrane . . . Character 3
Nonmechanical . . . Character 4
Pulsatile compression . . . Character 5
Other pump . . . Character 6
Continuous Positive Airway Pressure (CPAP) . . . Character 7
Intermittent Positive Airway Pressure (IPAP) . . . Character 8
Continuous Negative Airway Pressure (CNAP) . . . Character 9
Intermittent Negative Airway Pressure (INAP) . . . Character B
Supersaturated . . . Character C
Impeller Pump . . . Character D
No Qualifier . . . Character Z

LET'S CODE IT! SCENARIO

Mervin Maxwell, a 77-year-old male, was in the hospital for surgery on his leg. During Mervin's admission, Dr. Wilton ordered a CPAP machine to treat Mervin's obstructive sleep apnea, only at night.

Let's go through the steps of coding for ICD-10-PCS and determine the code or codes that should be reported for this encounter between Dr. Wilton and Mervin Maxwell for the CPAP treatment.

> **Character 1: Section: Extracorporeal Assistance and Performance . . . Character 5**
>
> **Character 2: Body Region: Physiological Systems . . . Character A**
>
> **Character 3: Root Operation: Assistance . . . Character 0**
>
> **Character 4: Body System: Respiratory . . . Character 9**
>
> **Character 5: Duration: Less than 24 consecutive hours . . . Character 3**
>
> **Character 6: Function: Ventilation . . . Character 5**
>
> **Character 7: Qualifier: Continuous Positive Airway Pressure . . . Character 7**

The ICD-10-PCS code you will report is

5A09357 CPAP ventilation, less than 24 consecutive hours
Good job!

Extracorporeal Therapies Section

LO 18.1 Character Definitions

The meanings for the Extracorporeal Therapies section characters are

Character Position	Character Meaning
1	Section of the ICD-10-PCS book
2	Physiological systems
3	Root operation
4	Body system
5	Duration
6	Qualifier, if applicable
7	Qualifier, if applicable

For the most part, the character positions for the Extracorporeal Therapies section have similar meanings as the other sections about which you have already learned. The difference between the procedures reported from this section and those from the Extracorporeal Assistance and Performance section is that these therapies do not involve the process of assisting a physiological function or performing that function for the body.

LO 18.2 Character Position 1: Extracorporeal Therapies Section 6

6
Section

Procedures reported from the Extracorporeal Therapies section will all begin with the number 6.

LO 18.3 Character Position 2: Physiology Systems

6	A	
Section	Physiology System	

There is only one option for the second character:

Physiological Systems . . . Character A

LO 18.4 Character Position 3: Root Operation

6	A	0–9
Section	Physiology System	Root Operation

There are 10 root operation terms used to report procedures in this section:

Atmospheric Control: Extracorporeal control of atmospheric pressure and composition . . . Character 0

Decompression: Extracorporeal elimination of undissolved gas from body fluids . . . Character 1

This root operation term is specific to a hyperbaric chamber used for treating decompression sickness, also known as the bends.

Electromagnetic Therapy: Extracorporeal treatment by electromagnetic rays . . . Character 2

Hyperthermia: Extracorporeal raising of body temperature . . . Character 3

When a hyperthermic procedure is used to treat a temperature imbalance, this is the section from which to report the code. However, if hyperthermia is used as an adjunct radiation treatment for a malignancy, this procedure is reported from the Radiation Oncology section (D).

Hypothermia: Extracorporeal lowering of body temperature . . . Character 4

Pheresis: Extracorporeal separation of blood products . . . Character 5

This procedure, pheresis, is used primarily for two purposes: (1) to treat a condition during which too much of a specific blood component is produced by the body (such as leukemia) and (2) to remove a blood product from donor blood for purposes of transfusion to another patient, such as platelets.

Phototherapy: Extracorporeal treatment by light rays . . . Character 6

The phototherapy process removes blood from the patient into a machine that exposes that blood to light rays, recirculates it, and then returns this blood to the body.

Shock Wave Therapy: Extracorporeal treatment by shock waves . . . Character 9

Note that this is placed in the tables section in numerical order (the last table for number 9) and not in alphabetic order.

Ultrasound Therapy: Extracorporeal treatment by ultrasound . . . Character 7

Ultraviolet Light Therapy: Extracorporeal treatment by ultraviolet light . . . Character 8

LO 18.5 Character Position 4: Body System

6	A	0–9	0–5, Z
Section	Physiology System	Root Operation	Body System

The specific body system being supported by these procedures are

Skin . . . Character 0

Urinary . . . Character 1

Central nervous . . . Character 2

Musculoskeletal . . . Character 3

Circulatory . . . Character 5

None . . . Character Z

Therapies such as atmospheric control, hyperthermia, and hypothermia are performed on the entire body and, therefore, have a body system of None Z.

LO 18.6 Character Position 5: Duration

6	A	0–2	0–5, Z	0–1
Section	Physiology System	Root Operation	Body System	Duration

The fifth character position will report the length of time, or the number of times, the patient received this treatment:

Single . . . Character 0 (one time or one session)

Multiple . . . Character 1 (more than one time or one session)

LO 18.7 Character Position 6: Qualifier

6	A	0–2	0–5, Z	0–1	Z
Section	Physiology System	Root Operation	Body System	Duration	Qualifier

In this character position, the only option is No Z.

LO 18.8 Character Position 7: Qualifier

6	A	0–2	0–5, Z	0–1	Z	0–7, T–Z
Section	Physiology System	Root Operation	Body System	Duration	Qualifier	Qualifier

When pheresis is performed, the Qualifier will specify what was used:

Erythrocytes . . . Character 0

Leukocytes . . . Character 1

Platelets . . . Character 2

Plasma . . . Character 3

Stem Cells, Cord Blood . . . Character T

Stem Cells, Hematopoietic . . . Character V

Ultrasound therapies performed on the circulatory system will utilize a Qualifier character to identify which specific vessels are being treated, when applicable:

Head and Neck Vessels . . . Character 4

Heart . . . Character 5

Peripheral Vessels . . . Character 6

Other Vessels . . . Character 7

No Qualifier . . . Character Z

All other root operation terms (therapies) reported from this section have no qualifier (Z).

LET'S CODE IT! SCENARIO

Teddy Emmerson, a 16-year-old male, was out walking near the ski resort where he was vacationing. He fell into a soft bed of snow and could not get out. The ski patrol took 5 hours to find him. At the hospital, Dr. Gelder used hyperthermia to warm his body gently back to normal temperature. A single treatment was sufficient.

Let's Code It!

Let's go through the steps of coding for ICD-10-PCS and determine the code or codes that should be reported for this encounter between Dr. Gelder and Teddy Emmerson for this therapy.

Character 1: Section: Extracorporeal Therapies . . . Character 6

Character 2: Body Region: Physiological Systems . . . Character A

Character 3: Root Operation: Hyperthermia . . . Character 4

Character 4: Body System: None . . . Character Z

Character 5: Duration: Single . . . Character 0

Character 6: Qualifier: None . . . Character Z

Character 7: Qualifier: None . . . Character Z

The ICD-10-PCS code you will report is

6A4Z0ZZ Hyperthermia for temperature imbalance

Good job!

Osteopathic Section

LO 18.1 Character Definitions

The meanings for the Osteopathic section characters are

Character Position	Character Meaning
1	Section of the ICD-10-PCS book
2	Anatomical regions
3	Root operation term
4	Body region
5	Approach
6	Method
7	Qualifier, if applicable

The Osteopathic section is very direct and straightforward.

LO 18.2 Character Position 1: Osteopathic Section 7

7
Section

Procedures reported from the Osteopathic section will all begin with the number 7.

LO 18.3 Character Position 2: Physiology System

7	W
Section	Anatomical Regions

There is only one option for the second character:

Anatomical Regions . . . Character W

LO 18.4 Character Position 3: Root Operation

7	W	0
Section	Anatomical Regions	Root Operation

There is only one root operation used when reporting osteopathic services:

<u>Treatment:</u> Manual treatment to eliminate or alleviate **somatic** dysfunction and related disorders . . . Character 0

somatic
Related to the body, especially separate from the brain or mind.

EXAMPLE

7W03X2Z General mobilization of the lumbar region

LO 18.5 Character Position 4: Body Region

7	W	0	0–9
Section	Anatomical Regions	Root Operation	Body Region

The specific body regions supported by osteopathic services are

Head . . . Character 0　　　Lower extremities . . . 6

Cervical . . . 1　　　Upper extremities . . . 7

Thoracic . . . 2　　　Rib cage . . . 8

Lumbar . . . 3　　　Abdomen . . . 9

Sacrum . . . 4

Pelvis . . . 5

EXAMPLE

7W06X8Z Isotonic muscle energy application to lower extremities

LO 18.6 Character Position 5: Approach

7	W	0	0–9	X
Section	Anatomical Regions	Root Operation	Body Region	Approach

All osteopathic services use an external approach, reported with character X.

LO 18.7 Character Position 6: Method

7	W	0	0–9	X	0–9
Section	Anatomical Regions	Root Operation	Body Region	Approach	Method

In this character position, you will identify the specific method used by the doctor during this session:

Articulatory—raising . . . Character 0

Facial release . . . Character 1

General mobilization . . . Character 2

High velocity–low amplitude . . . Character 3

Indirect . . . Character 4

Low velocity–high amplitude . . . Character 5

Lymphatic pump . . . Character 6

Muscle energy—isometric . . . Character 7

Muscle energy—isotonic . . . Character 8

Other method . . . Character 9

EXAMPLE

7W05X4Z Indirect treatment of the pelvic region

LO 18.8 Character Position 7: Qualifier

7	W	0	0–9	X	0–9	Z
Section	Anatomical Region	Root Operation	Body Region	Approach	Method	Qualifier

There are no options for this character in the Osteopathic section:

No Qualifier . . . Z

LET'S CODE IT! SCENARIO

Elayne Mariotti, a 41-year-old female, came to see Dr. Underwood for a treatment of her Bell's palsy. He performed a facial release.

Let's go through the steps of coding for ICD-10-PCS and determine the code or codes that should be reported for this encounter between Dr. Underwood and Elayne Mariotti for this treatment.

Character 1: Section: Osteopathic . . . Character 7

Character 2: Anatomical Regions . . . Character W

Character 3: Root Operation: Treatment . . . Character 0

Character 4: Body System: Head . . . Character 0

Character 5: Approach: External . . . Character X

Character 6: Method: Facial release . . . Character 1

Character 7: Qualifier: None . . . Character Z

The ICD-10-PCS code you will report is

7W00X1Z Facial release

Good job!

Other Procedures Section

LO 18.1 Character Definitions

The meanings for the Other Procedures section characters are

Character Position	Character Meaning
1	Section of the ICD-10-PCS book
2	Body system
3	Root operation term
4	Body region
5	Approach
6	Method
7	Qualifier, if applicable

For the most part, the character positions for the Other Procedures section have similar meanings as the other sections about which you have already learned.

LO 18.2 Character Position 1: Other Procedures Section 8

8
Section

Procedures reported from the Other Procedures section all begin with the number 8.

LO 18.3 Character Position 2: Physiology System

8	C or E
Section	Body System

There are only two options for the second character:

Indwelling device . . . Character C

Physiological Systems and Anatomical Regions . . . Character E

LO 18.4 Character Position 3: Root Operation

8	C or E	0
Section	Body System	Root Operation

There is just one root operation term used to report procedures in this section.

Other Procedures: Methodologies that attempt to remediate or cure a disorder or disease . . . Character 0

EXAMPLE

8C01X6J Collection of cerebrospinal fluid

LO 18.5 Character Position 4: Body Region

8	C or E	0	0–9, H–Y
Section	Physiology System	Root Operation	Body Region

There are several body regions represented in this section.

EXAMPLE

Nervous System . . . Character 1
Circulatory System . . . Character 2
Head and Neck Region . . . Character 9
Integumentary System and Breast . . . Character H
Lower Extremity . . . Character Y

LO 18.6 Character Position 5: Approach

8	C or E	0	0–9, H–Y	0–9, X
Section	Physiology System	Root Operation	Body Region	Approach

The fifth character position, reporting the approach, will provide you with options with which you have become familiar: Open (0), Percutaneous (3), Percutaneous Endoscopic (4), Via Natural or Artificial Opening (7), Via Natural or Artificial Opening Endoscopic (8), and External (X).

EXAMPLE

8E0W8CZ Procedure on trunk region, via natural or artificial opening endoscopic, robotic-assisted

LO 18.7 Character Position 6: Method

8	C or E	0	0–9, H–Y	0–9, X	0–6, B–Y
Section	Physiology System	Root Operation	Body Region	Approach	Method

In this character position, you will identify the method employed during this procedure:

Acupuncture . . . Character 0

Therapeutic Massage . . . Character 1

Collection . . . Character 6

Computer Assisted Procedure . . . Character B

Robotic Assisted Procedure . . . Character C

Near Infrared Spectroscopy . . . Character D

Other Method . . . Character Y

LO 18.8 Character Position 7: Qualifier

8	C or E	0	0–9, H–Y	0–9, X	0–6, B–Y	0–9, A–Z
Section	Physiology System	Root Operation	Body Region	Approach	Method	Qualifier

The Qualifier will provide additional details as available or necessary.

LET'S CODE IT! SCENARIO

Gabrielle Contucci, a 29-year-old female, just gave birth via c-section. The nurse provided a pump so that Gabrielle could collect breast milk for the baby.

You Code It!

Let's go through the steps of coding for ICD-10-PCS and determine the code or codes that should be reported for this procedure.

Character 1: Section: Other Procedures . . . Character 8

Character 2: Physiological Region: Physiological System and Anatomic Regions . . . Character E

Character 3: Root Operation: Other procedures . . . Character 0

Character 4: Body System: Integumentary System and Breast . . . Character H

Character 5: Approach: External . . . Character X

Character 6: Method: Collection . . . Character 6

Character 7: Qualifier: Breast milk . . . Character 2

The ICD-10-PCS code you will report is

8E0HX62 Collection of breast milk

Good job!

Chiropractic Section

LO 18.1 Character Definitions

The meanings for the Chiropractic section characters are

Character Position	Character Meaning
1	Section of the ICD-10-PCS book
2	Anatomical regions
3	Root operation term
4	Body region
5	Approach
6	Method
7	Qualifier, if applicable

The Chiropractic section is very direct and straightforward.

LO 18.2 Character Position 1: Chiropractic Section 9

9
Section

Procedures reported from the Chiropractic section will all begin with the number 9.

LO 18.3 Character Position 2: Anatomical Regions

9	W
Section	Anatomical Regions

There is only one option for the second character:

Anatomical Regions . . . Character W

LO 18.4 Character Position 3: Root Operation

9	W	B
Section	Anatomical Regions	Root Operation

There is only one root operation used when reporting chiropractic services:

Manipulation: Manual procedure that involves a directed thrust to move a joint past the physiological range of motion, without exceeding the anatomical limit . . . Character B

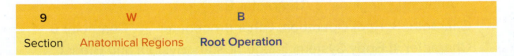

EXAMPLE

9WB1XBZ Non-manual manipulation of the cervical region

LO 18.5 Character Position 4: Body Region

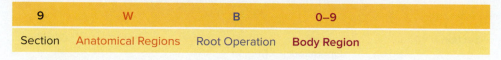

9	W	B	0–9
Section	Anatomical Regions	Root Operation	Body Region

The specific body regions supported by chiropractic services are

Head . . . Character 0   Lower extremities . . . 6

Cervical . . . 1   Upper extremities . . . 7

Thoracic . . . 2   Rib cage . . . 8

Lumbar . . . 3   Abdomen . . . 9

Sacrum . . . 4

Pelvis . . . 5

EXAMPLE

9WB7XK Manipulation of upper extremities, externally, with mechanical assistance

LO 18.6 Character Position 5: Approach

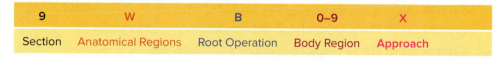

9	W	B	0–9	X
Section	Anatomical Regions	Root Operation	Body Region	Approach

All chiropractic services use an external approach, reported with Character X.

LO 18.7 Character Position 6: Method

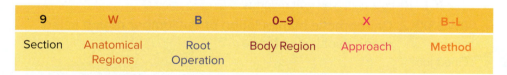

9	W	B	0–9	X	B–L
Section	Anatomical Regions	Root Operation	Body Region	Approach	Method

In this character position, you will identify the specific method used by the doctor during this session:

Non-manual . . . Character B

Indirect Visceral . . . Character C

Extra-Articular . . . Character D

Direct Visceral . . . Character F

Long Lever Specific Contact . . . Character G

Short Level Specific Contact . . . Character H

Long and Short Lever Specific Contact . . . Character J

Mechanically Assisted . . . Character K

Other Method . . . Character L

EXAMPLE

9WB4XFZ Manipulation of sacrum, external direct visceral method

LO 18.8 Character Position 7: Qualifier

9	W	B	0–9	X	B–L	Z
Section	Anatomical Region	Root Operation	Body Region	Approach	Method	Qualifier

There are no options for this character in the Chiropractic section:

No Qualifier . . . Z

LET'S CODE IT! SCENARIO

Keran McCarthey, a 53-year-old male, works in a warehouse and hurt his back. Dr. Ventia performed mechanically assisted manipulation on his lumbar region.

You Code It!

Let's go through the steps of coding for ICD-10-PCS and determine the code or codes that should be reported for this encounter between Dr. Ventia and Keran McCarthey.

Character 1: Section: Chiropractic . . . Character 9

Character 2: Body Region: Anatomical Regions . . . Character W

Character 3: Root Operation: Manipulation . . . Character B

Character 4: Body Region: Lumbar . . . Character 3

Character 5: Approach: External . . . Character X

Character 6: Method: Mechanically Assisted . . . Character K

Character 7: Qualifier: None . . . Character Z

The ICD-10-PCS code you will report is

9WB3XKZ Chiropractic manipulation of the lumbar region using mechanical assistance

Good job!

Chapter Summary

This chapter has given you the opportunity to walk through the Obstetrics (1), Placement (2), Administration (3), Measurement and Monitoring (4), Extracorporeal Assistance and Performance (5), Extracorporeal Therapies (6), Osteopathic (7), Other Procedures (8), and Chiropractic (9) sections of ICD-10-PCS. You have seen how each character position is important to reporting all of the pertinent details of a procedure, service, or treatment. You have learned that, in each section, the same character can have a different meaning. However, you always have the tables there to provide the options and their meanings to build the accurate code.

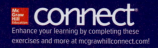

Using Terminology

Match each key term to the appropriate definition.

_____ **1.** LO 18.1 Outside of the body.

_____ **2.** LO 18.8 A drug used to induce an abortion.

_____ **3.** LO 18.4 Related to the body, especially separate from the brain or mind.

_____ **4.** LO 18.2 The zygote, embryo, or fetus, as well as the amnion, umbilical cord, and placenta.

_____ **5.** LO 18.8 Thin sticks of special seaweed, used to dilate the cervix, that can induce abortive circumstance during the first 3 months of pregnancy.

A. Abortifacient

B. Extracorporeal

C. Laminaria

D. Products of conception

E. Somatic

Checking Your Understanding

Choose the most appropriate answer for each of the following questions.

1. LO 18.1/18.6 Within the Obstetric section, character position 5 represents which of the following?

   a. body system.
   b. root operation term.
   c. approach.
   d. device.

2. LO 18.2 All of the codes reporting an Obstetrics procedure will begin with which section number?

   a. 5.
   b. 4.
   c. 2.
   d. 1.

3. LO 18.2 The products of conception include

   a. zygote and embryo.
   b. amnion and umbilical cord.
   c. placenta.
   d. all of these.

4. LO 18.4 All of the following are root operation terms in the Obstetrics section *except*

   a. abortion.
   b. delivery.
   c. irrigation.
   d. inspection.

5. LO 18.6 Within the Obstetrics section, character position 5 Approach, the approach to an intrauterine cordocentesis would be which of the following?

   a. via natural or artificial opening.
   b. percutaneous endoscopic.
   c. external.
   d. open.

6. LO 18.2 Within the Placement section, character position 2 Body System, Anatomical Orifices, is identified by which character?

   a. Y.
   b. W.
   c. X.
   d. Z.

7. LO 18.4 Within the Placement section, character position 3 Root Operation, Putting pressure on a body region (identified with number 1), is which of the following?

   a. dressing.
   b. immobilization.
   c. compression.
   d. traction.

8. LO 18.5 Within the Placement section, character position 4 Body Regions, the upper extremity, right is identified by which character or number?

   a. A.
   b. 8.
   c. C.
   d. 9.

9. LO 18.6 Within the Placement section, character position 5 Approach, which is the correct approach?

   a. open.
   b. percutaneous.
   c. via natural or artificial opening.
   d. external.

10. LO 18.7 Johnny was playing at school and fractured his left arm. Dr. Keller applied a cast to Johnny's left arm. Within the Placement section, character position 6 Device, what number identifies the cast?

    a. 1.
    b. 2.
    c. 3.
    d. 4.

11. LO 18.2 All procedures reported from the Administration section will begin with which section number?

    a. 1.
    b. 2.
    c. 3.
    d. 4.

12. LO 18.3 Within the Administration section, character position 2 Physiology System, an indwelling device would be identified with which character or number?

    a. 0.
    b. C.
    c. E.
    d. X.

13. LO 18.2 A blood transfusion would be reported from which section?

    a. Obstetrics.
    b. Placement.
    c. Administration.
    d. Measurement and Monitoring.

14. LO 18.5 Within the Administration section, character position 4 Body System/Region, when an irrigating substance (such as saline solution) is administered into an indwelling device (reported as body system Indwelling Device . . . C), the body system/region will be reported with which character?

    a. Z.
    b. X.
    c. C.
    d. G.

15. LO 18.8 Within the Administration section, character position 7 Qualifier, Oxazolidinones is reported with which character or number?

    a. 1.
    b. Z.
    c. 8.
    d. X.

16. LO 18.7 Within the Measurement and Monitoring section, character position 6 represents which of the following?

    a. physiological system.
    b. body system.
    c. function/device.
    d. qualifier.

17. LO 18.3 Within the Measurement and Monitoring section character position 2, a physiological device would be represented by which of the following characters or numbers?

    a. A.
    b. 1.
    c. B.
    d. 2.

18. LO 18.4 Within the Measurement and Monitoring section, character position 3 Root Operation, determining the level of a physiological or physical function repetitively over a period of time (identified by number 1) is known as

    a. an abortifacient.
    b. monitoring.
    c. measurement.
    d. laminaria.

19. LO 18.7 Within the Measurement and Monitoring section, character position 6, measuring a patient's temperature would be reported with which character?

    a. F.
    b. S.
    c. Q.
    d. K.

20. LO 18.7 Within the Measurement and Monitoring section, character position 6, a sleep study would be reported with which character?

    a. B.
    b. Q.
    c. X.
    d. Z.

21. LO 18.7 Within the Extracorporeal Assistance and Performance section, character position 6 represents which of the following?

    a. body system.
    b. root operation term.
    c. duration.
    d. function.

22. LO 18.1 Which of these is a term meaning "outside the body"?

    a. abortifacient.
    b. extracorporeal.
    c. laminaria.
    d. somatic.

23. LO 18.2 All of the Extracorporeal Assistance and Performance procedures will begin with which section number?

    a. 5.
    b. 4.
    c. 2.
    d. 1.

24. LO 18.4 Within the Extracorporeal Assistance and Performance section, character position 3 Root Operation, all of the following are root operation terms *except*

    a. assistance.
    b. performance.
    c. manipulation.
    d. restoration.

25. LO 18.6 Within the Extracorporeal Therapies section, character position 5 represents which of the following?

    a. body system.
    b. root operation term.
    c. duration.
    d. function.

26. LO 18.4 Within the Extracorporeal Therapies section, character position 3 Root Operation, which of the following is/are a root operation term(s)?

    a. atmospheric control.
    b. hypothermia.
    c. pheresis.
    d. all of these.

27. LO 18.5 Within the Extracorporeal Therapies section, character position 4 Body System, number 3 represents which of the following?

  a. urinary.
  b. central nervous.
  c. musculoskeletal.
  d. circulatory.

28. LO 18.8 Within the Extracorporeal Therapies section, character position 7 Qualifier, ultrasound therapies performed on the circulatory system, peripheral vessels would be reported with which character or number?

  a. 6.
  b. X.
  c. 5.
  d. Z.

29. LO 18.7 Within the Osteopathic section, character position 6 represents which of the following?

  a. anatomical region.
  b. method.
  c. body region.
  d. qualifier.

30. LO 18.2 All of the Osteopathic section procedures will begin with which section number?

  a. 5.
  b. 4.
  c. 7.
  d. 1.

31. LO 18.4 Within the Osteopathic section, which of the following is an option for character position 3 Root Operation?

  a. treatment.
  b. manipulation.
  c. phototherapy.
  d. electromagnetic therapy.

32. LO 18.7 Within the Osteopathic section, character position 6 Method, which number identifies low velocity–high amplitude?

  a. 0.
  b. 3.
  c. 5.
  d. 8.

33. LO 18.2 All of the Other Procedures section procedures will begin with which section number?

  a. 5.
  b. 8.
  c. 7.
  d. 9.

34. LO 18.3 Within the Other Procedures section, character position 2 Physiology System, an indwelling device is identified with which of the following characters?

a. H.

b. E.

c. Y.

d. C.

35. LO 18.6 Within the Other Procedures section, character position 5 Approach, a procedure performed via natural or artificial opening is identified with which character or number?

a. 7.

b. 3.

c. 8.

d. X.

36. LO 18.7 Within the Other Procedures section, character position 6 Method, acupuncture would be identified with which character or number?

a. B.

b. 6.

c. 0.

d. D.

37. LO 18.2 All of the Chiropractic section procedures will begin with which section number?

a. 5.

b. 8.

c. 7.

d. 9.

38. LO 18.3 Within the Chiropractic section, character position 2 Anatomical Regions, you have one option for the second character. Which of the following represents the anatomical regions?

a. B.

b. W.

c. X.

d. Z.

39. LO 18.6 Within the Chiropractic section, character position 5 Approach, you have one option for the fifth character. Which of the following represents the approach?

a. open.

b. percutaneous.

c. via natural or artificial opening.

d. external.

40. LO 18.7 Within the Chiropractic section, character position 6 Method, a long and short lever specific contact will be reported with which character?

a. G.

b. F.

c. J.

d. L.

Applying Your Knowledge

1. LO 18.1 List the seven Obstetrics section character positions of an ICD-10-PCS code, including each character's meaning. _____

   _____

2. LO 18.2 All of the codes reporting an obstetrics procedure will begin with what section number? _____

   _____

3. LO 18.2 List the products of conceptions. _____

   _____

4. LO 18.3 In the Obstetrics section, character position 2 Body System is represented with which number? Include the character description. _____

   _____

5. LO 18.4 Explain the difference between delivery and extraction, and include the character that represents each. _____

   _____

6. LO 18.4 Explain what a cesarean section procedure is, and include the root operation term used in ICD-10-PCS. _____

   _____

7. LO 18.4 Explain the process of in vitro fertilization, including the ICD-10-PCS root operation term. _____

   _____

8. LO 18.5 The Obstetrics section character position 4 focuses on three body parts, which are not specific anatomical sites. List the three body parts, including the character that identifies each. _____

   _____

9. LO 18.6 In the Obstetrics section, which character position identifies the approach? What does the approach explain? _____

   _____

10. LO 18.6 List the six approaches used in the Obstetrics section of ICD-10-PCS. Explain each approach, and include the character that identifies each approach. _____

_____

11. LO 18.7 Explain the differences between internal and external fetal monitoring. _____

_____

12. LO 18.8 What does the Obstetrics section 7th character position present? Is it required? _____

_____

13. LO 18.1 List the seven Placement section character positions of an ICD-10-PCS code, including each character's meaning. _____

_____

14. LO 18.2 Character position 1 in the Placement section of the ICD-10-PCS manual is represented by what section number? _____

_____

15. LO 18.4 What are the two body system options available in the Placement section, character position 2? Include the character that identifies each. _____

_____

16. LO 18.4 List the seven root operation terms used in the Placement section, character position 3. Explain each root operation term, and include the character that identifies each. _____

_____

17. LO 18.5 Within the Placement section, character position 4 Body Region, anatomical region "Back" would be identified by what character? _____

_____

18. LO 18.6 Within the Placement section, character position 5 Approach would be represented by what character? _____

_____

19. LO 18.7 Within the Placement section, character position 6: Device, a brace would be identified by what character?

_____

20. LO 18.8 Within the Placement section, character position 7 Qualifier, what are the options? _____

_____

21. LO 18.1 List the seven Administration section character positions of an ICD-10-PCS code, including each character's meaning. _____

_____

22. LO 18.2 Within the Administration section, character position 1 Administration section is identified by what section number? _____

_____

23. LO 18.3 Within the Administration section, character position 2 Physiology System, what are the three options? Include each identifying character. _____

_____

24. LO 18.4 Within the Administration section, character position 3 Root Operation, what are the three root operation terms? Include the descriptions and each identifying character. _____

_____

25. LO 18.5 Within the Administration section, character position 4 Body System/Region, there is an exception. What is that exception? _____

_____

26. LO 18.7 Within the Administration section, character position 6 Substance, what does this position identify? _____

_____

27. LO 18.2 Within the Measurement and Monitoring section, character position 1 is identified by what section number?_____

_____

28. LO 18.3 Within the Measurement and Monitoring section, character position 2 Physiology System, what are the two options for the position, including the character identifiers? _____

_____

29. LO 18.4 Within the Measurement and Monitoring section, character position 3 Root Operation, what are the root operation terms? Include the descriptions and character identifiers. _____

_____

30. LO 18.5 Within the Measurement and Monitoring section, character position 4 Body Systems/Regions, the respiratory system is identified by what character? _____

_____

31. LO 18.7 Within the Measurement and Monitoring section, character position 6 Function/Device, a defibrillator is identified by what character? _____

_____

32. LO 18.1 List the seven Extracorporeal Assistance and Performance section character positions, including each character's meaning. _____

_____

33. LO 18.2 within the extracorporeal assistance and performance section, character position 1 is identified by what section number? _____

_____

34. LO 18.3 Within the Extracorporeal Assistance and Performance section, character position 2 Physiology System, what are the options, including the character identifiers? _____

_____

35. LO 18.4 Within the Extracorporeal Assistance and Performance section, character position 3 Root Operation, list the three root operation terms, including the description and character identifier for each. _____

_____

36. LO 18.5 Within the Extracorporeal Assistance and Performance section, character position 4 Body Systems/Regions, the biliary system is identified by what character? _____

_____

37. LO 18.6 Within the Extracorporeal Assistance and Performance section, character position 5 Duration, *continuous, non-stop* would be represented what character? _____

_____

38. LO 18.7 Within the Extracorporeal Assistance and Performance section, character position 6 Function, oxygenation would be identified by what character? _____

_____

39. LO 18.8 Within the Extracorporeal Assistance and Performance section, character position 7 Qualifier, Pulsatile compress would be identified by what character? _____

_____

40. LO 18.1 List the seven Extracorporeal Therapies section character positions, including each character's meaning.

_____

41. LO 18.2 Within the Extracorporeal Therapies section, character position 1 is identified by what section number?

_____

42. LO 18.3 Within the Extracorporeal Therapies section, character position 2 Physiology System, what are the options, including the character identifiers? _____

_____

43. LO 18.4 Within the Extracorporeal Therapies section, character position 3 Root Operation, list the 10 root operation terms, including the description and character identifier for each. _____

_____

44. LO 18.5 Within the Extracorporeal Therapies section, character position 4 Body System, circulatory would be identified by what character? _____

_____

45. LO 18.6 Within the Extracorporeal Therapies section, character position 5 Duration, multiple sessions would be identified by what character? _____

_____

46. LO 18.8 Within the Extracorporeal Therapies section, character position 7 Qualifier, stem cells, hematopoietic would be identified by what character? _____

_____

47. LO 18.1 List the seven Osteopathic section character positions, including each character's meaning. _____

_____

48. LO 18.2 Within the Osteopathic section, character position 1 is identified by what section number? _____

_____

49. LO 18.4 Within the Osteopathic section, character position 3 Root Operation, list the root operation term, including the description and character identifier. _____

_____

50. LO 18.5 Within the Osteopathic section, character position 4 Body Region, the rib cage would be identified by what character? _____

_____

51. LO 18.6 Within the Osteopathic section, character position 5 Approach, what approach do all osteopathic services use? Include the character identifier. _____

_____

52. LO 18.7 Within the Osteopathic section, character position 6 Method, general mobilization would be identified by what character? _____

_____

53. LO 18.1 List the seven Other Procedures section character positions, including each character's meaning. _____

_____

54. LO 18.2 Within the Other Procedures section, character position 1 is identified by what section number? _____

_____

55. LO 18.5 Within the Other Procedures section, character position 4 Body region, Integumentary system and breast would be identified by what character? _____

_____

56. LO 18.7 Within the Other Procedures section, character position 6 Method, robotic assisted procedure would be identified by what character? _____

_____

57. LO 18.1 List the seven Chiropractic section character positions, including each character's meaning. _____

_____

58. LO 18.2 Within the Chiropractic section, character position 1 is identified by what section number? _____

_____

59. LO 18.4 Within the Chiropractic section, character position 3: Root Operation, list the root operation term, including the description and character identifier. _____

_____

60. LO 18.6 Within the Chiropractic section, character position 5 Approach, what options are available? Include character identifiers. _____

_____

61. LO 18.7 Within the Chiropractic section, character position 6 Method, extra-articular would be identified by what character? _____

_____

Using the techniques described in this chapter, carefully read through the case studies and determine the most accurate ICD-10-PCS code(s) for each case study.

1. Meagan Moss, a 28-year-old female, is G2 P1, at 40 weeks' gestation and is in labor. Meagan is admitted into Barton Hospital. The infant is in a breech position; Dr. Hanson performs a classical cesarean section.

   _____

2. Latoya Roberts, a 26-year-old female, is G1 P0, 8 weeks' gestation. Latoya requests an abortion due to genetic problems in the fetus. She is admitted into the hospital, where a vacuum abortion is performed, via natural or artificial opening.

   _____

3. Kimberly Hanks, a 32-year-old female, is admitted into Barton Hospital at 12 weeks' gestation. Dr. Adams performs a repair to the fetus's urinary system via natural or artificial opening, endoscopic approach.

   _____

4. Hank Willis, a 68-year-old male, is admitted into the hospital with a deep laceration to the forehead. Dr. Hancock applies a pressure dressing to his head to control the bleeding.

   _____

5. Anthony Charles, an 18-year-old male, has a nose bleed that will not stop. Dr. Lindsay packed his nasal cavity, external approach.

   _____

6. Henry Medlin, a 43-year-old male, is admitted into the hospital with a hemoglobin of 5.6 g/dL. Dr. Wallace performs a red blood cell transfusion, peripheral vein, percutaneous, non-autologous.

   _____

7. Samantha Jones, a 52-year-old female, has been in the hospital for 3 days with a peritoneal cavity indwelling device. Dr. Walker performs an irrigation of the device with irrigation substance, percutaneous approach.

   _____

8. Candy Watson, a 6-year-old female, is admitted into Barton Hospital with an unexplained high fever. Dr. Molnar measures Candy's temperature.

   _____

9. William Stevens, a 19-year-old male, wanted to join his college's football team. The team physical examination revealed a cardiac abnormality. William is admitted into Barton Hospital, where Dr. Allison monitors William's total cardiac activity under stress.

   _____

10. Angela Hamilton, a 73-year-old female, presents today with shortness of breath and a dry cough. Dr. Cooper admits Angela into the hospital and monitors her respiratory capacity, external approach.\

    _____

11. Robert Mason, a 55-year-old male, has been hospitalized for a week. Robert's lungs were not performing; he was placed on a respiratory ventilator 5 days ago.

    _____

12. Jane Morgan, a 48-year-old female, presents today in cardiac dysrhythmia. Dr. Robertson admits Jane into Barton Hospital and restores Jane's normal sinus rhythm.

    _____

13. Annie Bowens, a 21-year-old female, presents today for treatment of plantar fasciitis. Dr. Ransom performs extracorporeal shockwave therapy, right heel, single treatment.

    _____

14. Gerry Dunham, a 58-year-old male, has been diagnosed with urinary incontinence. Gerry presents today for a single treatment of electromagnetic therapy.

    _____

15. Latonya Garrison, a 52-year-old female, has lower back pain. She presents today for an osteopathic treatment, lumbar region, low velocity–high amplitude, external approach.

    _____

16. Benjamin Niles, a 16-year-old male, had his left arm immobilized by a cast following a fracture. Ben presents today for isometric muscle energy osteopathic treatment, left arm, external approach.

    _____

17. Marvin Sutton, a 25-year-old male, has been married 1 year. The couple is having infertility issues. Marvin presents today for collection of sperm, external approach.

    _____

18. Twanda Sumwalt, a 34-year-old female, diagnosed with trigeminal neuralgia (TGM), presents today for an acupuncture treatment, integumentary system, percutaneous approach, no qualifier.

_____

19. A. C. Tumbokon, a 16-year-old male, is having severe neck pain. Dr. Bell performs a chiropractic manipulation of the cervical region, mechanically assisted, external approach.

_____

20. Kwakita Chapman, a 37-year-old female, is having chronic hip pain. Dr. Dugan performs a chiropractic manipulation of the pelvic region with long and short lever specific contact, external approach.

_____

IMAGING THROUGH SUBSTANCE ABUSE TREATMENT SECTIONS (B–H)

19

Learning Outcomes *After completing this chapter, the student should be able to:*

LO 19.1 Recognize the details reported in other sections of ICD-10-PCS beyond the Medical and Surgical section.

LO 19.2 Evaluate the details to determine the section from which to code.

LO 19.3 Determine the body system or region being treated.

LO 19.4 Interpret the procedure to determine the accurate root operation or procedure term.

LO 19.5 Utilize knowledge of anatomy to determine the body part treated.

LO 19.6 Identify the approach used to access the body part.

LO 19.7 Distinguish the type of device implanted, or other qualifier, when applicable.

LO 19.8 Select the appropriate qualifier character.

The last six sections of ICD-10-PCS focus on coding for services provided by imaging professionals, rehabilitation specialists, audiologists, and mental health/behavioral health professionals.

Imaging Section

LO 19.1 Character Definitions

The meanings for the Imaging section characters are

Character Position	Character Meaning
1	Section of the ICD-10-PCS book
2	Body system
3	Root type
4	Body part (specific anatomical site)
5	Contrast, if applicable
6	Qualifier
7	Qualifier

Key Terms

Densitometry

High Osmolar

Intravascular Optical
Coherence

Low Osmolar

You might have noticed that these are the same meanings as for those in the Medical and Surgical section. You learned a lot about imaging services earlier, so you have a bit of a head start for these procedures.

LO 19.2 Character Position 1: Imaging Section B

B
Section

All of the codes from this section will begin with the letter *B*.

LO 19.3 Character Position 2: Body System

B	0–9, A-Y
Section	**Body System**

The body systems are very similar to those you learned about for the Medical and Surgical section:

Central Nervous System . . . Character 0
Heart . . . 2
Upper Arteries . . . 3
Lower Arteries . . . 4

Remember that the dividing line between Upper and Lower is the diaphragm.

Veins . . . 5
Lymphatic system . . . 7
Eye . . . 8
Ears, Nose, Mouth, and Throat . . . 9
Respiratory system . . . B
Gastrointestinal system . . . D
Hepatobiliary system . . . F
Endocrine system . . . G
Skin, Subcutaneous Tissue and Breast . . . H
Connective Tissue . . . L
Skull and Facial Bones . . . N
Non-Axial Upper Bones . . . P
Non-Axial Lower Bones . . . Q
Axial skeleton, except skull and facial bones . . . R

Remember, the axial skeleton is the torso (the body) and the appendicular (non-axial) skeleton is comprised of the extremities.

Urinary System . . . T
Female reproductive System . . . U
Male reproductive System . . . V
Anatomical regions . . . W
Fetus and obstetrical . . . Y

LO 19.4 Character Position 3: Root Type

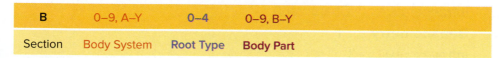

B	0–9, A–Y	0–4
Section	Body System	Root Type

The root type describes the type of imaging technology being used:

Plain Radiography (x-ray) . . . Character 0
Fluoroscopy . . . 1
Computerized Tomography (CT scan) . . . 2
Magnetic Resonance Imaging (MRI) . . . 3
Ultrasonography . . . 4

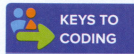

KEYS TO CODING

Review Chap. 9 in this text for more details on imaging modalities.

LO 19.5 Character Position 4: Body Part

B	0–9, A–Y	0–4	0–9, B–Y
Section	Body System	Root Type	Body Part

From the brain to the toes, each body part is listed, specific to the body system in conjunction with the root type.

EXAMPLES

Brain . . . Character 0 under Central Nervous System, CT Scan
Coronary Artery, Single . . . Character 0 under Heart, Fluoroscopy
Thoracic Aorta . . . Character 0 under Upper Arteries, Plain Radiography
Abdominal Aorta . . . Character 0 under Lower Arteries, MRI
Epidural Veins . . . Character 0 under Veins, Plain Radiography

LO 19.6 Character Position 5: Contrast

B	0–9, A–Y	0–4	0–2	0, 1, Y, Z
Section	Body System	Root Type	Body Part	Contrast

As you learned in Chap. 9, there are several types of imaging procedures performed with contrast materials. These materials may be barium or an iodine dye that is injected to highlight or make the visceral organs and body parts more clearly seen in the image.

High Osmolar . . . Character 0
Low Osmolar . . . 1
Other Contrast . . . Y
None . . . Z

high osmolar
An ionic water-soluable iodinated contrast medium.

low osmolar
A non-ionic water-soluable iodinated contrast medium.

LO 19.7 Character Position 6: Qualifier

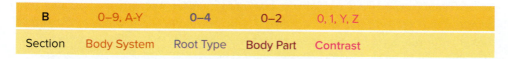

B	0–9, A–Y	0–4	0–2	0, 1, Y, Z	0–2, Z
Section	Body System	Root Type	Body Part	Contrast	Qualifier

As you can see, a character placed in the sixth position will identify an additional detail specific to that table.

Unenhanced and Enhanced . . . Character 0

Laser . . . 1

Intravascular Optical Coherence . . . 2

None . . . Z

intravascular optical coherence
A high-resolution, catheter-based imaging modality used for the optimized visualization of coronary artery lesions.

LO 19.8 Character Position 7: Qualifier

B	0–9, A-Y	0–4	0–2	0–9, X	0–2, Z	0–4, A, Z
Section	Body System	Root Type	Body Part	Contrast	Qualifier	Qualifier

The seventh character is required and may enable you to share additional details about this specific imaging procedure:

Intraoperative . . . Character 0

Densitometry . . . 1

Intravascular . . . 3

Transesophageal . . . 4

Guidance . . . A

None . . . Z

densitometry
The process used to measure bone density, most often done to assess the patient's risk for osteopenia or osteoporosis.

EXAMPLE

B212Y10 Intraoperative fluoroscopy of single coronary artery bypass graft, using laser, other contrast

LET'S CODE IT! SCENARIO

Sadie Polansky, a 63-year-old female, has a family history of osteoporosis and was admitted into the hospital with a hairline fracture of the right hip. Dr. Berringer took a plain radiographic densitometry of her right hip to see if osteoporosis was an underlying cause of the fracture.

Let's Code It!

Let's go through the steps of coding for ICD-10-PCS and determine the code or codes that should be reported for the procedure that was performed.

Character 1: Section: Imaging . . . Character B

Character 2: Body System: Non-Axial Lower Bones . . . Character Q

Character 3: Root Operation: Plain Radiography . . . Character 9

Character 4: Body Part: Hip, right . . . Character 0

Character 5: Contrast: None . . . Character Z

Character 6: Qualifier: None . . . Character Z

Character 7: Qualifier: Densitometry . . . Character 1

Nuclear Medicine Section

LO 19.1 Character Definitions

The meanings for the Nuclear Medicine section characters are

Character Position	Character Meaning
1	Section of the ICD-10-PCS book
2	Body system
3	Root type
4	Body part
5	Radionuclide
6	Qualifier
7	Qualifier

LO 19.2 Character Position 1: Nuclear Medicine Section C

C
Section

The procedures reported with codes from this section describe the use of radioactive material administered into the patient's body to enable the creation of an image for further study. This modality is beneficial as a diagnostic tool for the assessment of metabolic functions and/or a therapeutic tool for the treatment of pathologic conditions.

Note: When radioactive materials are used to treat malignancies, the procedure is reported from the Radiation Oncology section, discussed later in this chapter.

LO 19.3 Character Position 2: Body System

C	0–9, B–W
Section	Body System

The character descriptors of body systems in this section are those with which you have become familiar in this code set.

EXAMPLES

Central nervous system . . . Character 0
Lymphatic and Hematologic System . . . 7
Respiratory System . . . B
Urinary System . . . T

LO 19.4 Character Position 3: Root Type

C	0–9, B–W	0–7
Section	Body System	Root Type

The codes from the Placement section only report procedures that are noninvasive, meaning that the outer layer of the skin is not punctured and no incision is made.

Planar Nuclear Medicine Imaging: Introduction of radioactive materials into the body for single-plane display of images developed from the capture of radioactive emissions . . . Character 1

Tomographic (Tomo) Nuclear Medicine Imaging: Introduction of radioactive materials into the body for three-dimensional display of images developed from the capture of radioactive emissions . . . Character 2

Positron Emission Tomographic (PET) Imaging: Introduction of radioactive materials into the body for three-dimensional display of images developed from the simultaneous capture, 180 degrees apart, of radioactive emissions . . . Character 3

Nonimaging Nuclear Medicine Uptake: Introduction of radioactive materials into the body for measurements of organ function, from the detection of radioactive emissions . . . Character 4

Nonimaging Nuclear Medicine Probe: Introduction of radioactive materials into the body for the study of distribution and fate of certain substances by the detection of radioactive emissions; or alternatively, measurement of absorption of radioactive emissions from an external source . . . Character 5

Nonimaging Nuclear Medicine Assay: Introduction of radioactive materials into the body for the study of body fluids and blood elements, by the detection of radioactive emissions . . . Character 6

Systemic Nuclear Medicine Therapy: Introduction of unsealed radioactive materials into the body for treatment . . . Character 7

LO 19.5 Character Position 4: Body Part

C	0–9, B–W	0–7	0–9, A–W
Section	Body System	Root Type	Body Part

This list of body parts or systems is similar to the list shown in the Imaging section. Combination descriptors—such as Ear, Nose, Mouth, and Throat—as well as regions—such as Lower Extremity Veins, Right—are included along with specific body parts, such as thyroid gland and spleen.

LO 19.6 Character Position 5: Radionuclide

C	0–9, B–W	0–7	0–9, A–W	0–9, A–Z
Section	Body System	Root Type	Body Part	Radionuclide

The options in this list include the descriptors of radioactive materials—the source of the radiation. Be careful—some of these are very similar.

Technetium 99m (Tc-99m) . . . Character 1

Cobalt 58 (C0-58) . . . 7

Samarium 153 (Sm-153) . . . 8

Krypton (Kr-81m) . . . 9

Carbon 11 (C-11) . . . B

Cobalt 57 (Co-57) . . . C

Indium 111 (In-111) . . . D

Iodine 123 (I-123) . . . F

Iodine 131 (I-131) . . . G

Iodine 125 (I-125) . . . H

Fluorine 18 (F-18) . . . K

Gallium 67 (Ga-67) . . . L

Oxygen 15 (O-15) . . . M

Phosphorus 32 (P-32) . . . N

Strontium 89 (Sr-89) . . . P

Rubidium 82 (Rb-82) . . . Q

Nitrogen 13 (N-13) . . . R

Thallium 201 (Tl-201) . . .S

Xenon 127 (Xe-127) . . . T

Xenon 133 (Xe-133) . . . V

Chromium (Cr-51) . . . W

Other Radionuclide . . . Y

This option is available to report any newly approved radionuclides. It is recommended to append documentation to the claim using this character to explain the specific radiation source utilized on the patient.

None . . . Z

> **KEYS TO CODING**
>
> If the documentation shows that more than one radiopharmaceutical is used during one encounter, report a separate code for each identified substance.

LO 19.7 Character Position 6: Qualifier

C	0–9, B–W	0–7	0–9, A–W	0–9, A–Z	Z
Section	Body System	Root Type	Body Part	Radionuclide	Qualifier

This section has only one option for the character reported in the sixth position: None . . . Character Z.

LO 19.8 Character Position 7: Qualifier

C	0–9, B–W	0–7	0–9, A–W	0–9, A–Z	Z	Z
Section	Body System	Root Type	Body Part	Radionuclide	Device	Qualifier

There are no details reported by the Qualifier position, so None . . . Character Z is the only option.

Ralph Bennett, 71-year old male, was admitted into the hospital with dyspnea and chest pain. Dr. Wallace did a PET scan of his lungs and bronchi, using Fluorine 18.

Let's Code It!

Let's go through the steps of coding for ICD-10-PCS and determine the code or codes that should be reported for this encounter between Dr. Wallace and Ralph Bennett.

Character 1: Section: Nuclear Medicine . . . Character C

Character 2: Body System: Respiratory System . . . Character B

Character 3: Root Type: Positron Emission Tomographic (PET) imaging . . . Character 3

Character 4: Body Part: Lungs and Bronchi . . . Character 2

Character 5: Radionuclide: Fluorine 18 . . . Character K

Character 6: Qualifier: None . . . Character Z

Character 7: Qualifier: None . . . Character Z

The ICD-10-PCS code you will report is

CB32KZZ PET imaging of lungs and bronchi, with Fluorine 18

Good job!

Radiation Oncology Section

LO 19.1 Character Definitions

The meanings for the Radiation Oncology section characters are

Character Position	Character Meaning
1	Section of the ICD-10-PCS book
2	Body system
3	Root type
4	Treatment site
5	Modality qualifier
6	Isotope
7	Qualifier

LO 19.2 Character Position 1: Radiation Oncology Section D

D
Section

Procedures reported from the Radiation Oncology section will all begin with the letter *D*.

LO 19.3 Character Position 2: Body System

D	0–9, B–W
Section	Body System

Again, this list is very similar to other sections for body system.

LO 19.4 Character Position 3: Root Type

D	0–9, B–W	0–2, Y
Section	Body System	Root Type

There are only four root types used to describe the modality of these procedures:

<u>Beam Radiation:</u> Character 0
<u>Brachytherapy:</u> Character 1
<u>Stereotactic Radiosurgery:</u> Character 2
<u>Other Radiation:</u> Character Y

LO 19.5 Character Position 4: Treatment Site

D	0–9, B–W	0–2, Y	0–9, A–Z
Section	Body System	Root type	Treatment Site

Consistent with other sections, these anatomical sites are very specific. *Note:* The same character is used to identify different body parts throughout this section. It changes from body system to body system.

EXAMPLES

Brain stem . . . Character 1 under Central and Peripheral Nervous System
Thymus . . . Character 1 under Lymphatic and Hematologic System
Nose . . . Character 1 under Ear, Nose, Mouth, and Throat
Bronchus . . . Character 1 under Respiratory System

LO 19.6 Character Position 5: Modality Qualifier

D	0–9, B–W	0–2, Y	0–9, A–Z	0–9, B–K
Section	Body System	Root Type	Treatment Site	Modality Qualifier

This character will provide additional detail about the modality.

Photons <1 MeV . . . Character 0
Photons 1–10 MeV . . . 1
Photons >10 MeV . . . 2
Electrons . . . 3
Heavy Particles (Protons, Ions) . . . 4

Neutrons . . . 5

Neutron Capture . . . 6

Contact Radiation . . . 7

Hyperthermia . . . 8

High Dose Rate (HDR) . . . 9

Low Dose Rate (LDR) . . . B

Intraoperative Radiation Therapy (IORT) . . . C

Stereotactic Other Photon Radiosurgery . . . D

Plaque Radiation . . . F

Isotope Administration . . . G

Stereotactic Particulate Radiosurgery . . . H

Stereotactic Gamma Beam Radiosurgery . . . J

Laser Interstitial Thermal Therapy . . . K

LO 19.7 Character Position 6: Isotope

D	0–9, B–W	0–2, Y	0–9, A–Z	0–9, B–K	7–9, B–Z
Section	Body System	Root Type	Treatment Site	Modality Qualifier	Isotope

In this character position, you will identify the specific radioactive substance used during this procedure.

Cesium 137 (Cs-137) . . . Character 7

Iridium 192 (Ir-192) . . . 8

Iodine 125 (I-1250 . . . 9

Palladium 103 (Pd-103) . . . B

Californium 252 (Cf-252) . . . C

Iodine 131 (I-131) . . . D

Phosphorus 32 (P-32) . . . F

Strontium 89 (Sr-89) . . . G

Strontium 90 (Sr-90) . . . H

Other Isotope . . . Y

None . . . Z

LO 19.8 Character Position 7: Qualifier

D	0–9, B–W	0–2, Y	0–9, A–Z	0–9, B–K	7–9, B–Z	0 or Z
Section	Body System	Root Type	Treatment Site	Modality Qualifier	Isotope	Qualifier

This character will report that this radiation treatment was provided during a surgical procedure—or not.

Intraoperative . . . Character 0

No Qualifier . . . Z

Dr. Tucci performed brachytherapy on DeeAnna Unger's stomch using Cesium 137, High dose rate.

Let's Code It!

Let's go through the steps of coding for ICD-10-PCS and determine the code or codes that should be reported for this encounter between Dr. Tucci and DeeAnna Unger.

Character 1: Section: Radiation Oncology . . . Character D

Character 2: Body System: Gastrointestinal System . . . Character D

Character 3: Root Type: Brachytherapy . . . Character 1

Character 4: Treatment Site: Stomach . . . Character 1

Character 5: Modality Qualifier: High Dose Rate . . . Character 9

Character 6: Isotope: Cesium 137 (Cs-137) . . . Character 7

Character 7: Qualifier: None . . . Character Z

The ICD-10-PCS code you will report is

DD1197Z Brachytherapy, stomach, high dose rate, Cs-137

Good job!

Physical Rehabilitation and Diagnostic Audiology Section

LO 19.1 Character Definitions

The meanings for the Physical Rehabilitation and Diagnostic Audiology section characters are

Character Position	Character Meaning
1	Section of the ICD-10-PCS book
2	Section qualifier
3	Root type
4	Body system & region
5	Type qualifier
6	Equipment
7	Qualifier

For the most part, these character positions have different meanings than the other sections you have already learned about.

LO 19.2 Character Position 1: Physical Rehabilitation and Diagnostic Audiology Section F

F
Section

Procedures reported from the Physical Rehabilitation and Diagnostic Audiology section begin with the letter *F.*

LO 19.3 Character Position 2: Section Qualifier

F	0 or 1
Section	Section Qualifier

There are only two options for the second character:

Rehabilitation . . . Character 0
Diagnostic Audiology . . . Character 1

LO 19.4 Character Position 3: Root Type

F	0 or 1	0–9, B–F
Section	Section Qualifier	Root Type

The root type terms are unique to report procedures in this section.

Speech Assessment . . . Character 0
Monitor and/or Nerve Function Assessment . . . Character 1
Activities of Daily Living Assessment . . . Character 2
Hearing Assessment . . . Character 3
Hearing Aid Assessment . . . Character 4
Vestibular Assessment . . . Character 5
Speech Treatment . . . Character 6
Motor Treatment . . . Character 7
Activities of Daily Living Treatment . . . Character 8
Hearing Treatment . . . Character 9
Cochlear Implant Treatment . . . Character B
Vestibular Treatment . . . Character C
Device Fitting . . . Character D
Caregiver Training . . . Character F

LO 19.5 Character Position 4: Body System & Region

F	0 or 1	0–9, B–F	0–9, A–Z
Section	Section Qualifier	Root Type	Body Region

The specific body system being assessed or rehabilitated will be identified in this character position. In some cases, these may not be specified, such as with some speech assessment procedures or caregiver training. These are reported with a body system of None . . . Character Z.

EXAMPLES

Neurological system—whole body . . . Character 3
Circulatory system—Upper back/Upper extremity . . . 5
Genitourinary system . . . N

LO 19.6 Character Position 5: Type Qualifier

F	0 or 1	0–9, B–F	0–9, A–Z	0–8, X
Section	Section Qualifier	Root Type	Body Region	Type Qualifier

The character placed in this position will provide additional detail about the root type.

LO 19.7 Character Position 6: Equipment

F	0 or 1	0–9, B–F	0–9, A–Z	0–8, X	0–9, A–Z
Section	Section Qualifier	Root Type	Body Region	Type Qualifier	Equipment

In this character position, you will report any equipment that was used during the assessment or treatment.

LO 19.8 Character Position 7: Qualifier

F	0 or 1	0–9, B–F	0–9, A–Z	0–8, X	0–9, A–Z	Z
Section	Section Qualifier	Root Type	Body Region	Type Qualifier	Equipment	Qualifier

The only option in this position is None . . . Character Z.

LET'S CODE IT! SCENARIO

Isaac Mulrohney, a 77-year-old male, was admitted after having a stroke (CVA). Renee Ruderman, a certified physical therapist, is working with him on functional ambulation due to right side hemiplegia.

Let's Code It!

Let's go through the steps of coding for ICD-10-PCS and determine the code or codes that should be reported for this encounter between Renee Ruderman and Isaac Mulrohney.

Character 1: Section: Physical Rehabilitation & Diagnostic Audiology . . . Character F

Character 2: Section Qualifier: Rehabilitation . . . Character 0

Character 3: Root Type: Motor Treatment . . . Character 7

Character 4: Body Region: None . . . Character Z

Character 5: Type Qualifier: Gait Training/Functional Ambulation . . . Character 9

Character 6: Equipment: None . . . Character Z

Character 7: Qualifier: None . . . Character Z

The ICD-10-PCS code you will report is

F07Z9ZZ Gait training/functional ambulation

Good job!

Mental Health Section

LO 19.1 Character Definitions

The meanings for the Mental Health section characters are

Character Position	Character Meaning
1	Section of the ICD-10-PCS book
2	Body system
3	Root type
4	Type qualifier
5	Qualifier
6	Qualifier
7	Qualifier

LO 19.2 Character Position 1: Mental Health Section G

G
Section

Procedures reported from the Mental Health section will begin with the letter *G*.

LO 19.3 Character Position 2: Body System

G	Z
Section	Body System

There is only one option for the second character: None . . . Character Z.

LO 19.4 Character Position 3: Root Type

G	Z	0–2
Section	Body System	Root Type

There are 12 root types used in this section.

Psychological tests: Include developmental, intellectual, psychoeducational, neurobehavioral, cognitive, neuropsychological, personality, and/or behavioral testing . . . Character 1

Crisis Intervention: Includes defusing, debriefing, counseling, psychotherapy, and/or coordination of care with other providers or agencies . . . Character 2

Medication Management . . . Character 3

Individual Psychotherapy: Includes behavior, cognitive, interactive, interpersonal, psychoanalysis, psychodynamic, psychophysiological, and/or supportive . . . Character 5

Counseling: Exploration of vocational interest, aptitudes, and required adaptive behavior skills to develop and carry out a plan for achieving a successful vocational placement, enhancing work-related adjustment, and/or pursuing viable options in training education or preparation . . . Character 6

Family Psychotherapy: Remediation of emotional or behavioral problems presented by one or more family members when psychotherapy with more than one family member is indicated . . . Character 7

Electroconvulsive Therapy: Includes appropriate sedation and other preparation of the individual . . . Character B

Biofeedback: Includes electroencephalogram (EEG), blood pressure, skin temperature, or peripheral blood flow, electrocardiogram (ECG), electrooculogram, electromyogram (EMG), respirometry or capnometry, galvanic skin response (GSR) or electrodermal response (EDR), perineometry to monitor and regulate bowel or bladder activity and electrogastrogram to monitor and regulate gastric motility . . . Character C

Hypnosis . . . Character F

Narcosynthesis . . . Character G

Group Psychotherapy . . . Character H

Light Therapy . . . Character J

LO 19.5 Character Position 4: Type Qualifier

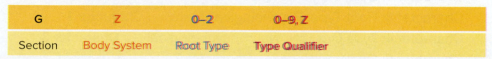

G	Z	0–2	0–9, Z
Section	Body System	Root Type	Type Qualifier

This character will explain whether the procedure was educational or vocational, providing more detail about the encounter. The descriptor presenting these additional details will be represented by the same character in different sections.

LO 19.6 Character Position 5: Qualifier

G	Z	0–2	0–9, Z	Z
Section	Body System	Root Type	Type Qualifier	Qualifier

The only option in this position is None . . . Z.

LO 19.7 Character Position 6: Qualifier

G	Z	0–2	0–9, Z	Z	Z
Section	Body System	Root Type	Type Qualifier	Qualifier	Qualifier

The only option in this position is None . . . Z.

LO 19.8 Character Position 7: Qualifier

G	Z	0–2	0–9, Z	Z	Z	Z
Section	Body System	Root Type	Body System	Qualifier	Qualifier	Qualifier

The only option in this position is None . . . Z.

LET'S CODE IT! SCENARIO

While in the hospital for repair of a stomach ulcer, Brandon Uninne, a 41-year-old male, was behaving oddly. Dr. Kingston performed some neuropsychological testing.

You Code It!

Let's go through the steps of coding for ICD-10-PCS and determine the code or codes that should be reported for this encounter between Dr. Kingston and Brandon Uninne.

Character 1: Section: Mental Health . . . Character G
Character 2: Body Region: None . . . Character Z
Character 3: Root Type: Psychological Tests . . . Character 1
Character 4: Type Qualifier: Neuropsychological . . . Character 3
Character 5: Qualifier: None . . . Character Z
Character 6: Qualifier: None . . . Character Z
Character 7: Qualifier: None . . . Character Z

The ICD-10-PCS code you will report is

GZ13ZZZ Neuropsychological testing

Good job!

Substance Abuse Treatment Section

LO 19.1 Character Definitions

The meanings for the Substance Abuse section characters are

Character Position	Character Meaning
1	Section of the ICD-10-PCS book
2	Body systems
3	Root type
4	Type qualifier
5	Qualifier
6	Qualifier
7	Qualifier

LO 19.2 Character Position 1: Substance Abuse Section H

H
Section

Procedures reported from the Substance Abuse Treatment Section section will all begin with the letter *H*.

LO 19.3 Character Position 2: Body Systems

H	Z
Section	**Body System**

There is only one option for the second character: None . . . Character Z.

LO 19.4 Character Position 3: Root Type

H	Z	2–9
Section	Body System	Root Type

There are seven root operation terms used to report procedures in this section:

<u>Detoxification Services:</u> Not a treatment modality but helps the patient stabilize physically and psychologically until the body becomes free of drugs and the effects of alcohol . . . Character 2

Individual Counseling: Comprising several techniques, which apply various strategies to address drug addiction . . . Character 3

Group Counseling: Provides structured group counseling sessions and healing power through the connection with others . . . Character 4

Individual Psychotherapy: . . . Character 5

Family Counseling: Provides support and education for family members of addicted individuals. Family member participation seen as critical to substance abuse treatment . . . Character 6

Medication Management: . . . Character 8

Pharmacotherapy: . . . Character 9

LO 19.5 Character Position 4: Type Qualifier

H	Z	2–9	0–9, B–Z
Section	Body System	Root Type	Type Qualifier

This character will add detail to the description of the Root Type.

EXAMPLES

12-Step . . . Character 3 for Root Type: Individual Counseling

Interactive . . . Character 5 for Root Type: Individual Psychotherapy

Nicotine Replacement . . . Character 0 for Root Type: Pharmacotherapy

LO 19.6 Character Position 5: Qualifier

H	Z	2–9	0–9, B–Z	Z
Section	Body System	Root Type	Type Qualifier	Qualifier

In this character position, the only option is None . . . Character Z.

LO 19.7 Character Position 6: Qualifier

H	Z	2–9	0–9, B–Z	Z	Z
Section	Body System	Root Type	Type Qualifier	Qualifier	Qualifier

In this character position, the only option is None . . . Character Z.

LO 19.8 Character Position 7: Qualifier

H	Z	2–9	0–9, B–Z	Z	Z	Z
Section	Body System	Root Type	Type Qualifier	Qualifier	Qualifier	Qualifier

In this character position, the only option is None . . . Character Z.

Dr. Oppenheim meets with Carter Ellison for medication management with his methadone maintenance treatment plan.

Let's Code It!

Let's go through the steps of coding for ICD-10-PCS and determine the code or codes that should be reported for this encounter between Dr. Oppenheim and Carter Ellison.

- Character 1: Section: Substance Abuse . . . Character H
- Character 2: Body System: None . . . Character Z
- Character 3: Root Type: Medication Management . . . Character 8
- Character 4: Type Qualifier: Methadone Maintenance . . . Character 1
- Character 5: Qualifier: None . . . Character Z
- Character 6: Qualifier: None . . . Character Z
- Character 7: Qualifier: None . . . Character Z

The ICD-10-PCS code you will report is

HZ81ZZZ Medication management for methadone maintenance

Good job!

Chapter Summary

This chapter has given you the opportunity to walk through the Imaging (B), Nuclear Medicine (C), Radiation Oncology (D), Physical Rehabilitation and Diagnostic Audiology (F), Mental Health (G), and Substance Abuse Treatment (H) sections of ICD-10-PCS. You have seen how each character position is important to reporting all of the pertinent details of a procedure, service, or treatment. You have learned that, in each section, the same character can have a different meaning. However, you always have the tables there to provide the options and their meanings to build the accurate code.

CHAPTER **19** REVIEW
Imaging through Substance Abuse Treatment Sections (B–H)

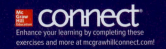
Enhance your learning by completing these exercises and more at mcgrawhillconnect.com!

Using Terminology

Match each key term to the appropriate definition.

_____ **1.** LO 19.6 A non-ionic water-soluable iodinated contrast medium.

_____ **2.** LO 19.7 A high-resolution, catheter-based imaging modality used for the optimized visualization of coronary artery lesions.

_____ **3.** LO 19.8 The process used to measure bone density, most often done to assess the patient's risk for osteopenia or osteoporosis.

_____ **4.** LO 19.6 An ionic water-soluable iodinated contrast medium.

A. Densitometry
B. High Osmolar
C. Intravascular Optical Coherence
D. Low Osmolar

Checking Your Understanding

Choose the most appropriate answer for each of the following questions.

1. LO 19.6 Within the Imaging section, character position 5 represents which of the following?

   a. body system.
   b. contract.
   c. device.
   d. qualifier.

2. LO 19.2 All of the codes reporting an Imaging section procedure will begin with what section letter?

   a. A.
   b. B.
   c. D.
   d. F.

3. LO 19.4 All of the following would be found within the Imaging section, character position 3 Root Type, *except*

   a. x-ray.
   b. CT scan.
   c. PET.
   d. MRI.

4. LO 19.7 Within the Imaging section, character position 6 Qualifier, which of the following are available options?

   a. unenhanced and enhanced.
   b. laser.
   c. intravascular optical coherence.
   d. all of these.

5. LO 19.2 Within the Nuclear Medicine section, character position 1 is identified by which of the following section letters?

   a. E.
   b. B.
   c. D.
   d. C.

6. LO 19.6 Within the Nuclear Medicine section, which character position represents the radioactive materials—the source of the radiation being used?

a. 5.
b. 4.
c. 3.
d. 2.

7. LO 19.4 Introduction of radioactive materials into the body for three-dimensional display of images developed from the capture of radioactive emissions identified by the character 2 is known as

a. positron emission tomographic (PET) imaging.
b. planar nuclear medicine imaging.
c. nonimaging nuclear medicine uptake.
d. tomographic (tomo) nuclear medicine imaging.

8. LO 19.4 Within the Radiation Oncology section, which character position describes the modality of the procedure?

a. 5.
b. 4.
c. 3.
d. 2.

9. LO 19.7 Californium would be classified as

a. a treatment site.
b. an isotope.
c. a modality.
d. a qualifier.

10. LO 19.8 Within the Radiation Oncology section, character position 7 Qualifier, which of the following characters represents the radiation treatment provided during a surgical procedure?

a. Z.
b. 0.
c. X.
d. 1.

11. LO 19.7 Within the Physical Rehabilitation and Diagnostic Audiology section, character position 6 represents which of the following?

a. section qualifier.
b. type qualifier.
c. equipment.
d. qualifier.

12. LO 19.3 Within the Physical Rehabilitation and Diagnostic Audiology section, character position 2 Section Qualifier, which of the following characters represents diagnostic audiology?

a. 0.
b. 1.
c. 2.
d. 3.

13. LO 19.4 Within the Physical Rehabilitation and Diagnostic Audiology section, character position 3 Root Type, which of the following characters represents a hearing aid assessment?

   a. B.
   b. 2.
   c. D.
   d. 4.

14. LO 19.2 All of the codes reporting a Mental Health section procedure will begin with which section letter?

   a. G.
   b. H.
   c. I.
   d. J.

15. LO 19.4 Within the Mental Health section, character position 3 Root Type, the encounter documents *Includes behavior, cognitive, interactive, interpersonal, psychoanalysis, psychodynamic, psychophysiological, and/or supportive,* identified by the character 5. This encounter is known as

   a. psychological tests.
   b. individual psychotherapy.
   c. counseling.
   b. crisis intervention.

16. LO 19.5 Within the Mental Health section, which character position identifies whether the procedure was educational or vocation?

   a. 2.
   b. 3.
   c. 4.
   d. 5.

17. LO 19.2 All of the codes reporting a Substance Abuse section procedure will begin with which section letter?

   a. F.
   b. H.
   c. J.
   d. K.

18. LO 19.4 Within the Substance Abuse section, the encounter documents *Not a treatment modality but helps the patient stabilize physically and psychologically until the body becomes free of drugs and the effects of alcohol,* represented by the character 2. This is known as

   a. individual psychotherapy.
   b. medication management.
   c. pharmacotherapy.
   d. detoxification services.

19. LO 19.5 Within the Substance Abuse section, what character position adds detail to the description of the Root Type?

   a. 4.
   b. 5.
   c. 6.
   d. 7.

20. LO 19.7 Within the Substance Abuse section, character position 6 Qualifier, what is the available character option?

    a. X.

    b. Z.

    c. Y.

    d. W.

Applying Your Knowledge

1. LO 19.1 List the seven Imaging section character positions of an ICD-10-PCS code, including each character's meaning. _____

_____

2. LO 19.2 All of the codes reporting an Imaging section procedure will begin with what section letter? _____

_____

3. LO 19.3 What is the dividing line between the Upper and Lower body systems? _____

_____

4. LO 19.3 Explain the difference between the axial skeleton and the appendicular skeleton. _____

_____

5. LO 19.4 List the five root types found within the Imaging section, character position 3. Include the character that identifies each. _____

_____

6. LO 19.6 List the types of contrast found in the Imaging section, character position 5. Include the character that identifies each. _____

_____

7. LO 19.7 List the types of qualifiers found in the Imaging section, character position 6 Qualifier. Include the character that identifies each. _____

_____

8. LO 19.8 List the types of qualifiers found in the Imaging section, character position 7 Qualifier. Include the character that identifies each. _____

_____

9. LO 19.1 List the seven Nuclear Medicine section character positions of an ICD-10-PCS code, including each character's meaning. _____

_____

10. LO 19.2 All of the codes reporting a Nuclear Medicine section procedure will begin with which section letter? ____

_____

11. LO 19.2 When radioactive materials are used to treat malignancies, the procedure is reported from which ICD-10-PCS section? _____

_____

12. LO 19.4 List the seven root types found in the Nuclear Medicine section, character position 3. Include the description and character that identifies each. _____

_____

13. LO 19.6 Within the Nuclear Medicine section, character position 5 Radionuclide, what do these descriptors explain?

_____

14. LO 19.7 Within the Nuclear Medicine section, character position 6 Qualifier, what is/are the option(s)? Include the character that identifies each. _____

_____

15. LO 19.1 List the seven Radiation Oncology section character positions of an ICD-10-PCS code, including each character's meaning. _____

_____

16. LO 19.2 All of the codes reporting a Radiation Oncology section procedure will begin with what section letter? ___

_____

17. LO 19.4 List the root types found within the Radiation Oncology section, character position 3. Include the character that identifies each. _____

_____

18. LO 19.6 Within the Radiation Oncology section, character position 5 Modality Qualifier, what do these descriptors provide? Include an example. _____

_____

19. LO 19.7 Within the Radiation Oncology section, character position 6 Isotope, what does this character position identify? Include an example. _____

_____

20. LO 19.8 Within the Radiation Oncology section, character position 7 Qualifier, what does this character position identify? Include the character that identifies each. _____

_____

21. LO 19.1 List the seven Physical Rehabilitation and Diagnostic Audiology section character positions of an ICD-10-PCS code, including each character's meaning. _____

_____

22. LO 19.2 All of the codes reporting a Physical Rehabilitation and Diagnostic Audiology section procedure will begin with what section letter? _____

_____

23. LO 19.3 List the Physical Rehabilitation and Diagnostic Audiology section, character position 2 Section Qualifier options, including the character that identifies each. _____

_____

24. LO 19.5 Within the Physical Rehabilitation and Diagnostic Audiology section, character position 4 Body System and Region, if the encounter is for caregiver training, what would be the character assignment to represent the encounter? _____

_____

25. LO 19.6 Within the Physical Rehabilitation and Diagnostic Audiology section, character position 5 Type Qualifier, what does this character position identify? Include an example. _____

_____

26. LO 19.7 Within the Physical Rehabilitation and Diagnostic Audiology section, character position 6 Equipment, what does this character position identify? _____

_____

27. LO 19.1 List the seven Mental Health Section character positions of an ICD-10-PCS code, include each character's meaning. _____

_____

28. LO 19.2 All of the codes reporting a Mental Health section procedure will begin with what section letter? _____

_____

29. LO 19.4 List six Mental Health section, character position 3 Root Type options, including the description and the character that identifies each. _____

_____

30. LO 19.5 Within the Mental Health section, character position 4 Type Qualifier, what does this character position explain? _____

_____

31. LO 19.1 List the seven Substance Abuse section character positions of an ICD-10-PCS code, including each character's meaning. _____

_____

32. LO 19.2 All of the codes reporting a Substance Abuse section procedure will begin with what section letter? _____

_____

33. LO 19.4 List the seven Substance Abuse section, character position 3 Root Type options, including the description and the character that identifies each. _____

_____

34. LO 19.5 Within the Substance Abuse section, character position 4 Type Qualifier, what does this character position identify? Include an example with description. _____

_____

35. LO 19.8 Within the Substance Abuse section, character position 7 Qualifier, what is/are the option(s)? Include the character that identifies each. _____

_____

YOU CODE IT! Practice

Chapter 19: Imaging through Substance Abuse Treatment Sections (B–H)

Using the techniques described in this chapter, carefully read through the case studies and determine the most accurate ICD-10-PCS code(s) for each case study.

1. Dale Harkey, a 23-year-old male, was riding his dirt bike and fell off, hurting his left ankle. Dale presents to Barton Hospital, where Dr. Allen takes an x-ray, without contrast, of the ankle.

   _____

2. Linda Bossard, a 14-year-old female, complains of urinary dribbling and feels like her bladder is still full after voiding. Dr. Clarke performs an ultrasound of Linda's urethra.

   _____

3. Harrison Bowman, a 58-year-old male, is having difficulty with his right knee. He presents to Barton Hospital for an MRI, without contrast, of his right knee.

   _____

4. Glenn Dorsey, a 16-year-old male, is diagnosed with Graves disease and presents to the hospital for a planar nuclear medicine imaging procedure of his thyroid gland, Iodine 123 (I-123).

   _____

5. Marie Cutis, a 42-year-old female, presents to the hospital for a tomographic nuclear medicine imaging procedure of her parathyroid glands, radionuclide— Technetium 99m (Tc-99m).

   _____

6. Lauren Butler, a 38-year-old female, presents today for a positron emission tomographic (PET) imaging procedure of the lungs and bronchi, radionuclide— Fluorine 18 (F-18).

   _____

7. Brain Clarivy, a 64-year-male, has been diagnosed with esophageal cancer. He presents to Barton Hospital for beam radiation therapy to the esophagus, Photons 1-10MeV.

   _____

8. James Fitch, a 45-year-old male, has been diagnosed with lymphatic cancer. James presents to Barton Hospital for brachytherapy of the inguinal lymphatic nodes, low dose rate, Iridium 192 (Ir-192).

_____

9. Joe Fredrick, a 27-year-old male, presents to Barton Hospital for stereotactic gamma beam radiosurgery on his eye.

_____

10. Harris Gibbons, a 63-year-old male, has been in Barton Hospital for a week and is showing signs of deteriorating speech. Dr. Housing performs a bedside swallowing and oral function speech assessment, no equipment.

_____

11. Carolyn Lewis, an 18-year-old female, was in an automobile accident and suffered left hemiplegia. Dr. Anderson performs an ADL home management assessment using assistive, adaptive, supportive, and protective equipment.

_____

12. Ben McCray, an 8-month-old male, has been diagnosed with severe sensorineural hearing loss. Ben has a multiple channel cochlear implant. Dr. Sauls performs a cochlear implant rehabilitation treatment today.

_____

13. Patty McCord, a 23-year-old female, has been diagnosed with tinnitus. Dr. Jackson fits a tinnitus masker, no equipment used.

_____

14. Susan Nally, a 56-year-old female, diagnosed with generalized anxiety disorder, presents today for an individual interpersonal psychotherapy session.

_____

15. Ozie Deas, a 14-year-old male, has been diagnosed with major depression. Ozie and his family participate in a family psychotherapy session led by Dr. Fluharty.

_____

16. Jeff Glover, age unknown, male, was found wondering the streets with no memory or ability to reason. A card with a name was found in one of his pockets. He was admitted into Barton Hospital, where Dr. Hatfield performed a cognitive status psychological test.

_____

17. Hugo Huggins, a 13-year-old male, is brought to Barton Hospital by his parents. Hugo's parents have noticed a dramatic personality change recently, as well as unexplained anger. Dr. Abrams completes a physical examination and finds Hugo has a substance abuse issue. Dr. Abrams admits Hugo into Barton Hospital and begins detoxification treatment.

_____

18. Hazel Abbott, a 34-year-old female, has been smoking cigarettes since she was 16 years old and is in the process of trying to stop smoking. Dr. Barbato manages her nicotine replacement medication.

_____

19. Phoebe Baker, a 56-year-old female, had been diagnosed as an alcoholic. She presents today for a 12-step individual psychotherapy session.

_____

20. Edward Eaddy, a 21-year-old male, has been diagnosed with human immunodeficiency virus (HIV). Edward attends a post-test group counseling session held by Dr. Dyson at Barton Hospital.

_____

PART IV

APPLICATION

Chapter 20   **Procedure Coding Application**

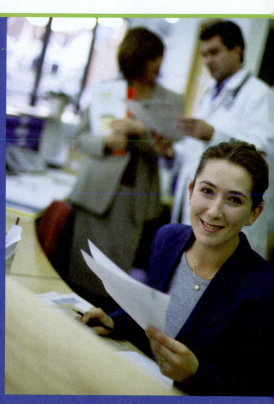

© Mark Thornton/Getty Images

20 PROCEDURE CODING APPLICATION

Learning Outcomes *After completing this chapter, the student should be able to:*

LO 20.1 Interpret the physician's notes carefully.

LO 20.2 Correctly abstract physicians' notes and operative reports.

LO 20.3 Identify any missing or unclear documentation and query the doctor.

LO 20.4 Assign the best, most accurate CPT and/or HCPCS Level II code(s) and modifier(s), if appropriate, for each patient encounter.

LO 20.5 Confirm the encounter has been accurately and completely coded.

The following pages include selections from actual physicians' notes and operative reports that document services and treatments performed for patients at various health care facilities.

Abstract the reports, and determine the most accurate CPT, HCPCS Level II and ICD-10-PCS code(s) and modifier(s), if appropriate, for each case study.

In the real world, you would code only one portion of a patient's chart, because you would be working for only one of the facilities or professionals. However, to benefit the most from this chapter, *you should code for the person who signed the encounter or report:*

- Attending physician
- Surgeon
- Anesthesiologist
- Radiologist
- Pathologist
- Physical therapist
- Chiropractor
- Facility

By coding for everyone, you will practice all types of medical coding and will be prepared to work for any type of facility.

The names of the facilities, health care professionals, and patients have all been changed to protect the privacy and confidentiality of all concerned in all case scenarios and physicians' notes contained in this textbook. Any similarities to actual persons or places are purely coincidental. The cases are to be used for educational purposes only.

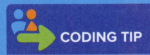

CODING TIP

In this application, HCPCS level II codes and modifiers are accepted by insurance carriers.

CIPHER, VICTORS & ASSOCIATES
A Complete Health Care Facility
234 MAIN STREET • ANYTOWN, FL 32711 • 407-555-1234

PATIENT: HUMPHREY, DONALD
ACCOUNT/EHR #:   HUMPDO01
DATE: 08/23/2018

Procedure Performed: Neurosurgical evaluation

Physician: Patrick B. Reynoso, MD

This is the first visit for this 79-year-old right-handed male, who comes for evaluation of possible normal pressure hydrocephalus. The patient's family has been noting that the patient has symptoms consistent with normal pressure hydrocephalus and apparently was made aware of this in recent publications. The patient has had mental deterioration. He has a history of urinary urgency and has been seen by Dr. Jackson for this. He has problems with his gait, which he describes as "vertigo in the legs," and he "minces his steps." His primary care physician is Dr. Thomas.

    The patient has allergies to pollen and hay fever. His medications include Plavix, aspirin, Lipitor, Avodart, Uroxatral, Hyzaar, calcium 600 + vitamin D, and multivitamins.

PERTINENT MEDICAL HISTORY: The patient does not smoke cigarettes or drink alcohol.

SOCIAL HISTORY: He is married and is a retired dentist.

FAMILY HISTORY: His mother died at the age of 96 of "dementia" and possible stroke. His father died at the age of 96 of an unknown cause.

REVIEW OF SYSTEMS: The patient had several transient ischemic attacks in January, April, and July. He is status post cataract surgery. He is status post a syncopal episode in January. He has a history of hypertension, asthma, and bronchitis, and he has a history of bilateral inguinal hernia repairs 45 years ago. In January, he had a urinary tract infection and had a cardiac evaluation, which was negative. Otherwise, his review of systems is negative for cardiac, pulmonary, gastrointestinal, genitourinary, or musculoskeletal disease.

PHYSICAL EXAMINATION: This is a well-developed, well-nourished elderly white male in no acute distress who appears to be awake, alert, and oriented. His blood pressure is 170/70. His pulse is 70. His respiration is 16. His head is atraumatic, normocephalic. He is status post cataracts. He has dentures. His neck is subtle without jugular venous distention or bruits. His lungs are clear to auscultation. His heart is regular rhythm. His abdomen is soft. His extremities are without clubbing, cyanosis, or edema. Examination of his spine does not demonstrate any direct cervical spine tenderness. The patient has kyphoscoliosis of the thoracolumbar spine. Neurological examination of cranial nerves II–XII demonstrate a decrease in upward gaze and a decrease in hearing. He wears hearing aids. Otherwise, the nerves appear to be grossly unremarkable. Motor function is 5/5 = in all major motor groups. Examination of sensory system appears to be grossly intact in all extremities. Deep tendon reflexes are 0 = for the biceps, triceps, and brachioradialis. In the lower extremities, the patellars, suprapatellars, and hamstrings are 0 =. The right Achilles is 2+, the left is absent. The toes are downgoing bilaterally. The patient's cerebellar testing is intact for finger to nose function. On regular gait testing, the patient has a magnetic/shuffling gait. Station testing does not demonstrate any drift or Romberg's sign.

(Continued)

REVIEW: There are no x-rays available for review.

IMPRESSION: The patient has possible normal pressure hydrocephalus verses ischemic cerebrovascular disease.

RECOMMENDATIONS: The patient will have an MRI scan, MR angiogram of the brain, and MR angiogram of the carotid and vertebral arteries and then return to see me in the office.

Patrick B. Reynoso, MD

PBR/mg   D: 08/23/18 09:50:16   T: 08/25/18 12:55:01

Determine the most accurate CPT and/or HCPCS Level II code(s) and modifier(s), if appropriate.

_____

_____

_____

CIPHER, VICTORS & ASSOCIATES
A Complete Health Care Facility
234 MAIN STREET • ANYTOWN, FL 32711 • 407-555-1234

PATIENT: HUMPHREY, DONALD
ACCOUNT/EHR #:   HUMPDO01
DATE: 08/25/2018

Procedure Performed: MRI, brain, no contrast
                                    MRA, brain, no contrast
                                    MRA, neck, no contrast

Radiologist: Michelle H. McNair, MD

Clinical Information: Evaluate for VP shunt
                                    No prior studies available for a comparison

TECHNICAL INFORMATION: The examination was performed without the use of intravenous contrast material.

INTERPRETATION: Evaluation of the posterior fossa demonstrates hydrocephalus versus low pressure communicating hydrocephalus.

Michelle H. McNair, MD

MHM/mg   D: 08/25/18 09:50:16   T: 08/27/18 12:55:01

Determine the most accurate CPT and/or HCPCS Level II code(s) and modifier(s), if appropriate.

_____

_____

_____

CIPHER, VICTORS & ASSOCIATES
A Complete Health Care Facility
234 MAIN STREET • ANYTOWN, FL 32711 • 407-555-1234

PATIENT: HUMPHREY, DONALD
ACCOUNT/EHR #:   HUMPDO01
DATE: 09/15/2018

Procedure Performed: Test evaluation

Physician: Patrick B. Reynoso, MD

The patient was last seen on August 23. The MRI scan of the brain demonstrates that the patient has hydrocephalus with transependymal edema.

IMPRESSION: The patient has either normal pressure hydrocephalus or a low pressure communicating hydrocephalus.

RECOMMENDATIONS: In either case, he requires a ventricular shunt placement. I have explained to the patient and his family the shunt procedure and its indications, risks, benefits, and alternatives in detail including the risk of bleeding, infection, and injury to the brain tissue with hemorrhages, stroke, paralysis, blindness, coma, or even death. All of their questions have been answered. No guarantees have been given. I have advised that the patient will need to have medical clearance from his primary care physician, Dr. Roger Thomas, 407-555-9899. Once we have the medical clearance, we can schedule him for surgery. Chest x-rays, 2 views, are taken to confirm patient is OK for surgery.

Patrick B. Reynoso, MD

PBR/mg   D: 09/15/18 09:50:16   T: 09/20/18 12:55:01

Determine the most accurate CPT and/or HCPCS Level II code(s) and modifier(s), if appropriate.

_____

_____

_____

CIPHER, VICTORS & ASSOCIATES
A Complete Health Care Facility
234 MAIN STREET • ANYTOWN, FL 32711 • 407-555-1234

PATIENT:	HUMPHREY, DONALD
ACCOUNT/EHR #:	HUMPDO01
Admission Date:	09/17/2018
Discharge Date:	09/19/2018

Operative Report:

Preoperative Diagnosis:	Normal pressure hydrocephalus
Postoperative Diagnosis:	Normal pressure hydrocephalus
Operation:	Right parieto-occipital ventriculoperitoneal shunt placement with cerebrospinal fluid manometry and Hakim valve programming
Surgeon:	Patrick B. Reynoso, MD
Assistant:	None
Anesthesia:	General endotracheal
Anesthesiologist:	Carter H. Beauman, MD
Estimated Blood Loss:	Less than 10 cc
COMPLICATIONS:	

PROCEDURE: This 79-year-old gentleman had progressive urinary, gait, and memory problems with MRI study demonstrating significant ventriculomegaly consistent with normal pressure hydrocephalus. Because of the patient's deterioration, he was offered the option of ventriculoperitoneal shunt placement to try to stop the downward deterioration of his mental faculties.

Following the obtaining of informed consent, the patient was taken to the operating table for the procedure.

The patient was placed supine on the operating table, inducted under general anesthesia, and intubated. His right parieto-occipital scalp was shaved, and then the scalp, neck, chest, and abdomen on the right side were washed with alcohol and prepped with DuraPrep solution and then draped with sterile drapes with additional ioban dressing. The skin incision was marked out with a skin marker for the right parieto-occipital scalp, centered on a point approximately 3 cm lateral to and 8 to 9 cm rostral to the inion, and in the right upper quadrant of the abdomen at the midcostal line. These incisions were then infiltrated with 0.5% lidocaine with 1:200,000 epinephrine solution. The skin incision was then made in the scalp with a #10 blade, and hemostasis was obtained with Bovie cauterization. A pneumatic perforator was used to drill a hole in the cranium, and then the margins of the bur hole were waxed with bone wax for hemostasis. Blunt dissection of the occipital scalp was used to create a subcutaneous cul-de-sac for placement of the valve system, and following this, a subcutaneous passer was used to create a track for passing the distal Bactocill peritoneal catheter between the two incisions. The abdominal incision was also opened with a #10 blade to facilitate passage.

Once the distal catheter was in place, the dura was cauterized using the Bovie cautery bayonet technique, and then a ventricular catheter was passed into the ventricles without difficulty. The cerebrospinal fluid pressure was measured to be approximately 9 cm of water, and cerebrospinal fluid was also sent for routine culture and Gram stain. Once the cerebrospinal fluid pressure had been measured, the Hakim valve was programmed to a pressure resistance of 60 mm of water. The valve was

(Continued)

then connected to the ventriculostomy catheter, which was 10 cm in length. A Bactocill catheter was used for this also. The connection was made with a 2-0 silk ligature. The valve was also connected to the distal peritoneal catheter with a 2-0 silk ligature. The valve was then pulled underneath the scalp and anchored to the pericranium with 3-0 Prolene anchoring sutures to prevent migration of the valve. There was good spontaneous flow of cerebrospinal fluid from the distal portion of the peritoneal catheter. Excess length of the peritoneal cavity was removed, and then several slits were made in the sides of the peritoneal catheter to provide additional egress points for cerebrospinal fluid as needed.

Once this was done, the abdominal incision was opened further with a Bovie cautery and cutting current. The anterior abdominal fascia was divided with a Bovie cautery, and then blunt dissection with a hemostat was used to split the fibers of the rectus abdominus muscles. The posterior abdominal fascia was then identified and lifted up with hemostats and then divided with Metzenbaum scissors. The peritoneum was then identified, lifted up with hemostats, and again divided with Metzenbaum scissors. Following this, the peritoneal cavity was easily visualized. A hemostat and then a peritoneal trocar were able to be passed into the peritoneal cavity without difficulty. Following this, the distal portion of the ventriculoperitoneal shunt was passed into the peritoneal cavity without difficulty, after once again ascertaining that there was spontaneous flow of spinal fluid. Once the catheter was in the peritoneal cavity, #0 Vicryl sutures were used to reapproximate the posterior abdominal fascia, and then the anterior abdominal fascia. The Scarpa's fascia was then closed with #0 Vicryl interrupted sutures with inverted knots. Gelfoam soaked in thrombin was placed overlying the point of insertion of the ventriculostomy catheter, and then the galea was closed with #0 Vicryl interrupted sutures with inverted knots. The areas were irrigated with bacitracin irrigation solution during the closure process, and then the skin incisions were closed with 3-0 nylon simple running sutures with good skin approximation. The skin incisions were then washed again with bacitracin irrigation solution, and then dressed with triple antibiotic ointment and coverlet dressings. The patient was awakened from general anesthesia, extubated, and taken to the recovery room for further observation. Estimated blood loss from the entire procedure was less than 10 cc. The patient appeared to have tolerated the procedure well.

Patrick B. Reynoso, MD

PBR/mg   D: 09/17/18 12:50:14   T: 09/21/18 11:02:01

Determine the most accurate CPT and/or HCPCS Level II code(s) and modifier(s), if appropriate.

_____

_____

_____

CIPHER, VICTORS & ASSOCIATES
A Complete Health Care Facility
234 MAIN STREET • ANYTOWN, FL 32711 • 407-555-1234

PATIENT: HUMPHREY, DONALD
ACCOUNT/EHR #: HUMPDO01
Admission Date: 09/17/2018
Discharge Date: 09/19/2018

Operative Report:
Preoperative Diagnosis: Normal pressure hydrocephalus
Postoperative Diagnosis: Normal pressure hydrocephalus
Operation: Right parieto-occipital ventriculoperitoneal shunt placement with cerebrospinal fluid manometry and Hakim valve programming
Surgeon: Patrick B. Reynoso, MD
Assistant: None
Anesthesia: General endotracheal
Anesthesiologist: Carter H. Beauman, MD

PROCEDURE: This 79-year-old gentleman had progressive urinary, gait, and memory problems with MRI study demonstrating significant ventriculomegaly consistent with normal pressure hydrocephalus. Because of the patient's deterioration, he was offered the option of ventriculoperitoneal shunt placement to try to stop the downward deterioration of his mental faculties.

Following the obtaining of informed consent, the patient was taken to the operating table for the procedure. The patient was placed supine on the operating table, inducted under general anesthesia, and intubated. His right parieto-occipital scalp was shaved, and then the scalp, neck, chest, and abdomen on the right side were washed with alcohol and prepped with DuraPrep solution and then draped with sterile drapes with additional Ioban dressing.

Vital signs were maintained at appropriate level.

The patient was awakened from general anesthesia, extubated, and taken to the recovery room for further observation. Estimated blood loss from the entire procedure was less than 10 cc. The patient appeared to have tolerated the procedure well.

_____

Carter H. Beauman, MD

CHB/mg   D: 09/17/18 12:50:14   T: 09/21/18 11:02:01

Determine the most accurate CPT and/or HCPCS Level II code(s) and modifier(s), if appropriate.

_____

_____

_____

CIPHER, VICTORS & ASSOCIATES
A Complete Health Care Facility
234 MAIN STREET • ANYTOWN, FL 32711 • 407-555-1234

PATIENT: HUMPHREY, DONALD
ACCOUNT/EHR #:   HUMPDO01
DATE: 09/18/2018

Procedure Performed: Subsequent inpatient visit

Physician: Patrick B. Reynoso, MD

The patient was admitted for surgery on September 17, 2016, and underwent a right parieto-occipital ventricular peritoneal shunt placement with a Hakim valve, which was programmed to 60 mm after CSF manometry demonstrated higher pressures. The procedure was uneventful. Postoperatively, the patient was awake, alert, and conversant. His postoperative CT scan demonstrated excellent position of the ventriculostomy catheter and the ventricles without the evidence of hemorrhage. The patient was noted to have a marked improvement in his gait according to his family within 12 hours of surgery. He had no headaches, and he was felt to be sufficiently stable. He was able to be discharged home for outpatient follow-up. His condition at discharge was stable/improved.

RECOMMENDATIONS: Patient to be seen in the office in one week for removal of external sutures.

_____

Patrick B. Reynoso, MD

PBR/mg   D: 09/18/18 09:50:16   T: 09/20/18 12:55:01

Determine the most accurate CPT and/or HCPCS Level II code(s) and modifier(s), if appropriate.

_____

_____

_____

CIPHER, VICTORS & ASSOCIATES
A Complete Health Care Facility
234 MAIN STREET • ANYTOWN, FL 32711 • 407-555-1234

PATIENT: HUMPHREY, DONALD
ACCOUNT/EHR #:   HUMPDO01
DATE: 09/18/2018

Procedure Performed: CT brain w/o contrast
Radiologist: Michelle H. McNair, MD
Clinical Information: Evaluate for VP shunt, postsurgical

No prior studies available for a comparison

TECHNICAL INFORMATION: Contiguous 3-mm-thick axial images were obtained through the skull base and posterior fossa structures followed by 7-mm-thick axial images through the remainder of the brain. The examination was performed without the use of intravenous contrast material.

INTERPRETATION: Evaluation of the posterior fossa demonstrates bilateral vertebral artery calcification. No abnormal intra- or extra-axial collections are noted. There is no evidence of midline shift.

   Analysis of the region of the sella turcica demonstrates calcification, likely atherosclerotic involving the cavernous carotid arteries bilaterally seen on series 2 image 7.

   Supratentorially, the lateral ventricles are prominent in size. A ventriculostomy catheter is seen coursing from the region of the postcentral sulcus with its distal tip terminating within the frontal horn of the right lateral ventricle abutting the septum pellucidum. Hypodensity is seen within the periventricular white matter particularly abutting the frontal horns of the lateral ventricles bilaterally. There is a mild degree of cerebral volume loss. No abnormal intra- or extra-axial collections are noted.

   Evaluation of the visualized skull and paranasal sinuses demonstrates a right parietal burr hole defect for placement of the patient's ventriculostomy catheter. A subcutaneous ventriculostomy valve is seen on series 2 image 23.

RECOMMENDATIONS: There is mild prominence of the lateral ventricles bilaterally without evidence of dilation of the cerebral aqueduct or fourth ventricle.

_____

Michelle H. McNair, MD

MHM/mg   D: 09/18/18 09:50:16   T: 09/20/18 12:55:01

Determine the most accurate CPT and/or HCPCS Level II code(s) and modifier(s), if appropriate.

_____

_____

_____

CIPHER, VICTORS & ASSOCIATES
A Complete Health Care Facility
234 MAIN STREET • ANYTOWN, FL 32711 • 407-555-1234

PATIENT: VANCE, NICOLE
ACCOUNT/EHR #:   VANCNI01
Admission Date: 09/01/2018

Procedure Performed: Newborn evaluation

Attending Physician: Pravdah H. Jeppard, MD

The patient is a female, gestational age 39 weeks, 4 days, born vaginally in this facility, 09/01/18, 02:35.

IMPRESSION: Neonate was of a single birth, BWT 2,857 grams without significant OR procedures with a normal newborn diagnosis. 19″ long. Head circumference: 32 cm. Amniotic fluid: clear. Cord: 3 vessels. Evidence of a benign tumor of blood vessels due to malformed angioblastic tissues (vascular hamartomas) at right groin. Appears pale with poor skin turgor, mucousy, and transitional stool.
   Apgar Score: 1 min = 9; 5 min = 9. Heart rate: >100; Respiratory effort: Good, Muscle tone: Active, Response to catheter in nostril: Cough, Color: Body pink, extremities blue

MATERNAL HISTORY: 30 years old, G1, blood type O+, spontaneous labor, 16 h, 24 min, epidural anesthesia, HIV tested during pregnancy: neg

ADMINISTRATIONS: Hepatitis B, Peds Vaccine (Recomb) 5 mcg/0.5 mL given: 9/2/18 Newborn hearing screening: passed.

RECOMMENDATIONS: Follow-up in office 2 days

_____

Pravdah H. Jeppard, MD

PHJ/mg   D: 09/01/18 09:50:16   T: 09/05/18 12:55:01

Determine the most accurate CPT and/or HCPCS Level II code(s) and modifier(s), if appropriate.

_____

_____

_____

CIPHER, VICTORS & ASSOCIATES
A Complete Health Care Facility
234 MAIN STREET • ANYTOWN, FL 32711 • 407-555-1234

PATIENT: VANCE, NICOLE
ACCOUNT/EHR #:   VANCNI01
Procedure Date: 09/01/2018

Procedure Performed: Newborn routine pathological evaluation

Laboratory Technician: Constance L. Hall

Attending Physician: Pravdah H. Jeppard, MD

GENERAL CHEMISTRY:
     BILI TOTAL   7.1   (0.0–10.0)   M
     BILIRUBIN DIRECT   0.6   (0.0–0.6)   M

SEROLOGY/IMMUNOLOGY STUDIES:
     SYPHILIS   RPR   NON-REAC   (NON-REAC)

BLOOD BANK:
     ANTIBODY SCREENING AND TESTING   DIRECT ANTIGLOB   NEG

CORD BLOOD EVALUATION, COOMBS TEST:
     DIRECT ANTIGLOB   NEGATIVE

Constance L. Hall

CLH/mg   D: 09/01/18 09:50:16   T: 09/05/18 12:55:01

Determine the most accurate CPT and/or HCPCS Level II code(s) and modifier(s), if appropriate.

_____

_____

_____

CIPHER, VICTORS & ASSOCIATES
A Complete Health Care Facility
234 MAIN STREET • ANYTOWN, FL 32711 • 407-555-1234

PATIENT: KLAUSING, CLARENCE
ACCOUNT/EHR #:   KLAUCL01
Admission Date: 10/15/2018

Attending Physician: Tracy R. Stover, MD
Location: Emergency Department visit

HISTORY OF PRESENT ILLNESS: The patient is a 37-year-old white male with underlying acquired immunodeficiency syndrome, whom we initially evaluated in the emergency room this past Friday with complaints of right-sided back pain radiating to the anterior abdominal wall. On examination, blisters were noted compatible with the diagnosis of herpes zoster. The patient was started on oral Zovirax at a dose of 800 mg five times a day, plus Percocet for pain.

   Over the weekend, the patient began complaining of nausea, vomiting, and inability to continue taking the medications, accompanied by constipation. The patient called in today with these complaints, and we asked the patient to come in to the hospital for admission for intravenous therapy and management of this problem.

PAST MEDICAL HISTORY: He has been human immunodeficiency virus positive for 3½ years. The patient is originally from Chicago and has been 1½ years here. Currently, he is not being followed by any physician for his underlying problem. He cannot recall his last CD4 count.

   Prior medical problems include a history of oral candidiasis, but he denies any sexually transmitted diseases, PCP, or other opportunistic infections. At age 4, he had trauma to the left eye, causing his eye to be completely opacified. He has been previously treated with AZT and dD4T.

ALLERGIES: He has no known drug allergies.

SOCIAL HISTORY: He is divorced. He is currently living with a friend of many years. He has two children by his first wife, ages 10 and 8. He has smoked one pack of cigarettes per day for the last 15 years. He denies any alcohol use. He has a prior history of intravenous drug use—cocaine—but according to him, he has been clean for the last 3½ years. He has no pets. He has been disabled secondary to his eye trauma.

FAMILY HISTORY: The family history is essentially noncontributory.
PHYSICAL EXAM: Appearance: The patient is alert and oriented times three, complaining of pain.
HEAD: Normocephalic
EYES: The right eye pupil is reactive. The left eye is completely opacified secondary to prior trauma.
EARS: Unremarkable
NOSE: Unremarkable
MOUTH/TONGUE/PHARYNX: The patient has complete upper dentures. No oral lesions detected, i.e., candidiasis or oral hairy leukoplakia.
LUNGS: Clear to auscultation
CARDIOVASCULAR: The heart is rhythmic, with no murmurs or gallops.
ABDOMEN: His abdomen is flat, soft, nontender, with no palpable organomegaly.
GENITALIA: The examination is normal. He is circumcised. The testicles are bilaterally descended, with no lesions detected.

(Continued)

EXTREMITIES: Both lower extremities—good peripheral pulses and no edema
SKIN: He has numerous blisters and bullae on the right side of his body, approximately at the level of T10–T12, midline upper back going down to the anterior portion of the abdomen at the same level. Blisters with surrounding erythema. He has no other lesions.
NEUROLOGIC: Nonfocalized

DIAGNOSES:
1. Herpes zoster involving T10–T12 dermatome
2. Nausea/vomiting secondary to oral medications
3. History of being positive with the human immunodeficiency virus

PLAN/RECOMMENDATIONS:
1. Admit to the hospital for initiation of intravenous Acyclovir plus analgesics for pain management.
2. Domeboro compresses have also been ordered.

Tracy R. Stover, MD

TRS/mg   D: 10/15/18 09:50:16   T: 10/20/18 12:55:01

Determine the most accurate CPT and/or HCPCS Level II code(s) and modifier(s), if appropriate.

_____

_____

_____

CIPHER, VICTORS & ASSOCIATES
A Complete Health Care Facility
234 MAIN STREET • ANYTOWN, FL 32711 • 407-555-1234

PATIENT: KLAUSING, CLARENCE
ACCOUNT/EHR #:   KLAUCL01
Admission Date: 10/16/2018

Procedures/Testing: Pathology and lab

Laboratory Technician: Patrick Jensen

Attending Physician: Tracy R. Stover, MD

HEMATOLOGY:

WBC	4.2L	5.1	4.8–10.8 K/UL
RBC	5.12	5.15	4.7–6.1 M/UL
HGB	15.5	15.3	14–18 G/DL
HCT	44.9	43.8	42–52%
PLT	200,000/mm^3	200,000/mm^3	150,000–400,000/mm^3

IMMUNO/SEROL:

RPR	NR	NR = NON-REACTIVE
CMV IGM	PEND	NEG
TOXOPLASMOS IGM	PEND	NEG

Patrick Jensen

PJ/mg   D: 10/16/18 09:50:16   T: 10/16/18 12:55:01

Determine the most accurate CPT and/or HCPCS Level II code(s) and modifier(s), if appropriate.

_____

_____

_____

CIPHER, VICTORS & ASSOCIATES
A Complete Health Care Facility
234 MAIN STREET • ANYTOWN, FL 32711 • 407-555-1234

PATIENT: REILLY, BARBARA
ACCOUNT/EHR #:   REILBA01
Admission Date: 10/02/2018

Attending Physician: Charles L. Beckman, MD

HISTORY OF PRESENT ILLNESS: This is the first Barton Hospital admission for this 63-year-old female, with a known history of hypertension, depression, hypothyroidism, and kidney stones. The patient developed symptoms of frequency with dysuria for several days associated with mild flank discomfort. She has been taking cranberry juice, hoping for resolution of symptoms. The severe right flank pain occurred yesterday, associated with several bouts of vomiting. The patient presented to the emergency room, and at that time her evaluation included an IVP, which showed an obstructing calculus at the right ureterovesicular junction and with a urinalysis that was positive. The patient was admitted for intravenous fluid, pain control, and urologic evaluation.

PAST MEDICAL HISTORY: Includes hypertension, hypothyroidism, depression, and history of kidney stones—last bout several years ago. She has no history of myocardial infarction.

SOCIAL HISTORY: The patient is a truck driver. She is a heavy smoker with a 45-pack year history. She drinks daily.

REVIEW OF SYSTEMS: Negative for fever or chills. There is no hematuria, but there is dysuria and flank pain, as described in HPI. She has no chest pain, no exertional shortness of breath, no melena, no hematemesis, no headaches, or blurred vision.

PHYSICAL EXAM:

GENERAL: She is currently quite comfortable in bed. She is in no pain.

VITAL SIGNS: Blood pressure 120/80, she is afebrile, respirations 18 and not labored.

HEENT: Normocephalic, atraumatic. Pupils equal, round and reactive to light. Conjunctiva not injected.

Neck: Supple, no JVD, no carotid bruits Lungs: Clear

Cardiac: Normal S1, S2, without S3, S4, murmurs, gallops or rubs

Abdomen: Soft, normoactive bowel sounds. Negative hepatosplenomegaly.

Extremities: Without cyanosis, clubbing, or edema GU: Unremarkable

Lab Results: IVP report, as stated above. Her urinalysis is positive for white cells and red cells. Her electrolytes today showed a sodium of 136, potassium 3.6, chloride 97, bicarb 30, glucose 106, BUN 18, creatinine 1.5, calcium 8.5. White count 9.5

(Continued)

DIAGNOSES: Renal calculus with obstruction

ASSESSMENT:

1. This is a 63-year-old, who is presenting with a bout of renal calculus with obstruction, associated with a urinary tract infection. She has not passed a stone, as evidenced by repeat KUB, and she is tentatively scheduled for retrograde studies with laser lithotripsy in the a.m. by the urologist. In the interim, will continue with parenteral antibiotic coverage, IV fluid, and antibiotics.
2. Hypothyroidism. Will resume Synthroid replacement.
3. History of hypertension, currently controlled. Continue with antihypertensive therapy.
4. Perform an EKG and chest x-ray, 2 views, to complete pre-op evaluation.
5. NPO pending surgery.
6. Control patient's blood pressure with IV Aldomet until postoperatively.

Charles L. Beckman, MD

CLB/mg   D: 10/02/18 09:50:16   T: 10/05/18 12:55:01

Determine the most accurate CPT and/or HCPCS Level II code(s) and modifier(s), if appropriate.

_____

_____

_____

CIPHER, VICTORS & ASSOCIATES
A Complete Health Care Facility
234 MAIN STREET • ANYTOWN, FL 32711 • 407-555-1234

PATIENT: REILLY, BARBARA
ACCOUNT/EHR #:   REILBA01
DATE: 10/03/2018

Attending Physician: Charles L. Beckman, MD

Reason for Exam: Stent placement
Radiologist: Neal R. Williams, MD

EXAMINATION:
Abdomen Single View
Two films are submitted. Supine view of the abdomen including pelvis demonstrates contrast material within the urinary bladder, which is smooth in contour with no filling defects seen.
    Film #1: A nonspecific bowel gas pattern and faint calcification over the right hemipelvis.
    Film #2: A double pigtail ureteral stent has been placed. The proximal pigtail ureteral stent appears to be somewhat low in position and is likely in the proximal ureter. The stones have apparently been removed.

IMPRESSION: Contrast material has cleared the kidneys such that status of the right renal collecting structures again cannot be ascertained. Suggest a right renal sonogram in further evaluation of suspected right-sided hydronephrosis. A right retrograde pyelogram could also be obtained to determine the site of suspected ureteral obstruction.

Neal R. Williams, MD

NRW/mg   D: 10/03/18 09:50:16   T: 10/04/18 12:55:01

Determine the most accurate CPT and/or HCPCS Level II code(s) and modifier(s), if appropriate.

_____

_____

_____

CIPHER, VICTORS & ASSOCIATES
A Complete Health Care Facility
234 MAIN STREET • ANYTOWN, FL 32711 • 407-555-1234

PATIENT: REILLY, BARBARA
ACCOUNT/EHR #:   REILBA01
DATE: 10/03/2018

Attending Physician: Charles L. Beckman, MD

Reason for Exam: MD order—pre-op clearance
Radiologist: Neal R. Williams, MD

EXAMINATION:

1. Chest two views
   Chest—AP and lateral views.
   Clinical history states evaluation: kidney stone with obstruction.
   Slightly elongated thoracic aorta. Prominent left ventricle. No pulmonary vascular congestion. No acute inflammatory infiltrates in the lungs.
   There are orthopedic screws transfixing the acromioclavicular joint, probably related with old shoulder fracture.

2. ECG, 12 leads
   Unremarkable

Neal R. Williams, MD

NRW/mg   D: 10/03/18 09:50:16   T: 10/04/18 12:55:01

Determine the most accurate CPT and/or HCPCS Level II code(s) and modifier(s), if appropriate.

_____

_____

_____

CIPHER, VICTORS & ASSOCIATES
A Complete Health Care Facility
234 MAIN STREET • ANYTOWN, FL 32711 • 407-555-1234

PATIENT: REILLY, BARBARA
ACCOUNT/EHR #:   REILBA01
DATE: 10/03/2018

Attending Physician: Charles L. Beckman, MD

Reason for Exam: Groin pain
Radiologist: Neal R. Williams, MD

EXAMINATION: IVP with tomo
                                    Intravenous pyelogram

There are several calcifications of the pelvis. There is one that is somewhat triangular shaped and measures approximately 8.0 mm in length and approximately 5 mm in diameter in the region of the right side of the pelvis in the proximal course of the right ureter.

There is prompt function on the left side and prompt filling of a normal-appearing collecting system with dumping into the urinary bladder.

The right kidney has not begun functioning, even on the 30-minute delayed film. I suspect that this is because the calcification described above represents an obstructing distal right ureterovesical junction calculus.

We plan to obtain additional radiographs, and addendum reports will be issued.

_____

Neal R. Williams, MD

NRW/mg   D: 10/03/18 09:50:16   T: 10/04/18 12:55:01

Determine the most accurate CPT and/or HCPCS Level II code(s) and modifier(s), if appropriate.

_____

_____

_____

CIPHER, VICTORS & ASSOCIATES
A Complete Health Care Facility
234 MAIN STREET • ANYTOWN, FL 32711 • 407-555-1234

PATIENT: REILLY, BARBARA
ACCOUNT/EHR #:   REILBA01
DATE: 10/03/2018

Attending Physician: Charles L. Beckman, MD

Preoperative Diagnosis: Right ureteral calculus

Postoperative Diagnosis: Same

Operative Procedure: Cystoscopy, right retrograde pyelogram, ureteroscopy, Holmium laser lithotripsy, and double-J stent placement

Surgeon: Sarah Lyndale, MD

Assistant: None

Anesthesiologist: Lorenzo Garrett, MD Anesthesia: General

DESCRIPTION OF OPERATION: The patient was prepped and draped in the usual manner after induction of general anesthesia. Examination of the anterior urethra using a 21 French cystourethroscope revealed no anterior lesions or strictures. Examination of the bladder revealed normal bladder mucosa; however, bulging of the intramural ureter was prominent on the right side. After the bladder was examined, using the 30° and 70° lens of the cystoscope, a #8 French cone-tipped catheter was inserted in the right ureteral orifice. Under fluoroscopic control, the contrast material was instilled. Stone was noted to be impacted in the distal intramural ureter with proximal hydronephrosis. Next, a 0.35 glide wire followed by a guide wire introducer and a second glide wire were introduced under fluoroscopic and x-ray control. The balloon dilators were used, 4 cm in size, to dilate the intramural ureter. The miniureteroscope was then inserted under direct vision, and the stone was identified in the distal ureter, impacted in the wall. Using the Holmium dye laser, lithotripsy at 3–4 watts range for 414 seconds at 2,070 Hertz with a total joules of 489.2, the stone fragmented and most of the stone material washed out and could not be easily retrieved. The stone appeared to be uric acid in nature. At this point, although no stone fragments could actually be basketed, a 7 × 26 double-J ureteral stent was placed under fluoroscopic and x-ray control and noted to be in the proximal upper ureter, which was quite tortuous because of previous hydronephrosis, and in the bladder. The string was brought out externally. The bladder was then emptied. A #15 French Foley catheter was passed. The patient was brought to the recovery room in fair condition.

Sarah Lyndale, MD

SL/mg   D: 10/03/18 09:50:16   T: 10/04/18 12:55:01

Determine the most accurate CPT and/or HCPCS Level II code(s) and modifier(s), if appropriate.

_____

_____

_____

CIPHER, VICTORS & ASSOCIATES
A Complete Health Care Facility
234 MAIN STREET • ANYTOWN, FL 32711 • 407-555-1234

PATIENT: REILLY, BARBARA
ACCOUNT/EHR: REILBA01
DATE: 10/03/18

Attending Physician: Charles L. Beckman, MD

Preoperative Diagnosis: Right ureteral calculus

Postoperative Diagnosis: Same

Operative Procedure: Cystoscopy, right retrograde pyelogram, ureteroscopy, Holmium laser lithotripsy, and double-J stent placement

Surgeon: Sarah Lyndale, MD

Assistant: None

Anesthesia: General

Anesthesiologist: Lorenzo Garrett, MD

DESCRIPTION OF OPERATION: The patient was prepped and draped in the usual manner after induction of general anesthesia. Examination of the anterior urethra using a 21 French cystourethroscope revealed no anterior lesions or strictures. Examination of the bladder revealed normal bladder mucosa; however, bulging of the intramural ureter was prominent on the right side. After the bladder was examined, using the 30° and 70° lens of the cystoscope, a #8 French cone-tipped catheter was inserted in the right ureteral orifice. Under fluoroscopic control, the contrast material was instilled. Stone was noted to be impacted in the distal intramural ureter with proximal hydronephrosis. Next, a 0.35 glide wire followed by a guide wire introducer and a second glide wire were introduced under fluoroscopic and x-ray control. The balloon dilators were used, 4 cm in size, to dilate the intramural ureter. The miniureteroscope was then inserted under direct vision, and the stone was identified in the distal ureter, impacted in the wall. Using the Holmium dye laser, lithotripsy at 3–4 watts range for 414 seconds at 2,070 Hertz with a total joules of 489.2, the stone fragmented and most of the stone material washed out and could not be easily retrieved. The stone appeared to be uric acid in nature. At this point, although no stone fragments could actually be basketed, a 7 × 26 double-J ureteral stent was placed under fluoroscopic and x-ray control and noted to be in the proximal upper ureter, which was quite tortuous because of previous hydronephrosis, and in the bladder. The string was brought out externally. The bladder was then emptied. A #15 French Foley catheter was passed.

    Vital signs were maintained at appropriate level.

    The patient was awakened from the general anesthesia and brought to the recovery room in fair condition.

Lorenzo Garrett, MD

LG/mg D: 10/03/18 09:50:16   T: 10/04/18 12:55:01

Determine the most accurate CPT and/or HCPCS Level II code(s) and modifier(s), if appropriate.

_____

_____

_____

CIPHER, VICTORS & ASSOCIATES
A Complete Health Care Facility
234 MAIN STREET • ANYTOWN, FL 32711 • 407-555-1234

PATIENT: REILLY, BARBARA
ACCOUNT/EHR #:   REILBA01
DATE: 10/03/2018

Attending Physician: Charles L. Beckman, MD

Scheduled Medications: MD order

MEDICATIONS:
    Levofloxacin, 250 mg, IV
    Ciprofloxacin 500 mg, IV (Cipro)
    Compazine, 10 mg, IM
    Meperidine HCL 75 mg, IM
    Hydroxyzine HCL 100 mg, IM

David C. Samuels, RN

DCS/mg   D: 10/03/18 09:50:16   T: 10/04/18 12:55:01

Determine the most accurate CPT and/or HCPCS Level II code(s) and modifier(s), if appropriate.

_____

_____

_____

CIPHER, VICTORS & ASSOCIATES
A Complete Health Care Facility
234 MAIN STREET • ANYTOWN, FL 32711 • 407-555-1234

PATIENT:	FLEMINGTON, EUGENE
ACCOUNT/EHR #:	FLEMEU01
DATE:	11/11/2018
Attending Physician:	Pravdah H. Jeppard, MD
TRANSPORTATION:	Acute care—MD order
RECEIVING FACILITY:	Harrison Medical Center
SENDING FACILITY:	Barton Hospital
DIAGNOSIS:	Hyponatremia, hypopotassemia, fever, anemia
TRANSPORTATION PROTOCOL:	Pediatric ALS, nonemergency
PATIENT AGE:	17 months
MILEAGE:	12

Joleen L. Abernathy, EMT

JLA/mg   D: 11/11/18 09:50:16   T: 11/11/18 12:55:01

Determine the most accurate CPT and/or HCPCS Level II code(s) and modifier(s), if appropriate.

_____

_____

_____

CIPHER, VICTORS & ASSOCIATES
A Complete Health Care Facility
234 MAIN STREET • ANYTOWN, FL 32711 • 407-555-1234

PATIENT: FLEMINGTON, EUGENE
ACCOUNT/EHR #:   FLEMEU01
DATE: 11/11/2018

Attending Physician: Pravdah H. Jeppard, MD

HISTORY OF PRESENT ILLNESS: The patient is a 17-month-old male brought in by ambulance. Pt has fever over 101°, nonproductive cough, and vomiting for the past 6 days. He was seen by his primary care physician, Dr. Golden, and started on antibiotics for otitis media. Also, Dr. Golden notes that the child's abdomen has been getting distended.

    Patient is developmentally on track for age, with no signs of impairment. Since illness began, patient is noted to be lethargic. Decreased appetite 6 days, when started to get sick.

ALLERGIES: NKA

PHYSICAL EXAMINATION: Patient is alert and crying. Abdomen is distended. Tympanic membrane is diffused. Bowel sounds are hypoactive; last BM 6 days ago.
    Pupils are equal and reactive. Breath sounds are clear, breathing regular.
    Skin is warm, heart rhythm is regular, peripheral pulses normal, edema none.
    HR 174, R 36, T 100.4°

DIAGNOSIS: Hyponatremia, hypopotassemia, fever, anemia

TESTING/PROCEDURES: CBC, comprehensive metabolic panel performed. Results pending.

RECOMMENDATIONS: Admission to pediatric unit for observation

_____

Pravdah H. Jeppard, MD

PHJ/mg   D: 11/11/18 09:50:16   T: 11/11/18 12:55:01

Determine the most accurate CPT and/or HCPCS Level II code(s) and modifier(s), if appropriate.

_____

_____

_____

CIPHER, VICTORS & ASSOCIATES
A Complete Health Care Facility
234 MAIN STREET • ANYTOWN, FL 32711 • 407-555-1234

PATIENT: FLEMINGTON, EUGENE
ACCOUNT/EHR #:   FLEMEU01
DATE: 11/12/2018

Radiologist: Pedro L. Pacheco, MD

Attending Physician: Pravdah H. Jeppard, MD

EXAMINATION: Chest and abdomen
CLINICAL HISTORY: Fever

CHEST: AP supine and lateral films demonstrate no evidence of alveolar infiltrate or consolidation or pleural effusion. The mediastinal structures are not enlarged. There is very mild increase in central bronchovascular markings. There is no evidence of focal destructive bone lesion.

IMPRESSION: No infiltrate

ABDOMEN: Supine and erect films demonstrate mild to moderate dilatation of loops of small bowel with short air/fluid levels on the erect film. The large bowel is within normal limits in size but is visualized to the level of the splenic flexure. There is no air visualized in the remainder of the colon. The findings are not specific but consistent with ileus. Further clinical correlation is advised. There is no evidence of focal destructive bone lesion. There is no suspicious calcification in the upper abdomen.

IMPRESSIONS: Abdominal bowel pattern, not specific, consistent with ileus

---

Pedro L. Pacheco, MD

PLP/mg D: 11/12/18 09:50:16 T: 11/12/18 12:55:01

Determine the most accurate CPT and/or HCPCS Level II code(s) and modifier(s), if appropriate.

_____

_____

_____

CIPHER, VICTORS & ASSOCIATES
A Complete Health Care Facility
234 MAIN STREET • ANYTOWN, FL 32711 • 407-555-1234

PATIENT:	FLEMINGTON, EUGENE
ACCOUNT/EHR #:	FLEMEU01
DATE:	11/12/2018

Attending Physician: Pravdah H. Jeppard, MD

PATIENT SERVICES:
   IV fluid replacement for dehydration, intravenous, 58 minutes
   Continuous pulse oximetry
   Therapeutic warm water enema for intussusception

_____

Renee K. McDonald, RN

RKM/mg   D: 11/12/18 09:50:16   T: 11/12/18 12:55:01

Determine the most accurate CPT and/or HCPCS Level II code(s) and modifier(s), if appropriate.

_____

_____

_____

CIPHER, VICTORS & ASSOCIATES
A Complete Health Care Facility
234 MAIN STREET • ANYTOWN, FL 32711 • 407-555-1234

Patient Name: GERRERRA, RAUL
ACCOUNT/EHR #:   GERRRA01
DATE: 10/27/2018

Physical Therapist: Kevin Bryant

Attending Physician: Harvey Bradshaw, MD

DX: Postsurgical carpal tunnel (CT) release LT
TYPE OF THERAPY: Occupational therapy (hand) B. I. W. × 3 week

VISIT # 1/6:
Reported Pain Level: 5/10
Patient reports: "I am still having pain in my hand and fingers."

1. Ultrasound for 6 minutes, 3 MHz; 0.4 W/cm2 100% to scar at LT CT area
2. Massage: Retrograde, 3 minutes to LT hand
3. Manual therapy: soft tissue mobilization, 5 minutes to scar at LT wrist
4. AROM and stretching, 3 minutes
5. Therapeutic exercise: 12 minutes tendon glides, joint blocking, digit extension, median nerve glides and desensitization with cold towels (tolerated up until #6)

Pain level: 4–5/10. Pt still with heavy scar tissue adhesions in CT area. Pt still having pain in fingertips and numbness, reportedly up arm and into his neck.

_____

Kevin Bryant

KB/mg D: 10/27/18 09:50:16 T: 10/29/18 12:55:01

Determine the most accurate CPT and/or HCPCS Level II code(s) and modifier(s), if appropriate.

_____

_____

_____

CIPHER, VICTORS & ASSOCIATES
A Complete Health Care Facility
234 MAIN STREET • ANYTOWN, FL 32711 • 407-555-1234

Patient Name: GERRERRA, RAUL
ACCOUNT/EHR #:   GERRERA01
DATE: 11/03/2018

Physical Therapist: Kevin Bryant

Attending Physician: Harvey Bradshaw, MD

DX: Postsurgical carpal tunnel Release LT
TYPE OF THERAPY: Occupational therapy (hand) B. I. W. × 3 weeks

VISIT # 3/6
Reported pain level: 5/10
Patient reports: "The scar still feels very hard, and when I rest my palm on something, it is very uncomfortable."

1. Cold pack
2. Fluidotherapy (dry whirlpool): 15 minutes LT hand
3. Massage: Retrograde, 4 minutes to LT hand and wrist
4. Manual therapy: soft tissue mobilization, scar tissue 8 minutes MFR to scar at LT wrist
5. AROM, AAROM, PROM, and stretching: gentle carpal stretches, 4 minutes
6. Therapeutic exercise: 10 minutes of wrist AROM, joint blocking, place + hold FDS glides, rubber band–finger extensions, desensitizing (rods and rice bucket)

Pain level: 4/10. Pt demonstrated decreased scar tissue adhesions at wrist scar. Pt did not tolerate rubber band exercises well.

_____

Kevin Bryant

KB/mg   D: 11/03/18 09:50:16   T: 11/05/18 12:55:01

Determine the most accurate CPT and/or HCPCS Level II code(s) and modifier(s), if appropriate.

_____

_____

_____

CIPHER, VICTORS & ASSOCIATES
A Complete Health Care Facility
234 MAIN STREET • ANYTOWN, FL 32711 • 407-555-1234

Patient Name: PHELPS, MAXINE
ACCOUNT/EHR #:   PHELMA01
DATE: 12/13/2018

Attending Physician: Yamira E. Newadha, MD
Location: Office

HISTORY OF PRESENT ILLNESS: This is a 51-year-old female who a month ago noted a lump in her right breast (8 o'clock position of the right breast just outside the areola). This prompted bilateral screening mammography. The mammo demonstrated a linear area of increased density and architectural distortion at the 12 o'clock position in the right periareolar region.

    This was suspicious mammographically, and a biopsy of this was recommended. The patient had follow-up ultrasound as well. The ultrasound demonstrated a lobulated cyst of 3 mm at the 8 o'clock position corresponding to the patient's area of palpable abnormality. No other lesions were noted.

    Due to the mammogram, the patient has an incidental finding of an area of increased density at the 12 o'clock position and requires biopsy. This is not appreciable on examination and requires needle localization and excisional biopsy, for which she is here today.

    The patient has no family history of breast cancer. Age of menarche 13. She was pregnant three times with one child, first child born at age 20.

PAST MEDICAL HISTORY: No coronary disease, hypertension, or diabetes
PAST SURGICAL HISTORY: None
MEDICATIONS: None
ALLERGIES: None
SOCIAL HISTORY: The patient does not smoke, does not drink. No history of drug use.

PHYSICAL EXAMINATION:
Breasts: The patient examined in erect and supine. Both breasts are symmetric. There is no skin dimpling. There is no nipple inversion. There is no mass appreciated in either breast with careful attention paid to the right breast overlying the 8 o'clock region as well as the 12 o'clock region. Again, no mass was appreciated. She has no axillary, cervical, supraclavicular, or infraclavicular adenopathy notes.
Lungs: Clear
Heart: Regular rhythm
IMPRESSION: Right breast mass

This is a 51-year-old who has an incidental finding of an area of increased density at the 12 o'clock position of the right breast. This cannot be appreciated on physical examination. She will require needle loc/excisional biopsy. The indication, alternatives, and complications of the procedure have been discussed with this patient. She understands and wishes to proceed.

_____

Yamira E. Newadha, MD

YEM/mg   D: 12/13/18 12:55:01   T: 12/18/18 09:50:16

Determine the most accurate CPT and/or HCPCS Level II code(s) and modifier(s), if appropriate.

_____

_____

_____

CIPHER, VICTORS & ASSOCIATES
A Complete Health Care Facility
234 MAIN STREET • ANYTOWN, FL 32711 • 407-555-1234

PATIENT NAME: PHELPS, MAXINE
ACCOUNT/EHR #:   PHELMA01
DATE: 12/14/2018

Radiologist: Harry O. Leu, MD

Attending Physician: Yamira E. Newadha, MD

Examination of: Right breast needle localization

CLINICAL HISTORY: Ridge-like area of increased density in upper right periareolar region; for preoperative localization. A signed informed consent was obtained from the patient prior to the procedure, after an explanation of the relative benefits, risks, and potential side effects.

 After sterile preparation, a 3-mm Homer Mammalok needle/wire combination was advanced percutaneously via a superior approach, and its tips were localized at the site of a ridge-like density in the upper periareolar region; an alphanumeric grid was utilized. The wire was advanced through the needle and secured in place. Repeat views confirmed the localization of needle and wire tips to be at the site of the ridge-like density.

 The patient tolerated the procedure well, without immediate complications, and left the mammography suite with needle and wire secured in place.

IMPRESSION: Percutaneous needle/wire localization of ridge-like right upper periareolar density

---

Harry O. Leu, MD

HOL/mg D: 12/14/18 12:55:01 T: 12/18/18 09:50:16

Determine the most accurate CPT and/or HCPCS Level II code(s) and modifier(s), if appropriate.

_____

_____

_____

CIPHER, VICTORS & ASSOCIATES
A Complete Health Care Facility
234 MAIN STREET • ANYTOWN, FL 32711 • 407-555-1234

PATIENT NAME: PHELPS, MAXINE
ACCOUNT/EHR #:   PHELMA01
DATE: 12/15/2018

Preoperative Diagnosis: Right breast mass
Postoperative Diagnosis: Same (pending pathology)
Operation: Excision of right breast mass, intermediate wound closure—4 cm

Surgeon: Roweena L. Macomba, MD

Assistant: None
Anesthesiologist: Terence Abernathy MD
Anesthesia: MAC/1% lidocaine diluted 50% with bicarbonate (10 cc)

HISTORY: This is a 51-year-old female admitted to the minor surgery suite for excision of a 3-cm palpable nodule in the superficial aspect of the right breast in the 12 o'clock axis near the periphery. The indications, alternatives, and possible complications were reviewed, and consent was obtained.

PROCEDURE: With the patient in the supine position, the area in question was prepped and draped in the usual sterile fashion using Betadine. After adequate IV sedation, 1% lidocaine without epinephrine was used to infiltrate the soft tissues at that level to create a field block.

    An elliptical incision was made about the lesion itself, considering its intimate association with the overlying skin. The 4-cm incision was deepened into the subcutaneous space. The mass was excised in its entirety with a rim of normal appearing breast, fat, and surrounding skin. Adequate hemostasis was secured within the depths of the wound. The wound was closed in layers. The deeper breast tissue was approximated using interrupted 3-0 chromic sutures. The subcuticular layer was approximated using interrupted 4-0 Biosyn sutures. The skin edges were closed using 4-0 Vicryl in the subcuticular space in a continuous fashion. Mastisol and Steri-Strips were applied. A dressing was applied. The procedure was terminated. Needle, sponge, and instrument counts were correct. Estimated blood loss was minimal.

DISPOSITION: The patient tolerated the procedure and was discharged from the minor operating department in satisfactory condition.

Roweena L. Macomba, MD

RLM/mg   D: 12/15/18 12:55:01   T: 12/18/18 09:50:16

Determine the most accurate CPT and/or HCPCS Level II code(s) and modifier(s), if appropriate.

_____

_____

_____

CIPHER, VICTORS & ASSOCIATES
A Complete Health Care Facility
234 MAIN STREET • ANYTOWN, FL 32711 • 407-555-1234

PATIENT NAME: PHELPS, MAXINE
ACCOUNT/EHR #:   PHELMA01
DATE: 12/15/2018

Preoperative Diagnosis: Right breast mass
Postoperative Diagnosis: Same (pending pathology)
Operation: Excision of right breast mass, intermediate wound closure—4 cm

Surgeon: Roweena L. Macomba, MD

Assistant: None
Anesthesiologist: Terence Abernathy, MD
Anesthesia: MAC/1% lidocaine diluted 50% with bicarbonate (10 cc)

HISTORY: This is a 51-year-old female admitted to the minor surgery suite for excision of a 3-cm palpable nodule in the superficial aspect of the right breast in the 12 o'clock axis near the periphery. The indications, alternatives, and possible complications were reviewed, and consent was obtained.

PROCEDURE: With the patient in the supine position, the area in question was prepped and draped in the usual sterile fashion using Betadine. After adequate IV sedation, 1% lidocaine without epinephrine was used to infiltrate the soft tissues at that level to create a field block.
    Vital signs were maintained at an acceptable level.
    The patient tolerated the procedure and was discharged from the minor operating department in satisfactory condition.

Terence Abernathy, MD

TA/mg   D: 12/15/18 12:55:01   T: 12/18/18 09:50:16

Determine the most accurate CPT and/or HCPCS Level II code(s) and modifier(s), if appropriate.

_____

_____

_____

CIPHER, VICTORS & ASSOCIATES
A Complete Health Care Facility
234 MAIN STREET • ANYTOWN, FL 32711 • 407-555-1234

PATIENT NAME:	BATCHELDER, LINDA
ACCOUNT/EHR #:	BATCLI01
DATE:	11/29/18

Consulting Physician:	Robert R. Forester, MD
Attending Physician:	Giselle R. Usher, MD
Reason for Consultation:	Retroperitoneal abscess

HISTORY OF PRESENT ILLNESS: The patient is well known to me from her earlier hospitalization. This is a 73-year-old white female with a past history of metastatic follicular carcinoma of the thyroid who had been recently treated for superior vena cava syndrome and obstruction with anticoagulation. At that time, she developed a febrile illness, at which time infectious diseases department was consulted.

It turned out that an infectious disease workup was negative, and it was felt that she had an underlying autoimmune-type basis to her fever and was put on prednisone. On the prednisone, her fever resolved and all the other symptoms resolved, and she had been doing quite well.

In the interim, it was determined that she did have metastatic thyroid carcinoma disease, and so she was admitted on 11/29/18 for radioactive iodine therapy. However, during the physical examination at the clinic yesterday, Dr. Harrel discovered an abdominal mass. The patient had, totally, no symptoms from this mass. She denied any history of trauma; denied fevers, chills, sweats, or other systemic symptoms. She had been doing quite well actually since going home on low-dose maintenance prednisone therapy.

A CT was done that showed a retroperitoneal mass, and a CT-guided biopsy was done this morning that revealed rank pus. She subsequently underwent drainage of 500 cc of grossly purulent material, described as pea-green soup. We are now asked to consult to help with the antibiotic management. The fluid did not apparently appear to be foul smelling but did look green and thick.

The patient, again, continues to deny any fevers, chills, sweats, or systemic symptoms. At the time the subsequent drainage was done today, two drainage catheters were placed into the abscess. She experienced hypotension, nausea, and diaphoresis, which resolved with some fluid boluses. She is now in the intermediate care for further management because of the episode of hypotension and a concern of sepsis.

Again, on talking to the patient, she denies any history of trauma to the area. She denies any history of abdominal pain, fevers, chills, sweats, nausea, vomiting, diarrhea, or systemic symptoms. She has no past history of diverticulitis or diverticular disease. She has not had any diarrhea or abdominal pain.

The preliminary gram stain results show a few white blood cells; no organisms. Cultures are pending.

Her white count at this time was 12,800, with a left shift, but she is on oral prednisone. The sedimentation rate was 42. The PT was 12.4 and the PTT is 25. The chemistries are remarkable for a glucose of 115, albumin of 3.6, and cholesterol of 235; the liver function tests were normal.

PAST MEDICAL HISTORY: As stated, the past medical history is significant for follicular cell carcinoma of the thyroid, status post subtotal thyroidectomy, 10/08/08; status post right internal jugular repair from tumor invasion into the jugular; and biopsy of mediastinal metastatic disease. The patient also has a history of superior vena cava syndrome, status post her carcinoma. She is status post mastectomy for breast carcinoma in 07/05. She has post thoracotomy syndrome in 03/08, with fever and effusion, which resolved. She has a history of a small clot at the site of the venogram entry of the left leg. She had been on Coumadin and may possibly have had a retroperitoneal bleed. She also has a history of hypocalcemia secondary to her thyroidectomy and is on calcium maintenance.

(Continued)

MEDICATIONS: Her medications at this time include Nolvadex 10 mg po bid, Os-Cal 1,000 mg po tid, Rocaltrol 0.25 mcg po bid, and prednisone 10 mg po qam.

ALLERGIES: She is allergic to penicillin and sulfa.

REVIEW OF SYSTEMS: As stated, the review of systems is essentially unremarkable. She denies fevers, chills, sweats, abdominal pain, nausea, vomiting, and diarrhea. The fevers had resolved on the prednisone.

PHYSICAL EXAM: B/P: 100/60; P 90; T 98.4

APPEARANCE: Alert, oriented, 73-year-old female lying in bed, in no acute distress.
HEAD: Normocephalic, atraumatic.
EYES: Pupils are equal, round, and reactive to light and accommodation. Extraocular movements full.
MOUTH/TONGUE/PHARYNX: Throat clear, no thrush or exudates.
NECK: Supple. No stiffness.
LUNGS: Few crackles at both bases. Scattered rhonchi bilaterally. Good air exchange.
CARDIOVASCULAR: Regular rhythm. Normal S1 and S2. No murmurs.
ABDOMEN: Soft. Some tenderness in the right middle quadrant, with two drainage catheters in place and no definite mass appreciated at this time.
EXTREMITIES: No joint effusions or deformities. Trace edema of the ankles.
SKIN: Some scattered ecchymoses. No significant rashes or lesions noted.
NEUROLOGIC: Grossly normal. No focal deficits.

IMPRESSION:
1. Retroperitoneal mass appears to be an abscess; may have been secondary to a possible bleed that secondarily got infected. She has had no preceding systemic signs of infection or trauma to the area. Other etiologies would be some type of relationship to possible abdominal disease, but she has no history of diverticular disease and this would be less likely. The most likely organisms to consider, again, would be Staphylococcus, Streptococcus, anaerobes, and gut flora.
2. Penicillin allergic.
3. Metastatic thyroid follicular carcinoma; to receive radiation therapy.

PLAN/RECOMMENDATIONS:
1. Will start her empirically on IV antibiotic therapy with clindamycin and Cipro, which should cover Staphylococcus, Streptococcus, anaerobes, and gram-negatives, until more culture results are known.
2. Monitor vital signs carefully and supportive care if she becomes hypotensive again.
3. Will check blood cultures as well as urine culture.
4. Would not give radioactive iodine at this time until we have cleared up her infection.

Thanks for this consultation. Will follow.

Robert R. Forester, MD

RRF/mg   D: 11/29/18 12:55:01   T: 11/30/18 09:50:16

CC: Giselle R. Usher, MD

Determine the most accurate CPT and/or HCPCS Level II code(s) and modifier(s), if appropriate.

_____

_____

_____

CIPHER, VICTORS & ASSOCIATES
A Complete Health Care Facility
234 MAIN STREET • ANYTOWN, FL 32711 • 407-555-1234

PATIENT NAME: OSGOOD, BENITA
ACCOUNT/EHR #:   OSGOBE01
DATE: 09/15/2018

Attending Physician: Roland F. LaScala, MD

INTERVAL HISTORY: The patient is a 29-year-old female G1 P0 who presents at term with regular uterine contractions. The patient's antepartum course has been uncomplicated to date. Sonogram and amniocentesis were normal. GBS culture was negative.

PHYSICAL EXAMINATION:

HEENT:	Unremarkable
Neck:	Supple
Chest:	Clear
Abd:	Guarded, soft
Contractions:	Q3–4 minutes, 40–50 seconds duration
Membrane:	Ruptured @ 2:45 with clear fluids
Vaginal discharge:	"Show"
Vaginal exam:	3 cm dilated Eff: 80%, Sta: −2
Vital Signs:	T98.7, P82, R20, FHR 130s, Location LLQ
Fetal Status:	Reassuring
Assessment:	Term pregnancy, in spontaneous labor
PLAN:	Admit, expectant management for delivery

Roland F. LaScala, MD

RFL/mg   D: 09/15/2018 12:55:01   T: 09/17/2018 09:50:16

Determine the most accurate CPT and/or HCPCS Level II code(s) and modifier(s), if appropriate.

_____

_____

_____

CIPHER, VICTORS & ASSOCIATES
A Complete Health Care Facility
234 MAIN STREET • ANYTOWN, FL 32711 • 407-555-1234

PATIENT NAME: OSGOOD, BENITA
ACCOUNT/EHR #:   OSGOBE01
DATE: 09/15/2018

Attending Physician: Roland F. LaScala, MD

Admission to Labor and Delivery

PATHOLOGY AND LABORATORY:
CBC w/diff & PLT
Hold Clot
Urinalysis, qualitative

MEDICATIONS:
IV Ringer's Lactate, 1,000 ml @ 125 mL/hr
Oxytocin 10 units in 500 ml, D5W (premixed) to run via infusion device
Fentanyl 200 mcg/100 mL + Ropivacaine (naropin) 0.2% 100 mL premixed bag

_____

Roland F. LaScala, MD

RFL/mg   D: 09/15/2018 12:55:01   T: 09/17/2018 09:50:16

Determine the most accurate CPT and/or HCPCS Level II code(s) and modifier(s), if appropriate, for Pathology and Lab.

_____

_____

_____

CIPHER, VICTORS & ASSOCIATES
A Complete Health Care Facility
234 MAIN STREET • ANYTOWN, FL 32711 • 407-555-1234

Patient Name: OSGOOD, BENITA
ACCOUNT/EHR #:   OSGOBE01
DATE: 09/15/2018

Attending Physician: Roland F. LaScala, MD

ANESTHESIA:	Epidural
TYPE OF DELIVERY:	NSVD
CONDITION OF PERINEUM:	MLE
EPISIOTOMY:	Midline preformed
VAGINA/CERVIX:	Intact
DELIVERED:	Live, single born, female, weight 6 lb, 4 oz
TYPE OF STIMULATION:	Mouth suction
CONDITION:	Good
BIRTH INJURY:	None
APGAR RATING:	1 min = 9
	5 min = 9

Roland F. LaScala, MD

RFL/mg   D: 09/15/2018 12:55:01   T: 09/20/2018 09:50:16

Determine the most accurate CPT and/or HCPCS Level II code(s) and modifier(s), if appropriate.

_____

_____

_____

CIPHER, VICTORS & ASSOCIATES
A Complete Health Care Facility
234 MAIN STREET • ANYTOWN, FL 32711 • 407-555-1234

PATIENT NAME: OSGOOD, BENITA
ACCOUNT/EHR #:   OSGOBE01
DATE: 09/15/2018

Anesthesiologist: Sabine Suwani, MD

Anesthesia: Epidural
TYPE OF DELIVERY: NSVD
CONDITION OF PERINEUM: MLE
EPISIOTOMY: Midline preformed
VAGINA/CERVIX: Intact
DELIVERED: Live, single born, female, weight 6 lb, 4 oz
TYPE OF STIMULATION: Mouth suction
CONDITION: Good
BIRTH INJURY: None
APGAR RATING: 1 min = 9
     5 min = 9

Sabine Suwani, MD

SS/mg   D: 09/15/2018 12:55:01   T: 09/20/2018 09:50:16

Determine the most accurate CPT and/or HCPCS Level II code(s) and modifier(s), if appropriate.

_____

_____

_____

CIPHER, VICTORS & ASSOCIATES
A Complete Health Care Facility
234 MAIN STREET • ANYTOWN, FL 32711 • 407-555-1234

PATIENT NAME: COOKE, CARLEEN
ACCOUNT/EHR #:   COOKCA01
DATE: 01/05/2018

Indications: Ulcerative enterocolitis
Procedure: Colonoscopy

Attending Physician: Dean Sing, MD

Instrument: Olympus video colonoscope CF 100L
Anesthesia: Versed 4 mg; Demerol 75 mg MAC $<$ 30 min

HISTORY: This is a 71-year-old female admitted to the ambulatory surgical center for a colonoscopy. Due to her chronic enterocolitis, she is at high risk for a malignancy of the colon, and therefore, this screening is being done. She has been informed of the nature of the procedure, the risks, and the consequences, as well as told of alternative procedures. She consents to the procedure.

PROCEDURE: The patient is placed in the left lateral decubitus position. The rectal exam reveals normal sphincter tone and no masses. A colonoscope is introduced into the rectum and advanced to the distal sigmoid colon. Due to a marked fixation and severe angulation of the rectosigmoid colon, the scope could not be advanced any further and the procedure was aborted.

On withdrawal, no masses or polyps are noted, and the mucosa is normal throughout. Retroflexion in the rectal vault is unremarkable.

DISPOSITION: The patient tolerated the procedure and was discharged from the minor operating department in satisfactory condition.

IMPRESSIONS: Normal colonoscopy, only to the distal sigmoid colon

PLAN: Strong recommendation for a barium enema

_____

Dean Sing, MD

DS/mg   D: 01/05/18 12:55:01   T: 01/08/18 09:50:16

Determine the most accurate CPT and/or HCPCS Level II code(s) and modifier(s), if appropriate.

_____

_____

_____

CIPHER, VICTORS & ASSOCIATES
A Complete Health Care Facility
234 MAIN STREET • ANYTOWN, FL 32711 • 407-555-1234

PATIENT: MAGOO, MARGARET
ACCOUNT/EHR #:   MAGOMA01
Date of Operation: 06/17/18

Preoperative Diagnosis: Nuclear sclerosis 2+ with a 2+ posterior subcapsular cataract,
                                 right eye
Postoperative Diagnosis: Same
Operation: Phacoemulsification of cataract with posterior chamber
                                 intraocular lens implantation, right eye

Surgeon: Mark C. Marcus, MD

Assistant: Ralph Malphini, MD
Anesthesia: Local

DESCRIPTION OF OPERATIVE PROCEDURE: Local anesthesia was obtained with retrobulbar and
modified Van Lint injection using a 50-50 mixture of 4% lidocaine and 0.75% Marcaine with Wydase.
A Honan balloon was placed for approximately 15 minutes. The patient was positioned, prepped, and
draped in the usual sterile fashion. A wire lid speculum was inserted, and the operating microscope
was brought into position. A temporal limbal corneal incision was made with a 2.75 mm keratome, and
Viscoat was injected into the anterior chamber. Using a cystotome and Utrata forceps, a continuous
tear capsulorrhexis was performed. A limbal paracentesis stab incision was made at 6 o'clock with a
diamond blade. Hydrodissection and hydrodelineation of the lens was accomplished with balanced salt
solution via cannular injection. Phacoemulsification of the lens proceeded as the lens was sectioned into
quadrants with each quadrant removed. Residual lens cortex was removed with irrigation and aspiration.
The posterior capsule was polished with an irrigating Graether collar button. Viscoat was injected into
the capsular bag, and the cataract incision was opened with the keratome. Using lens-folding forceps,
an Alcon, model MA60VM, 6.0 mm optic, 21.5 diopter posterior chamber intraocular lens was inserted
into the capsular bag. A Sinskey hook was used to facilitate rotation and centration of the lens. Residual
anterior chamber Viscoat was removed with irrigation and aspiration. Balanced salt solution was injected
into the anterior chamber, and the wound was observed to be watertight. Subconjunctival Celestone
and Cefazolin were injected. Topical Iopidine solution and Maxitrol ophthalmic ointment were instilled.
Dressing included eye pad and Fox shield. The patient tolerated the procedure well without complications.

Mark C. Marcus, MD

MCM/mg   D: 06/17/18 09:50:16   T: 06/19/18 12:55:01

Determine the most accurate CPT and/or HCPCS Level II code(s) and modifier(s), if appropriate.

_____

_____

_____

CIPHER, VICTORS & ASSOCIATES
A Complete Health Care Facility
234 MAIN STREET • ANYTOWN, FL 32711 • 407-555-1234

PATIENT: MAGOO, MARGARET
ACCOUNT/EHR #:   MAGOMA01
Date of Operation: 06/17/18

Preoperative Diagnosis: Nuclear sclerosis 2+ with a 2+ posterior subcapsular cataract, right eye

Postoperative Diagnosis: Same

Operation: Phacoemulsification of cataract with posterior chamber intraocular lens implantation, right eye

Surgeon: Mark C. Marcus, MD

Assistant: Ralph Malphini, MD
Anesthesia: Local

DESCRIPTION OF OPERATIVE PROCEDURE: Local anesthesia was obtained with retrobulbar and modified Van Lint injection using a 50-50 mixture of 4% lidocaine and 0.75% Marcaine with Wydase. A Honan balloon was placed for approximately 15 minutes. The patient was positioned, prepped, and draped in the usual sterile fashion. A wire lid speculum was inserted, and the operating microscope was brought into position. A temporal limbal corneal incision was made with a 2.75 mm keratome, and Viscoat was injected into the anterior chamber.

   Using a cystotome and Utrata forceps, a continuous tear capsulorrhexis was performed. A limbal paracentesis stab incision was made at 6 o'clock with a diamond blade. Hydrodissection and hydrodelineation of the lens was accomplished with balanced salt solution via cannular injection. Phacoemulsification of the lens proceeded as the lens was sectioned into quadrants with each quadrant removed. Residual lens cortex was removed with irrigation and aspiration. The posterior capsule was polished with an irrigating Graether collar button. Viscoat was injected into the capsular bag, and the cataract incision was opened with the keratome. Using lens-folding forceps, an Alcon, model MA60VM, 6.0 mm optic, 21.5 diopter posterior chamber intraocular lens was inserted into the capsular bag. A Sinskey hook was used to facilitate rotation and centration of the lens. Residual anterior chamber Viscoat was removed with irrigation and aspiration. Balanced salt solution was injected into the anterior chamber, and the wound was observed to be watertight. Subconjunctival Celestone and Cefazolin were injected. Topical Iopidine solution and Maxitrol ophthalmic ointment were instilled. Dressing included eye pad and Fox shield. The patient tolerated the procedure well without complications.

_____

Ralph Malphini, MD

RM/mg   D: 06/17/18 09:50:16   T: 06/19/18 12:55:01

Determine the most accurate CPT and/or HCPCS Level II code(s) and modifier(s), if appropriate.

_____

_____

_____

CIPHER, VICTORS & ASSOCIATES
A Complete Health Care Facility
234 MAIN STREET • ANYTOWN, FL 32711 • 407-555-1234

PATIENT: DOE-SMITH, JANE
ACCOUNT/EHR #:   DOESJA01
Date of Operation: 11/09/2018

Preoperative Diagnosis: Hallux limites, right foot
Postoperative Diagnosis: Same
Operation: Shortening, osteotomy, first metatarsal, right foot, with screw fixation and cheilectomy, first metatarsal head, right foot

Surgeon: Allen Roberston, DPM

Assistant: N/A
Anesthesia: IV sedation with local anesthesia

DESCRIPTION OF OPERATIVE PROCEDURE: Following the customary sterile preparation and draping, the right limb was elevated approximately 5 minutes in order to facilitate circulatory drainage, at which time the pneumatic cuff, which had previously been placed on her right ankle, was inflated to a pressure of 250 mmHg. The right limb was then placed in the operative position. The operative site was injected with 2% Xylocaine mixed with 0.5% Marcaine. Upon having achieved anesthesia, a curvilinear incision was created on the plantar medial aspect of the first metatarsophalangeal joint of the right foot. The incision was deepened with sharp dissection; traversing veins were cauterized. Capsule was identified on the medial and dorsomedial aspect. Capsule was longitudinally incised on the dorsomedial aspect and meticulously dissected to expose the head of the first metatarsal into the operative site. At this point, it was noted that the cartilage of the first metatarsal head was healthy; however, there was distinct irritation to the dorsal portion of the metatarsal head with an apparent flattening of the metatarsal head secondary to the hallux limites. Using a rongeur, the hypertrophic exuberant portion of the first metatarsal head was resected, and the remaining surface was rasped smooth in order to recreate a ball joint. Using an oscillating saw, an osteotomy was performed from medial to lateral in a V-shaped fashion with the apex centrally located and the dorsal arm longer than the plantar arm. A segment of bone was removed from the dorsal arm in order to shorten and plantar flex the metatarsal head. Upon having done so, two 2.0-mm screws were obliquely driven into the osteotomy site; following range of motion was noted that the osteotomy remained stable. At this point, the hallux had approximately 90 degrees of motion to the metatarsal shaft. The area was copiously irrigated with sterile saline. The capsular tissue was repaired using 4-0 Vicryl; subcutaneous tissue was repaired using 5-0 Vicryl. Operative site was injected with dexamethasone; Betadine-soaked Adaptic was applied to the incision site, along with sterile gauze and Kling. The pneumatic cuff was deflated. Normal color, circulation was noted to return to all digits immediately. The patient tolerated the surgery well. Vital signs remained stable throughout the entire procedure. The patient returned to the recovery room in good condition.

Allen Robertson, DPM

AR/mg   D: 11/09/18 09:50:16   T: 11/12/18 12:55:01

Determine the most accurate CPT and/or HCPCS Level II code(s) and modifier(s), if appropriate.

_____

_____

_____

CIPHER, VICTORS & ASSOCIATES
A Complete Health Care Facility
234 MAIN STREET • ANYTOWN, FL 32711 • 407-555-1234

PATIENT:	HUNTER, ASHLEY
ACCOUNT/EHR #:	HUNTAS01
Admission Date:	09/07/2018
Discharge Date:	09/08/2018
DATE:	09/07/2018

Preoperative Dx:	Stenotic cervical os with hematometrium
Postoperative Dx:	Same
Operation:	Cervical dilatation with release of old blood. This was done under ultrasound guidance followed by endometrial curettage.
Surgeon:	Rodney L. Cohen, MD
Assistant:	None
Anesthesia:	General by LMA
Complications:	None
Findings:	See body of dictation
Specimens:	Endometrial curettings to pathology
Disposition:	Stable to recovery room

PROCEDURE: The patient was taken to the OR, where she was placed in the supine position and administered general anesthesia per LMA. She was then placed in candy-cane stirrups and prepped and draped in the usual sterile fashion. A weighted speculum was placed in the vagina, and with the aid of a Deaver retractor, the anterior portion of the cervix was grasped with single-toothed tenaculum. There were no evident holes or dimples or scenes suggestive of where the external cervical os might be, as the cervix had completely agglutinated across the entire surface. Using lacrimal ducts and gentle tension, the area of suspicion was gently poked until a perforation gave way. This tract was followed with serial dilators until, ultimately, brown old blood was released, ensuring that I was in the right place. This was done with the aid of abdominal ultrasound guidance, for the risk of false tracking and missing the endocervical canal uterus was real. The uterus was emptied. The cervix was dilated up to approximate 8 mm. This allowed for free flow of the contained old blood. This was followed by sharp curette of all the uterine lining surfaces. This specimen was captured and sent to pathology. Lastly a small 7 size suction catheter was inserted to ensure the remainder of any old captured blood that may be sitting in the deep recesses of this severely retroverted uterus was obtained, and this concluded the case. The instruments were removed. The patient was taken down from cane stirrups. The patient was awakened from anesthesia and taken to the recovery room in stable condition.

Rodney L. Cohen, MD

RLC/mg   D: 09/07/2018 11:47:39   T: 09/09/2018 09:50:16

Determine the most accurate CPT and/or HCPCS Level II code(s) and modifier(s), if appropriate.

_____

_____

_____

CIPHER, VICTORS & ASSOCIATES
A Complete Health Care Facility
234 MAIN STREET • ANYTOWN, FL 32711 • 407-555-1234

PATIENT: KLOTSKY, STACY
ACCOUNT/EHR #:   KLOTST01
Admission Date: 10/05/2018
Discharge Date: 10/05/2018
DATE: 10/05/2018

Preoperative Dx: Rule out bladder tumor
Postoperative Dx: Same
Procedure: Cystoscopy, biopsy, and fulguration of bladder

Surgeon: Leonard Dupont, MD

Assistant: None
Anesthesia: Spinal

INDICATIONS: The patient is a 73-year-old female with a history of grade II superficial transitional cell carcinoma of the bladder. Cystoscopy showed a suspicious erythematous area on the right trigone. She presented today for cystoscopy, biopsy, and fulguration. Findings—the urethra was normal, the bladder was 1+ trabeculated, the mid and right trigone areas were slightly erythematous and hypervascular. No papillary tumors were noted; no mucosal abnormalities were noted.

PROCEDURE: The patient was placed on the table in supine position. Satisfactory spinal anesthesia was obtained. She was placed in dorsolithotomy position. She was prepped sterilely with Hibiclens and draped in the usual manner. A #22 French cystoscopy sheath was passed per urethra in atraumatic fashion. The bladder was resected with the 70-degree lens with findings as noted above. Cup biopsy forceps were placed, and three biopsies were taken of the suspicious areas of the trigone. These areas were fulgurated with the Bugby electrode; no active bleeding was seen. The scope was removed; the patient was returned to recovery, having tolerated the procedure well. Estimated blood loss was minimal.

PATHOLOGY REPORT: Chronic cystitis (cystica) with squamous cell metaplasia

Leonard Dupont, MD

LD/mg   D: 10/05/2018 11:47:39   T: 10/07/2018 09:50:16

Determine the most accurate CPT and/or HCPCS Level II code(s) and modifier(s), if appropriate.

_____

_____

_____

CIPHER, VICTORS & ASSOCIATES
A Complete Health Care Facility
234 MAIN STREET • ANYTOWN, FL 32711 • 407-555-1234

PATIENT:	DENNISON, DANIEL
ACCOUNT/EHR #:	DENNDA01
DATE:	11/23/2018
Procedure Performed:	Vasectomy
Physician:	Sunil Kaladuwa, MD
INDICATIONS:	Elective sterilization
PROCEDURE:	The patient was given Versed for anxiety, and local anesthesia was administered. Removal of a segment of the deferent duct was accomplished bilaterally. Patient tolerated the procedure well.
IMPRESSION:	Successful outcome
PLAN:	Postoperative semen examination is scheduled for 1 week.

Sunil Kaladuwa, MD

SK/mg   D: 11/23/18 09:50:16   T: 11/25/18 12:55:01

Determine the most accurate CPT and/or HCPCS Level II code(s) and modifier(s), if appropriate.

_____

_____

_____

CIPHER, VICTORS & ASSOCIATES
A Complete Health Care Facility
234 MAIN STREET • ANYTOWN, FL 32711 • 407-555-1234

PATIENT: KLACKSON, KEVIN
ACCOUNT/EHR #:   KLACKE01
DATE: 09/15/2018

Diagnosis: Primary cardiomyopathy with chest pain
Procedure: Arterial catheterization

Physician: Frank Vincent, MD

Anesthesia: Local

PROCEDURE: The patient was placed on the table in supine position. Local anesthesia was
administered. Once we were assured that the patient had achieved no nervous stimuli, the incision was
made and the catheter was introduced percutaneously. The incision was sutured with a simple repair.
The patient tolerated the procedure well and was transferred to the recovery room.

_____

Frank Vincent, MD

FV/mg   D: 09/15/18 09:50:16   T: 09/15/18 12:55:01

Determine the most accurate CPT and/or HCPCS Level II code(s) and modifier(s), if appropriate.

_____

_____

_____

CIPHER, VICTORS & ASSOCIATES
A Complete Health Care Facility
234 MAIN STREET • ANYTOWN, FL 32711 • 407-555-1234

PATIENT: GIRALDI, MELODY
ACCOUNT/EHR #:   GIRAME01
DATE: 10/02/2018

Diagnosis: Lumbar stenosis, sciatica
Procedure: CMT; traction, manual

Physician: Roxan K. Paschal, DC

PROCEDURE: The patient was placed on the table.
Chiropractic manipulative treatment: spinal, thoracic
Chiropractic manipulative treatment: lower extremity, left
Manual traction: cervical & lumbar regions × 30 minutes

Roxan K. Paschal, DC

RKP/mg   D: 10/02/18 09:50:16   T: 10/05/18 12:55:01

Determine the most accurate CPT and/or HCPCS Level II code(s) and modifier(s), if appropriate.

_____

_____

_____

Barton Hospital
239 Main Street • Anytown, FL 32711 • 407-555-1243

PATIENT: GREGORAN, ERIC
ACCOUNT/EHR #:   GREGER001
DATE: 09/20/18

Diagnosis: Ruptured eyeball, left

Attending Physician: Julio Yearlin, MD

Pt is a 23-year-old male who was involved in a fistfight at a local bar the previous evening. He was admitted to the hospital today complaining of an ache in the area of his left eye as well as severe pain around his right ear. The patient is taken to the OR and a repair of the left eye rupture is performed.

_____

Julio Yearlin, MD

JY/mg   D: 09/20/18 09:50:16   T: 09/22/18 12:55:01

Determine the most accurate ICD-10-PCS code(s).

_____

_____

_____

Barton Hospital
239 Main Street • Anytown, FL 32711 • 407-555-1243

PATIENT: OLIVETTE, HARRISON
ACCOUNT/EHR #:   OLIVHA001
DATE: 10/05/18

Diagnosis: Cervical sprain C1–C7; lumbar strain L4–L5; multiple subluxation of cervical spine

Attending Physician: Terrence Fontaine, MD

This 23-year-old male was admitted after being involved in a two-car MVA 2 weeks ago. He saw his family physician, Dr. Ashley Proctor, after experiencing constant neck pain radiating into the shoulders. Pain medication and rest (no movement) provided temporary relief. Dr. Proctor suggested admission for further evaluation.

In addition to neck pain, Pt states pain radiating across the lower back area beginning approximately 2 hours after the MVA. He states it hurts to move, bend, and walk. Pt denies similar pain in back or neck before.

BP 122/85. P60. After review of patient history questionnaire, PE indicates general appearance is age appropriate with average build and a protective gait. Normal lymph nodes: cervical; axillae; groin. Upper and lower extremities appear normal with the exception of muscle strength in both arms and left leg. Toe-walk exam rates 3 of 5. Limited-to-no ROM with pain C1–C7 and L4–L5. Pt exhibits spinal tenderness: cervical, dorsal, and lumbar. Evidence of edema: cervical and lumbar regions. Muscle spasms evident: scalenes, traps, lat, and paraspinal.

Patient sent to Radiology for x-rays: cervical and lumbar. Radiologic results show multiple subluxations of the cervical vertebrae with pain on movement. Dens and spinous process are intact. No breaks or fractures. Lumbar spine is intact with no breaks or fractures.

_____

Terrence Fontaine, MD

TF/mg   D: 10/05/18 09:50:16   T: 10/07/18 12:55:01

Determine the most accurate ICD-10-PCS code(s).

_____

_____

_____

Barton Hospital
239 Main Street • Anytown, FL 32711 • 407-555-1243

PATIENT: MOSURE, DENISE
ACCOUNT/EHR #: MOSUDE001
DATE: 09/20/2018

Diagnosis: Nosebleed

Attending Physician: Daniel Vickmann, MD

Pt is a 33-year-old female who was having a nosebleed and went to see Dr. Vickmann immediately. She is admitted to the hospital.

The patient was taken to the OR, where an extensive cautery in the anterior portion of her right nasal passage, open approach, was performed to control the bleeding.

_____

Daniel Vickmann, MD

DV/mg   D: 09/20/18 09:50:16   T: 09/22/18 12:55:01

Determine the most accurate ICD-10-PCS code(s).

_____

_____

_____

Barton Hospital
239 Main Street • Anytown, FL 32711 • 407-555-1243

PATIENT: COOPER, KATY
ACCOUNT/EHR #:   COOPKA001
DATE: 10/05/18

Diagnosis: Deviated septum, nasal

Attending Physician: Jacob Zorman, MD

Pt is a 4-year-old female who is having difficulty breathing; also has had several sinus infections recently and snores. Her pediatrician, Dr. Zorman, admits her into the hospital.

    The patient is taken to the OR, where Dr. Zorman performs a septoplasty, open approach, with cartilage scoring.

___

Jacob Zorman, MD

JZ/mg   D: 10/05/18 09:50:16   T: 10/07/18 12:55:01

Determine the most accurate ICD-10-PCS code(s).

___

___

___

Barton Hospital
239 Main Street • Anytown, FL 32711 • 407-555-1243

PATIENT: MORIARITY, CALVIN
ACCOUNT/EHR #:   MORICA001
DATE: 10/10/18

Diagnosis: Stab wound, abdomen

Attending Physician: Richard Neilson, MD

Calvin Moriarity, a 25-year-old male, was walking home through the park, where he was mugged and stabbed in the abdomen. Calvin was rushed to Barton's emergency department. After Dr. Neilson examines Calvin he is taken to the OR to do an exploration of the abdominal wound, which penetrated the peritoneal cavity.

_____

Richard Neilson, MD

RN/mg   D: 10/10/18 09:50:16   T: 10/12/18 12:55:01

Determine the most accurate ICD-10-PCS code(s).

_____

_____

_____

Barton Hospital
239 Main Street • Anytown, FL 32711 • 407-555-1243

PATIENT: DUBOIS, DOROTHY
ACCOUNT/EHR #:   DUBIDO001
DATE: 10/20/18

Diagnosis: Renal calculus

Attending Physician: Julio Yearlin, MD

Pt is a 73-year-old female who was admitted into the hospital with hematuria, nausea, and vomiting. A routine ECG is taken in preparation for her surgery, which is scheduled for tomorrow.

Julio Yearlin, MD

JY/mg   D: 10/20/18 09:50:16   T: 10/22/18 12:55:01

Determine the most accurate ICD-10-PCS code(s).

_____

_____

_____

_____

Barton Hospital
239 Main Street • Anytown, FL 32711 • 407-555-1243

PATIENT: NEIMAN, ROSA
ACCOUNT/EHR #:   NEIMRO001
DATE: 10/21/18

Diagnosis: Appendicitis

Attending Physician: Richard Neilson, MD

Rose Neiman, a 39-year-old female, was admitted into the hospital with suspected appendicitis. An ultrasound of the abdomen was performed.

_____

Richard Neilson, MD

RN/mg   D: 10/21/18 09:50:16   T: 10/23/18 12:55:01

Determine the most accurate ICD-10-PCS code(s).

_____

_____

_____

Barton Hospital
239 Main Street • Anytown, FL 32711 • 407-555-1243

PATIENT: FRIENZE, ALEXANDER
ACCOUNT/EHR #:   FRIEAL001
DATE: 10/25/18

Diagnosis: Concussion

Attending Physician: Jacob Zorman, MD

Pt is a 52-year-old male admitted to the hospital with a concussion. A skull x-ray without contrast and brain MRI without contrast are both performed.

_____

Jacob Zorman, MD

JZ/mg   D: 10/25/18 09:50:16   T: 10/27/18 12:55:01

Determine the most accurate ICD-10-PCS code(s).

_____

_____

_____

Forms

Claim Forms

Virtually all claims submitted by a health care provider are done so electronically. On a rare occasion, a paper claim is used. The CMS-1500 (used to report physician and outpatient services) and the CMS-4500 (used by facilities) are included here to help you understand the details and information required, as they are comparable to the electronic claim format.

As stated on Medicare's website:

"Claims may be electronically submitted to a Medicare Administrative Contractor (MAC) from a provider using a computer with software that meets electronic filing requirements as established by the HIPAA claim standard and by meeting CMS requirements contained in the provider enrollment & certification category area of this web site and the EDI Enrollment page in this section of the web site. Providers that bill institutional claims are also permitted to submit claims electronically via direct data entry (DDE) screens."

CMS-1500 Claim Form

CMS-1500 is used for reporting the provision of outpatient and physician services.

HEALTH INSURANCE CLAIM FORM

APPROVED BY NATIONAL UNIFORM CLAIM COMMITTEE (NUCC) 02/12

CARRIER

☐☐ PICA   PICA ☐☐☐

1. MEDICARE ☐ (Medicare#)   MEDICAID ☐ (Medicaid#)   TRICARE ☐ (ID#/DoD#)   CHAMPVA ☐ (Member ID#)   GROUP HEALTH PLAN ☐ (ID#)   FECA BLK LUNG ☐ (ID#)   OTHER ☐ (ID#)   1a. INSURED'S I.D. NUMBER   (For Program in Item 1)

2. PATIENT'S NAME (Last Name, First Name, Middle Initial)

3. PATIENT'S BIRTH DATE MM DD YY   SEX M ☐ F ☐

4. INSURED'S NAME (Last Name, First Name, Middle Initial)

5. PATIENT'S ADDRESS (No., Street)

6. PATIENT RELATIONSHIP TO INSURED   Self ☐ Spouse ☐ Child ☐ Other ☐

7. INSURED'S ADDRESS (No., Street)

CITY   STATE

8. RESERVED FOR NUCC USE

CITY   STATE

ZIP CODE   TELEPHONE (Include Area Code) ( )

ZIP CODE   TELEPHONE (Include Area Code) ( )

9. OTHER INSURED'S NAME (Last Name, First Name, Middle Initial)

10. IS PATIENT'S CONDITION RELATED TO:

11. INSURED'S POLICY GROUP OR FECA NUMBER

a. OTHER INSURED'S POLICY OR GROUP NUMBER

a. EMPLOYMENT? (Current or Previous) ☐ YES ☐ NO

a. INSURED'S DATE OF BIRTH MM DD YY   SEX M ☐ F ☐

b. RESERVED FOR NUCC USE

b. AUTO ACCIDENT? ☐ YES ☐ NO   PLACE (State)

b. OTHER CLAIM ID (Designated by NUCC)

c. RESERVED FOR NUCC USE

c. OTHER ACCIDENT? ☐ YES ☐ NO

c. INSURANCE PLAN NAME OR PROGRAM NAME

d. INSURANCE PLAN NAME OR PROGRAM NAME

10d. CLAIM CODES (Designated by NUCC)

d. IS THERE ANOTHER HEALTH BENEFIT PLAN? ☐ YES ☐ NO *If yes*, complete items 9, 9a, and 9d.

READ BACK OF FORM BEFORE COMPLETING & SIGNING THIS FORM.

12. PATIENT'S OR AUTHORIZED PERSON'S SIGNATURE I authorize the release of any medical or other information necessary to process this claim. I also request payment of government benefits either to myself or to the party who accepts assignment below.

SIGNED _____ DATE _____

13. INSURED'S OR AUTHORIZED PERSON'S SIGNATURE I authorize payment of medical benefits to the undersigned physician or supplier for services described below.

SIGNED _____

PATIENT AND INSURED INFORMATION

14. DATE OF CURRENT ILLNESS, INJURY, or PREGNANCY (LMP) MM DD YY   QUAL.

15. OTHER DATE QUAL.   MM DD YY

16. DATES PATIENT UNABLE TO WORK IN CURRENT OCCUPATION MM DD YY FROM TO MM DD YY

17. NAME OF REFERRING PROVIDER OR OTHER SOURCE   17a.   17b. NPI

18. HOSPITALIZATION DATES RELATED TO CURRENT SERVICES MM DD YY FROM TO MM DD YY

19. ADDITIONAL CLAIM INFORMATION (Designated by NUCC)

20. OUTSIDE LAB? ☐ YES ☐ NO $ CHARGES

21. DIAGNOSIS OR NATURE OF ILLNESS OR INJURY Relate A-L to service line below (24E)   ICD Ind.

A. ____ B. ____ C. ____ D. ____
E. ____ F. ____ G. ____ H. ____
I. ____ J. ____ K. ____ L. ____

22. RESUBMISSION CODE   ORIGINAL REF. NO.

23. PRIOR AUTHORIZATION NUMBER

24. A. DATE(S) OF SERVICE From MM DD YY To MM DD YY	B. PLACE OF SERVICE	C. EMG	D. PROCEDURES, SERVICES, OR SUPPLIES (Explain Unusual Circumstances) CPT/HCPCS MODIFIER	E. DIAGNOSIS POINTER	F. $ CHARGES	G. DAYS OR UNITS	H. EPSDT Family Plan	I. ID. QUAL.	J. RENDERING PROVIDER ID. #
1									NPI
2									NPI
3									NPI
4									NPI
5									NPI
6									NPI

PHYSICIAN OR SUPPLIER INFORMATION

25. FEDERAL TAX I.D. NUMBER   SSN ☐ EIN ☐

26. PATIENT'S ACCOUNT NO.

27. ACCEPT ASSIGNMENT? (For govt. claims, see back) ☐ YES ☐ NO

28. TOTAL CHARGE $

29. AMOUNT PAID $

30. Rsvd for NUCC Use

31. SIGNATURE OF PHYSICIAN OR SUPPLIER INCLUDING DEGREES OR CREDENTIALS (I certify that the statements on the reverse apply to this bill and are made a part thereof.)

SIGNED _____ DATE _____

32. SERVICE FACILITY LOCATION INFORMATION

a. NPI   b.

33. BILLING PROVIDER INFO & PH # ( )

a. NPI   b.

NUCC Instruction Manual available at: www.nucc.org   **PLEASE PRINT OR TYPE**   APPROVED OMB-0938-1197 FORM 1500 (02-12)

UB-04 Claim Form (CMS 1450)

UB-04 is the new form used for reporting the provision of inpatient services. This replaced the UB-92.

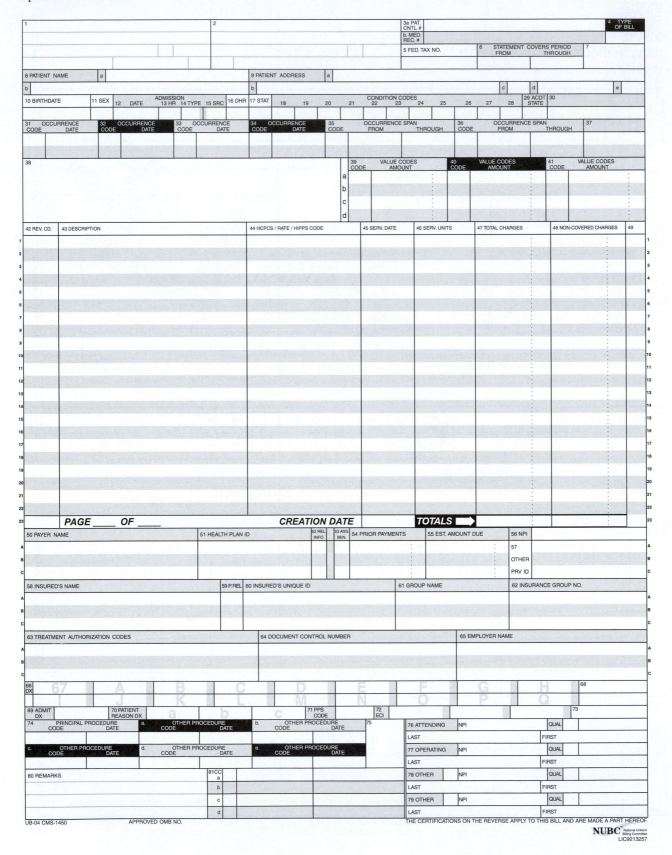

Place of Service Codes for Professional Claims

Database (updated November 1, 2012)

Listed below are place of service codes and descriptions. These codes should be used on professional claims to specify the entity where service(s) were rendered. Check with individual payers (e.g., Medicare, Medicaid, other private insurance) for reimbursement policies regarding these codes. If you would like to comment on a code(s) or description(s), please send your request to posinfo@cms.hhs.gov.

The code set is annotated with the effective dates for all codes added on and after January 1, 2003. Codes without effective dates are long-standing and in effect on and before January 1, 2003.

Place of Service Code(s)	Place of Service Name	Place of Service Description
01	Pharmacy**	A facility or location where drugs and other medically related items and services are sold, dispensed, or otherwise provided directly to patients.
02	Unassigned	N/A
03	School	A facility whose primary purpose is education.
04	Homeless Shelter	A facility or location whose primary purpose is to provide temporary housing to homeless individuals (e.g., emergency shelters, individual or family shelters).
05	Indian Health Service Free-standing Facility	A facility or location, owned and operated by the Indian Health Service, which provides diagnostic, therapeutic (surgical and nonsurgical), and rehabilitation services to American Indians and Alaska Natives who do not require hospitalization.
06	Indian Health Service Provider-based Facility	A facility or location, owned and operated by the Indian Health Service, which provides diagnostic, therapeutic (surgical and nonsurgical), and rehabilitation services rendered by, or under the supervision of, physicians to American Indians and Alaska Natives admitted as inpatients or outpatients.

(Continued)

Place of Service Code(s)	Place of Service Name	Place of Service Description
07	Tribal 638 Free-standing Facility	A facility or location, owned and operated by a federally recognized American Indian or Alaska Native tribe or tribal organization under a 638 agreement, which provides diagnostic, therapeutic (surgical and nonsurgical), and rehabilitation services to tribal members who do not require hospitalization.
08	Tribal 638 Provider-based Facility	A facility or location, owned and operated by a federally recognized American Indian or Alaska Native tribe or tribal organization under a 638 agreement, which provides diagnostic, therapeutic (surgical and nonsurgical), and rehabilitation services to tribal members admitted as inpatients or outpatients.
09	Prison/ Correctional Facility	A prison, jail, reformatory, work farm, detention center, or any other similar facility maintained by either Federal, State, or local authorities for the purpose of confinement or rehabilitation of adult or juvenile criminal offenders.
10	Unassigned	
11	Office	Location, other than a hospital, skilled nursing facility (SNF), military treatment facility, community health center, state or local public health clinic, or intermediate care facility (ICF), where the health professional routinely provides health examinations, diagnosis, and treatment of illness or injury on an ambulatory basis.
12	Home	Location, other than a hospital or other facility, where the patient receives care in a private residence.
13	Assisted Living Facility	Congregate residential facility with self-contained living units providing assessment of each resident's needs and on-site support 24 hours a day, 7 days a week, with the capacity to deliver or arrange for services including some health care and other services.
14	Group Home*	A residence, with shared living areas, where clients receive supervision and other services such as social and/or behavioral services, custodial service, and minimal services (e.g., medication administration).
15	Mobile Unit	A facility/unit that moves from place to place and is equipped to provide preventive, screening, diagnostic, and/or treatment services.
16	Temporary Lodging	A short-term accommodation such as a hotel, camp ground, hostel, cruise ship, or resort where the patient receives care and that is not identified by any other POS code.
17	Walk-in Retail Health Clinic	A walk-in health clinic, other than an office, urgent care facility, pharmacy, or independent clinic and not described by any other Place of Service code, that is located within a retail operation and provides, on an ambulatory basis, preventive and primary care services. (This code is available for use immediately, with a final effective date of May 1, 2010.)
18	Place of Employment—Worksite	A location, not described by any other POS code, owned or operated by a public or private entity where the patient is employed, and where a health professional provides on-going or episodic occupational medical, therapeutic or rehabilitative services to the individual. (This code is available for use effective January 1, 2013 but no later than May 1, 2013)
19	Unassigned	N/A

Place of Service Code(s)	Place of Service Name	Place of Service Description
20	Urgent Care Facility	Location, distinct from a hospital emergency room, an office, or a clinic, whose purpose is to diagnose and treat illness or injury for unscheduled, ambulatory patients seeking immediate medical attention.
21	Inpatient Hospital	A facility, other than psychiatric, that primarily provides diagnostic, therapeutic (both surgical and nonsurgical), and rehabilitation services by, or under the supervision of, physicians to patients admitted for a variety of medical conditions.
22	Outpatient Hospital	A portion of a hospital that provides diagnostic, therapeutic (both surgical and nonsurgical), and rehabilitation services to sick or injured persons who do not require hospitalization or institutionalization.
23	Emergency Room—Hospital	A portion of a hospital where emergency diagnosis and treatment of illness or injury is provided.
24	Ambulatory Surgical Center	A free-standing facility, other than a physician's office, where surgical and diagnostic services are provided on an ambulatory basis.
25	Birthing Center	A facility, other than a hospital's maternity facilities or a physician's office, that provides a setting for labor, delivery, and immediate postpartum care as well as immediate care of newborn infants.
26	Military Treatment Facility	A medical facility operated by one or more of the Uniformed Services. Military Treatment Facility (MTF) also refers to certain former U.S. Public Health Service (USPHS) facilities now designated as Uniformed Service Treatment Facilities (USTF).
27–30	Unassigned	N/A
31	Skilled Nursing Facility	A facility which primarily provides inpatient skilled nursing care and related services to patients who require medical, nursing, or rehabilitative services but does not provide the level of care or treatment available in a hospital.
32	Nursing Facility	A facility which primarily provides to residents skilled nursing care and related services for the rehabilitation of injured, disabled, or sick persons or, on a regular basis, health-related care services above the level of custodial care to other than mentally retarded individuals.
33	Custodial Care Facility	A facility which provides room, board, and other personal assistance services, generally on a long-term basis, and that does not include a medical component.
34	Hospice	A facility, other than a patient's home, in which palliative and supportive care for terminally ill patients and their families is provided.
35–40	Unassigned	N/A
41	Ambulance—Land	A land vehicle specifically designed, equipped, and staffed for lifesaving and transporting the sick or injured.
42	Ambulance—Air or Water	An air or water vehicle specifically designed, equipped, and staffed for lifesaving and transporting the sick or injured.
43–48	Unassigned	N/A

(Continued)

Place of Service Code(s)	Place of Service Name	Place of Service Description
49	Independent Clinic	A location, not part of a hospital and not described by any other Place of Service code, that is organized and operated to provide preventive, diagnostic, therapeutic, rehabilitative, or palliative services to outpatients only (effective 10/1/03).
50	Federally Qualified Health Center	A facility located in a medically underserved area that provides Medicare beneficiaries preventive primary medical care under the general direction of a physician.
51	Inpatient Psychiatric Facility	A facility that provides inpatient psychiatric services for the diagnosis and treatment of mental illness on a 24-hour basis, by or under the supervision of a physician.
52	Psychiatric Facility— Partial Hospitalization	A facility for the diagnosis and treatment of mental illness that provides a planned therapeutic program for patients who do not require full-time hospitalization but who need broader programs than are possible from outpatient visits to a hospital-based or hospital-affiliated facility.
53	Community Mental Health Center	A facility that provides the following services: outpatient services, including specialized outpatient services for children, the elderly, individuals who are chronically ill, and residents of the CMHC's mental health services area who have been discharged from inpatient treatment at a mental health facility; 24-hour-a-day emergency care services; day treatment, other partial hospitalization services, or psychosocial rehabilitation services; screening for patients being considered for admission to state mental health facilities to determine the appropriateness of such admission; and consultation and education services.
54	Intermediate Care Facility/Mentally Retarded	A facility that primarily provides health-related care and services above the level of custodial care to mentally retarded individuals but does not provide the level of care or treatment available in a hospital or SNF.
55	Residential Substance Abuse Treatment Facility	A facility that provides treatment for substance (alcohol and drug) abuse to live-in residents who do not require acute medical care. Services include individual and group therapy and counseling, family counseling, laboratory tests, drugs and supplies, psychological testing, and room and board.
56	Psychiatric Residential Treatment Center	A facility or distinct part of a facility for psychiatric care that provides a total 24-hour therapeutically planned and professionally staffed group living and learning environment.
57	Nonresidential Substance Abuse Treatment Facility	A location that provides treatment for substance (alcohol and drug) abuse on an ambulatory basis. Services include individual and group therapy and counseling, family counseling, laboratory tests, drugs and supplies, and psychological testing.
58–59	Unassigned	N/A
60	Mass Immunization Center	A location where providers administer pneumococcal pneumonia and influenza virus vaccinations and submit these services as electronic media claims or paper claims or by using the roster billing method. This generally takes place in a mass immunization setting, such as, a public health center, pharmacy, or mall, but may include a physician office setting.

Place of Service Code(s)	Place of Service Name	Place of Service Description
61	Comprehensive Inpatient Rehabilitation Facility	A facility that provides comprehensive rehabilitation services under the supervision of a physician to inpatients with physical disabilities. Services include physical therapy, occupational therapy, speech pathology, social or psychological services, and orthotics and prosthetics services.
62	Comprehensive Outpatient Rehabilitation Facility	A facility that provides comprehensive rehabilitation services under the supervision of a physician to outpatients with physical disabilities. Services include physical therapy, occupational therapy, and speech pathology services.
63–64	Unassigned	N/A
65	End-Stage Renal Disease Treatment Facility	A facility other than a hospital, which provides dialysis treatment, maintenance, and/or training to patients or caregivers on an ambulatory or home-care basis.
66–70	Unassigned	N/A
71	Public Health Clinic	A facility maintained by either state or local health departments that provides ambulatory primary medical care under the general direction of a physician.
72	Rural Health Clinic	A certified facility which is located in a rural medically underserved area that provides ambulatory primary medical care under the general direction of a physician.
73–80	Unassigned	N/A
81	Independent Laboratory	A laboratory certified to perform diagnostic and/or clinical tests independent of an institution or a physician's office.
82–98	Unassigned	N/A
99	Other Place of Service	Other place of service not identified above.

GLOSSARY

A

Ablation The destruction or eradication of tissue.

Abortifacient A drug used to induce an abortion.

Abstracting The process of identifying the relevant words or phrases in healthcare documentation in order to determine the best, most appropriate code(s).

Adjunct code The equivalent of CPT's add-on code. This code may not be reported alone or as a first-listed code.

Advanced life support (ALS) Life-sustaining, emergency care provided, such as airway management, defibrillation, and/or the administration of drugs.

Allotransplantation The relocation of tissue from one individual to another (both of the same species) without an identical genetic match.

Alphanumeric Containing both letters and numbers.

Ambulatory surgery center (ASC) A facility specially designed to provide surgical treatments without an overnight stay; also known as a *same-day surgery center.*

Anesthesia The loss of sensation, with or without consciousness, generally induced by the administration of a particular drug.

Anesthesiologists Physicians specializing in the administration of anesthesia.

Angiography The imaging of blood vessels after the injection of contrast material.

Anticipatory guidance Recommendations for behavior modification and/or other preventive measures.

Approach The specific technique used for the procedure.

Arrhythmia An irregular heartbeat.

Arthrodesis The immobilization of a joint using a surgical technique.

Arthrography The recording of a picture of an anatomical joint after the administration of contrast material into the joint capsule.

B

Basic life support (BLS) The provision of emergency CPR, stabilization of the patient, first aid, control of bleeding, and/or treatment of shock.

Basic personal services Services that include washing/bathing, dressing and undressing, and assistance in taking medications and getting in and out of bed.

Bilateral Both sides.

Body part The anatomical site upon which the procedure was performed.

Body system The physiological system, or anatomical region, upon which the procedure was performed.

C

Cannula A tube that is inserted into the body to either deliver or extract fluid, such as a nasogastric tube.

Care plan oversight services E/M of a patient, reported in 30-day periods, including infrequent supervision along with preencounter and postencounter work, such as reading test results and assessment of notes.

Category I codes The codes listed in the main text of the CPT book, also known as CPT codes.

Category II codes Codes for performance measurement and tracking.

Category III codes Codes for emerging technology.

Catheter A thin, flexible tube, inserted into a body part, used to inject fluid, to empty fluid, or to keep a passage open.

Caudal Near the hind part, or tail, of the body; the sacrum and coccyx areas.

Certified registered nurse anesthetist (CRNA) A registered nurse (RN) who has taken additional, specialized training in the administration of anesthesia.

Character: A letter or number component of an ICD-10-PCS code.

Chelation therapy The use of a chemical compound that binds with metal in the body so that the metal will lose its toxic effect. It might be done when a metal disc or prosthetic is implanted in a patient, eliminating adverse reactions to the metal itself as a foreign body.

Class A finding Nontraumatic amputation of a foot or an integral skeletal portion.

Class B finding Absence of a posterior tibial pulse; absence or decrease of hair growth; thickening of the nail, discoloration of the skin, and/or thinning of the skin texture; and/or absence of a posterior pedal pulse.

Class C finding Edema, burning sensation, temperature change (cold feet), abnormal spontaneous sensations in the feet, and/or limping.

Clinical Laboratory Improvement Amendment (CLIA) Federal legislation created for the monitoring and regulation of clinical laboratory procedures.

Closed treatment A fracture treated without surgically opening the affected area.

Code for coverage To choose a code by the insurance company's rules of what it will pay for, rather than a code that accurately reflects the truth about the encounter.

Completeness Structure that allows all procedures, services, and treatments to be represented by a code.

Complex closure A method of sealing an opening in the skin involving a multilayered closure and a reconstructive procedure such as scar revision, debridement, or retention sutures.

Computed tomography (CT) A specialized computer scanner with very fine detail that records imaging of internal anatomical sites; also known as computerized axial tomography (CAT).

Computed tomography angiography (CTA) A CT scan using contrast materials to visualize arteries and veins all over the body.

Conscious sedation The use of a drug to reduce stress and/or anxiety.

Consultation An encounter for purposes of a second physician's opinion or advice, requested by another physician, regarding the management of a patient's specific health concern. A consultation is planned to be a short-term relationship between a healthcare professional and a patient.

Covered entities Healthcare providers, health plans, and healthcare clearinghouses—businesses that have access to the personal health information of patients.

CPT code modifier A two-character code that may be appended to a code from the main portion of the CPT book to provide additional information.

Critical care services Services for a patient who has a life-threatening condition expected to worsen.

Customary clinical documentation The usual contents of the notes and reports written after a healthcare encounter.

Cytology The investigation and identification of cells.

D

Decubitus ulcer A bedsore, or wound created by lying in the same position, on the same irritant without relief.

Densitometry The process used to measure bone density, most often done to assess the patient's risk for osteopenia or osteoporosis.

Device The identification of any materials or appliances that may remain in or on the body after the procedure is completed.

Diagnosis A physician's determination of a patient's condition, illness, or injury.

Disclosure The sharing of information between healthcare professionals working in separate entities, or facilities, in the course of caring for the patient.

DMEPOS Durable medical equipment, prosthetic, and orthotic supplies.

Donor area (site) The area or part of the body from which skin or tissue is removed with the intention of placing that skin or tissue in another area or body.

Duplex scan An ultrasonic scanning procedure to determine blood flow and pattern.

Durable medical equipment (DME) Apparatus and tools that help individuals accommodate physical frailties, deliver pharmaceuticals, and provide other assistance that will last for a long time and/or be used to assist multiple patients over time.

Durable medical equipment regional carrier (DMERC) A company designated by the state or region to act as the fiscal intermediary for all DME claims.

E

Early and Periodic Screening, Diagnostic, and Treatment (EPSDT) A Medicaid preventive health program for children under 21.

End-stage renal disease (ESRD) Chronic, irreversible kidney disease requiring regular treatments.

Enteral Within, or by way of, the gastrointestinal tract.

Established patient A person who has received professional services within the last 3 years from either this provider or another provider of the same specialty belonging to the same group practice.

Ethical behaviors Actions that are in agreement with society's concept of right and wrong.

Etiology The study of the causes of disease.

Evaluation and management (E/M) Specific characteristics of a face-to-face meeting between a healthcare professional and a patient.

Excision The full-thickness removal of a lesion, including margins; includes (for coding purposes) a simple closure.

Expandability Structure that includes room for growth.

Experimental A procedure or treatment that has not yet been accepted by the healthcare industry as the standard of care.

Extracorporeal Outside of the body.

F

Fascia lata graft The transplanting of a connective tissue that encases the thigh muscles.

Fiscal intermediary (FI) A company that administers the day-to-day operation of reviewing and reimbursement of claims for state Medicare programs.

Fluoroscope A piece of equipment that emits x-rays through a part of the patient's body onto a fluorescent screen, causing the image to identify various aspects of the anatomy by density.

Fraud Using inaccurate information or other dishonest actions to wrongly gain money or other benefit.

Full-thickness A measure that extends from the epidermis to the connective tissue layer of the skin.

G

General anesthesia The administration of a drug in order to induce a loss of consciousness in the patient, who is unable to be aroused even by painful stimulation.

Global period The length of time allotted for postoperative care included in the surgical package, which is generally accepted to be 90 days for major surgical procedures and up to 10 days for minor procedures.

Global surgery package A group of services already included in the code for the operation and not reported separately.

Gross examination The visual study of a specimen (with the naked eye).

H

Harvesting The process of taking skin or tissue (on the same body or another).

HCPCS Level II modifier A two-character alphabetic or alphanumeric code that may be appended to a code from the main portion of the CPT book or a code from the HCPCS Level II book.

High Osmolar An ionic water-soluble iodinated contrast medium.

HIPAA's Privacy Rule A portion of HIPAA that ensures the availability of patient information for those who should see it while protecting that information from those who should not.

Hospice An organization that provides services to terminally ill patients and their families.

Hospital A facility that provides diagnostic, therapeutic (both surgical and nonsurgical), and rehabilitation services by, or under the supervision of, physicians to patients admitted for a variety of medical conditions; also known as acute care facility.

I

Immunization To make someone resistant to a particular disease by vaccination.

Incontinence The inability to control urination or fecal expulsion.

Infusion The introduction of a fluid into a blood vessel.

Injection Compelling a fluid into tissue or cavity.

Inpatient An individual admitted for an overnight or longer stay in a hospital.

Intermediate closure A multilevel method of sealing an opening in the skin involving one or more of the deeper layers of the skin. Single-layer closure of heavily contaminated wounds that required extensive cleaning or removal of particulate matter also constitutes intermediate closure.

Internal fixation The process of placing plates and screws or pins, or other devices, directly onto or around a fractured bone, inside of the patient.

Interval The time measured between one point and another, such as between physician visits.

Intervention Action taken to change or prevent something that is happening, most often to stop or prevent something undesirable.

Intravascular Optical Coherence A high-resolution, catheter-based imaging modality used for the optimized visualization of coronary artery lesions.

Invalid Not an acceptable code for reporting any procedure, service, or treatment.

L

Laboratory A location with scientific equipment designed to perform experiments and tests.

Laminaria Thin sticks of kelp-related seaweed, used to dilate the cervix, that can induce abortive circumstance during the first 3 months of pregnancy.

Laminectomy The surgical removal of a vertebral posterior arch.

Laterality Relating to the side or sides of the body, *unilateral* meaning one side and *bilateral* meaning both sides.

Level of patient history The amount of detail involved in the documentation of patient history.

Level of physical examination The extent of a physician's clinical assessment and inspection of a patient.

Liters per minute (LPM) The measurement of how many liters of a drug or chemical are provided to the patient in 60 seconds.

Local anesthesia The injection of a drug to prevent sensation in a specific portion of the body; includes local infiltration anesthesia, digital blocks, and pudendal blocks.

Locum tenens physician A physician that fills in, temporarily, for another physician.

Low Osmolar A non-ionic water-soluble iodinated contrast medium.

M

Magnetic resonance arthrography (MRA) MR imaging of an anatomical joint after the administration of contrast material into the joint capsule.

Magnetic resonance imaging (MRI) A three-dimensional radiologic technique that uses nuclear technology to record pictures of internal anatomical sites.

Manipulation The attempted return of the fracture or dislocation to its normal alignment manually by the physician.

Medical decision making (MDM) The level of knowledge and experience needed by the provider to determine the diagnosis or to decide what to do next.

Medical exclusion criteria Medical reasons a patient's data should not be reported with a certain code.

Medical necessity The assessment that the provider was acting according to standard practices in providing a procedure or service for an individual with a specific diagnosis.

Medicare code edit (MCE) A computerized system that identifies coding errors and/or concerns regarding medical necessity; part of the Correct Coding Initiative.

Microscopic examination The study of a specimen using a microscope (under magnification).

Modifier A two-character code that affects the meaning of another code; a code addendum that provides more meaning to the original code.

Monitored anesthesia care (MAC) The administration of sedatives, anesthetic agents, or other medications to relax but not render the patient unconscious while under the constant observation of a trained anesthesiologist; also known as "twilight" sedation.

Multiaxial Consistent use of characters and elements throughout a book.

Mutually exclusive codes Codes that are identified as those that are not permitted to be used on the same claim form with other codes.

N

New patient A person who has not received any professional services within the past 3 years from either the provider or another provider of the same specialty who belongs to the same group practice.

Not otherwise specified (NOS) An indication that more detailed information is not available from the physician's notes.

Nuclear medicine Treatment that includes the injection or digestion of isotopes.

Nursing home A facility that provides skilled nursing treatment and attention along with limited medical care for its (usually long-term) residents, who do not require acute care services (hospitalization).

O

Open treatment Surgically opening the fracture site, or another site in the body nearby, in order to treat the fractured bone.

Ophthalmologist A physician qualified to diagnose and treat eye disease and conditions with drugs, surgery, and corrective measures.

Optional At your discretion; not required.

Optometrist A professional qualified to carry out eye examinations and to prescribe and supply eyeglasses and contact lenses.

Orthotic A device used to correct or improve an orthopedic concern.

Ostomy An artificial opening made in the body surgically.

Otorhinolaryngology The study of the human ears, nose, and throat systems.

Outpatient A patient treated without being kept overnight.

P

Parenteral By way of anything other than the gastrointestinal tract, such as intravenous, intramuscular, intramedullary, or subcutaneous.

Parenteral enteral nutrition (PEN) Nourishment delivered using a combination of means other than the gastrointestinal tract (such as IV) in addition to via the gastrointestinal tract.

Pathology The study of the nature, etiology, development, and outcomes of disease.

Patient population A group with common traits among patients using the same healthcare facility or healthcare provider.

Percutaneous skeletal fixation The insertion of fixation instruments (such as pins) placed across the fracture site. It may be done under x-ray imaging for guidance purposes.

Performance measure Criteria for gathering specific data to study.

Personnel modifier A modifier adding information about the professional(s) attending to the provision of this procedure or treatment to the patient during this encounter.

PFSH An acronym for *past*, *family*, and *social history*.

Physical status modifier A two-character alphanumeric code used to describe the condition of the patient at the time anesthesia services are administered.

Preventive A type of action or service that stops something from happening or from getting worse.

Procedure A treatment or service provided by a healthcare professional.

Products of conception The zygote, embryo, or fetus, as well as the amnion, umbilical cord, and placenta.

Prosthetic A fabricated artificial replacement for a damaged or missing part of the body.

Protected health information (PHI) Any patient-identifiable health information regardless of the form in which it is stored (paper, computer file, etc.).

Push The delivery of an additional drug via an intravenous line over a short period of time.

Q

Qualifier Any additional feature of the procedure, if applicable.

Qualitative The determination of character or essential element(s).

Quantitative The counting or measurement of something.

Query To ask.

R

Radiation The high-speed discharge and projection of energy waves or particles.

Recipient area The area, or site, of the body receiving a graft of skin or tissue.

Regional anesthesia The administration of a drug in order to interrupt the nerve impulses without loss of consciousness.

Regional blocks Anesthesia for a large, limited part of the body; neuroaxial blocks include epidural and spinal anesthesia; plexus blocks include brachial plexus blocks and single nerve blocks; also known as axillary, bier, retrobulbar, peribulbar, interscalene, subarachnoid, supraclavicular, and infraclavicular blocks.

Reimbursement Payment for services provided.

Relationship The level of familiarity between provider and patient.

Risk factor reduction intervention Action taken by the attending physician to stop or reduce a behavior or lifestyle that is predicted to have a negative affect on the individual's health.

Root operation term The category or classification of a particular procedure, service, or treatment.

S

Saphenous vein Either of the two major veins in the leg that run from the foot to the thigh near the surface of the skin.

Self-administer To give medication to oneself, such as a diabetic giving herself an insulin injection.

Service-related modifier A modifier relating to a change or adjustment of a procedure or service provided.

Simple closure A method of sealing an opening in the skin (epidermis or dermis), involving only one layer. It includes the administration of a local anesthesia and/or chemical or electrocauterization of a wound not closed.

Somatic Related to the body, especially separate from the brain or mind.

Sonogram The use of sound waves to record images of internal organs and tissues; also called an *ultrasound*.

Specialty care transport (SCT) Continuous care provided by one or more health professionals in an appropriate specialty area, such as respiratory care or cardiovascular care, or by a paramedic with additional training.

Specimen A small part or sample of any substance obtained for analysis and diagnosis.

Standardized terminology One established meaning for each term used in code descriptions.

Standard of care The accepted principles of conduct, services, or treatments that are established as the expected behavior.

Structural integrity The structure of the codes individually, and the system in total, can be maintained while still expanding the set to include new technology.

Superbill A form preprinted with the diagnosis codes and procedure codes most frequently used in a particular facility.

Supplemental report A letter or report written by the attending physician or other healthcare professional to provide additional clarification or explanation.

Supporting documentation The paperwork in the patient's file that corroborates the codes presented on the claim form for a particular encounter.

Surgical approach The methodology or technique used by the physician to perform the procedure, service, or treatment.

Surgical pathology The study of tissues removed from a living patient during a surgical procedure.

Synchronous Simultaneous; occurring at the same time.

T

Topical anesthesia The application of a drug to the skin to reduce or prevent sensation in a specific area temporarily.

Transcutaneous electrical nerve stimulators (TENS) The use of electricity to agitate the skin to relieve pain.

Transfer of care When a physician gives up responsibility for caring for a patient, in whole or with regard to one specific condition, and another physician accepts responsibility for the care of that patient.

Transplantation The transfer of tissue from one site to another.

U

Unbundling Coding individual parts of a specific procedure rather than one combination, or bundle, that includes all the components.

Unique definitions ICD-10-PCS codes are constructed of individual values that stay consistent throughout the code set.

Unlisted codes Codes shown at the end of each subsection of the CPT used as a catch-all for any procedure not represented by an existing code.

Upcoding Using a code on a claim form that indicates a higher level of service than that which was actually performed.

Urea reduction ratio (URR) A formula to determine the effectiveness of hemodialysis treatment.

Use The sharing of information between people working in the same healthcare facility for purposes of caring for the patient.

V

Venography The imaging of a vein after the injection of contrast material.

W

Willful ignorance Purposely avoiding learning about a law to excuse not following that law.

nuclear medicine section
  body part, 540
  body system, 539
  character definitions, 539
  qualifier, 541
  radionuclide, 540–541
  root type, 540
  section C, 541
physical rehabilitation and diagnostic
    audiology section, 545–546
  body system & region, 546
  character definitions, 545
  equipment, 547
  qualifier, 547
  root type, 546
  section F, 545–546
  section qualifier, 546
  type qualifier, 547
radiation oncology section
  body system, 543
  character definitions, 542
  isotope, 544
  modality qualifier, 543–544
  qualifier, 544
  root type, 543
  section D, 542
  treatment site, 543
substance abuse section
  body systems, 551
  character definitions, 551
  qualifier, 552
  root type, 551–552
  section H, 551
  type qualifier, 552
Substance abuse treatment services, 360
Substance, administration section,
    499–500
Successful reporting, definition of, 336
Superbill, **33**
  ultrasound services coded from, 256
Superscript numbers, for performance
    measures, 331, 332, 334
Supplemental reports, modifiers, 67–68
Supplies; *see also* Durable medical
    equipment; *specific item*
  HCPCS Level II modifiers, 387
  medical, 352, 355, 408–415
  pharmaceutical, 418–421
  surgical, 168, 171
Supporting documentation, **14**, **33**
Surgeons
  anesthesia by, 149
  multiple, 172–173
Surgery; *see also specific organ or*
    procedure
  anesthesia care during
      (*see* Anesthesia)
  related procedure, 169
  repeat, 169, 170
  staged, 169, 185
  unrelated procedure, 170

Surgery coding, 165–188, 199–234
  auditory system, 231–233
  cardiovascular system, 207–215
  digestive system, 215–219
  eye and ocular adnexa, 229–231
  guidelines, 174–176
  integumentary system, 176–188
  musculoskeletal system, 199–204
  nervous system, 226–229
  respiratory system, 205–207
  scope of, 199
  urinary system, 219–222
Surgery package, 167–171
  services always included in, 168
  services not included in, 168–171
Surgical anesthesia; *see* General anesthesia
Surgical approach, **166**, 166–167
Surgical care only modifier, 172
Surgical pathology, **281**, 281–283, 282*f*
Surgical procedures, types of, 166–167
Surgical supplies, 168, 171
SV modifier, 387
Symbols, 41–43; *see also specific symbol*
  conscious sedation, 318
  HCPCS, 362–363

T

T codes
  deletion of, 339
  national, for state Medicaid agencies,
      360–361
  transportation services, 423
Table of Drugs (HCPCS), 358, 368, 419
Tabular listing; *see also* Numerical listing
  ICD-10-PCS codes, 446–449, 446*t*
Tax Relief and Health Care Act of 2006
    (TRHCA), 330
TCD (transcranial Doppler), 310
Technical component, radiology services,
    247–248
Telephone E/M services, 317
Temporary codes, 359, 360, 423
Temporary National Codes category, 360
Temporary procedures, 358
TEMPR (transcutaneous electrical
    modulation pain reprocessing), 228
TENS (transcutaneous electrical nerve
    stimulators), **416**
Terminology, standardized, **439**
Therapeutic procedures, surgical, 166
Third-party payers; *see* Insurance carriers
Thoracotomy, 200
Three-dimensional computer-generated
    reconstruction, in radiation
    oncology, 259
Throat, 306
Thyroid uptake scans, 259
Time
  acupuncture, 314–315
  conscious sedation, 148

drug administration, 300
  extracorporeal assistance and
      performance section, 505
  extracorporeal therapies section, 509
  postoperative care (global period),
      168, 171
  radiation oncology, 259
  transportation services, 425, 425*t*
  unusual, special rates for, 396
Time reporting, anesthesia services, **146**
Tissue transfer, adjacent, 183–184
Tobacco use intervention, 334–336, 335*f*
Topical anesthesia, 141, **142**, 168
TOS (type of service), 368
Training, for self-management, 317
Transcatheter procedures, radiologic, 255
Transcranial Doppler (TCD), 310
Transcutaneous electrical modulation pain
    reprocessing (TEMPR), 228
Transcutaneous electrical nerve stimulators
    (TENS), **416**
Transfer of care, 82, **83**
Transfers, 96
Transitional care management services,
    preventive medicine, 128–130
Transplantation, **206**; *see also* Donor;
    Grafts
  heart/lung, 209–210
  kidney, 219–221
  liver, 217–218
  lung, 205–206
  pancreas, 218–219
Transportation services, 355, 421–426;
    see also Ambulance services
  codes in other sections, 423–424
  coding components, 422–423
  HCPCS Level II modifiers, 391
  location modifier, 424, 425*b*
Transurethral surgery, 222–223
Trauma; *see* Wounds
Treatment; *see also* Procedure(s);
    Service(s); *specific treatment*
  unusual, 173–174
Treatment, payment, and/or operations
    (TPO), 7
Treatment site, radiation oncology
    section, 543
TRHCA (Tax Relief and Health Care Act
    of 2006), 330
Tunneled catheter, 215
Tympanostomy, 232–233
Type of service (TOS), 368

U

UB-04 claim form, 624
Ulcer, decubitus, **416**
Ultrasound (sonogram), 248, 255–257
Unbundling, **15**
  example of, 299
  panels and, 273